Developmental Neuropathology

Reinhard L. Friede

Springer-Verlag
New York Wien

Reinhard L. Friede, M.D.

Professor of Neuropathology
Case Western Reserve University
Cleveland, Ohio

presently

Professor of Neuropathology
University of Zurich
Switzerland

Printed in Austria by Adolf Holzhausens Nfg., Wien

With 163 Figures

Library of Congress Cataloging in Publication Data. Friede, Reinhard L. Developmental neuropathology. Includes bibliographies and index. 1. Pediatric neurology. 2. Developmental neurology. 3. Metabolism, Inborn errors of. I. Title. [DNLM: 1. Nervous system diseases—Pathology. 2. Nervous system diseases—In infancy and childhood. 3. Metabolism, Inborn errors. WS340 F899d] RJ486.F69. 618.9'28'047. 75-37563.

ISBN 0-387-81325-X Springer-Verlag New York — Wien
ISBN 3-211-81325-X Springer-Verlag Wien — New York

Preface

The present text was envisioned as a supplement to existing texts on human neuropathology, covering only those aspects of pediatric neuropathology which pertain to and are peculiar of the immature nervous system. No coverage—or only brief comment—is given to diseases commonly found in adults which may, on occasion, occur in childhood or infancy as well. The subject matter is divided into three main categories: 1. The "acquired" lesions dating to the fetal, perinatal or early postnatal periods, 2. the malformations, and 3. the heritable metabolic defects. The first 6 chapters (2–7) are reserved to the lesions most intimately linked to the circumstances of birth. There is some inherent ambiguity in distinguishing between "acquired" lesions and malformations, as, indeed, no sharp distinction can be made between one and the other. Many malformations result from diseases acquired during fetal life and their peculiarity resides in the fact that the organ becomes affected before its development terminates and in such a way that its subsequent development becomes deranged or partly abrogated. A variety of causes acting at the same developmental period or over a common pathogenetic mechanism may produce the same type of derangement, including chemical, physical, infectious or genetic factors, as pointed out repeatedly in the text. Consequently, the definition of a malformation, as differing from an "acquired" residual lesion was made dependant on evidence for the derangement of developmental processes subsequent to the acquisition of the disease. The hemispheric defects of porencephaly, for example, are described among the acquired lesions (chapter 11) while the polymicrogyria that often fringes these defects is described among the malformations (chapter 29) as it clearly results from deranged development of the affected cortex subsequent to the formation of the main lesion. This distinction is carried to a fine point in listing the aplasia of the cerebellar granular layer among the malformations of the cerebellar cortex (chapter 30): recent experimental evidence clearly identified the lesion with a developmental failure subsequent to a destruction of the superficial granular layer of the cortex. In this peculiar instance a derangement of development may still be induced postnatally, at least in the rat. In reporting on the "acquired" lesions and the malformations relatively great weight was given to the original reports and the older literature, as the detailed morphologic accounts published during the nineteenth and early present century often left only details to be covered to later authors. The number of references cited had to be restricted severely for obvious reasons, but it is hoped that those given will suffice for locating the remainder of the literature. Knowledge on the inherited metabolic defects, covered in the third part, has progressed by leaps and bounds during the past two decades, and much of the labours of generations of morphologists have been negated in the process. Consequently less attention is paid to the older literature, concentrating on the recent insights and the resultant reclassification of diseases. The third part also includes a number of entities of unknown etiology, listed among the inherited metabolic defects according to their morphologic similarities but without pretent of prejudging their true nature.

Completion of this book would have been impossible without the generous help and advice of many colleagues and associates, particularly without the untiring help of Mrs. Frida Wallenstein in preparing and editing the manuscript. The author is also indebted to Dr. Angevine for editing Table 1, and to Drs. Anzil, Barson, Blinzinger, Carpenter, Powell, Lampert, Lindenberg, and Schochet who kindly permitted use of their illustrations.

Zurich, October 1975 R. L. Friede

Contents

1. Gross and Microscopic Development of the Central Nervous System

This chapter concerns mainly the gross and microscopic aspects of normal cerebral development during the second half of gestation, that is the period usually encountered by the pathologist. Its purpose is to provide a frame of reference for assessing normalcy in the brain of the fetus and of the newborn, to point out changes of borderline significance, and to establish base lines for the evaluation of gross or microscopic pathologic changes. The chapter does not provide an extensive review of normal embryology of the human central nervous system; developmental principles are cited only to the extent to which they are of help in interpreting abnormal tissue structure, and pertinent data are generally included in the respective chapters of the text.

Timing of Origin of Various Neuronal Groups. The time of origin of the neurons of various nuclear groups can be determined from the incorporation of labelled thymidine into the nuclei of dividing cells, as shown by radioautography. The central nervous system of the mouse has been studied in greatest detail, and Table 1 provides a "calendar" of neuronal development in the mouse brain. The timing of origin of neurons in the human brain has not been determined with similar accuracy, but Table 1 permits reasonable extrapolation as to the order in which the various groups form during early fetal development. O'Rahilly and Gardner (1971) tabulated staged timing of developmental events in the central nervous system during the first 8 weeks of fetal life.

Mass Growth of the Brain. The growth of the central nervous system is exceptionally rapid during the early fetal period; for example, the increase in its volume between the 2nd and 3rd month amounts to 416 percent, while it amounts to only 42 percent at the end of gestation (Mikhailets, 1952). The rapid initial growth of the CNS is precocious when compared with other body tissues; its weight comprises 21 percent of body weight at the 6th month, 15 percent at term, and 3 percent in the adult (Wilmer, 1940). The overall growth of the CNS is the composite product of different growth rates for its main portions. The increase in the volume of the cerebral hemispheres is slow and steady between the 2nd and early 6th month and accelerates thereafter. The brain stem grows most rapidly between the 2nd and the end of the 6th month, less rapidly thereafter. The cerebellum grows slowly between the 2nd and 5th month; then an exceptionally rapid increase in volume begins and continues until the 6th postnatal month (Dunn, 1921). The main portions of the brain thus constitute different fractions of total weight at different phases of development. For example, cerebral hemispheres, cerebellum and

Table 1. *Timing of Origin of Neurons in Mouse Brain*

Nucleus	Site of Origin	Time of Origin (days)	Author
Brain stem (most nuclei completed by day 14)			
Cranial motor nuclei	Primitive ependyma	10 and earlier	Taber, 1963, 1964
Secondary sensory neurons	Primitive ependyma	10 and 11	Taber, 1963, 1964
Reticular formation	Ependyma and rhombic lip	10 and earlier	Taber, 1963, 1964
Inferior olivary nucleus	Rhombic lip, caudal	10	Taber, 1963, 1964
Pontine gray matter	Rhombic lip, caudal	10–16	Taber Pierce, 1966
Nucleus reticularis tegmenti	Mostly primitive ependyma of pons	12–13	Taber Pierce, 1966
Cochlear nucleus	Rhombic lip, middle portion	Large neurons, 10–12; medium and small, 11–13; granular cells, 12–18	Taber Pierce, 1967
Cerebellum			
Purkinje cells and roof nuclei	Subependymal germinal layer (direct outward migration)	10–13	Uzman, 1960 Miale and Sidman, 1961
Golgi II neurons of granular layer	Subependymal germinal layer (direct outward migration)	10–15	Miale and Sidman, 1961
Superficial granular layer	Rhombic lip, migrates to cerebellar surface	Beginning of migration, 13 days; continued division	Miale and Sidman, 1961
Granule cells	From superficial granular layer by inward migration	Late embryo to 15 days postnatal	Miale and Sidman, 1961
Small cells of roof nuclei		13 days to 1st postnatal week	Miale and Sidman, 1961
Cerebral Hemispheres			
Thalamus: ventral lateral, zona incerta, dorsal lateral, geniculate, posterior pretectal, lateral, posterior ventral	Primitive ependyma of third ventricle; general gradients in timing caudal-rostral, ventral-dorsal, lateral-medial	10–15	Angevine, 1970
Thalamus: anterior group; paratenial, paraventricular, reuniens, rhomboides		10–15	Angevine, 1970
Habenula	Ventricular matrix	10–16	Angevine, 1970
Amygdaloid nucleus	Ventricular matrix	10; peak 12	Sidman and Angevine, 1962

Basal cortical nuclei and claustrum	Ventricular matrix	10; peak 12–13	Sidman and Angevine, 1962
Caudate nuclei and putamen	Ventricular matrix	10; peak 12–13	Sidman and Angevine, 1962
Medial septal nuclei	Ventricular matrix	12–15	Sidman and Angevine, 1962
Olfactory bulb:			
Triangular cells	Local matrix	10–11	Hinds, 1966
Mitral cells		11–13	Hinds, 1966
Rest of cells (inside out order)		11–20	Hinds, 1966
Granule cells		11–20 postnatal	Hinds, 1966
Hippocampal region:			
Entorhinal, subicular region, hippocampal sector CA_2		11–15	Angevine, 1965
Hippocampal sector CA_1, CA_3		Continues to day 19 (birth)	
Granule cells of fascia denta (outside in order)		Until 20 days postnatal	Angevine, 1965
Convexity cortex:			
Deep layers	Periventricular matrix	11	Angevine and Sidman, 1962
Upper layers	Periventricular matrix	13–15	Angevine and Sidman, 1962
Most superficial layers	Periventricular matrix	17	Angevine and Sidman, 1962

Table 2. *Brain Weight Related to Gestational Age* (Modified, Gruenwald and Minh, 1960)

Gestational Age (weeks/days)	Brain Weight (gm)	Body Weight (gm)	Body Length (cm)	Number of Cases
23/5 ± 2/3	70 ± 18	500	29.4 ± 2.5	317
26/0 ± 2/6	107 ± 27	750	32.9 ± 3.0	311
27/5 ± 3/1	143 ± 34	1,000	35.6 ± 3.1	295
29/0 ± 3/0	174 ± 38	1,250	38.4 ± 3.0	217
31/3 ± 2/3	219 ± 52	1,500	41.0 ± 2.7	167
32/4 ± 2/6	247 ± 51	1,750	42.6 ± 3.1	148
34/6 ± 3/2	281 ± 56	2,000	44.9 ± 2.8	140
36/4 ± 3/0	308 ± 49	2,250	46.3 ± 2.9	124
38/0 ± 3/2	339 ± 50	2,500	47.3 ± 2.3	120
39/2 ± 2/2	362 ± 48	2,750	48.7 ± 2.9	138
40/0 ± 2/1	380 ± 55	3,000	50.0 ± 2.9	144
40/4 ± 1/6	395 ± 53	3,250	50.7 ± 2.6	133
40/4 ± 1/5	411 ± 55	3,500	51.8 ± 3.0	106
40/6 ± 2/3	413 ± 55	3,750	52.1 ± 2.3	57
41/4 ± 1/3	420 ± 62	4,000	52.4 ± 2.7	31
41/2 ± 2/1	415 ± 38	4,250	53.2 ± 2.5	15

brain stem respectively constitute 88.6, 3.1, and 8.3 percent of total brain weight at the 3rd month, 92.7, 5.8, and 1.5 percent at birth, and 88.0, 10.1, and 1.9 percent at the age of 20 years. The weight of the whole brain more than doubles during the first 9 months after birth and reaches over 90 percent of the adult weight by the 6th year (Scammon, 1933). The postnatal increase in cranial circumference serves as a convenient clinical parameter of normalcy in cranial development (Silver and Diemer, 1948; Nellhaus, 1968; Kantero and Tiisala, 1971).

Cerebral Cortex. The development of the cerebral hemispheric surface proceeds gradually from the flat (lissencephalic) brain of the fetus to the gyral pattern of adults. The Sylvian fissure is apparent at approximately 14 weeks gestation, forming a shallow indentation into the smooth hemispheric surface. The opercula are formed by the growing cortex next to the Sylvian fissure eventually concealing the insula. Indentations of the cortical surface leading to the formation of the Rolandic and calcarine fissures appear between 24 and 26 weeks, followed by the demarcation of the superior temporal and the pre- and postcentral gyri. Formation of the cortical gyri proceeds rapidly at the 30th week of gestation, and the entire hemispheric surface is gyrated by approximately 32 weeks; the gyri, however, are less numerous than in the adult brain. Pryse-Davies and Beard (1973) demonstrate that the gestational age can be estimated by counting the number of convolutions crossed by a line from the frontal to the occipital pole above the insula and adding 21 to the gyral count; this gyral index is most reliable between 28 and 37 weeks, less reliable between 37 weeks and term. The cortical surface area of the newborn measures approximately 679 cm^2, of which 61 per cent is intrasulcal (Hessdoerffer and Scammon, 1935). The hemispheric surface more than doubles during postnatal growth, to reach an adult value of approximately

1,600 m^2. This growth is accompanied with an increase in the size and number of gyri, so that the intrasulcal portion of the adult cortex is about the same as that in the newborn. The adult cortical surface is reached by the 2nd year of life.

The development of the laminar architecture of the cerebral cortex has been studied extensively, and only the most essential features are reviewed here. During early embryogenesis (the 5th to 6th week) the hemispheric wall consists of an inner layer of matrix tissue (the germinal layer) and a superficial, acellular zone (the Randschleier). The cerebral cortex separates from the matrix tissue by the 7th week, as neuroblasts migrate from the matrix to the surface of the tissue. A layer of low cell density forms between cortex and matrix tissue, increasing subsequently in width to become the white matter. The cortical cell population is fed by the continued proliferation of matrix cells located in the periventricular tissue, reaching the cortex by their successive migration across the white matter. Autoradiographic studies (Table 1) have shown that the cortical layers develop from inside out from successive waves of neuroblasts, the first one forming the deep cortical layer and the later waves migrating sequentially past their predecessors to the cortical surface (Angevine and Sidman, 1961; Sidman and Angevine, 1962). In the rat, the 5th and 6th cortical layers form at the 16th and 17th days, the fourth layer on the 18th day, and the second and third layers on the 19th to 21st days (Berry and Rogers, 1965). The observations of Rakić (1972) suggest that the migration of neuroblasts toward the cortex is guided by their movement along ependymo-glia processes which extend from the ventricular walls across the white matter to the cortical surface. The speed of migration of neuroblasts was estimated as 15 to 30 μ, that is once or twice the length of the cell body, per hour (Hicks and D'Amato, 1968). Altman (1966) determined speeds of 50 to 750 μ per day in rat olfactory bulb and cerebellum.

The cerebral cortex of the 5-month-old fetus shows a molecular and a cell layer; the latter is divided into a thin outer portion of high cell density and a thick inner portion of low cell density. The six-layered neocortex begins to emerge from this pattern by the 6th month, first with a gradual differentiation of the fifth and sixth layers. The first neurons to mature are the pyramids of the deep cortical layers; they exhibit, with conventional staining methods, large cytoplasmic perikarya and vesicular nuclei when most of the remainder of the neuronal population is still in the neuroblast stage. Illustrations of typical cortical profiles at various stages of fetal development were published by Larroche (1962). The changes in cortical laminar architecture are accompanied with a corresponding redistribution in the activity of several oxydative enzymes (Friede, 1966).

The rearrangement of cortical layering is accompanied with a progressive decrease in the packing density of nerve cells, a universal feature of maturation of gray matter. It results from the increase in the volume of neuropil, which, in turn, is due to the dentritic growth and to the ramification of afferent processes in the tissue between the neuronal perikarya. The growth in the thickness of the cerebellar and hippocampal molecular layers is equivalent to the growth of neuropil in cerebral cortex.

A peculiar aspect of cerebral cortical development is the transient appearance of a superficial granular layer in the form of a thin lamina of matrix cells immediately underneath the leptomeninges. This layer appears first at the 12th to 13th week of gestation in the basal allocortical zones, where it derives from columns of cells ascending from the periventricular matrix (Brun, 1965). It spreads into the isocortex during the 13th to 14th week and covers the entire convexity by the 16th to 18th week, reaching greatest thickness by 22 weeks. Subsequent involution of the superficial granular layer seems to result from the migration of cells into the cerebral cortex. The layer disappears in the insula and anterior cingular cortex by 27 to 29 weeks, in the precentral cortex by 32 weeks, in the calcarine cortex by 33 weeks, in the postcentral and posterior cingular cortex at 36 weeks, and in the frontal and occipital cortex at 39 weeks. Remnants of the superficial granular layer persist in term infants at the inferior temporal and orbital cortex. Brun thought that persistence of the superficial granular layer in certain malformations, such as in polymicrogyria, constitutes a marker of the teratogenetic determination period; he also considered the layer the source of various types of abnormal cellular hyperplasias of the cortical surface (Chapter 29).

The Ammon's horn is generally considered a phylogenetically old portion of the cerebral cortex, but radioautographic studies have shown that at least part of its neurons originate late in development (Angevine, 1965). A peculiar aspect of the maturation of the Ammon's horn are marked differences in the rate of maturation of the neurons in its sectors. The neurons of the so-called "resistant sector" mature first, followed closely by those in the "endplate". In term infants, these neurons have vesicular nuclei and significant cytoplasmic bodies; whereas, those in Sommer's sector are still neuroblasts (Fig. 1). Development of the cells in Sommer's sector progresses from outside in, starting in the outermost portion of the cell layer; maturation is concluded by about the 2nd year. The immaturity of the Sommer's sector in newborns is a potential source of error in identifying perinatal asphyctic lesions. The segmental differences in cellular maturation may well explain patterns of selective vulnerability of the Ammon's horn characteristic of kernicterus (Chapter 8) or of pontosubicular neuronal necrosis (Chapter 7).

White Matter. The hemispheric white matter grows slower than the cortical gray matter during fetal development, but the growth of white matter continues postnatally long after the gray matter has reached its definite volume. The growth of the cortex subsides by the 2nd year of life; that of the hemispheric white matter continues until after the first decade because of continued accumulation of myelinated fibers and increase in their calibers (Scammon, 1933). Because of the differences in the rate and the timing of growth of gray and white matter, their proportions change during development. Between the 6th and 18th postnatal month for example, the volume of white matter is relatively small when compared with the nearly fully developed, deeply gyrated cortex. This normal aspect of cerebral development should not be mistaken for hypoplasia of white matter, but it may persist in certain diseases (Chapter 41).

The microscopic structure of the developing cerebral white matter is determined to a large extent by two successive events occurring with considerable overlap. The passing of waves of migrating neuroblasts on their way to the cortex is the dominant feature of early fetal white matter. It is superseded and replaced toward the end of gestation by the proliferation of glial tissue associated with myelination (myelination gliosis). The following sections refer to these two events.

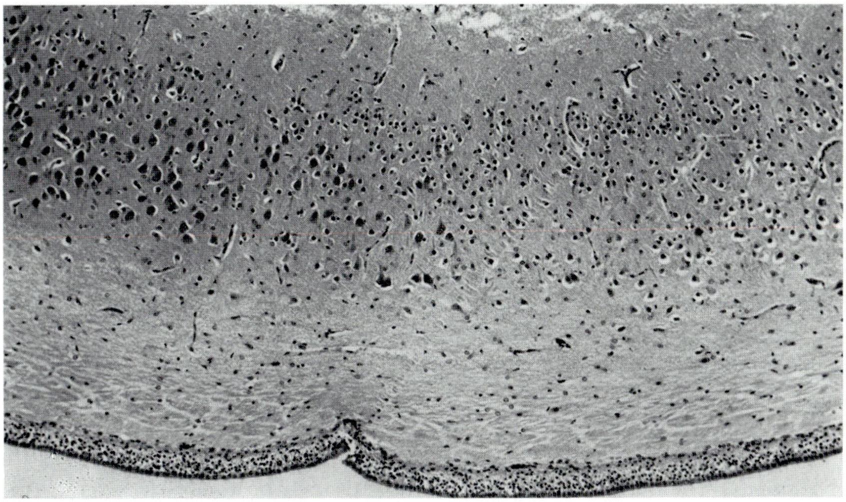

Fig. 1. Difference in neuronal maturation between Sommer's and resistant sectors of the Ammon's horn in a term newborn; H & E ×80

Periventricular Matrix Tissue. The matrix tissue of the lateral ventricles forms a subependymal layer of tightly packed immature cells extending over the entire ventricular wall up to 30 weeks of gestation. At this time, the layer begins to thin out and it loses continuity first at the fornix and the corpus callosum, the dissolution progressively extending toward the corners of the lateral ventricles where the solid layer breaks into islands of cells by the 36th to 39th week. Matrix cells often persist longest in perivascular tissue. Term infants show only scattered islands of tightly packed matrix cells in the ventricular wall, except for a thick cushion at the ganglionic eminence between the thalamus and the caudate nucleus. This cushion becomes fragmented during the first 3 postnatal months, and nearly all of the matrix tissue normally disappears by the first year of life. Nests of matrix cells also occur in the basal portions of the frontal lobe, off the ventricular surface.

Waves of migrating cells may produce a marked layering of cell density in the early fetal white matter. This pattern persists longest in the occipital lobe, where a concentric periventricular halo of increased cell density may encompass the occipital horn, being separated from the subependymal matrix tissue by a zone of lower cell density. Undifferentiated cells are scattered throughout the hemispheric white matter up to and shortly after the dissolution of the periventricular matrix. The presence of these cells needs to be considered when assessing pathologic changes in the newborn white matter, as they are superficially similar to migrating microglia. The identification of necrobiotic changes in migrating cells is also difficult as their nuclei are normally small and dense and their cytoplasm is too sparse to allow evaluation with conventional stains.

Myelin Formation, Fine Structure. Myelin formation, in a narrow sense, consists of the helical wrapping of surface membranes of Schwann cells, or of oligodendroglia, respectively, around axons (Geren, 1954). This phase of sheath formation, however, merely constitutes the end product of a series of cellular and chemical events involving the sheath cell population as well as the axon during the myelination period.

Prior to the onset of myelination there are few sheath cells in the white matter, both in terms of their number per volume tissue or of their number per density of nonmyelinated axons. Proliferation of sheath cells is initiated before the onset of sheath formation and may reach its peak before myelinated fibers become discernible by light and electron microscopic methods (Schonbach *et al.*, 1968). The proliferating sheath cells contact the axons and engulf the axis cylinder with their cytoplasm. Formation of the sheath begins with the wrapping of the mesaxon of the sheath cell around the axis cylinder, first in the form of a loose spiral of alternating layers of cytoplasm and of cell membranes. This wrapping is followed by obliteration of the intracellular compartment; the inner surfaces of the cell membranes fuse and form the major dense line of the sheath by their coalescence (Peters and Muir, 1959). The process of sheath formation is associated with metabolic activation of the sheath cells, evident from radioautographic and enzyme histochemical data and from changes in the density of cytoplasmic organelles. Attachment of the sheath cell to the axon occurs with the onset of axonal growth and may be triggered by initial axon enlargement; it is, however, not rigidly linked to a specific dimension of the axon (Matthews and Duncan, 1971). The mechanism responsible for the initial contact between sheath cells and axis cylinder and for triggering the formation of the initial turns of the sheath cell membranes around the fiber are not known. The subsequent deposition of additional turns of myelin sheaths occurs in proportion to the growth of the axon (Friede and Samorajski, 1968; Samorajski and Friede, 1968); axon growth, in turn, occurs in proportion to the growth of the perikarya of the neurons (Martinez and Friede, 1970). Experimental data suggest that the amount of myelin formed by the sheath cell is controlled by the rate of expansion of the growing axis cylinder (Friede, 1972).

The basic aspects of myelin formation are similar for peripheral and central nerve fibers, but there are differences in the types of relations established between the sheath cell and the axon. A Schwann cell in a peripheral nerve attaches its perikaryon to one given fiber, and forms a sheath only around the engulfed segment of this one fiber. An oligodendroglia cell projects processes to a number of axons which it myelinates; estimates of the number of fibers myelinated by a given oligodendroglia cell vary considerably, from 4 or 5 (McFarland and Friede, 1971) to more than 50 (Matthews and Duncan, 1971).

Regional Timing of Myelination. Myelination of any given fiber system involves all the events described above, but different fiber tracts myelinate at different developmental periods; even the component populations of a given tract may differ in timing (Matthews and Duncan, 1971). Myelination of tracts proceeds, generally speaking, in a caudo-cranial order earlier in the spinal cord than in the cranial portions of the CNS. The schedule of myelination was first elaborated by Flechsig (1876), and useful reviews were published by Lucas Keene and Hewer (1931) and, more recently, by Riggs and Rorke (1969).

The following fiber systems begin to show myelin sheaths by 14 weeks gestation: Posterior and anterior spinal roots, tractus cuneatus (Burdach), direct cerebellar tracts, Gower's tracts, anterior ground bundle, medial longitudinal bundle, and all cranial nerves except the cochlear, the optic and the sensory trigeminal.

At 22 to 24 weeks, myelination is also seen in the tractus gracilis (Goll), the lateral and posterior ground bundles, the connecting fibers of the gray matter in the cord, the olivary and cerebellar connections, the tractus retroflexus, ansa lenticularis, and the cochlear and sensory trigeminal nerves.

Just before birth, myelination commences in Lissauer's bundle, the cortico- and rubrospinal tracts, the external arcuate fibers, the pontine fibers, corticocerebellar fibers, striothalamic bundles, Meynert's commissure, and the optic nerve and radiation. Myelination of the hemispheric white matter commences gradually during the first 2 postnatal years and continues to juvenile age; postnatal myelination by the 5th to 9th postnatal month is also observed in the retroflex tract, the olivo-spinal tract and the fornix.

Myelination of peripheral nerves generally occurs during fetal life, at about 14 to 16 weeks in the brachial and sciatic plexus; its electron microscopic features in human fetuses (Cravioto, 1965) resemble those known from the examination of laboratory animals. The peripheral portion of the nerve root beyond the glia-Schwann cell border stains much more intensely with conventional myelin stains than its central portion. The difference is due to the different proteolipid-protein composition of peripheral and central myelin; it may give the misleading impression of a much earlier onset of myelination in the distal portion of the root.

Myelination Gliosis. The stage of myelination can be assessed in routine sections of white matter, even without myelin stains, from the extent of proliferation and the density of glia cells, or myelination gliosis (Roback and Scherer, 1935). Counts in the human internal capsule show a more than six-fold higher density of glia cells per volume tissue at term than at the 6th fetal month; similar but smaller differences are found in the hemispheric white matter (Friede, 1961). Maximum cell density at the peak of myelination gliosis may be greater than in the adult brain for some tracts as the glia cells become dispersed later on by the growth in the caliber of the myelinating fibers.

The proliferating glial cells of myelination gliosis have not acquired the morphologic features of mature oligodendroglia cells and show enlarged, somewhat vesicular nuclei and eccentric cytoplasmic bodies staining slightly basophilic (Roback and Scherer, 1935). At this stage, the cells are best referred to as "myelination glia"; they should not be mistaken for reactive astrocytes. The physiologic phenomenon of myelination gliosis renders it very difficult to assess the extent of a pathologic reactive gliosis in the white matter of the newborn brain, unless the latter is focal. The significance of droplets of neutral fat in myelinating fiber tracts is discussed in Chapter 5.

Basal Ganglia. The time of origin of neurons in various nuclear groups of mouse basal ganglia is shown in Table 1. The origin of thalamic neurons in the mouse occurs in three overall gradients extending across the thalamic nuclei. There is a ventro-medial gradient, a caudo-rostral gradient, and a latero-medial, or outside-in, gradient; the latter is opposite to the inside-out gradient in the neuron formation of cerebral cortex (Angevine, 1970). Large neurons generally originate earlier than small neurons. The formation of the human thalamus differs from that of mouse thalamus in the development of a large pulvinar commencing at the 13th week and reaching greatest growth between the 16th and 37th week. The neurons of the pulvinar evidently do not originate from the germinal layer in the wall of the third ventricle, from which the rest of the thalamus originates, since this germinal layer dissolves at approximately 9½ weeks (Dekaban, 1954). The origin of the pulvinar has been traced to the cushion of matrix tissue in the ganglionic eminence (Rakić and Sidman, 1969). This is of particular interest as the subependymal hemorrhages in the ganglionic eminence (Chapter 2) were erroneously claimed to be causes of mental retardation.

There are marked differences in the timing of the cellular maturation in the different nuclei of the basal ganglia (Richter, 1965). The cells of the pallidum mature very early, having substantial cytoplasmic bodies by the 24th week of gestation. At this time, most thalamic nuclear groups have been laid out and the large neurons begin to acquire cytoplasmic bodies (Dekaban, 1954), though they are usually less advanced than those in the pallidum. All of the cells of the striatum are still at the neuroblast stage; their development begins with the maturation of the large cells at the 28th to 30th week, when all of the small cells are still in the neuroblast stage. The maturation of the small cells is protracted, commencing at the 33rd to 36th week, though undifferentiated cells remain for several months after birth. Swelling of the large cells, reminiscent of central chromatolysis, is often observed during this period, apparently as a normal developmental phenomenon. The definite cellular architecture of the striatum is essentially established by the end of the first year. The great developmental spread in the maturation of the neuronal perikarya corresponds to similar differences in the timing of myelin formation in basal ganglia; the myelination of pallidum precedes that of the striatum by as much as 5 months (Richter, 1965).

Micronodular mineralization (Fig. 2) is a fairly common alteration of the developing striatum, but it has received little attention in the literature. The change consists of focal deposits of basophilic granular material in the gray matter, either free in the neuropil or in the proximity of blood vessels.

The basophilic granules may be at the core of a small microglial nodule; other granules show only a few glial nuclei in their proximity or are without any reactive glial change. The granules stain positive with the periodic acid Schiff reaction and with Kossa's stain and negative with iron stains (Gilles and Murphy, 1969).

Micronodular mineralization has a predilection for putamen and caudate nucleus, but it may be observed in the adjacent white matter and other nuclei. Gilles and Murphy (1969) found it in 66 percent of abnormal and 9.6 percent of control brains. Testing a series of 69 unselected newborn autopsies in the present author's material, micronodular mineralization was found in 26,

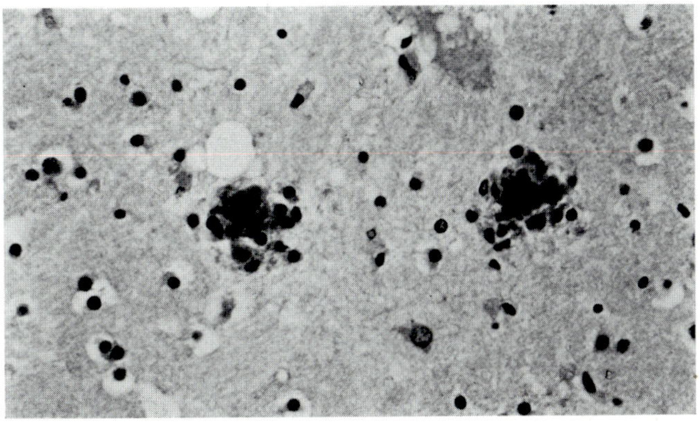

Fig. 2. Micronodular mineralization (putamen); H & E ×275

ranging from one or two to many nodules per section. Micronodular mineralization is not diagnostic of cerebral damage, nor is there any known clinical significance, and its usefulness as an index of perinatal anoxia or leukencephalopathy (Brack, 1973; Murofushi, 1974) is doubtful. However, some brains having definite lesions elsewhere may show an unusual degree of micronodular mineralization in the basal ganglia and in adjacent white matter. In these instances micronodular mineralization may be confused with focal scarring from encepholoclastic processes. Micronodular mineralization resembles the mineralization seen in the pallidum at advanced age, but the latter differs in its regional distribution and in the absence of glial nodular response.

Ventricular System. The developmental changes in the configuration of the fetal cerebral ventricles are determined mainly by the gradual narrowing of the lumen of the brain vesicle upon growth and increase in the thickness of its walls (Barbe, 1938). The ventricles of prematures, accordingly, are larger than those of term infants whose ventricles are usually quite narrow and slit shaped. A cavum septi pellucidi is present in all newborns and its walls lack ependymal lining; its relation to the cavum Vergae is described in Chapter 28. The cavum septi pellucidi usually obliterates during the first 2 years of life, as it is often absent in children of 2 years or older and is found in only 20 percent of adults (Schwidde, 1952).

Coarctations of the ventricular walls (Davidoff, 1946) are variants in the shape of the lateral ventricles due to unilateral or bilateral fusion of their angles between the corpus callosum and the head of the caudate nucleus. Bates and Netsky (1955) used the term „coaptation“ if the ventricular walls were merely in close contact, and "fusion" if they were merged by glial tissue. Coarctations are found in approximately one-sixth of all adult brains (Davidoff, 1946; Morel and Wildi, 1954; Westergaard, 1970), but they are absent in newborns.

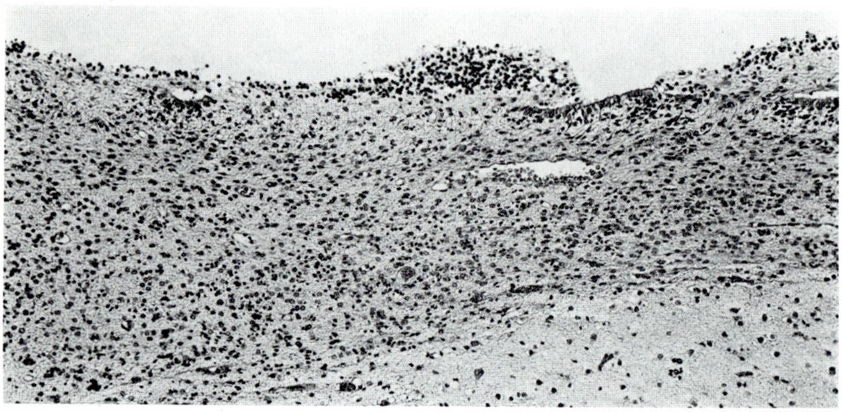

Fig. 3. Ependymal defects and gliosis in the wall of the lateral ventricles, seen often in otherwise normal infants; H & E ×80

Focal defects of the ependyma of the lateral ventricles are common in newborns (Fig. 3); in an unselected series of test cases they were found in 38 (74 percent) of 51 consecutive autopsies. These defects have been mentioned by Haymaker *et al.* (1961) as presumably unrelated findings in a series on kernicterus and by Banker and Larroche (1962) who emphasized their proximity to periventricular infarcts. Ependymal defects occur in the lateral ventricles, with the greatest frequency at the surface of the corpus callosum and near the corners of the lateral ventricles; they are generally absent from the walls of the third and fourth ventricles. Their *in vivo* origin is evident from slight proliferative changes in the subependymal glia, which may fill the defect to the level of the ependymal surface or may form a thin protruding cushion. The matrix tissue underneath the defect may be rarefied. The glial response in the subependymal tissue is usually very slight regardless of the degree of maturity of the newborn. Conceivably, ependymal defects may form upon deformation of the ventricles and compression of the skull upon birth; one may also speculate that they may induce coarctation of the ventricular corners upon healing.

Excrescences of matrix tissue consist of small nodules or mushroom shaped protrusions extending through breaches in the ependyma into the ventricle (Fig. 4). There are no reactive or inflammatory changes in the adjacent ventricular walls. Excrescences differ from reactive gliosis in being composed almost entirely of matrix tissue rather than of subependymal glia. Occasionally, capillaries may extend into the excrescence. Rydberg (1932) considered excrescences normal features of the ventricular walls of newborns, evidently referring to small protrusions of matrix tissue into the ependymal defects described above. If excrescences are defined more rigidly (a pedunculated mass composed mainly of matrix tissue and joined with the subependymal matrix by a narrow transependymal stalk in the absence of larger ependymal defects), they are rather uncommon and, in the present author's experience, seen only

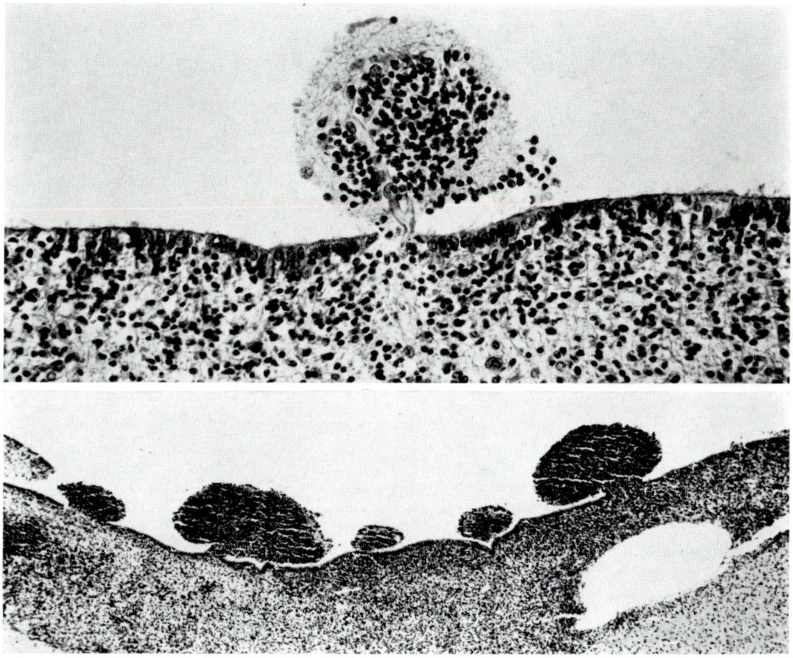

Fig. 4. Excrescences of matrix tissue over the caudate nucleus; H & E ×36, ×200

on occasion in malformed brain or in brains having destructive lesions elsewhere. Bergel (1928) reported a matrix excrescence into the spinal canal of a 16.5 mm fetus with doubling of the central canal. Seeding of cells from excrescences into the CSF may be considered a possible mode of formation of heterotopias of neural tissue in the leptomeninges.

Brain Stem Nuclei. The basic organization of the nuclear groups of midbrain, pons and medulla oblongata is established in the young fetus (Table 1), and most nuclei show well developed nerve cells by the 2nd half of gestation. The cell population of the pontine gray matter matures relatively late and may still be mainly neuroblastic by the 25th to 26th week. No matrix tissue is found in the medulla oblongata at this stage, except for occasional small residual nests in the cochlear nucleus, which corresponds to its protracted period of neurogenesis (Table 1). Little is known about the timing of biochemical and functional maturation of the various nuclear groups of the brain stem in man. Histochemical data for laboratory animals show that oxydative enzyme activity increases at different periods in different nuclear groups; for example, the cranial motor nuclei of rat mature early, while the superior and inferior colliculi mature late (Friede, 1966).

A peculiar aspect of the maturation of the brain stem is the deposition of melanin in the neurons of the substantia nigra and nucleus coerulus, as well as in the dorsal vagal nucleus and in a few other cell groups not discernible to the naked eye. These cells are not pigmented in the newborn;

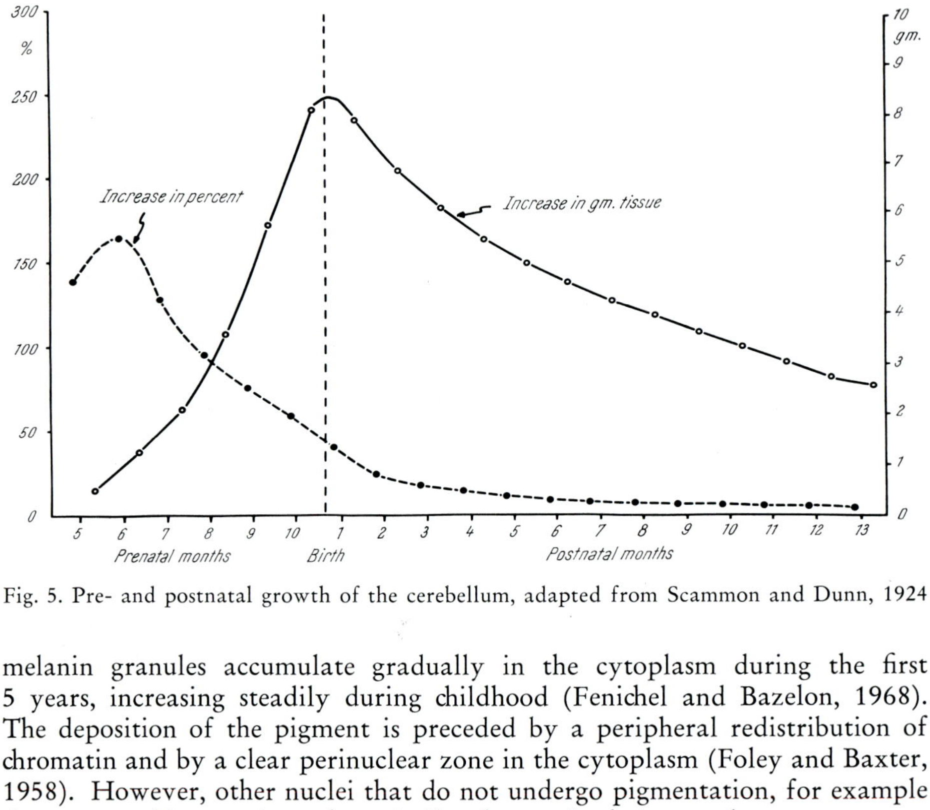

Fig. 5. Pre- and postnatal growth of the cerebellum, adapted from Scammon and Dunn, 1924

melanin granules accumulate gradually in the cytoplasm during the first 5 years, increasing steadily during childhood (Fenichel and Bazelon, 1968). The deposition of the pigment is preceded by a peripheral redistribution of chromatin and by a clear perinuclear zone in the cytoplasm (Foley and Baxter, 1958). However, other nuclei that do not undergo pigmentation, for example the supratrochlear nucleus, show similar changes in their cytoplasm.

Pigmentation of brain stem nuclei is not disturbed in albinism (Foley and Baxter, 1958). Children succumbing to chronic diseases have been reported to show less than normal pigmentation for age (Spence and Gilles, 1971). These observations are difficult to interpret: There is considerable variance in the rate of melanin deposition in normal children, and the quantity of melanin per cell is difficult to assess.

Cerebellum. The rate of cerebellar growth is less than that of cerebral hemispheres until the 5th month of pregnancy (Fig. 5). The adult proportions of cerebellar and cerebral hemispheres result from an accelerated increase in cerebellar volume from the 5th month on; normal proportions of the cerebellum are attained by or before the age of 18 months (Scammon and Dunn,

1924). The cerebellar weight expressed as a percentage of brain weight is only 5.7 percent in the newborn, 7.4 percent at 2 months, 8.5 percent at 4 months, 10 percent at 9 months, and 10.6 percent at 18 months, equal to the adult value (Ellis, 1920). The tissue content of DNA, a measure of the total number of nuclei, increases in the human cerebellum throughout gestation in a straight line relationship with age; whereas, the increase in cerebral hemispheric DNA diminishes exponentially toward the end of gestation (Howard *et al.*, 1969). The growth in cerebellar weight, or in total cerebellar

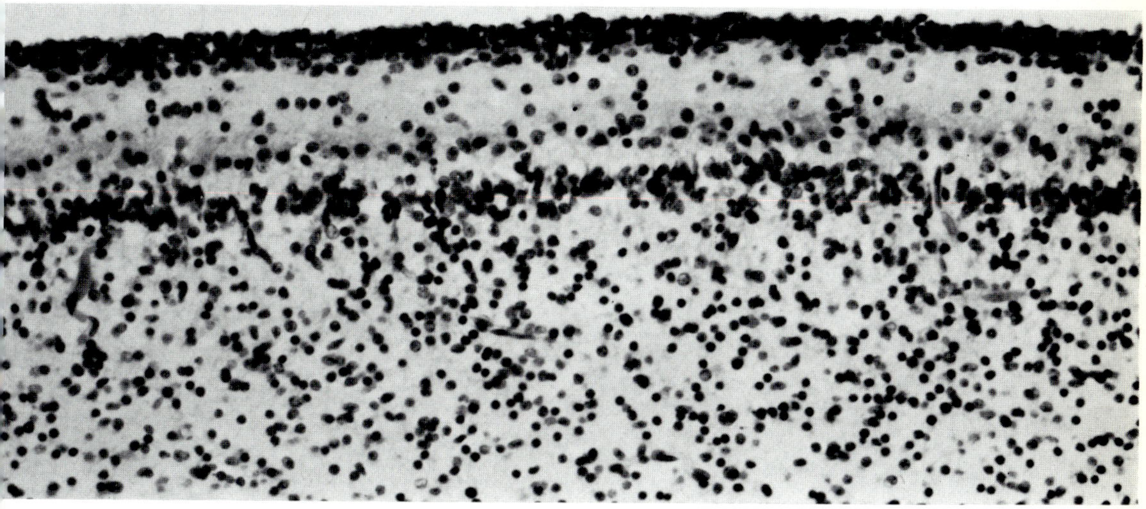

Fig. 6. Cerebellar cortex at 25 weeks gestation; H & E ×320

cell number, is the product of several successive and overlapping processes in cortex and white matter, and some of these can be timed with considerable accuracy.

The cerebellar Purkinje cells form early in embryonal life in the periventricular matrix and migrate directly to their definite cortical sites. Although Purkinje cells form at the same time as the neurons of the cerebellar roof nuclei, they mature much later, residing in the cortex in an undifferentiated stage until the development of cortical architecture has advanced. The superficial granular layer forms from matrix cells of the rhombic lip, which migrate during the early fetal period to the cortical surface where they continue to proliferate long after the periventricular matrix tissue has disappeared (Uzman, 1960; Miale and Sidman, 1961). The cerebellar granular layer forms from the proliferating cells in the superficial granular layer; the descent of matrix cells toward the deeper portions of the cortex appears to be guided by the processes of glia cells (Rakić, 1971). Further details on cerebellar cortical maturation are given in Chapter 31.

The following cortical layers are discernible in the cerebellum of the 25-week-fetus (Fig. 6): The superficial granular layer underneath the pia mater is composed of round or elongate matrix cells; it covers a thin molecu-

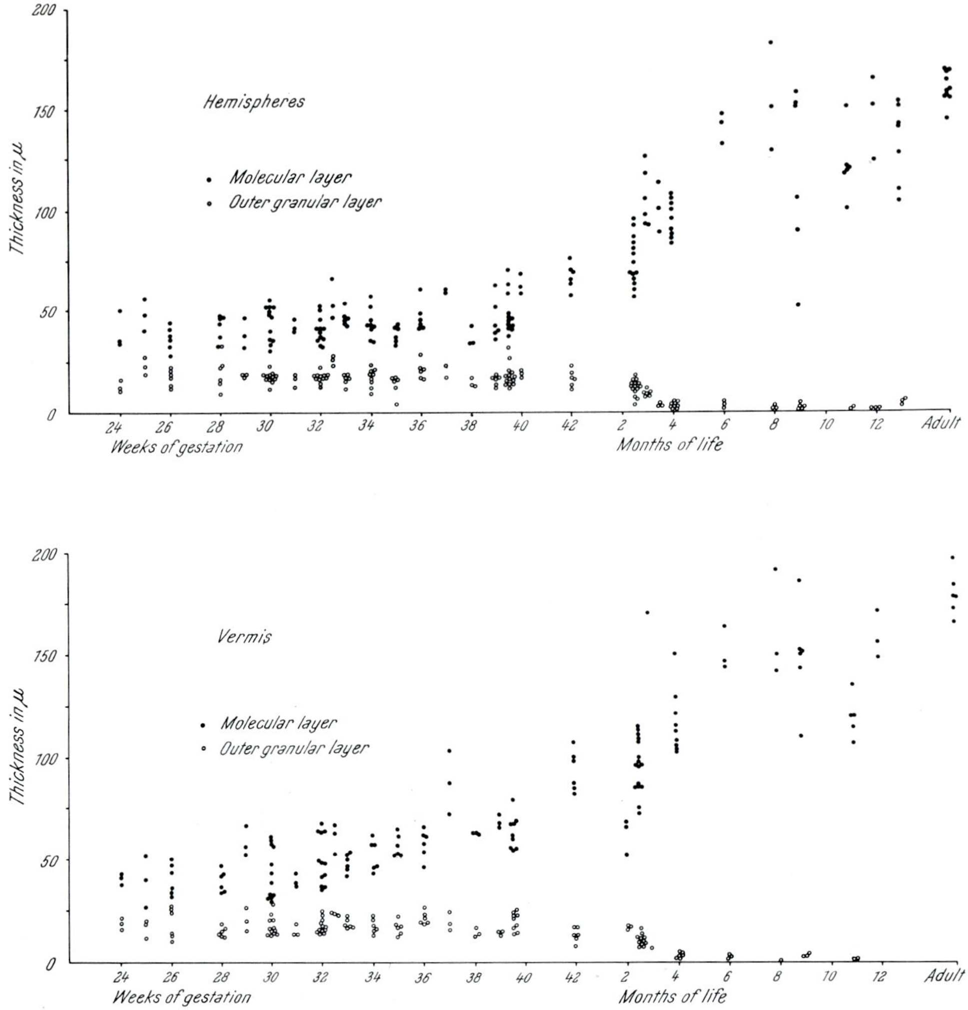

Fig. 7. Growth of cerebellar cortical layers (Friede, 1973)

lar layer. The Purkinje cells cannot be identified by conventional staining methods, but their precursors form a thin lamina of cells separated from the rudimentary granular layer by a clear zone, the lamina dissecans (Rakić and Sidman, 1970). The dates given for the following events refer to vermis and cerebellar hemispheres respectively (Friede, 1973). The lamina dissecans disappears at 28 and 32 weeks of gestation, at which time the Purkinje cells first become discernible. The latter change from a diploid to a tetraploid state between the 32nd week and term (Lapham, 1966). The inner granular layer begins to increase in thickness by the 30th and 32nd weeks and becomes sharply delineated from the white matter at 30 weeks and at term. The thickness of the molecular changes little until 30 and 38 weeks, at which time an increase in thickness commences, leading to adult thickness at approxi-

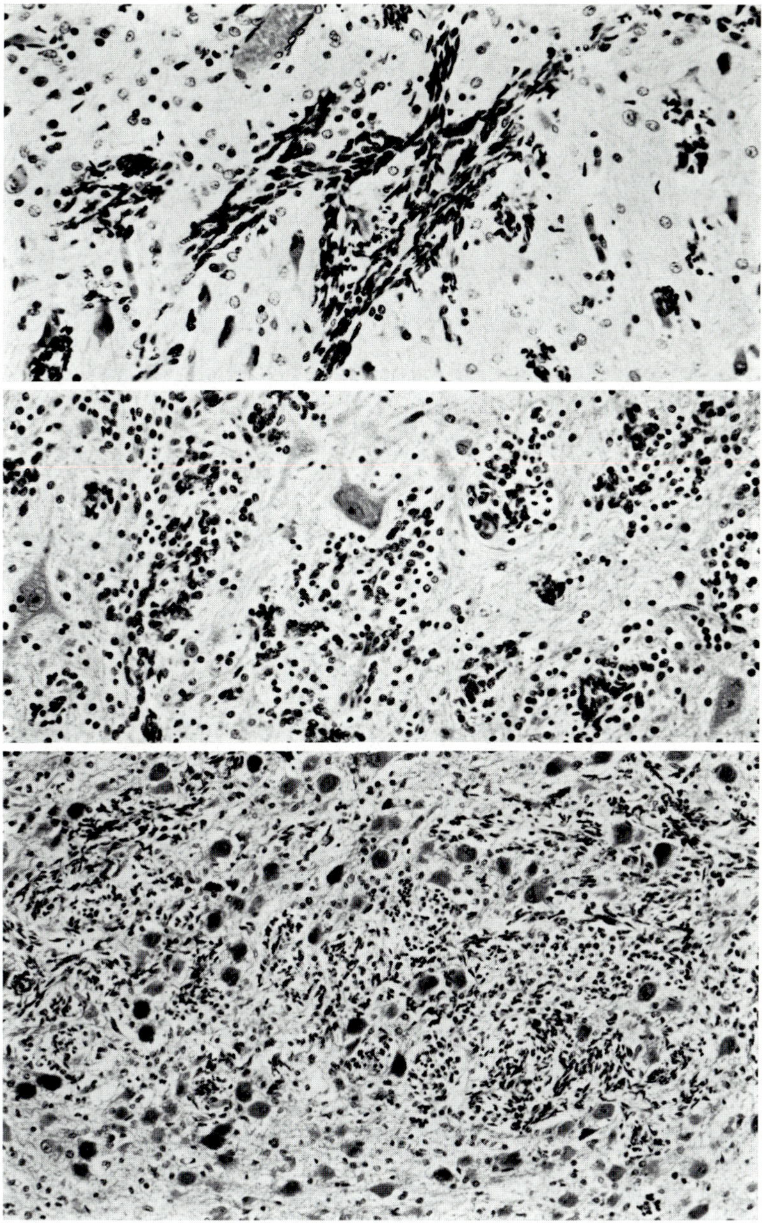

Fig. 8. Residual matrix tissue in the dentate nucleus (top and middle, ×200) and in the cochlear nucleus (bottom, ×135, H & E)

mately the 8th to 12th postnatal month (Ellis, 1920; Raaf and Kernohan, 1944). The growth of the molecular layer represents an approximate measure of the growth of Purkinje dendrites; dendritic growth is difficult to determine in other grisea in which the dendrites are not in register. The superficial granular layer persists to the 2nd and 4th postnatal month, at which time a fairly rapid involution sets in; the last remnants of the layer disappear by

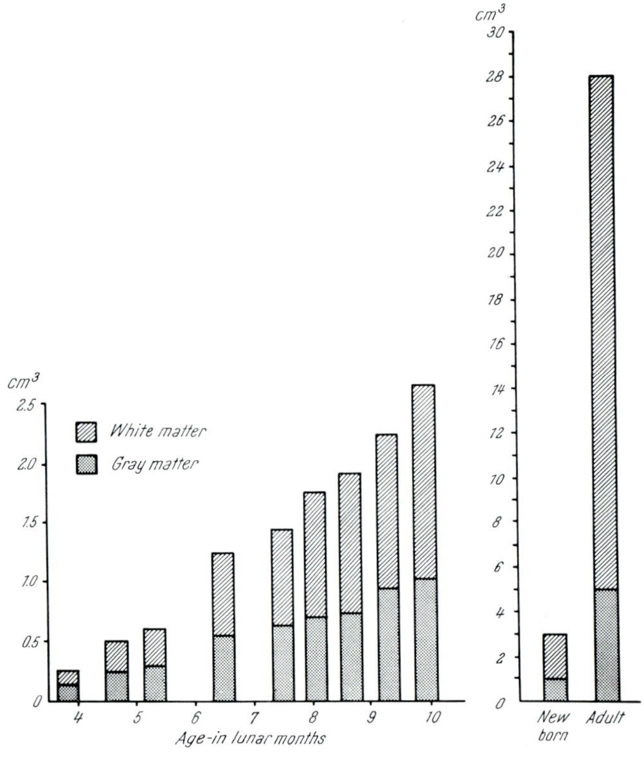

Fig. 9. Pre- and postnatal growth of the gray and white matter of human spinal cord; adapted from Lasseck and Rasmussen, 1938, 1939

the 9th and 13th month (Berliner, 1905; Ellis, 1920; Friede, 1973). Delayed involution of the superficial granular layer was described by Biach (1909) who found a persistent layer to up to 2 years of age in hydrocephalic or brain-damaged children. Brun (1917–18) also mentions persistence of the superficial granular layer in a 2½-year-old pachygyric child. Generally, there is no consistent relationship between the late involution of the superficial granular layer and specific disease processes (Fig. 7).

The cerebellar roof nuclei of newborn infants frequently show scattered nests or strands of round or spindle shaped matrix cells in the neuropil or in perivascular distribution (Fig. 8). These cell nests are most common in the dentate nucleus but are seen in other roof nuclei as well. Berard-Badier *et al.* (1965) considered them of dysgenetic origin, but they are more likely variants of normal development. They are found in 28 percent of infants less than 4 months and undergo involution without residual lesions thereafter (Friede, 1973; Jellinger, 1974). Normal newborns also often show foci of cerebellar cortical disorganization, or heterotopic nests of cortical tissue, or heterotopic groups of large neurons in the cerebellar white matter (Chapter 31). These minor focal disorganizations found in normal newborns need to be distinguished from the similar but larger lesions found in 13–15 trisomy (Chapter 33).

Spinal Cord. The studies of Lassek and Rasmussen (1938, 1939) show that the length of the spinal cord increases 9.9 times between 16 weeks and term. The length of the spinal cord of the newborn averages 15.4 cm; its postnatal growth amounts to 2.7 times the length at birth, the increase being greatest in the thoracic region. The growth in the length of the cord is associated with changes in the proportion of its gray and white matter (Fig. 9). The increase in the volume of white matter is considerably greater than that of gray matter and extends over a longer period, presumably due to the continued growth of myelinated fibers. These changes are similar to the developmental changes in the proportions of gray and white matter in general, as described above for the cerebral hemispheres.

The growth of the spinal column was studied by Calkins and Scammon (1927, 1932). The postnatal growth of the spine exceeds that of the cord, so that the caudal end of the cord moves from the level of the third lumbar vertebra at birth to the level of the first lumbar vertebra in adults. The spinal roots, accordingly, take a descending, caudal course. However, ascending roots are found in the mid and upper thoracic regions of adults in as much as 71 percent of autopsies (Reid, 1960). Variation in the course of roots probably results from differences in the relative growth rate of vertebral and spinal segments; it has not been described for newborns.

Basic Reactions. The customary section, or chapter, on basic reactions has not been included at this point. Instead, the subject matter is discussed at various points throughout the text, wherever most pertinent to the lesions described. The peculiarities of necrosis and organization of immature fetal tissue, for example, are discussed in Chapter 11 as an introduction to fetal encephaloclastic lesions. Metabolic astrocytosis and its differentiation from nonspecific reactive astrocytosis is described in Chapter 45 along with the disease processes most likely to induce metabolic astrocytosis. Age-dependent differences in the manifestations of neuronal necrosis are described in Chapter 9, and axon pathology in general in Chapter 43, as a preface to the axonal dystrophies. This approach was considered preferable because the introductory materials provide continuity into the description and assessment of the respective lesions of the immature brain.

References

Altman, J.: Autoradiographic and histological studies of postnatal neurogenesis. J. comp. Neurol. 128: 431—474, 1966.

Angevine, J. B., Jr.: Time of neuron origin in the hippocampal region. Exp. Neurol. Suppl. 2: 1—70, 1965.

Angevine, J. B., Jr.: Time of neuron origin in the diencephalon of the mouse. An autoradiographic study. J. comp. Neurol. 139: 129—188, 1970.

— Sidman, R. L.: Autoradiographic study of cell migrations during histogenesis of cerebral cortex in the mouse. Nature 192: 766—768, 1961.

— — Autoradiographic study of histogenesis in the cerebral cortex of the mouse. Anat. Rec. 142: 210—210, 1962.

Banker, B. Q., Larroche, J.-C.: Periventricular leukomalacia of infancy. Arch. Neurol. 7: 386—410, 1962.

Barbe, A.: Recherches sur l'embryologie du système nerveux central de l'homme. Paris: Masson & Cie. 1938.

Bates, I. J., Netsky, M. G.: Developmental anomalies of the horns of the lateral ventricles. J. Neuropath. exp. Neurol. 14: 316—325, 1955.

Bérard-Badier, M., Colmant, H.-J., Jacob, H., Solcher, H.: Über die Spindel- und Rundzelldysgenesien im Dendatumvlies und ihre Genese. Acta Neuropath. 5: 243—251, 1965.

Bergel, A.: Über ein tumorähnliches Knötchen der Seitenwand des Rückenmarkes bei einem menschlichen Embryo von 16,5 größter Länge. Z. Neur. 116: 687—691, 1928.

Berliner, K.: Beiträge zur Histologie und Entwicklungsgeschichte des Kleinhirns. Arch. mikr. Anat. 66: 220—270, 1905.

Berry, M., Rogers, A. W.: The migration of neuroblasts in the developing cerebral cortex. J. Anat. 99: 691—711, 1965.

Biach, P.: Zur normalen und pathologischen Anatomie der äußeren Körnerschicht des Kleinhirns. Arb. neurol. Inst. Univ. Wien 18: 13—30, 1909—1910.

Brack, M.: Perinatal telencephalic leucoencephalopathy in chimpanzees (Pan troglodytes). Acta Neuropath. (Berlin) 25: 307—312, 1973.

Brun, A.: Zur Kenntnis der Bildungsfehler des Kleinhirns. Schweiz. Arch. Neurol. Psychiat. 1: 61—123; 2: 48—105; 3: 13—88, 1917—1918.

— The subpial granular layer of the foetal cerebral cortex in man. Its ontogeny and significance in congenital cortical malformations. Acta Path. Microbiol. Scand., Suppl. 179, 1965.

Calkins, L. A., Scammon, R. E.: The growth of the spinal axis of the human body in prenatal life. Proc. Soc. exp. Biol. Med. 24: 300—303, 1927.

— — The growth of the individual vertebrae of the human spine in prenatal life. Anat. Rec. 52: 6—7, 1932.

Cravioto, H.: The role of Schwann cells in the development of human peripheral nerves. An electron microscopic study. J. Ultrastruct. Res. 12: 634—651, 1965.

Davidoff, L. M.: Coarctation of the walls of the lateral angles of the lateral cerebral ventricles. J. Neurosurg. 3: 250—256, 1946.

Dekaban, A.: Human thalamus. II. Development of the human thalamic nuclei. J. comp. Neurol. 100: 63—97, 1954.

Dunn, H. L.: The growth of the central nervous system in the human fetus as expressed by graphic analysis and empirical formulae. J. comp. Neurol. 33: 405—491, 1921.

Ellenberger, C., Hanaway, J., Netzky, M. G.: Embryogenesis of the inferior olivary nucleus in the rat: a radioautographic study and a re-evaluation of the rhombic lip. J. comp. Neurol. 137: 71—79, 1969.

Ellis, R. S.: Norms for some structural changes in the human cerebellum from birth to old age. J. comp. Neurol. 32: 1—35, 1920.

Fenichel, M. D., Bazelon, M.: Studies on neuromelanin. II. Melanin in the brainstems of infants and children. Neurology 18: 817—820, 1968.

Fleschsig, P.: Die Leitungsbahnen im Gehirn und Rückenmark des Menschen. Leipzig: Engelmann 1876.

Foley, J. M., Baxter, D.: On the nature of pigment granules in the cells of the locus coeruleus and substantia nigra. J. Neuropath. exp. Neurol. 17: 586—598, 1958.

Friede, R. L.: A histochemical study of DPN-diaphorase in human white matter; with some notes on myelination. J. Neurochem. 8: 17—30, 1961.

— Control of myelin formation by axon caliber (with a model of the control mechanism). J. comp. Neurol. 144: 233—252, 1972.

— Dating the development of human cerebellum. Acta Neuropath. (Berl.) 23: 48—58, 1973.

Friede, R. L., Samorajski, T.: Myelin formation in the sciatic nerve of rat. A quantitative electron microscopic, histochemical and radioautographic study. J. Neuropath. exp. Neurol. 27: 546—571, 1968.

Geren, B. B.: The formation from the Schwann cell surface of myelin in the peripheral nerves of chick embryos. Exp. Cell Res. 7: 558—562, 1954.

Gilles, F. H., Murphy, S. E.: Perinatal telencephalic leucoencephalopathy. J. Neurol. Neurosurg. Psychiat. 32: 404—413, 1969.

Hanaway, J., McConnell, J. A., Netsky, M. G.: Histogenesis of the substantia nigra, ventral tegmental area of Tsai and interpeduncular nucleus: an autoradiographic study in the mesencephalon in the rat. J. comp. Neurol. 142: 59—73, 1971.

Haymaker, W., Margoles, C., Pentschew, A., Jacob, H., Lindenberg, R., Sáenz Arroyo, L., Stochdorph, O., Stowens, D.: Pathology of kernicterus and posticteric encephalopathy. Presentation of 87 cases, with a consideration of pathogenesis and etiology. In: Kernicterus and its Importance in Cerebral Palsy, pp. 21—228. Springfield, Ill.: Ch. C Thomas 1961.

Hesdorffer, H., Scammon, R. E.: Growth of human nervous system. Proc. Soc. exp. Biol. 33: 415—421, 1935.

Hicks, S. P., D'Amato, C. J.: Cell migrations to the isocortex in the rat. Anat. Rec. 160: 619—634, 1968.

Hinds, J. W.: Autoradiographic study of histogenesis in the olfactory bulb and accessory olfactory bulb in the mouse. Anat. Rec. 154: 358—359, 1966.

Howard, E., Granoff, D. M., Bujnovszky, P.: DNA, RNA, and cholesterol increase in cerebrum and cerebellum during development of human fetus. Brain Res. 14: 697—706, 1969.

Jellinger, K.: Persistent matrix cell nests in human cerebellar nuclei. Neuropädiatrie 5: 28—33, 1974.

Kantero, R.-L., Tiisala, R.: Growth of head circumference from birth to 10 years. Acta Paed. Scand., Suppl 220: 27—32, 1971.

Lapham, L. W.: The tetraploid DNA content of normal human Purkinje cells and its development during the perinatal period. Proc. Vth Internat. Congr. Neuropath. Zurich. Excerpta Med. Found. 1966, pp. 445—449.

Larroche, J. C.: Quelques aspects anatomiques du development cerebral. Biol. Neonat. 4: 126—153, 1962.

Lassek, A. M., Rasmussen, G. L.: A quantitative study of the newborn and adult spinal cords of man. J. comp. Neurol. 69: 371—379, 1938.

— — A regional volumetric study of the gray and white matter of the human prenatal spinal cord. J. comp. Neurol. 70: 137—151, 1939.

Lucas Keene, M. F., Hewer, E. E.: Some observations on myelination in the human central nervous system. J. Anat. 66: 1—13, 1931.

McFarland, D. E., Friede, R. L.: Number of fibers per sheath cell and internodal length in cat cranial nerves. J. Anat. 109: 169—176, 1971.

Martinez, A. J., Friede, R. L.: Changes in nerve cell bodies during the myelination of their axons. J. comp. Neurol. 138: 329—338, 1970.

Matthews, M. A., Duncan, D.: A quantitative study of morphological changes accompanying the initiation and progress of myelin production in the dorsal funiculus of the rat spinal cord. J. comp. Neurol. 142: 1—22, 1971.

Miale, I. L., Sidman, R. L.: An autoradiographic analysis of histogenesis in the mouse cerebellum. Exp. Neurol. 4: 277—296, 1971.

Mikhailets, V. V., 1952: Quoted in: The Human Brain in Figures and Tables (Blinkov, S. M., Glezer, I. I.), p. 334. New York: Plenum Press 1968.

Morel, F., Wildi, E.: Les ventricules cérébraux dans la démence précoce. Mschr. Psychiat. Neurol. 127: 1—10, 1954.

Murofushi, K.: Symmetrischer Pseudokalk in Stammganglien und Großhirnmark mit diskreter Leukencephalopathie bei Downschem Syndrom. Neuropädiatrie 1: 103—108, 1974.

Nellhaus, G.: Head circumference from birth to eighteen years. Practical composite international and interracial graphs. Pediatrics 41: 106—114, 1968.

O'Rahilly, R., Gardner, E.: The timing and sequence of events in the development of the human nervous system during the embryonic period proper. Z. Anat. Entwickl.-Gesch. 134: 1—12, 1971.

Peters, A., Muir, A. R.: The relationship between axons and Schwann cells during development of peripheral nerves in the rat. Quart. J. exp. Physiol. 44: 117—130, 1959.

Pryse-Davies, J., Beard, R. W.: A necropsy study of brain swelling in the newborn with special reference to cerebellar herniation. J. Path. 109: 51—73, 1973.

Raaf, J., Kernohan, J. W.: A study of the external granular layer in the cerebellum. Amer. J. Anat. 75: 151—172, 1944.

Rakić, P.: Neuron-glia relationship during granule cell migration in developing cerebellar cortex. A Golgi and electron-microscopic study in macacus rhesus. J. comp. Neurol. 141: 283—312, 1971.

— Mode of cell migration to the superficial layers of fetal monkey neocortex. J. comp. Neurol. 145: 61—84, 1972.

— Sidman, R. L.: Telencephalic origin of pulvinar neurons in the fetal human brain. Z. Anat. Entwickl.-Gesch. 129: 53—82, 1969.

— — Histogenesis of cortical layers in human cerebellum, particularly the lamina dissecans. J. comp. Neurol. 139: 473—500, 1970.

Reid, J. D.: Ascending nerve roots. J. Neurol. Neurosurg. Psychiat. 23: 148—155, 1960.

Richter, E.: Die Entwicklung des Globus pallidus und des Corpus subthalamicum. Monogr. Neurol. Psychiat. (Berl.) 108: 1—131, 1965.

Riggs, H. E., Rorke, L. B.: Myelination of the Brain in the Newborn. Philadelphia: Lippincott 1969.

Roback, H. N., Scherer, J. J.: Über die feinere Morphologie des frühkindlichen Hirnes unter besonderer Berücksichtigung der Gliaentwicklung. Virchow Arch. path. Anat. 294: 365—413, 1935.

Rydberg, E.: Cerebral injury in new-born children consequent on birth trauma; with an inquiry into the normal and pathological anatomy of the neuroglia. Acta Path. Microbiol. Scand., Suppl. 10: 1—247, 1932.

Samorajski, T., Friede, R. L.: A quantitative electron microscopic study of myelination in the pyramidal tract of rat. J. comp. Neurol. 134: 323—338, 1968.

Scammon, R. E.: Growth and Development of the Child. Part II, Anatomy and Physiology. The central nervous system. In: White House Conference on Child Health and Protection, pp. 176—190. New York-London: The Century Co. 1933.

— Dunn, H. L.: On the growth of the human cerebellum in early life. Proc. Soc. exp. Biol. Med. 21: 217—221, 1924.

Schonbach, J., Hu, K. H., Friede, R. L.: Cellular and chemical changes during myelination. Histologic, autoradiographic and biochemical data on myelination in the pyramidal tract and corpus callosum of rat. J. comp. Neurol. 134: 21—38, 1968.

Schwidde, J. T.: Incidence of cavum septi pellucidi and cavum vergae in 1,032 human brains. Arch. Neurol. Psychiat. 67: 625—632, 1952.

Sidman, R. L., Angevine, J. B., Jr.: Autoradiographic analysis of time of origin of nuclear versus cortical components of mouse telecephalon. Anat. Rec. 142: 326—327, 1962.

Silver, H. K., Diemer, W. C.: Graphs of the head circumference of the normal infant. J. Pediat. 33: 167—171, 1948.

Solcher, H.: Zur Neuroanatomie und Neuropathologie der Frühfetalzeit. Monogr. Neurol. Psychiat. (Berl.) 127: 1—78, 1968.

Spence, A. M., Gilles, F. H.: Underpigmentation of the substantia nigra in chronic disease in children. Neurology 21: 386—390, 1971.

Taber, E.: Histogenesis of brain stem neurons studied autoradiographically with thymidine-H^3 in the mouse. Anat. Rec. 145: 291—291, 1963.

— Histogenesis of brain stem neurons studied autoradiographically with thymidine-H^3 in the mouse. Anat. Rec. 148: 344—344, 1964.

Taber Pierce, E.: Histogenesis of the nuclei griseum pontis, corporis pontobulbaris and reticularis tegmenti pontis (Bechterew) in the mouse. An autoradiographic study. J. comp. Neurol. 126: 219—239, 1966.

Taber, Pierce, E.: Histogenesis of the dorsal and ventral cochlear nuclei in the mouse. Neurol. 131: 27—54, 1967.

Uzman, L. L.: The histogenesis of the mouse cerebellum as studied by thymidine uptake. J. comp. Neurol. 114: 137—159, 1960.

Westergaard, E.: The Lateral Cerebral Ventricles and Ventricular Walls. Odense: Andelsbogtrykkeriet 1970.

Wilmer, H. A.: Changes in structural components of the human body from six lunar months to maturity. Proc. Soc. exp. Biol. Med. 43: 545—547, 1940.

Part 1. Acquired Lesions in Newborns and Infants

2. Hemorrhages Characteristic of Asphyxiated Premature Infants

Intracranial hemorrhages, in particular subependymal, intraventricular and leptomeningeal hemorrhages, are the most common autopsy findings in the brain of asphyxiated premature infants. The incidence of intraventricular hemorrhage has been reported at approximately 1.1 per 1,000 live births (Fedrick and Butler, 1970), but the figure is of limited significance as some degree of subependymal bleeding is extremely common in the newborn succumbing to prematurity. The relationship of these hemorrhages to prematurity was recognized early (Couvelaire, 1903; Ylppö, 1919) and was confirmed in numerous later autopsy series (Hausbrandt and Meier, 1936; Craig, 1939; Gröntoft, 1953, Leech and Kohnen, 1974). Intraventricular hemorrhage also correlates with other factors related to prematurity, such as maternal disease, social factors, primiparity and lower than average birth weight (Fedrick and Butler, 1970; Harcke *et al.*, 1972).

Most infants are found to be abnormal at birth, showing cyanosis, apnea and lethargy, some requiring resuscitation. A downhill course with progressive respiratory distress ensues, and many of the infants die within 40 hours after birth. Small subependymal hemorrhages may be asymptomatic, or their manifestations clouded by the general distress. Large intraventricular hematomas cause coma, flaccid quadruparesis and respiratory arrest either precipitous or in the form of a fluctuating deterioration. A drop in hematocrit may signal massive bleeding. Hemorrhages may develop ante-, sub- or postpartum, but investigations using chromium-labelled erythrocytes have shown that the onset of bleeding usually occurs after the first 6 hours postpartum (for 22 of 28 infants; Dyer *et al.*, 1971), at a median age of 38 hours (36 infants, Tsiantos *et al.*, 1974).

Hyaline membrane disease of the lungs is frequently found in babies with intraventricular hemorrhage, and a causal relation between the two processes has been considered (Leech and Kohnen, 1974). However, no support for their interdependence comes forth from statistical studies: Infants having intraventricular hemorrhage but no hyaline membrane disease are of lower birth weight and lower gestational age than those having intraventricular hemorrhage and hyaline membrane disease (Spears *et al.*, 1969); also, hyaline membrane disease occurs with maximum frequency 6 to 48 hours after birth, which is not paralleled by the incidence of intraventricular hemorrhages (Fedrick, 1972).

Subependymal and Intraventricular Hemorrhages. Scattered case reports on these hemorrhages are found in the older literature, but the first systematic studies based on series of more than 100 cases were reported by Schwartz and Fink (1925) and Schwartz (1927). Subependymal hemorrhages originate in the subependymal matrix tissue in the region of the terminal vein (vena thalamostriata) between the thalamus and caudate nucleus. The most common site of bleeding is just posterior to the foramen of Monroe where the terminal vein turns down toward the foramen. The terminal vein receives its tributaries from the basal ganglia and the periventricular white matter. Near the foramen of Monroe it joins with the vena septi pellucidi and the choroid vein to form the internal cerebral veins which take an occipital course and form, by their junction, the great vein of Galen (vena cerebri magna) entering into the straight sinus. The subependymal hemorrhages near the foramen of Monroe are usually bilateral, though not necessarily of equal size, ranging from pinpoint petechiae to hematomas bulging into the lateral ventricle being covered by a thin layer of ependyma. Larger hematomas may dissect along the stria terminalis parallel to the caudate nucleus; they usually do not invade the grey matter of the caudate nucleus or the thalamus. Less frequent sites of bleeding are at the tributaries of the terminal vein, such as the lateral ventricular veins in the occipital horn or the subependymal veins in the temporal horns. The internal cerebral veins or the great vein of Galen are not typical sites of bleeding.

Subependymal hematomas readily disrupt the delicate layer of ependymal tissue. The site of disruption may not be apparent on inspection with the naked eye, even though large amounts of blood may escape into the lateral ventricles. Hematomas may spread from one or both lateral ventricles into the third and fourth ventricles with complete tamponade of the entire ventricular system. Their presence in the uncut brain is usually announced by a clot emerging from the cerebellar foramina or one filling the entire basal cisterns. It extends from there along the spinal subarachnoid space; whereas, extension along the central canal of the cord is less common. If the acute phase of bleeding is survived for hours to days, the flow of CSF may flush most of the blood from the lateral ventricles into the fourth and into the basal cisterns, and little, if any, blood is seen in the lateral ventricles where the bleeding had originated.

Microscopic examination discloses that the hemorrhages originate almost invariably within the thick layer of matrix tissue at the stria terminalis (Fig. 10), as first emphasized by Ruckensteiner and Zöllner (1929) who thought that the blood vessels burst because the soft matrix tissue provides only insufficient mechanical support; other authors (Gruenwald, 1951; Ross and Dimmette, 1965) speculated on primary changes in the matrix tissue triggering the bleeding. The matrix tissue shows congested, thin walled veins with recent hemorrhages, often multifocal and in a perivenous distribution around the stem or the tributaries of the terminal vein. Bursted veins can be seen in fortuitous sections. The hematomas enlarge by confluence and dissect along the path of least resistance, disrupting the matrix tissue and the thin layer of ependyma. There is no objective evidence of necrosis of matrix tissue antedating the hemorrhage. Thrombosis of subependymal veins is observed infrequently in association with subependymal hemorrhages and probably is a secondary change or complication. Towbin's (1968) claim that phlebothrombosis with resultant matrix infarction is generally responsible for intraventricular hemorrhages lacks convincing histologic documentation. Definite fibrinous thrombi in dilated veins were documented in isolated instances by Larroche (1954) and Ross and Dimmette, 2 of 30 cases, (1965) and were observed occasionally in the present author's material. These cases, however, consistute only a small fraction of all intraventricular hemorrhages; the thrombi may develop in reaction to the hemorrhage (Claireaux, 1959), or upon prolonged stasis in the congested vessels.

Subependymal and intraventricular hemorrhages may coexist with periventricular infarcts (Chapter 4) in as many as one-third to one-fourth of the cases (Larroche, 1964; Ross and Dimmette, 1965). Schwartz (1924) considered the infarcts secondary to terminal vein hemorrhages in his first pertinent publication, but he gave separate descriptions of the two types of lesions in his later papers (1927). A relatively small percentage of periventricular infarcts may develop secondary hemorrhages into the necrotic tissue (Armstrong and Norman, 1974). On gross inspection these lesions present as multiple hemorrhages into softened white matter around the corners of the lateral ventricles, more dorsal than the typical site of bleeding near the terminal vein. Cases of this type may lead to the erroneous conclusion that all subependymal hemorrhages are caused by hemorrhagic infarction of periventricular tissue, unless a careful histologic examination of the ventricular walls discloses the coexistence of two types of lesions.

Another cause of atypical distribution of hemorrhages about the corners of the lateral ventricles is from the distension and disruption of the ventricular walls by very large hematomas filling one or both lateral ventricles or causing tamponade of the entire ventricular system (Rydberg, 1932). In assessing the degree of ventricular distension, one needs to keep in mind that the ventricles of prematures are normally much larger than those of term infants (Chapter 1). Large intraventricular hematomas in the adult brain, or projectiles traversing the ventricles, are known to cause bursting and laceration of the walls of lateral ventricles (Harris *et al.*, 1968). Such bursting characteristically occurs at the corners of the lateral ventricles, in the occipital and temporal horns. Similar disruption of the ventricular corners in infants is accompanied with petechial hemorrhages and extension of the intraventricular hematoma into the white matter (Larroche, 1964). The pathogenesis of these lesions may not be evident from the examination of microscopic sections if the large hematomas had been removed from the ventricles when the brain was cut. Bursting of ventricles or secondary hemorrhages into periventricular infarcts probably account for the majority of instances in which subependymal hemorrhages are found at sites other than their typical occurrence near the terminal vein (Fig. 11).

Massive hematomas occluding the aqueduct or the basal cisterns may cause acute or subacute ventricular distension from obstruction of the flow of CSF; this effect is usually more evident after a few days survival, when

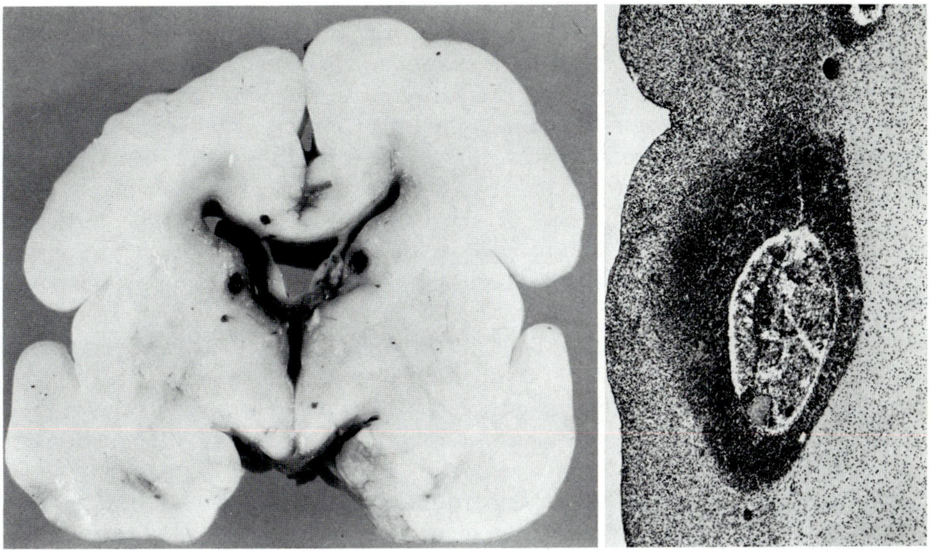

Fig. 10. Subependymal and intraventricular hemorrhages; microscopic examination of small hemorrhages demonstrates involvement—often multifocal—of perivenous matrix tissue; H & E ×40

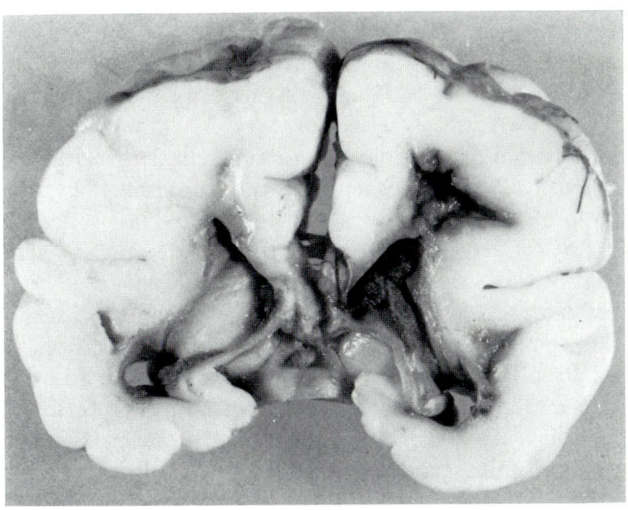

Fig. 11. Extension of intraventricular hemorrhage into a liquefying periventricular infarct. A similar infarct on the left side is ischemic and lacks communication with the ventricle

much of the blood has been washed into the basal cisterns. Ventricular distension was illustrated for a $5^1/_2$-day-old infant by Rydberg (1932) and for one of 21 days of age by Ross and Dimmette (1965). Direct transition into posthemorrhagic hydrocephalus may ensue, as the obstruction of CSF spaces becomes sustained by the fibrous organization of the hematoma.

Choroid Plexus Hemorrhage. Massive intraventricular hemorrhages rarely originate from the choroid plexus (Fig. 12). Entrapment of blood in the villi of the plexus or extreme congestion of its blood vessels may give a false impression of a high incidence of choroid plexus hemorrhages. Gröntoft (1963) observed only one case of definite choroid plexus hemorrhage causing intraventricular hemorrhage in his series and concluded that the plexus is not a significant factor for the production of intraventricular bleeding. In the present author's material of histologically verified cases only 13 choroid plexus hemorrhages were found for 174 cases of subependymal hemorrhages. This 7 percent incidence, however, includes relatively small bleedings in the choroid plexus stroma, only a few of which were thought accountable for an intraventricular hematoma.

Subarachnoid Hemorrhage. Subarachnoid hemorrhage may result from the spreading of an intraventricular hematoma into the subarachnoid spaces of the basal cisterns and the cerebellar meninges. In addition, subarachnoid hemorrhages frequently arise independently in the leptomeninges, with or without concurrent intraventricular hemorrhages. Ylppö (1919) emphasized the occurrence of subarachnoid hemorrhages in 17 of 20 premature infants and Craig (1939) in 29 of 36. The predilection of subarachnoid hemorrhage for prematures is inverse to the predilection of subdural hemorrhages for mature infants (Craig, 1939). According to Glaser (1928), the presence of small numbers of red blood cells is a physiologic phenomenon in the spinal fluid of premature infants.

Subarachnoid hemorrhages may occur anywhere over the cerebral hemispheres, but they are most frequent over the parietal and occipital lobes, ranging from thin effusions to substantial hematomas of several mm thickness. They probably originate from capillary diapedesis since the leptomeningeal veins are usually intact (Schwartz and Fink, 1925).

Subpial Hemorrhages. The existence of subpial hemorrhages as distinct from subarachnoid hemorrhages has received little attention, although they were mentioned by Glaser (1928) and Courville (1971). Subpial hemorrhages constitute approximately 15 percent of all perinatal intracranial hemorrhages (Friede, 1972). They are, strictly speaking, intracerebral hemorrhages, as the bleeding occurs in the superficial subpial layer of glial processes which are disrupted by the expanding hemorrhage, lifting the pia-arachnoid with some adherent glial remnants off the brain surface (Fig. 13). Subpial hemorrhage may occur in the absence of subarachnoid hemorrhage, or both may combine. It is most frequent over temporal and parietal lobes and over the cerebellar hemispheres. Cerebellar subpial hemorrhages often show a characteristic straight and sharp boundary from one gyrus to the next, as the hematoma has to extend along the sulcal cortical surface to reach the next gyrus; whereas, a subarachnoid hemorrhage readily reaches the next gyrus by crossing the

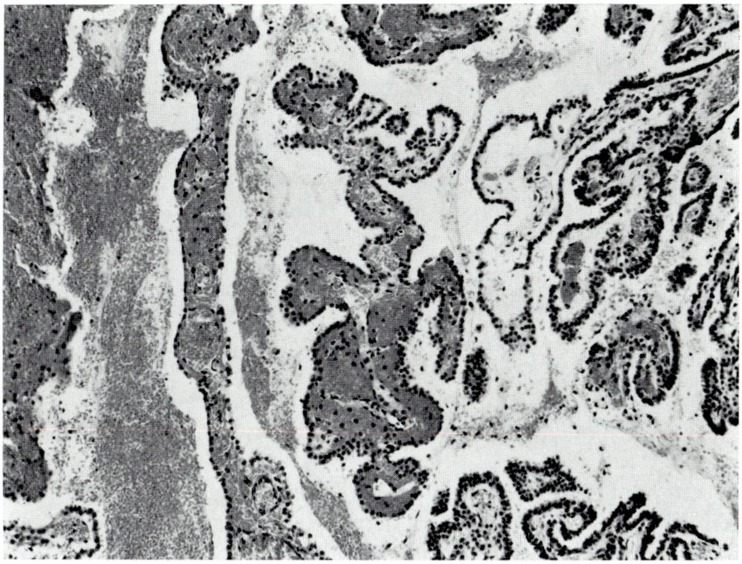

Fig. 12. Choroid plexus and intraventricular hemorrhage; H & E ×85

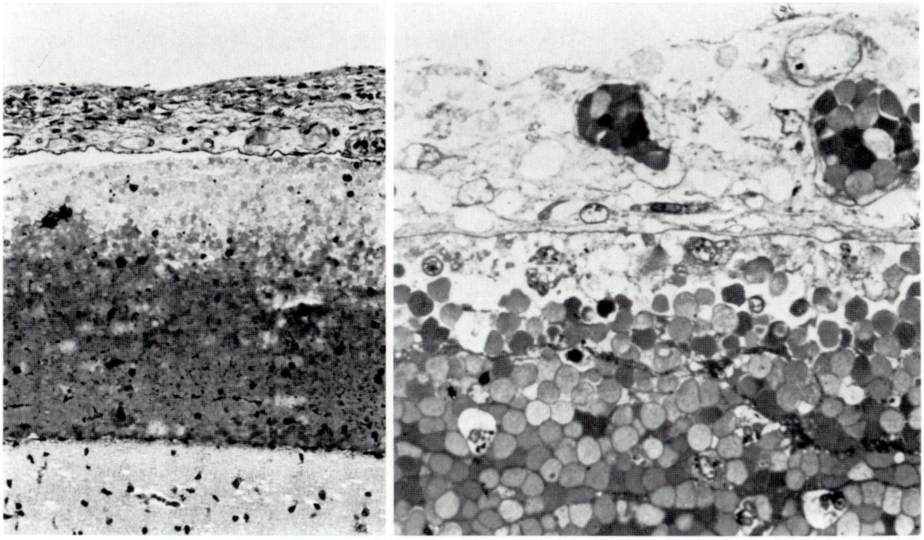

Fig. 13. Subpial hemorrhage, left; H & E ×150. Right: Thick section of plastic-embedded material shows residua of glial tissue at the inner surface of the basement membrane which adhers to the leptomeninges; there is no hemorrhage into the leptomeninges

subarachnoid space. Subpial hemorrhages disturb the structural integrity of the tissue much more than do subarachnoid hemorrhages.

Hemorrhages into the Falx. It is customary to consider the leptomeningeal hemorrhages in prematures as asphyctic and the hemorrhages into the falx and tentorium as traumatic (Chapter 3). However, small petechiae into the falx and tentorium are so common in mature as well as in premature babies that their attribution to birth trauma is debatable; it is more likely that many are of asphyctic origin (Fig. 14).

Cerebellar and Other Parenchymal Hemorrhages. Intracerebral hematomas are rare in premature infants except for the cerebellum where they occur at high frequency (Schwartz and Fink, 1925). These cerebellar hemorrhages are nearly always multifocal, originating within the cortex or subcortical white matter, most commonly at the tentorial surface or at the outer convexity of the cerebellar hemispheres. There may be multiple small hematomas, some dissecting between the layers of the cerebellar cortex, some breaking locally through its surface and forming small subpial effusions (Fig. 15). Considerable destruction of cerebellar tissue results from the extension and confluence of these hematomas. Large infratentorial clots may form; these are easily mistaken for hemorrhages arising from rupture of the great vein of Galen unless the blood clot is examined with the microscope, which almost invariably reveals embedded fragments of cerebellar cortex.

Large hematomas in the cerebral hemispheres of newborns are rare; if present, they suggest mechanical trauma, embolic infarcts (Chapter 12), phlebothrombosis (Chapter 13) or other concurrent disease processes (Chapter 46). Microscopic extravasations of blood may be seen in all portions of the brain, but their significance is doubtful. Hemsath and Canavan (1932) observed petechiae in 54 percent of one or two sections taken at random from the brain stem, and Hirvensalo (1949) found them in 37 percent of his cases but did not consider them of clinical significance. Craig (1939) observed major perivascular hemorrhages in only 6 of 126 cases, all of whom were larger children delivered at term under prolonged labor. Very young, aborted fetuses may show such hemorrhages with greater frequency, such as 63 of 65 (Solcher, 1968), including hemorrhages into the choroid plexus, ventricular walls and cerebral hemispheres.

Residual Lesions. The various types of hemorrhages described in the present chapter appear to develop most often during a critical phase close to the infant's demise, so that acute hemorrhages are seen much more often than residual lesions. Only 5 percent of the subependymal hemorrhages in the present author's series presented as residual lesions. The residual lesions are rather inconspicuous and easily overlooked. Minimal subependymal hemorrhages may leave only minute brownish spots near the terminal vein in infants a few weeks old, which seem to disappear completely later on. Microscopically they are seen best in sections stained for iron, disclosing focal deposition of hemosiderin throughout the tissue and in macrophages, as well as focal glial scarring and mineral deposits. More conspicuous lesions consist of smooth-walled subependymal cysts, situated bilateral near the foramen of Monroe at the same sites where the acute hemorrhages occur (Schwartz, 1927;

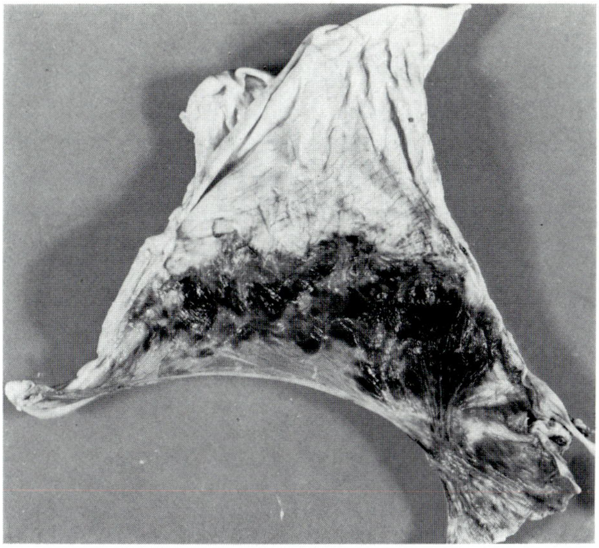

Fig. 14. Falcine hemorrhages

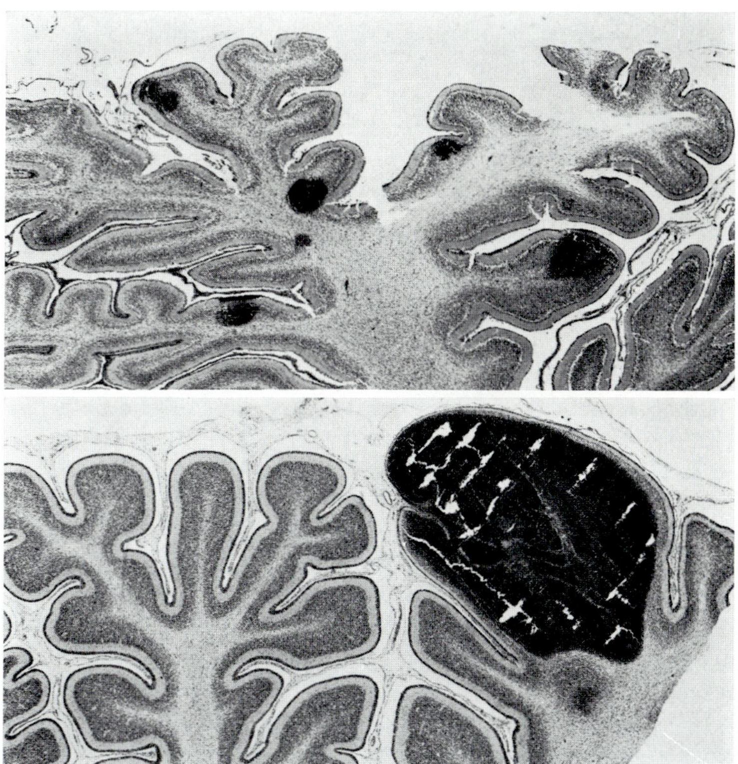

Fig. 15. Hemorrhages into cerebellar cortex; H & E ×11.5

Claireaux, 1959). These cysts may have a single lumen, or be loculated being traversed by delicate glial septae (Figs. 16, 17). In infants a few weeks old, they often show a characteristic budding of small nests of matrix tissue from the cyst wall or from the septae traversing the cyst (Larroche, 1972). There usually is very little gliosis near these cysts, and deposits of hemosiderin are

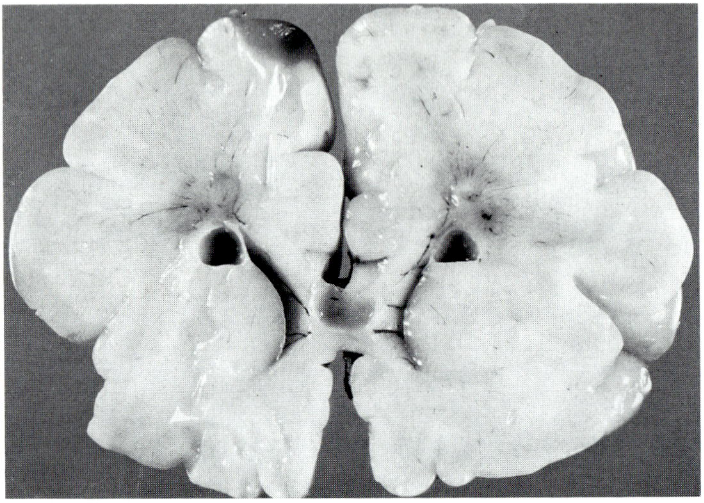

Fig. 16. Subependymal cysts residual to subependymal hemorrhage

sparse, and often altogether absent. However, a scrutiny of the leptomeninges in these instances often furthers evidence of past hemorrhage in the form of hemosiderin-laden macrophages and moderate fibrosis. The macrophages also stain brightly with the PAS reaction. Destruction of the head of the caudate nucleus with cavitation and hemosiderin-laden scars appears to be very rare and was reported for a 9-month-old child by Schwartz (1927) and was also mentioned by Norman (1969).

Hemorrhage into the subarachnoid space may cause obstructive hydrocephalus, either acutely from the direct obliteration of the basal cisterns by clots of blood or from the chronic effects of its organization (Fig. 18) with fibrosis of the subarachnoid space (Larroche, 1972; Chapter 22). Another mechanism of obstruction of the CSF spaces is from the organization of an intraventricular hematoma by way of reactive gliosis from the ventricular walls (Siegmund, 1955; Larroche, 1972). The latter mechanism appears to be much less common than fibrosis of the subarachnoid space, judging from the frequency at which either of these changes are encountered when scrutinizing the respective regions in infants who survived complicated birth for a few months. Lorber and Bassi (1965) evaluated 588 cases of hydrocephalus on basis of clinical criteria: 478 were associated with spina bifida cystica. Of the remaining 110 there were 43 with a definite history of postnatal acquisition: 20 postmeningitic, 19 posthemorrhagic.

There are remarkably few accounts of residual lesions of the cerebellar hemorrhages although the acute lesions are quite common in prematures. Schwartz (1927) reported pigmented residual cavities with marked hemosiderosis of their walls in the cerebellum. Instances of diffuse superficial hemosiderosis of the cerebellar hemispheres (Chapter 9) may be accounted for by cerebellar hemorrhages.

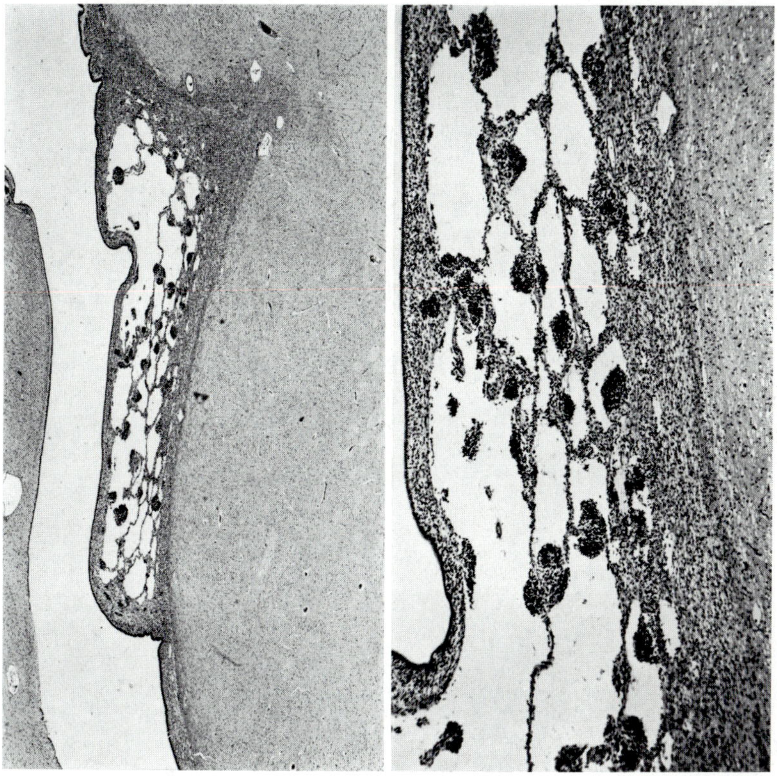

Fig. 17. Loculated subependymal cysts with characteristic budding of matrix tissue into their lumen; compare distribution with Fig. 10; H & E ×11.5, ×40

Pathogenetic Considerations. The pathogenesis of subependymal and intraventricular hemorrhages has been subject of much speculation, particularly in the older literature in which the relationship between these lesions and mechanical birth trauma is often discussed at great length. However, mechanical birth trauma is an unlikely cause of the bleeding since the hemorrhages have been found in aborted fetuses (Solcher, 1958), macerated fetuses (Gröntoft, 1953), or infants delivered by Cesarean section (Craig, 1939). Furthermore, the use of chromium-labelled erythrocytes has shown conclusively that hemorrhages develop hours after birth (Dyer *et al.*, 1971). The assumption of a hemorrhagic diathesis either on the basis of immaturity or precipitated by asphyxia has been popular for some time, but there is no similarity at all between the lesions described in the present chapter and those from established clotting disorders of infancy which either present as random intracerebral hematomas, or abundant, random petechiae (Chapter 46). The fragility of the fetal blood vessels or the poor mechanical support provided to them by the loose matrix tissue was blamed by other authors, but these factors cannot account for all of the typical regional

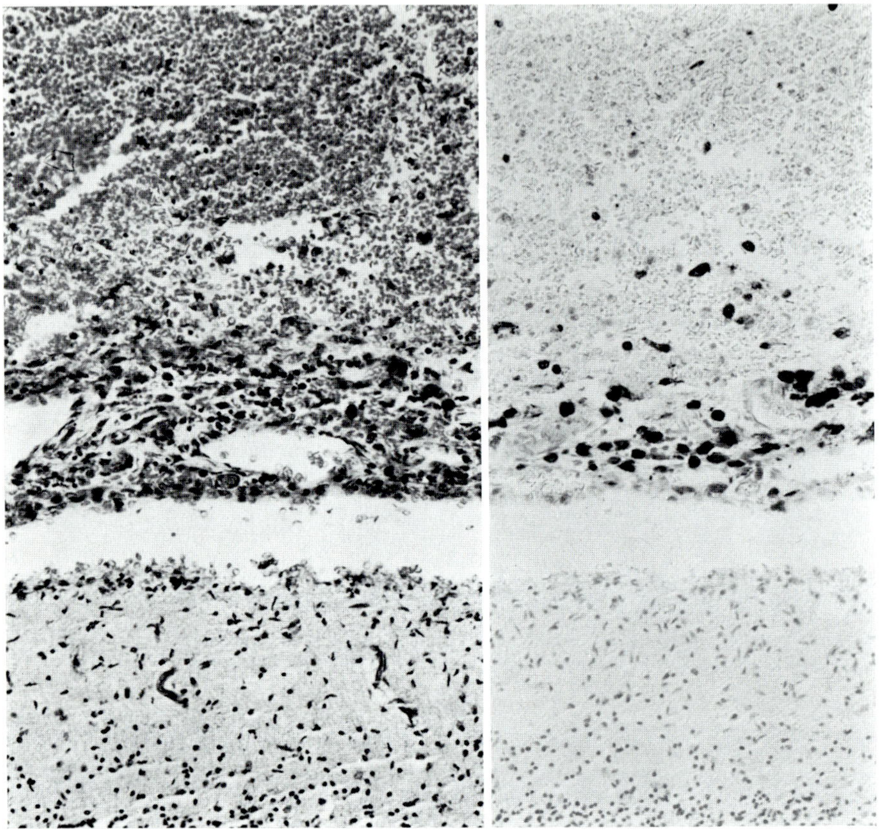

Fig. 18. Early organization of subarachnoid hemorrhage; H & E and iron stain ×150

patterns of these hemorrhages. Necrosis or retrogressive changes in the matrix tissue, or hemorrhagic infarction of periventricular tissue have also been implicated. The difficulties with these theories is the lack of corroborating histologic evidence. The most solid evidence comes from clinicopathologic correlations showing that prolonged, severe anoxia or asphyxia are the critical factors in causing the hemorrhages of prematures (Gröntoft, 1953; Harrison *et al.*, 1968). The experiments of Noell and Schneider (1942) on the effects of severe anoxia (dogs exposed to a nitrogen athmosphere) are important for the understanding of the neonatal lesions. Exposure to severe hypoxia for variable times, from a few minutes to near one hour, resulted in hypoxemic circulatory collapse which was heralded by a severe decrease in arterio-venous oxygen difference. During collapse the respiratory volume decreased to zero and pulse frequency to approximately half normal ("vagus pulse"). Blood pressure dropped and cerebral circulation decreased to negligible values even when a low blood pressure (approximately 40 mm Hg) was maintained for a while. Corresponding to these changes, the oxygen tension of the venous blood dropped to zero and a sharp increase in venous pressure (up to 25 mm Hg) was measured in the right auricle. The arterio-venous pressure difference, and cerebral perfusion, was minimized by the drop in arterial pressure combined with increase in venous pressure. The drop to zero in the oxygen tension in venous blood was considered the critical phenomenon in inducing these severe disturbances, depriving the brain tissue of all residual sources of oxygen. Resuscitation from collapse within 2 minutes was followed by tachycardia, a sharp rise in blood pressure to near twice normal and a compensatory increase in cerebral perfusion up to 200 percent; however, resuscitation was often slowed by persistent circulatory failure. Hence, cardiac failure needs to be considered critical in inducing cerebral damage, allthemore as the heart's tolerance to anoxia may vary independently from that of the brain (Miller, 1970). The sharp rise in venous pressure during anoxic circulatory collapse is probably the determining factor in inducing the various types of hemorrhages in the premature, possibly aided by vascular fragility and superimposed anoxic damage. Nearer to term, when the brain tissue is more mature, the same mechanisms may produce parenchymal lesions such as the ulegyria in watershed distribution (Chapter 6).

Animal experimentation has otherwise not contributed to the understanding of perinatal hemorrhages; subependymal and intraventricular hemorrhages comparable to those in humans have not been induced experimentally. Petechial cerebral hemorrhages were observed in asphyxiated guinea pigs (Bailey and Windle, 1959) but were never seen in subsequent experiments in monkeys which were sacrificed before reaching the state of terminal agony (Ranck and Windle, 1959). Dekaban and Windle (1962) concluded that asphyxiation may weaken capillary walls which then may be ruptured mechanically by excessive venous congestion resulting from terminal heart failure. Hemorrhages in the basal ganglia were produced experimentally in fetuses whose mothers had been given oxytocin or who had complicated delivery (Windle, 1970).

References

Armstrong, D., Norman, M. G.: Periventricular leucomalacia in neonates: complications and sequelae. Arch. Dis. Child. 49: 367—375, 1974.

Bailey, C. J., Windle, W. F.: Neurological, psychological, and neurobiological defects following asphyxia neonatorum in the guinea pig. Exp. Neurol. 1: 467—482, 1959.

Claireaux, E. E.: Cerebral pathology of newborns. Guy Hosp. Rep. 108: 2—20, 1959.

Courville, C. B.: Birth and Brain Damage. Pasadena: M. F. Courville 1971.

Couvelaire, A.: Hémorrhagies du système nerveux central des nouveau-nés. Ann. Gynec. Obstet. 59: 253—268, 1903.

Craig, W. W.: Intracranial hemorrhage in the newborn. Arch. Dis. Child. 13: 89—124, 1938.

Dekaban, A., Windle, W. F.: Hemorrhagic lesions in acute birth injuries. J. Neuropath. exp. Neurol. 21: 305—306, 1962.

Dyer, N., Brill, A. B., Gutberlat, R., *et al.:* Timing of intracranial bleeding in newborn infants. J. nuclear Med. 12: 353—354, 1971.

Fedrick, J.: Neonatal deaths. Time of death, maturity and lesion. Biol. Neonat. 18: 369—378, 1972.

— Butler, N. R.: Certain causes of neonatal death. II. Intraventricular hemorrhage. Biol. Neonat. 15: 257—290, 1970.

Friede, R. L.: Subpial hemorrhage in infants. J. Neuropath. exp. Neurol. 31: 548—556, 1972.

Glaser, J.: The cerebrospinal fluid of premature infants. Amer. J. Dis. Child. 36: 195—247, 1928.

Gröntoft, O.: Intracerebral and meningeal haemorrhages in perinatally deceased infants. I. Intracerebral haemorrhages. A pathologico-anatomical and obstetric study. Acta obstet. gynec. scand. 32: 308—333, 1953.

— Intracerebral and meningeal haemorrhages in perinatally deceased infants. II. Meningeal haemorrhages. A pathologico-anatomical and obstetric study. Acta obstet. gynec. scand. 32: 458—498, 1953.

Gruenwald, P.: Subependymal cerebral hemorrhage in premature infants and its relation to various injurious influences at birth. Amer. J. Obstet. Gynec. 61: 1285—1292, 1951.

Harcke, H. T., Jr., Naeye, R. L., Storch, A., Blanc, W. A.: Perinatal cerebral intraventricular hemorrhage. J. Pediat. 80: 37—42, 1972.

Harris, L. S., Roessmann, U., Friede, R. L.: Bursting of cerebral ventricular walls. J. Path. Bact. 1: 33—38, 1968.

Harrison, V. C., Heese, H., Klein, M.: Intracranial hemorrhage associated with hyaline membrane disease. Arch. Dis. Child. 43: 116—120, 1968.

Hausbrandt, F., Meier, A.: Zur Kenntnis der geburtstraumatischen und extrauterin erworbenen Schäden des Zentralnervensystems bei Neugeborenen. Frankfurt. Z. Path. 49: 21—62, 1936.

Hemsath, F. A., Canavan, M. M.: Microscopic cerebral hemorrhage in stillbirths and newborn deaths. Amer. J. Obstet. Gynec. 23: 471—478, 1932.

Hirvensalo, M.: On hemorrhages of the medulla oblongata and the pons and on respiratory disorders in premature infants. Acta Paediat. (Suppl. 1) 37: 1—112, 1949.

Larroche, J.-C.: Hémorrhagies cérébrales intraventriculaires chez le prématuré. Biol. Neonat. 7: 26—56, 1964.

— Post-haemorrhagic hydrocephalus in infancy. Anatomical study. Biol. Neonat. 20: 287—299, 1972.

— Sub-ependymal pseudocysts in the newborn. Biol. Neonat. 21: 170—183, 1972.

Leech, R. W., Kohnen, P.: Subependymal and intraventricular hemorrhages in the newborn. Am. J. Path. 77: 465—476, 1974.

Lorber, J., Bassi, U.: The aetiology of neonatal hydrocephalus. Develop. Med. Child Neurol. 7: 289—294, 1965.

Miller, J. A., Jr.: Prevention of brain damage during asphyxia. Proc. 2nd Cong. Int. Asso. Sci. Study Mental Deficiency, Poland, 1970, pp. 444—449.

Naeye, R. L., Burt, S., Wright, D. L., Blanc, A., Tatter, D.: Neonatal mortality, the male disadvantage. Pediatrics 48: 902—906, 1971.

Noell, W., Schneider, M.: Über die Durchblutung und die Sauerstoffversorgung des Gehirns im akuten Sauerstoffmangel. Pflügers Arch. ges. Physiol. 246: 181—249, 1942.

Norman, R. M.: Malformations of the nervous system, birth injury and diseases of early life. In: Greenfield's Neuropathology, Chapter 6, pp. 324—440. E. Arnold 1969.

Ranck, J. B., Windle, W. F.: Brain damage in the monkey, *Macaca mulatta,* by asphyxia neonatorum. Exp. Brain Res. 1: 130—154, 1959.

Ross, J. J., Dimmette, R. M.: Subependymal cerebral hemorrhage in infancy. Amer. J. Dis. Child. 110: 531—542, 1965.

Ruckensteiner, E., Zöllner, F.: Über die Blutungen im Gebiete der Vena terminalis bei Neugeborenen. Frankfurt. Z. Path. 37: 568—578, 1929.

Rydberg, E.: Cerebral injury in newborn children consequent on birth injury. Acta path. scand., Suppl. 10: 1—247, 1932.

Schwartz, P.: Erkrankungen des Zentralnervensystems nach traumatischer Geburtsschädigung. Z. Neurol. Psychiat. 90: 263—468, 1924.

Schwartz, P.: Die traumatischen Schädigungen des Zentralnervensystems durch die Geburt. Ergebn. inn. Med. Kinderheilk. 31: 165—372, 1927.

— Fink, L.: Morphologie und Entstehung der geburtstraumatischen Blutungen im Gehirn und Schädel des Neugeborenen. Z. Kinderheilk. 40: 427—474, 1925.

Siegmund, H.: Die geburtstraumatischen Veränderungen des Zentralnervensystems einschließlich der Encephalitis congenita. Virchows Handbuch Spec. Path. Anat. Histol. XIII/3: 239—287, 1955.

Solcher, H.: Zur Neuroanatomie und Neuropathologie der Frühfetalzeit. Monogr. Neurol. Psychiat. 127: 1—78. Berlin-Heidelberg-New York: Springer 1968.

Spears, R. L., Hodgman, J. E., Cleland, R. D., Tatter, D., Hanes, B.: Relationship between hyaline membrane disease and intraventricular hemorrhage as cause of death in low birthweight infants. Amer. J. Obstet. Gynec. 105: 1028—1031, 1969.

Towbin, A.: Cerebral intraventricular hemorrhage and subependymal matrix infarction in the fetus and premature newborn. Amer. J. Path. 52: 121—139, 1968.

Tsiantos, A., Victorin, L., Relier, J. P., *et al.*: Intracranial hemorrhage in the prematurely born infants. J. Pediat. 85: 854—859, 1974.

Windle, W. F.: Cerebral hemorrhage in relation to birth asphyxia. Science 167: 1000—1003, 1970.

Ylppö, A.: Pathologisch anatomische Studien bei Frühgeborenen. Z. Kinderheilk. 20: 212—431, 1919.

3. Cerebral Lesions from Physical Trauma

The types of hemorrhagic lesions characteristic of mature infants differ from those of prematures in distribution and pathogenesis. Hemorrhages in prematures are mainly subependymal and intraventricular, leptomeningeal, or in the cerebellar parenchyma, and are related to asphyxia. They become less frequent as the infant approaches maturity. The types of hemorrhages characteristic of the mature newborn are related to mechanical trauma, such as lacerations of tentorium, falx or large venous channels, subdural hematomas, or injuries of the spinal cord. In addition to these types of lesions, the present chapter also includes a discussion of herniations of intracranial contents of the newborn.

Intradural Hemorrhages. Lacerations of the tentorium or falx need to be distinguished from intrafalcine or intradural hemorrhages (Pott, 1911). Hemorrhages into the loose connective tissue of the immature falx or tentorium are quite common in term as well as premature infants. They are multicentric and range from small petechiae to large, confluent effusions, commonly involving the falx, particularly in the portion near the superior sagittal sinus. Larger hematomas, of 2 to 3 mm thickness, may cause the falx or the tentorium to bulge, penetrating to the very surface of the tissue. It is uncommon for these intradural hemorrhages to rupture into the subdural space and to cause substantial subdural hematomas (Ylppö, 1919). They are of no clinical significance; their attribution to either asphyxia or mechanical trauma is a matter of conjecture. Their resorption evidently occurs very quickly and without difficulty; infants a few months old rarely show organizing hematomas or pigmentation in falx or tentorium in spite of the great frequency at which acute hemorrhages are seen at these sites in newborns.

Lacerations of Tentorium and Falx. Lacerations of the tentorium are more serious lesions than the intradural hemorrhages and received wide recognition after having been described by Beneke (1910), who called attention to the need for a thorough inspection of the tentorium before its resection from the skull. A profusion of case reports and of large series of cases followed Beneke's publication, and the preoccupation with this type of lesion had evidently often distracted the authors from the identification of other sources of bleeding, particularly the common intraventricular hemorrhages in prematures.

The frequency of tentorial lacerations increases with gestational age or with birth weight. They are rare in prematures (Ylppö, 1919); only 17 cases of falx or tentorium hemorrhages were observed among 126 cases of intraventricular hemorrhage (Larroche, 1964). Conversely, two-thirds of the infants with tentorial lacerations were in the weight group of over 4,500 gms, compared with an incidence of only 4 percent in prematures (Gröntoft, 1953); similar statistics were obtained by Hausbrandt and Meier (1936), Goerttler and Draisbach (1963), and others.

Data on the general frequency of tentorial lacerations vary over a wide range. Holland (1921), for example, found them in 48 percent of 168 autopsies; whereas, Rohrbach (1953) observed them in only 2.7 percent of 402 autopsies. Nesbitt and Anderson (1956) report a frequency of deaths from dural laceration and resulting intracranial hemorrhage of 1 in 2,060 births. Several factors enter the great range of reported frequencies: There was often insufficient distinction between hemorrhages from dural lacerations and asphyctic hemorrhages in the older reports, in which all intracranial hemorrhages in newborns were considered traumatic. A high frequency also results from the pooling of lacerations of dura with intradural hemorrhages. There are also true changes in frequency as dural lacerations became rare with improved techniques of obstetric management, while, on the other hand, due to improvement in the management of prematures, asphyctic hemorrhages are now seen more frequently in autopsy material. In the present author's material from Rainbow Babies and Children's Hospital (Cleveland, Ohio), dural lacerations are extremely rare, while the various types of asphyctic hemorrhages are commonplace.

Lacerations of the tentorium occur most commonly at its free edge and may be complete or incomplete, affecting either the superior or the inferior leaf of the tentorial tissue. Ragged edges are seen in the torn tissue. Hemorrhages ensue from rupture of intratentorial blood vessels, and they attain major extent from the opening of larger venous channels. Extension of the tear in median direction opens the straight sinus, while lateral extension opens the transverse sinus (Holland, 1921). The vein of Galen may be torn off its insertion at the straight sinus, but this type of injury is rather rare and is often confused with large asphyctic cerebellar hematomas (Chapter 2). Subdural hemorrhages from the tearing of briding veins from the sagittal sinus are often mentioned, but well documented cases are difficult to find (Schipke *et al.*, 1954; Chapt. 19). Lacerations are much less frequent in the falx than in the tentorium and comprise between 4 and 12 percent of all lacerations (Holland, 1921; Schäfer, 1922; Goerttler and Draisbach, 1963). Even these figures on the frequency of falcine lacerations are exaggerated with cases in whom the fenestration of the falx that occurs as a normal developmental variant was thought to represent disruption. Other uncommon sources of hemorrhage are from rupture of the longitudinal sinus due to the overlapping of the parietal and occipital bones, from the tearing of bridging veins by the overriding of parietal bones, and from lacerations of the sigmoid sinus by occipital osteodiastesis (Schäfer, 1922; Hemsath, 1934; Craig, 1938). Lacerations of the tentorium appear to heal completely as there are no reports of residual lesions in adults.

Laceration of the dura is evidently caused by mechanical trauma during birth, as postulated by Beneke (1910) who thought that tentorial laceration is caused by bitemporal compression of the skull. Holland (1921) discussed the various types of deformation of falx and tentorium that result from deformation of the skull. Gröntoft (1953) concluded that the following circumstances are principally involved in causing tentorial lacerations: Rapid forcing of the fetal head through the birth canal, such as in precipitate labor, breech presentation or extraction; a disproportion between the fetal head and the pelvis; cranial trauma caused by forceps; rigidity of the soft parts of the birth canal.

Bleeding from dural lacerations causes subdural hematomas which are dealt with on p. 190 in Chapter 19. Resorption of these hematomas is slower than that of subarachnoid hemorrhages because of their larger size and because of the inherently slower resorption of fluids from the subdural space. Large organizing hematomas have been found attached to the tentorium in infants several months old. Subdural hematomas are a potential source of chronic subdural hematomas or hygromas, particularly of those of the inferior cerebral fossa.

Bone Injuries. Birth-related fractures of cranial bones in infants are presently rare. Impression fractures of the parietal bone have resulted from forced instrumental delivery (Capon, 1922). Osteodiastesis or fractures of the occipital bone at the posterior intraoccipital synchondrosis were observed upon breech or instrumental delivery (Hemsath, 1934); the high frequency reported by this author appears to have decreased substantially, and this type of injury is now rarely observed (Claireaux, 1959). Traumatic epidural hemorrhages, likewise, are quite rare in infants; only 4 were seen among 50,000 autopsies (Courville, 1971). In a series of 42 infants with severe head trauma at birth there were 15 depressed, 2 linear and 1 basal fractures; there were also 24 subdural hematomas, 1 intracerebral, 13 chronic subdural and no large epidural hematomes (Natelson and Sayers, 1973).

Lesions from Herniation of Cerebral Tissue. The manifestations of increased intracranial pressure in the newborn differ in principle from those in the adult because of the extreme pliability and elasticity of the infantile cranial vault. Increased intracranial pressure in the adult invariably forces cerebral tissue in the general direction of the foramen magnum which is the only major nonrigid portion of the cranial capsule; consequently, there are resultant herniations at the falx, the tentorial hiatus and the foramen magnum. The fontanels of infants permit distension of the cranium, thus diminishing or abrogating the force of caudal dislocation of the tissue. Indeed, some lesions of increased intracranial pressure in adults, for example the secondary midbrain hemorrhages, are virtually unknown in the newborn infant. Signs of increased intracranial pressure may be observed in the newborn, including flattening of gyri, or cerebellar tonsillar herniation, but they occur usually above a gestational age of 35 weeks (Pryse-Davies and Beard, 1973). Cerebellar herniation to the extent of causing acute tonsillar necrosis (Fig. 19) is an exceptionally rare complication of severe asphyctic lesions in the hemispheres. The relatively mild degree of herniations in the newborn may be conditioned not only by the mechanical properties of the skull but, also, by

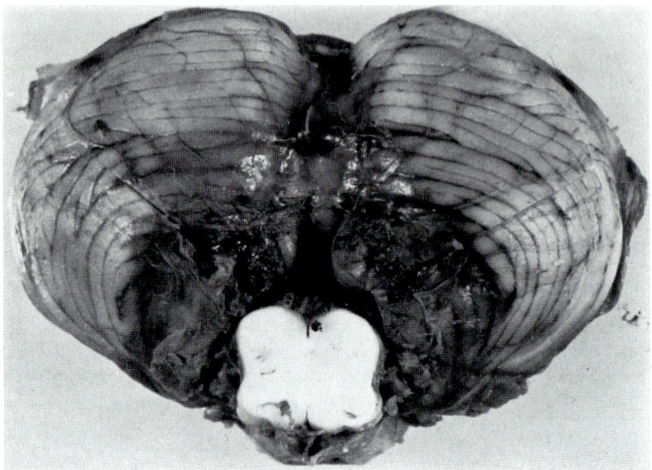

Fig. 19. Necrosis of cerebellar tonsils from herniation secondary to subtotal necrosis of the cerebral hemispheres

the lesser tendency of the immature brain tissue to develop edema (Go *et al.*, 1973).

The production of permanent cerebral damage from herniations caused by intrapartum molding of the head is controversial. Earle *et al.* (1953) attributed gliosis of the temporal lobes to "incisural sclerosis" from intrapartum molding of the head. Their conclusion was based on the presence of astrocytic gliosis in neurosurgical biopsies from the temporal lobes of 157 patients with temporal epilepsy, only 25 of whom had a history of difficult birth. They also reported model experiments, in which the heads of stillborn infants were tightly wrapped with rubber bands then frozen and cut, showing uncal herniation at the tentorium. This model is open to criticism as it ignores the intrauterine pressure transmitted onto the entire body contents of the infant when its head enters the cervical canal; further, the pressure gradient in the cranial vault is opposite to that produced in the experiment once the head of the infant emerges from the cervical canal. The parenchymal lesions of "incisural sclerosis" have never been demonstrated unequivocally in autopsy cases, except for controversial interpretations of postconvulsive sclerosis of the Ammon's horn.

Bilateral cerebellar sclerosis along a groove around the protruding tonsils has been reported as a residuum of swelling or displacement of the cerebellum in early life (McHenry *et al.*, 1964). This interpretation is based on conjecture, and the lesions are more consistent with the chronic tonsillar herniations described in Chapter 25. However, instrumental delivery with extreme compression of the cranium may cause excessive cerebellar tonsillar herniation with necrosis and sloughing of cerebellar fragments into the spinal canal (Towbin, 1964).

One has to conclude that the evidence for the production of permanent cerebral damage by intrapartum herniation of the cerebral tissue is at present unsatisfactory. There is also reason to believe that cerebral herniations from increased intracerebral pressure are generally less severe in infants than in children or adults.

Intracerebral Hemorrhages. Large hematomas of the cerebral hemispheres of newborns are infrequent. They may be caused by gross mechanical trauma, as attested by a number of dramatic reports in the older literature. Jaffe (1929), for example, described a pigmented cavity communicating with the lateral ventricle and with the surface of the occipital lobe in a 22-year-old subject who had been dropped 80 cms to the floor in the course of the excitement following his birth. Lesions of this type are rare, at least in terms of reported instances.

Indirect evidence of severe mechanical disruption of brain tissue by traumatic birth may be obtained from emboli of cerebral tissue in pulmonary blood vessels, as first observed by Runge (1879). Valdes-Dapena and Arey (1967) reviewed 4 occurrences including 2 cases of their own both having lacerations of the tentorium. The births had been considered uneventful, which may be taken as a reflection on the general value of clinico-pathologic correlations for severe birth trauma.

Hemorrhagic lesions of the cerebral hemispheres are also found in the absence of anatomic evidence of cranio-cerebral trauma; these occur in the subcortical white matter or as wedge-shaped hemorrhagic zones in the cortex (Siegmund, 1923; Schwartz and Fink, 1925). The interpretation of these lesions as cortical contusions is questionable. Microscopic examination of the cases available to the present author disclosed that the lesions were hemorrhagic infarcts rather than traumatic hemorrhages; they are considered further in Chapter 12.

Injuries of the Spinal Cord. The first report on spinal injury during delivery by Parrot (1870) was followed by a number of case reports. Larger series of cases were studied by Crothers (1923), Ford (1925), and Crothers and Putnam (1927), the latter with a comprehensive review of the literature. Since then, only scattered reports have been published, but the lesion has by no means disappeared from the scene of perinatal pathology. Most cord injuries are in the cervical and upper thoracic spinal cord and are caused by excessive traction during breech delivery. Cord injuries are uncommon upon cephalic delivery. Shulman *et al.* (1971) reviewed 15 cases of the latter; the lesions affected mostly the upper cervical cord, apparently in consequence of excessive rotation of the head. Hyperextension of the neck was suggested as another damaging mechanism by Hellström and Sallmander (1968), and it may cause cord injury in breech presentations even with careful obstetric management (Bresnan and Abroms, 1974). Spinal cord injuries are found mostly in mature infants.

The clinical symptoms consist of paraplegia from birth with spinal shock, flaccidity, atonic areflexia and excessive mobility of joints. Demonstration of a definite sensory level is important in distinguishing cord injury from paraplegia of other causes (Leventhal, 1960). Upon survival, there may be persistent flaccidity if the cord damage is extensive, or the flaccidity may change to spasticity within weeks or months. Neurologic recovery for cases of subtotal damage may be partial or complete.

The acute lesions consist of fractures of vertebral bodies and intervertebral joints, separation of the vertebral epiphysis, and direct crushing of the cord with large intraspinal hematomas (Couvelaire, 1903). Extreme stretching and disruption of the cord may be accompanied with laceration of the meninges, including complete separation of the spinal dura at the level of injury (Ford, 1925). The residual lesions in survivors show severe destruction of the cord with pigmentation, formation of glio-mesodermal scars, and dense adhesions between the residual cord tissue, the fibrotic leptomeninges and the dura (Vest, 1956; Stern and Rand, 1959; and others). The extent of damage to the spinal cord varies from complete destruction with minimal residual glial tissue to severe attenuation of the cord with gliosis, destruction of fiber tracts and loss of nerve cells. The cord may be replaced by a single large cyst, or there may be cavitation of cord tissue with numerous small cysts. There may be destruction of only part of the cross section of the cord with softening, gliosis and multiple cysts (Melchior and Tygstrup, 1963). Extensive cord necrosis from secondary circulatory changes was described by Jellinger and Schwingshackl (1973). The myelination of fiber tracts proximal to the lesions may be hindered as a consequence of the cord damage (Hedley-Whyte and Gilles, 1974).

Cord lesions of the types described above need to be distinguished from the often observed minor perivascular petechiae in the cord and from the extreme congestion or hemorrhagic imbibition of the epidural adipose tissue of newborns (Yates, 1959; Towbin, 1969). These findings are of uncertain clinical significance; their inclusion into the statistics on spinal injury in the newborn results in what seem to be unreasonably high incidences of perinatal damage (*e.g.*, more than 10 percent of all newborn necropsies; Towbin, 1969), considering the comparatively small number of cases having neurological deficits or documented residual lesions in the cord. Yates also commented on the frequency of hemorrhages into the adventitia of vertebral arteries and considered these a source of circulatory disturbances in the nervous parenchyma; this point, likewise, has not been proven in terms of documented parenchymal lesions.

References

Beneke, R.: Über Tentoriumzerreißungen bei der Geburt sowie die Bedeutung der Duraspannung für chronische Gehirnerkrankungen. Münch. med. Wschr. 57: 2125—2127, 1910.

Bresnan, M. J., Abroms, I. F.: Neonatal spinal cord transection secondary to intrauterine hyperextension of the neck in breech presentation. J. Pediat. 84: 734—737, 1974.

Capon, N. B.: Intracranial trauma in newborn. J. Obstet. Gynaec. Brit. Emp. 29: 572—590, 1922.

Claireaux, A. E.: Cerebral pathology of newborns. Guy Hosp. Rep. 108: 2—20, 1959.

Craig, W. S.: Intracranial hemorrhage in the newborn. Arch. Dis. Child. 13: 89—124, 1938.

Crothers, B.: Injury of the spinal cord in breech extraction as an important cause of fetal death and of paraplegia in childhood. Amer. J. med. Sci. 165: 94—110, 1923.

— Putnam, M. C.: Obstetrical injuries of the spinal cord. Medicine (Balt.) 6: 41—126, 1927.

Courville, C. B.: Birth and Brain Damage. Loma Linda, Calif.: M. F. Courville 1971.

Couvelaire, A.: Hémorrhagies du système nerveux central des nouveau-nés. Ann. Gynec. Obstet. 59: 253—268, 1903.

Earle, K. M., Baldwin, M., Penfield, W.: Incisural sclerosis and temporal lobe seizures produced by hippocampal herniation at birth. Arch. Neurol. Psychiat. (Chic.) 69: 27—42, 1953.

Ford, F. R.: Breech delivery in its possible relations to injury of the spinal cord. With special reference to infantile paraplegia. Arch. Neurol. Psychiat. (Chic.) 14: 742—750, 1925.

Go, K. G., Ebels, E. J., Van Woudenberg, F., Geerlings, T.: The development of oedema in the immature brain. A comparison of cold-induced oedema in young and adult cat brain. Psychiat. Neurol. Neurochir. 76: 427—437, 1973.

Goerttler, K., Draisbach, F. J.: On the genesis of tentorium ruptures and intracranial hemorrhages. Formal basis and patho-anatomical findings. Biol. Neonat. 5: 59—112, 1963.

Gröntoft, O.: Intracerebral and meningeal haemorrhages in perinatally deceased infants. II. Meningeal haemorrhages. A pathologico-anatomical and obstetric study. Acta obstet. gynec. scand. 32: 458—498, 1953.

Hausbrandt, F., Meier, A.: Zur Kenntnis der geburtstraumatischen und extrauterin erworbenen Schäden des Zentralnervensystems bei Neugeborenen. Frankfurt. Z. Path. 49: 21—62, 1936.

Hedley-Whyte, E. T., Gilles, F. H.: Observations on myelination of human spinal cord and some effects on parturitional transection. J. Neuropath. exp. Neurol. 33: 436—445, 1974.

Hellström, B., Sallmander, U.: Prevention of spinal cord injury in hyperextension of the fetal head. JAMA 204: 1041—1044, 1968.

Hemsath, F. A.: Birth injury of the occipital bone with a report of thirty-two cases. Amer. J. Obstet. Gynec. 27: 194—203, 1934.

Holland, E.: On cranial stress in the foetus during labour and on the effects of excessive stress on the intracranial contents; with an analysis of eighty-one cases of torn tentorium cerebelli and subdural cerebral hemorrhage. Trans. Edinb. obstet. Soc. 40: 112—143, 1921.

Jaffé, R. H.: Traumatic porencephaly. Arch. Path. 8: 797—799, 1929.

Jellinger, K., Schwingshackl, A.: Birth injury of the spinal cord. Report of two necropsy cases with several weeks survival. Neuropediatrie 4: 111—123, 1973.

Larroche, J. C.: Hémorrhagie cérébrales intraventriculaires chez le prématuré. Biol. Neonat. 7: 26—56, 1964.

Leventhal, H. R.: Birth injuries of the spinal cord. J. Pediat. 56: 447—453, 1960.

McHenry, L. C., Jr., Ewald, R. A., Talbert, W. M., Elwell, R. H.: Bilateral cortical cerebellar sclerosis. Residuum of cerebellar swelling or displacement early in life. Arch. Path. 78: 665—672, 1964.

Melchior, J. C., Tygstrup, I.: Development of paraplegia after breech presentation. Acta Paediat. 52: 171—176, 1963.

Natelson, E., Sayers, M. P.: The fate of children sustaining severe head trauma during birth. Pediatrics 51: 169—174, 1973.

Nesbitt, R. E. L., Anderson, G. W.: Perinatal mortality. Obstet. Gynec. 8: 50—60, 1956.

Parrot, M. J.: Note sur un cas de rupture de la moelle chez un nouveau-né, par suite de manœvres pendant l'accouchement. L'Union Medic. 9: 137—141, 1870.
Pott, R.: Über Tentoriumzerreißungen bei der Geburt. Z. Geburtsh. Gynäk. 69: 674—718, 1911.
Pryse-Davies, J., Beard, R. W.: A necropsy study of brain swelling in the newborn with special reference to cerebellar herniation. J. Path. 109: 51—73, 1973.
Rohrbach, H.: Gehirnventrikelblutungen als häufiger Sektionsbefund bei Feten und Frühgeburten. Zbl. Gynäk. 75: 1709—1712, 1953.
Runge, C.: Über cerebrale Embolie bei Neugeborenen. Z. Geburtsh. Gynäk. 4: 271—275, 1879.
Schäfer, P.: Über intracranielle Blutungen bei Neugeborenen. Z. Geburtsh. Gynäk. 84: 239—254, 1922.
Schwartz, P., Fink, L.: Morphologie und Entstehung der geburtstraumatischen Blutungen im Gehirn und Schädel des Neugeborenen. Z. Kinderheilk. 40: 427—474, 1925.
Schipke, R., Riege, D., Scoville, W. B.: Acute subdural hemorrhage at birth. Pediatr. 14: 468—473, 1954.
Shulman, S. T., Madden, J. D., Shanklin, D. R., Esterly, J. R.: Transection of spinal cord. A rare obstetrical complication of cephalic delivery. Arch. Dis. Child. 46: 291—294, 1971.
Siegmund, H.: Geburtsschädigungen des kindlichen Gehirns und ihre Folgen. Münch. med. Wschr. 70: 137—139, 1923.
Stern, W. E., Rand, R. W.: Birth injuries to the spinal cord. Amer. J. Obstet. Gynec. 78: 498—512, 1959.
Towbin, A.: Spinal cord and brain stem injury at birth. Arch. Path. 77: 620—632, 1964.
— Latent spinal cord and brain stem injury in newborn infants. Develop. Med. Child. Neurol. 11: 54—68, 1969.
Valdes-Dapena, M. A., Arey, J. B.: Pulmonary emboli of cerebral origin in the newborn. Arch. Path. 84: 643—646, 1967.
Vest, M.: Zur geburtstraumatisch bedingten Querschnittsläsion des Rückenmarkes (Hämatomyelie). Ann. Paediat. 186: 321—337, 1956.
Yates, P. O.: Birth trauma to the vertebral arteries. Arch. Dis. Child. 34: 436—441, 1959.
Ylppö, A.: Pathologisch-anatomische Studien bei Frühgeborenen. Z. Kinderheilk. 20: 212—431, 1919.

4. Periventricular Infarcts

Parrot (1868 a) gave a short but precise description of periventricular infarcts which he called "cerebral steatose" attributing them to malnutrition. A second paper (1868 b) contains a convincing illustration. He mentions the presence of cerebral steatose in several later articles dealing with other disease entities in infants. Parrot (1873) recognized the periventricular lesions as initial phases of "pale infarcts", distinguishing them from the red softenings caused by phlebothrombosis. He also emphasized that periventricular infarcts differed, in principle, from the diffuse fatty change described by Virchow (1867). Virchow (1867, 1868) is widely misquoted as being the first to describe periventricular infarcts. He really described diffuse fatty changes in the white matter of the brain and spinal cord (Chapter 5), although mentioning briefly that fatty cells may accumulate in certain places to the extent that they become recognizable to the naked eye. Sixteen years later Virchow (1883) distinguished diffuse fatty change from a focal form leading to softening; yet, he never detailed the appearance or distribution of these lesions, considering them merely a local intensification of diffuse fatty change.

Parrot (1873) refers to periventricular infarcts as yellowish or chalky plaques, 5 to 6 mm in diameter, occurring 1 to 15 mm from the ependymal surface. They affect preferentially the lateral corners of the ventricle while sparing the gray matter. The plaques later undergo softening, forming cavities filled with a milky fluid; these never communicate with the ventricle and are seen only exceptionally in portions of the brain other than the immediate periventricular tissue. His microscopic description refers to granular bodies, evidently macrophages, and stalactite-shaped bodies which may represent macrophages or mineralized swollen axons. Parrot's description,

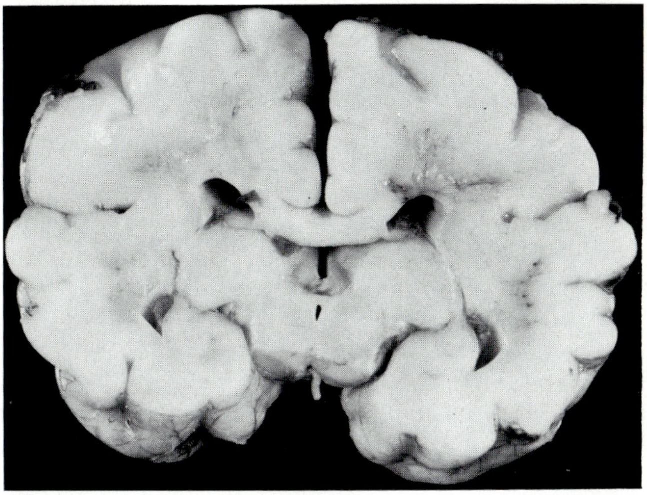

Fig. 20. Periventricular infarcts: Softening and dusky discoloration of periventricular white matter

to which later investigators had little to add, remained largely unnoticed for more than half a century. Periventricular infarcts were again described by Schwartz (1924), first without clear distinction from subependymal hemorrhages, later with due recognition of the morphologic differences between these lesions (Schwartz and Fink, 1925; Schwartz, 1927). A comprehensive study of periventricular infarcts by Banker and Larroche (1962) is based on 51 cases; they define for the first time the clinico-pathologic correlations for this type of lesion. The designation "periventricular leukomalacia", suggested by the authors is not adopted here as it suggests a diffuse, widespread affectation of white matter, and as the term infarct is preferable to malacia.

The frequency of periventricular infarcts in the series of Banker and Larroche (1962) was 18.8 percent of autopsies. There was equal distribution between sexes and 64 percent of the cases were prematures. Anoxia was present without exception. The anoxic episode was always severe and did not constitute a terminal event; resuscitation was required for the majority of infants. Clinical symptoms were lethargy, inactivity, hyperactivity, weak cry, poor suck and incomplete Moro reflex. Neurological signs were present upon the anoxic episode but were neither specific nor focal. Retardation and spasticity were observed in 2 of 3 infants surviving for more than 1 month.

Gross and Microscopic Features. Periventricular infarcts in newborns present as sharply circumscribed, pale areas in the subependymal tissue adjacent to the lateral ventricles. They range from pale to distinctly yellowish or chalky and the surrounding tissue tends to be dusky and soft (Fig. 20). The lesions are multiple, a few mm in diameter, variable in shape, and bilateral without exhibiting strict symmetry. There is a striking preference for the periventricular tissue, but the lesions always remain separated from the ventricles by a 1 to 2 mm layer of intact glial tissue. The most frequent localizations are anterior to the frontal horn, the lateral corners of the lateral ventricles, and the lateral surfaces of the occipital horn; extension to the subependymal tissue of the temporal horns is less frequent. The lesions occur rarely beyond 15 mm from the ventricular wall.

The earliest microscopic changes are inconspicuous and correspond to coagulation necrosis, with nuclear pyknosis and sponginess of the tissue. Banker and Larroche (1962) showed that the periodic acid-Schiff reaction helps in the demonstration of these early lesions which are outlined by meandering bands of bright red staining at their edges (Fig. 21). After a few days astrocytic proliferation sets in at the periphery of the infarcts and there are numerous varicose axon swellings. Microglia proliferates and lipid-laden macrophages accumulate in the infarcted tissue. The organizing lesions become well delineated by prominent proliferation and reactive gliosis at their edges. Cavitation sets in within a few weeks with formation of cysts having rough walls formed by moderately dense gliosis. Swollen axons mineralize quickly, during the organizing phase, and persist for many months in the walls of these cysts. The vast majority of the infarcts are ischemic and lack hemorrhages; few cases show a thrombosed vessel in or near an infarct, probably representing a secondary change, or a complication, since vasculo-occlusive changes are absent for the majority.

Periventricular infarcts may coexist with a variety of other perinatal lesions such as subependymal hemorrhages, kernicterus, cortical necrosis or pontosubicular neuronal necrosis; these lesions differ sufficiently from each other to allow their distinction when occurring together. There are also several reports in the literature in which periventricular infarcts were described as components of fetal infection with rubella or other organisms or with degenerative diseases. The association of these lesions must be considered coincidental, considering that periventricular infarcts are fairly common perinatal lesions.

Hemorrhages into Infarcts. Of particular interest are occasional cases in which hemorrhages are found in a distribution identical to that of periventricular infarcts. Noetzel and Jerusalem (1965) reported two such cases which they attributed to venous thrombosis although no thrombi were demonstrated microscopically. Armstrong and Norman (1974) have shown the derivation of these lesions from secondary hemorrhage into periventricular infarcts and stress that these hemorrhages may assume massive proportions.

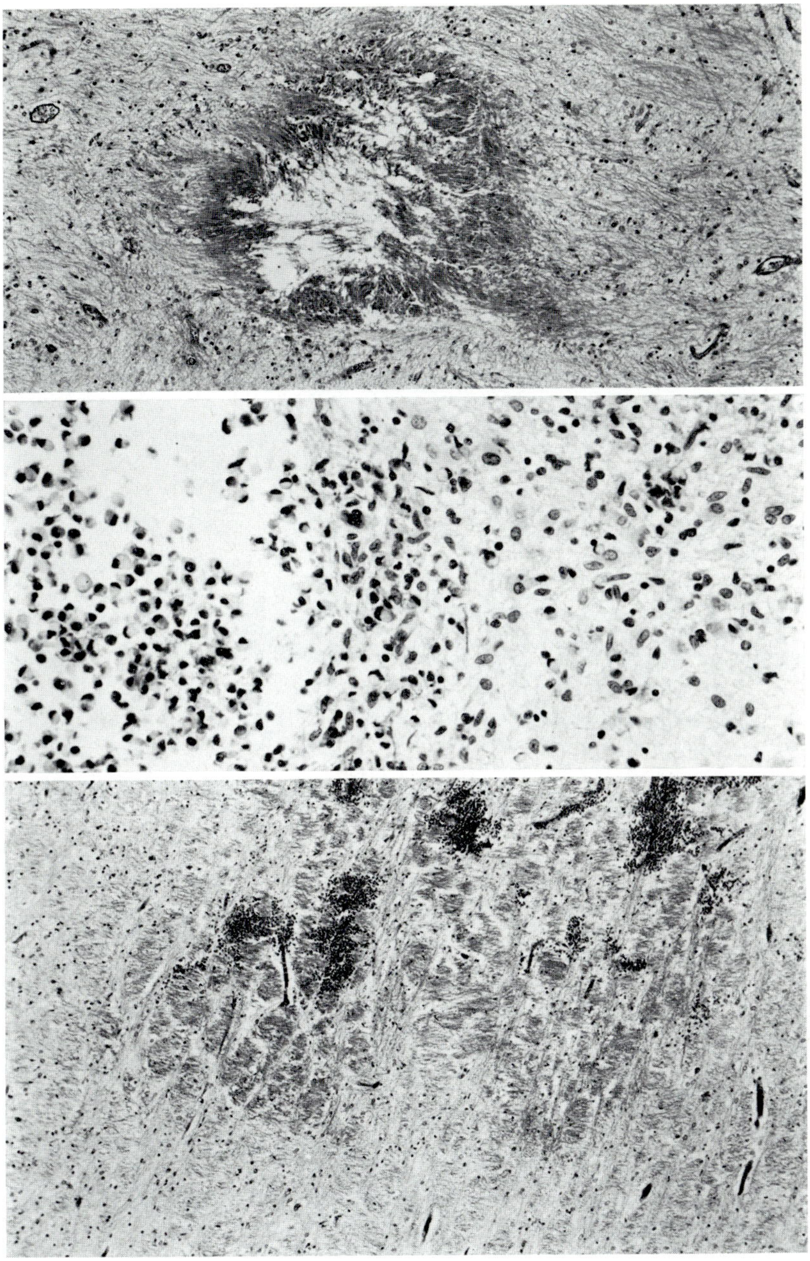

Fig. 21. Microscopic features of periventricular infarcts. Top: delineation of the acute lesions with PAS stain; ×80. Middle: gliosis and macrophages in an organizing periventricular infarct; H & E ×200. Bottom: foci of secondary hemorrhage within recent periventricular infarcts; PAS ×80

Another hemorrhagic lesion was described under the name of central hemorrhagic encephalopathy of early infancy (Courville, 1960), but its classification remains uncertain. The report pertains to 3 newborns who died 9 to 41 hours after birth; all had passed meconium and were in severe distress upon birth. The white matter of the cerebral hemisphere was extremely congested with numerous perivascular hemorrhages, inducing hemorrhagic necrosis in at least one of the cases. The changes in the white matter spread into its subcortical portions, but there was relative or complete sparing of the cerebral cortex. Similar lesions are known to be caused by phlebothrom-

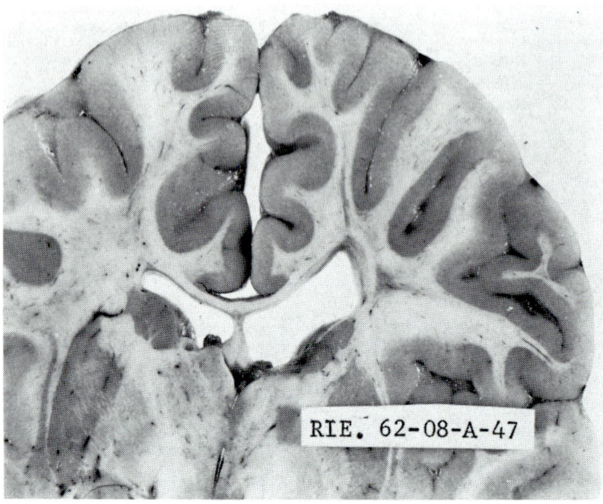

Fig. 22. Residual scarring of periventricular infarcts (courtesy Dr. Lindenberg)

bosis of internal cerebral veins (Chapter 13), but no evidence of thrombosis was found for these cases.

Residual Lesions. The residual lesions of periventricular infarcts are fairly common and have, indeed, been considered "hallmarks of birth injury" (Norman, 1969). Numerous articles on cerebral birth injury published during the first half of this century contained case reports highly suggestive of residual lesions of periventricular infarcts. Many are of little help in classifying pathologic entities as residual lesions of periventricular infarcts are reported intermingled with cases of porencephaly, hydranencephaly, local or diffuse cortical sclerosis or hemiatrophy; clinical data also are often incomplete.

The best descriptions of the residual lesions of periventricular infarcts were given by Norman (1949, 1953, 1969); his articles demonstrate multiple cavities clustering arround the corners of the lateral ventricles in a pattern conforming closely to the distribution of necrotic foci found in newborns (Fig. 22). Other authors were more impressed by cases with widespread cystic lesions in the centrum semiovale, which they called central porencephaly (Schwartz, 1924), cystic degeneration of white matter (Benda, 1945, 1952), or chronic central cystic degeneration (Courville, 1953).

The size of the brain may appear normal, or only slightly reduced, and the cerebral cortex may show remarkably little change on external inspection. Other cases may show focal or disseminated cortical atrophy, since ulegyria often coexists with periventricular infarcts. A reduction in the volume of hemispheric white matter with corresponding enlargement of the lateral ventricles is evident in the cut brain. The corpus callosum is abnormally thin. The periventricular tissue in the frontal lobes and at the corners of the lateral ventricle is grayish and loose in texture; it may contain only a few small cavities, or many of them clustered and scattered into the white matter at some distance from the ventricles. Delicate strands and septae of glial tissue are often seen within the cavities. Typical cases show an intact ventricular wall, composed of a very thin layer of subependymal tissue, and the basal ganglia are spared. Pigmentation of the walls of the cavities is not characteristic.

Microscopic examination shows fibrillary glial scar tissue in the walls of the cavities and strands or septae of glial tissue and occasional persisting blood vessels within. The extent of fibrillary gliosis usually is not extreme and mineralization is not a prominent feature. Myelinated fibers are greatly diminished or absent in the glial scars and are reduced in the adjacent white matter; however, the fiber tracts encompassing the basal ganglia are commonly spared. Periventricular cavitation may coexist with other perinatal lesions including status marmoratus of the basal ganglia (Norman, 1949) or with focal or widespread sclerosis of the cerebral cortex (Benda, 1945, 1952).

In extreme cases the entire white matter is transformed into a spongy tissue consisting of innumerable cystic cavities sparing only cortex and basal ganglia; the ventricular wall typically remains intact. The derivation of such widespread lesions from periventricular infarcts remains uncertain. For example, in a case reported by Sternberg (1930) the birth had lasted 32 hours; the baby was born without signs of life and had to be resuscitated for 90 minutes. On death at 16 months nearly the entire white matter was occupied by a spongy tissue with a delicate web of thin fibers; the basal ganglia and most of the cerebral cortex were spared except for foci of cortical sponginess and atrophy. The derivation of the lesions from severe perinatal asphyxia in this case is convincing, and the lesions may be considered an extreme form of periventricular infarcts. Extensive lesions of this type show transitions to multilocular cystic encephalopathy (Chapter 11) in which cortex as well as white matter is involved; indeed, Sternberg's case and others of similar extent have been ascribed to different entities by different authors. Benda (1952) suggested that the thin walls of the periventricular cysts may break down, forming large cysts with secondary communication with the ventricles.

Differential Diagnosis of Periventricular Cavitated Lesions. A number of cavitating disease processes of infancy show a striking predilection for the periventricular tissue. The following points may be of help in classifying the residual lesions. The residual defects of periventricular infarcts are identified by their bilateral distribution about the lateral corners of the ventricles, the clustering of multiple septated cavities and the integrity of ventricular walls. The basal ganglia, for typical cases, are spared from cavities, but status marmoratus may be present. The residual lesions of the infarcts complicating neonatal meningitis produce larger cavities in more random distribution, with scattering into basal ganglia as well as cerebral cortex (Chapter 17). There is obliteration of the ventricular walls by intense gliosis forming adhesions or loculations of the ventricles, ventricular diverticula, and destruction of periventricular tissue structures. Commonly associated lesions are meningeal fibrosis and obstructive hydrocephalus. There is no description in the literature of residual lesions subsequent to verified thrombosis of internal cerebral veins (Chapter 13). From the features of the acute lesions, one may expect large and widespread cavitation lacking the delicate septation of periventricular infarcts which originate from smaller and more restricted lesions. Residual pigmentation of the walls of the cavity would favor phlebothrombotic origin as these infarcts are nearly always hemorrhagic. Involvement of basal ganglia would be frequent. Pigmented periventricular cavities of uncertain origin were described by Malamud (1957). The residual lesions of subependymal hemorrhage in prematures are smooth-walled, relatively small cysts with very little, if any, gliosis. These cysts typically do not occupy the white matter near the corners of the lateral ventricles, but rather the subependymal glia tissue along the stria terminalis, where the acute hemorrhages occur in most instances (Chapter 2). They usually do not extend into the gray matter of the adjacent caudate nucleus or thalamus.

Pathogenetic Considerations. Several hypotheses on the causes of periventricular infarcts were proposed in the older literature, often compounding these lesions with other types of periventricular lesions of infancy. The investigations by Banker and Larroche (1962) identified severe perinatal anoxia necessitating resuscitation as the most important clinical factor. Lesions extremely similar to periventricular infarcts were produced in mature cats (Abramowicz, 1964) by experimental obliteration of the basilar artery and subsequent compression or closure of one or both carotid arteries. The similarity of these experimental lesions to periventricular infarcts in infants was ascribed to a similar vascular anatomy in terms of straight, long arteries penetrating deep into the white matter with few collaterals. These experiments suggest that perinatal anoxia may merely precipitate periventricular infarcts; a disturbance of circulation, such as shock, may play the decisive role in their formation. The appearance of the infarcts as sharply circumscribed zones of complete tissue necrosis, rather than as diffuse tissue damage, is consistent with this interpretation. When compared with lesions found in the adult brain, periventricular infarcts are more similar to those produced by vascular occlusion than to those of diffuse anoxic encephalopathy. De Reuck *et al.* (1972) attribute the lesions to the terminal distribution of arterial branches, or to interarterial border zones, respectively, a view shared by Armstrong and Norman (1974). The corners of the lateral ventricles are clearly shown to be a "watershed region" in the injected specimen of Fig. 9 in the paper of Hilal *et al.* (1971).

References

Abramowicz, A.: The pathogenesis of experimental periventricular cerebral necrosis and its possible relation to the periventricular leucomalacia of birth trauma. J. Neurol. Neurosurg. Psychiat. 27: 85—96, 1964.

Armstrong, D., Norman, M. G.: Periventricular leucomalacia in neonates: complications and sequelae. Arch. Dis. Child. 49: 367—375, 1974.

Banker, B. Q., Larroche, J.: Periventricular leukomalacia in infancy. Arch. Neurol. (Chic.) 7: 386—410, 1962.

Benda, C. E.: The late effects of cerebral birth injuries. Medicine 24: 71—110, 1945.

— Structural cerebral histopathology of mental deficiencies. In: Proceeding International Congress of Neuropathologists, Rome 1952. Turin: Rosenberg and Sellier 1952.

Courville, C. B.: Contributions to the study of cerebral anoxia. III. Neonatal asphyxia and its relation to certain degenerative diseases of the brain in infancy and childhood. Bull. Los Angeles neurol. Soc. 15: 155—195, 1950.

— Contributions to the Study of Anoxia. Los Angeles: San Lucas Press 1953.

— Central hemorrhagic encephalopathy of early infancy. Neurology (Minneap.) 10: 70—80, 1960.

De Reuck, J., Chattha, A. S., Richardson, E. P.: Pathogenesis and evolution of periventricular leukomalacia in infancy. Arch. Neurol. (Chic.) 27: 229—236, 1972.

Hilal, S. K., Solomon, G. E., Gold, A. P., Carter, S.: Primary cerebral arterial occlusive disease in children. Part I: Acute acquired hemiplegia. Radiology 99: 71—86, 1971.

Malamud, N.: Atlas of Neuropathology. Berkeley-Los Angeles: University of California Press 1957.

Noetzel, H., Jerusalem, F.: Die Hirnvenen- und Sinusthrombosen. Monogr. Neurol. Psychiat. (Berl.) 106: 1—63, 1965.

Norman, R. M.: Etat marbré of the thalamus following birth injury. Brain 72: 83—88, 1949.

— The pathology and etiology of infantile cerebral palsies. Proc. roy. Soc. Med. 46: 627—631, 1953.

— Cerebral birth injury. In: Greenfield's Neuropathology. London: E. Arnold 1969.

Parrot, M. J.: Sur la stéatose viscérale par inanition chez le nouveau-né. C. R. Acad. Sci. (Paris) 67: 412—414, 1868 a.

— Etude sur la stéatose interstitielle diffuse de l'encéphale chez le nouveau-né. Arch. Physiol. Norm. Path. (Paris) 1: 530—550; 622—642; 706—715, 1868 b.

— Etude sur le ramollissement de l'encéphale chez le nouveau-né. Arch. Physiol. Norm. Path. (Paris) 5: 59—73; 176—195; 283—303, 1973.

Schwartz, P.: Erkrankungen des Zentralnervensystems nach traumatischer Geburtsschädigung. Z. Neurol. Psychiat. 90: 263—468, 1924.

— Die traumatischen Schädigungen des Zentralnervensystems durch die Geburt. Erg. inn. Med. Kinderheilk. 31: 165—372, 1927.

— Fink, L.: Morphologie und Entstehung der geburtstraumatischen Blutungen im Gehirn und Schädel des Neugeborenen. Z. Kinderheilk. 40: 427—474, 1925.

Sternberg, C.: Multiple Höhlenbildungen im Großhirn (Markporencephalien) als Folge des Geburtstraumas. Beitr. Path. Anat. 84: 521—528, 1930.

Virchow, R.: Zur pathologischen Anatomie des Gehirns: 1. Congenitale Encephalitis und Myelitis. Virchow Arch. 38: 129—142, 1867.

— Über interstitielle Encephalitis. Virchow Arch. 44: 472—476, 1868.

— Encephalitis congenita. Berlin. klin. Wschr. 20: 705—709, 1883.

5. Diffuse Fatty Change of White Matter

The interpretation of diffuse fatty change of the white matter of newborns has been the subject of much controversy for more than a century, and the listing of this tissue alteration among the lesions of asphyctic and traumatic birth is open to challenge. Its description at this point of the text is merely a matter of concern for its overlap with the periventricular infarcts described in Chapter 4. Virchow (1867) described diffuse fatty change of the white matter of newborns under the title "Congenital Encephalitis and Myelitis". He considered it the result of fatty metamorphosis of glia cells of the white matter of brain and of the tracts of spinal cord, with a general sparing of gray matter. His study was made during an epidemic of smallpox, and he attributed fatty change to an infective process transmitted from the mother to the infant. The interpretation of Virchow's observations became embroiled in controversy from the very start, as other investigators noticed the near constant occurrence of fatty change in newborns. Hayem (1868) observed fatty change in all of 12 infants studied, but Virchow (1868, 1883) replied that it was often absent, particularly in stillborns and in infants who had not died upon birth. Jastrowitz (1871) observed fatty change in all but one of 37 newborns from 28 to 40 weeks gestation; it was sparse in 7 fetuses, 5 to 7 months old, and was generally absent in infants older than 6 months; similar results were obtained by Merzbacher (1910) for 26 normal newborns and fetuses. Tuthill (1938), studying 46 brains up to 2 years old, found fat in all of 21 less than 4 months old and considered the fat a waste product of myelination. Controversy continued in the voluminous literature as to whether fatty change is normal or a pathologic alteration. These publications, reviewed by Siegmund (1955), are concerned mainly with the interpretation and discussion of fatty change and do not add substantial new information. Indeed, it is difficult to find a concise description of the phenomenon under discussion.

Studies in which fatty change was searched for systematically in unselected newborn autopsies agree in that it is present for the majority of newborn infants, in excess of 80 percent even for the lowest reported series. It is found in mature as well as in premature infants but tends to be less intense in very young fetuses. The intensity of fatty change is maximum during the first months of life, and it diminishes in infants older than 5 or 6 months. There is no indication that diffuse fatty change relates to any clinical manifestation. Its high frequency in newborns and the virtual absence of subacute or residual lesions in older infants strongly suggest that the change, whatever its nature, is transient and reversible.

Gross dissection of the brain does not disclose characteristic alterations. Frozen sections stained with any of the conventional methods for neutral fat show a diffuse dusting of the white matter with innumerable droplets of fat; the gray matter is completely spared for most cases. The change affects all of the various fiber systems of the spinal cord, brain stem, and cerebral and cerebellar hemispheres, but its intensity varies considerably among tracts, to the extent that one may get the impression of selective sparing or selective affectation of a given fiber system.

In the spinal cord fatty change is most constant in the dorsal columns, often with preferential involvement of Goll's tract, and also in the lateral columns (Fig. 23). The corticospinal tract may be spared in very young prematures, or it may be heavily affected in older infants. Similar topographic differences are observed in the brain stem; in the pons the intensity of fatty

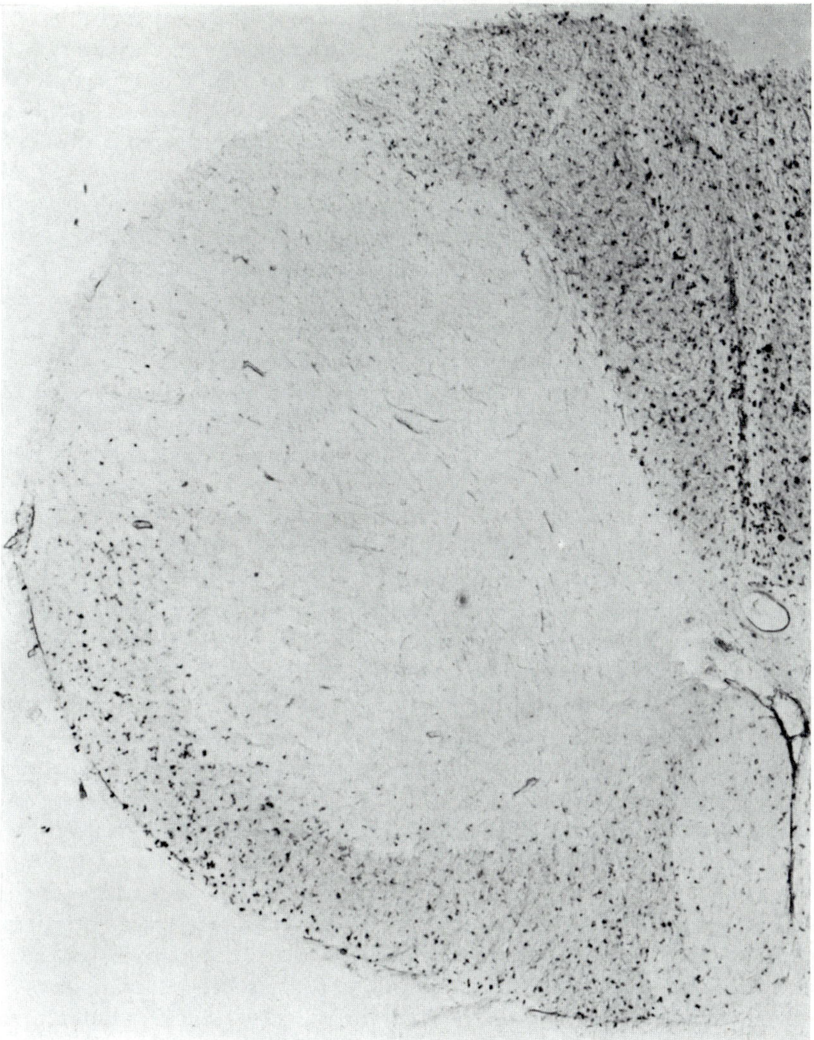

Fig. 23. Fatty change of spinal white matter of a premature infant; note the restriction of fat droplets to the white matter and the sparing of the corticospinal tracts which have not begun to myelinate; oil red O ×68

change may differ strikingly for the dorsal longitudinal fascile, the ponto-cerebellar fibers, and the corticospinal fibers. Fatty change is at times particularly intense in the corpus callosum and in the internal capsule of the cerebral hemispheres. Little fat may be found in the hemispheric white matter of prematures, but it is widespread in mature infants. Such variance in the patterns of affectation of different fiber systems suggest that fatty change is less likely to develop in a fiber system that has not yet begun to myelinate. It is difficult, however, to define a more precise relation between fatty change and myelination, as the overall intensity of the phenomenon varies considerably from case to case.

There is also considerable variance in the cellular distribution of fat droplets. They often accumulate in the perinuclear cytoplasm of glia cells, but columns of fat droplets may outline glial processes. Other droplets seem freely dispersed in the tissue without recognizable cytoplasmic localization. The majority of glial cells of a given fiber system are affected alike. Several studies in the older literature concerned themselves with cytological details and morphologic variants of the fatty cells, or with the problem of intra- or extracellular localization of the fat droplets (Rydberg, 1932), a problem beyond the resolving power of the methods available at the time. Of greater importance is Wohlwill's (1921) report drawing attention to the morphologic difference between fat-laden macrophages in necrotizing lesions and fatty change of the neuroglia, a difference which had been ignored in many of the earlier investigations. However, perivascular accumulations of lipid-laden macrophages are also a normal component of diffuse fatty change; they were found most often between the third and sixth month in 215 randomly selected brains (Jellinger *et al.*, 1971).

The very high frequency with which fatty change is seen in the white matter of newborn infants renders it near certain that it will be found coexistent with other more specific types of lesions. In particular, fatty change of white matter often coexists with periventricular infarcts (Chapter 4), and therein lies the difficulty and the sources of confusion concerning the identity of both processes. Numerous lipid-laden macrophages are found in organizing periventricular infarcts within the area of necrosis. Fat stains of white matter containing periventricular infarcts, accordingly, show focal clusters of macrophages at the lesions and macrophages dispersed among fat-containing glial cells at the edges of the lesion and fatty glial cells only at some distance with continuous blending of both cell populations. At later phases there may be also massive deposition of neutral fat in fiber tracts undergoing Wallerian degeneration. Periventricular infarcts, therefore, are often considered local intensifications of diffuse fatty change of white matter, an interpretation proposed by Virchow (1883) and accepted by many later investigators. This interpretation is difficult to accept if one considers the regional distribution of periventricular infarcts with that of diffuse fatty change. Periventricular infarcts are highly selective to the corners of the lateral ventricles and they never occur in brain stem or cord. Fatty change, on the other hand, affects the fiber tracts of brain stem and cord as well as the cerebral and cerebellar hemispheric white matter, but there is never any evidence of its aggravation to form necrotizing lesions in cerebellum, brain stem or cord. Diffuse fatty change in the white matter should also be considered in evaluating observations thought to represent a perinatal sudanophilic leukodystrophy (Sarnat and Adelman, 1973), an aspect particularly pertinent to Pelizaeus-Merzbacher disease (Chapter 41).

The controversy on the interpretation of diffuse fatty change is essentially a contest among three theories: 1. Fatty change is a pathologic lesion which differs only in intensity from periventricular infarcts (Virchow, 1883). 2. Fatty change is a normal feature of myelin formation (Jastrowitz, 1871), as recently restated by Mickel and Gilles (1970). 3. Fatty change is abnormal, and represents an acute derangement of glia involved in the process of myelination formation (Siegmund, 1923). The first of these hypotheses is not acceptable, as discussed above, as it is based on a coexistence of diffuse fatty change and periventricular infarcts. Controversy also arose in the older literature from confusing fatty change with foci of matrix cells, or with macrophages in organizing widespread lesions, as in diffuse cortical necrosis or diffuse softening of the hemispheres. The second hypothesis is difficult to accept in view of the absence of fat droplets in myelinating fiber tracts of animals, as reported by Staemmler (1928). His light microscopic observations are consistent with the more recent electron microscopic literature in which there is virtual consensus as to the absence of lipid droplets in the cytoplasm of normal myelin-forming glia cells. It is unlikely that myelination in man differs from all other animal species in this regard. The third hypothesis appears to be the least objectionable, but it leaves many questions unanswered. Siegmund (1923, 1955) thought that fatty change results from a derangement of myelin formation in the white matter induced by unknown factors, presumably related to birth. Myelinating white matter differs from adult white matter in that the myelin-forming sheath cells undergo considerable changes in metabolic activity (Schonbach *et al.*, 1969) with commensurate increases in the rate of lipid synthesis (Friede, 1972), The accelerated rate of metabolism may render the myelin-forming glia cells more susceptible to metabolic derangement or, perhaps, to subpathologic agonal changes. Sumi *et al.* (1972) recently reported on experimental induction of fatty change in the white matter of monkeys by anoxia induced by lowering maternal blood pressure. However, in the present author's experience it is difficult to induce fatty change in rats even with prolonged and repeated hypoxia. Mossakowski *et al.* (1968) had reported marked increase in glial glycogen in experimental perinatal hypoxia, but they did not comment at all on the occurrence of fat. One has to conclude that the appearance of fat droplets in glia cells in newborn brains is in some way conditioned by the process of myelin formation, but the precise causes of their appearance remain undisclosed. There has been recent revival of interest in the interpretation of diffuse fatty change. Larroche and Amakawa (1973) counted the number of fatty glial cells in a number of fiber tracts and found an increase with myelination, though not always in strict proportion to it. Leech and Alvord (1974), on the basis of similar counts, conclude that fatty change represents an abnormal response of the immature glia cell to hypoxic acidotic metabolic stress.

Perinatal Telencephalic Leukoencephalopathy. This term was used by Gilles and Murphy (1969) to describe hypertrophic astrocytes and pyknotic glial nuclei in the white matter of newborn infants; observations on the frequency of these changes in various perinatal conditions were reported in several subsequent publications. The significance of these reports is at present unclear. Reactive astrocytes in the newborn brain are difficult to distinguish from the cytoplasmic hypertrophy found normally in the so-called myelination glia (Roback and Scherer, 1936). Nuclear pyknosis also is difficult to assess as small nuclei of migrating neuroblasts abound in the white matter of infants. The contention by Gilles and Murphy (1969) that this change produces hypoplasia of the white matter as a residual lesion is difficult to accept on the basis of the available evidence. Leviton and Gilles (1974), in a more recent study, relate the frequency of white matter changes to that of congenital cardiac disease.

References

Friede, R. L.: Control of myelin formation by axon caliber (With a model of the control mechanism). J. comp. Neurol. 144: 233—252, 1972.

Gilles, F. H., Murphy, S. F.: Perinatal telencephalic leucoencephalopathy. J. Neurol. Neurosurg. Psychiat. 32: 404—413, 1969.

Hayem, G.: Etudes sur les diverses formes d'encéphalitis (Anatomie et Physiologie pathologiques). Thesis, Doctorate Medicine, Paris 1968.

Jastrowitz, M.: Studien über die Encephalitis und Myelitis des ersten Kindesalters. Arch. Psychiat. 3: 162—213, 1871.

Jellinger, K., Seitelberger, F., Kozik, M.: Perivascular accumulation of lipids in the infant human brain. Acta Neuropath. 19: 331—342, 1971.

Larroche, J. C., Amakawa, H.: Glia of myelination and fat deposit during early myelogenesis. Biol. Neonat. 22: 421—435, 1973.

Leech, R. W., Alvord, E. C., Jr.: Glial fatty metamorphosis: An abnormal response of premyelin glia frequently accompanying periventricular leukomalacia. Amer. J. Path. 74: 603—612, 1974.

Leviton, A., Gilles, F. H.: Astrocytosis without globules in infant cerebral white matter. An epidemiologic study. J. Neurol. Sci. 22: 329—340, 1974.

Merzbacher, L.: Untersuchungen über die Morphologie und Biologie der Abräumzellen im Zentralnervensystem. Histol. Histopath. Arb. Großhirnrinde 3: 1—142, 1910.

Mickel, H. S., Gilles, F. H.: Changes in glial cells during human telencephalic myelinogenesis. Brain 93: 337—346, 1970.

Mossakowski, M. J., Long, D. M., Myers, R. E., *et al.:* Early histochemical changes in perinatal asphyxia. J. Neuropath. exp. Neurol. 27: 500—516, 1968.

Roback, H. N., Scherer, J. J.: Über die feinere Morphologie des frühkindlichen Hirnes unter besonderer Berücksichtigung der Gliaentwicklung. Virchow Arch. 294: 365—413, 1935.

Rydberg, E.: Cerebral injury in newborn children consequent on birth injury. Acta path. scand., Suppl. 10: 1—247, 1932.

Sarnat, H. B., Adelman, L. S.: Perinatal sudanophilic leukodystrophy. Amer. J. Dis. Child. 125: 281—289, 1973.

Schonbach, J., Hu, K. H., Friede, R. L.: Cellular and chemical changes during myelination: Histologic, autoradiographic, histochemical and biochemical data on myelination in the pyramidal tract and corpus callosum of rat. J. comp. Neurol. 134: 21—38, 1968.

Siegmund, H.: Geburtsschädigungen des kindlichen Gehirns und ihre Folgen. Münch. med. Wschr. 70: 137—139, 1923.

— Die geburtstraumatischen Veränderungen des Zentralnervensystems einschließlich der Encephalitis congenita Virchow. Handbuch der Speziellen Pathol. Anat. Histol. XIII/3: 239—287, 1955.

Staemmler, M.: Über den Befund von Fettkörnchenzellen im Gehirn neugeborener Tiere. Münch. med. Wschr. 70: 1430—1431, 1928.

Sumi, S. M., Alvord, E. C., Parer, J., Eng, M., Ueland, K.: Accumulation of sudanophilic lipids in the cerebral white matter of premature primates. J. Neuropath. exp. Neurol. 31: 183, 1972.

Tuthill, C. R.: Fat in the infant brain in relation to myelin, blood vessels and glia. Arch. Path. 25: 336—346, 1938.

Virchow, R.: Zur pathologischen Anatomie des Gehirns: 1. Congenitale Encephalitis und Myelitis. Virchow Arch. 38: 129—142, 1867.

— Über interstitielle Encephalitis. Virchow Arch. 44: 472—476, 1868.

— Encephalitis congenita. Berl. klin. Wschr. 20: 705—709, 1883.

Wohlwill, F.: Zur Frage der sogenannten Encephalitis congenita (Virchow). Z. Neurol. 68: 360—415, 1921.

6. Perinatal Lesions of Cerebral and Cerebellar Cortex

Ulegyria. Bresler (1889) reported pathologic observations in 2 mentally defective patients, both showing focal narrowing of cortical gyri on gross inspection of the brain. In the first case there was a cleft in the region of the left Sylvian fissure, communicating with the ventricle, and small convoluted gyri were abundant in both frontal and anterior parietal lobes. The second showed foci of small gyri in approximately symmetrical distribution, parasagittal in the central regions and in the occipital lobes. Microscopic examination of the first case revealed numerous minute gyri with a dense population of nerve cells and radial and transverse myelinated fibers. In the second case the cortex was absent at the bottom of the sulci; the gyri appeared pedunculated on long stalks, their crowns containing irregular islands of cortical tissue separated by zones of dense gliosis having affinity for myelin stains. The different characteristics of the small gyri in these cases were documented with gross and microscopic illustrations. Bresler compared his cases with others in the literature—in particular his second case with the one reported by Köppen (1896)—and concluded that the two types of gyral atrophy differed in principle. He proposed to call the first type microgyria, the second ulegyria (gyral scarring). He emphasized that ulegyria differed from microgyria in the extent of glial proliferation, indicating scar formation.

Ulegyria was later described under the terms of atrophic sclerosis, mantle sclerosis, or sclerotic microgyria, but there is considerable variance among authors in the classification of the lesions and in the application of the above terms. Malamud *et al.* (1964), for example, classified ulegyria among "primary subcortical lesions", considering it merely an extension of periventricular infarcts; they distinguished ulegyria from primary cortical atrophy which affects all portions of the cortex in a diffuse manner. Benda (1945) used the term "mantle sclerosis" for large defects, presumably vasculo-occlusive, which he distinguished from cystic degeneration of white matter and from patchy cortical devastation; the latter evidently includes ulegyria. Courville (1954) used the term mantle sclerosis synonymous with ulegyria.

Although ulegyria may show transitions to other lesions, its morphologic features are sufficiently characteristic to be considered an entity (Norman, 1969). The relationship between ulegyria and birth injury was documented by relating the lesions to well documented clinical histories (Norman, 1944; Norman *et al.*, 1957) and is also evident from its frequent association with periventricular infarcts (Fig. 24) and marbled state of the basal ganglia. No data on the frequency of ulegyria are available, which is, at least in part, a reflection of its transition into and association with other types of cortical lesions.

Acute and Subacute Lesions. Only brief references to the acute lesions of ulegyria are found in the literature, which refer to a dark band accentuating the deep layers of the cortex (Banker, 1967) and, microscopically, to a diffuse or laminar pallor of the cortex in the depth of sulci (Banker and Larroche, 1962). The sparsity of data is a reflection on the rather indistinct features of the acute lesions which, in the present author's experience, are not evident on gross inspection of the cut brain. For 6 cases with acute lesions studied by the present author, all having a history of severe perinatal asphyctic distress, the lesions were discernable only on microscopic examination of large sections of the hemispheres by comparing sulci with gyri. The depth of the sulci shows a diffuse pallor of the cortex, compared with its normal staining at the crowns of gyri (Fig. 25). In the pale areas there is vacuolization and sponginess of the tissue, nuclear pyknosis, chromatolysis, and dissolution and

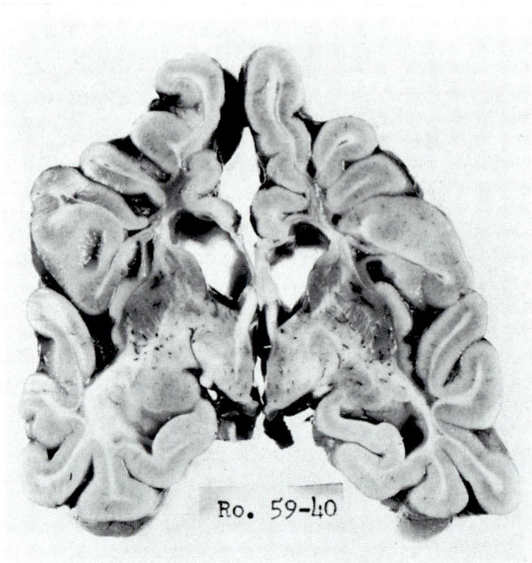

Fig. 24. Ulegyria combined with severe scarring of white matter (Courtesy Walsh and Lindenberg, Bull. Johns Hopkins Univ. 106, 100, 1961, The Johns Hopkins University Press)

dropping out of neurons. Eosinophilic degeneration of the cytoplasm or karyorrhexis, which are helpful in recognizing neuronal necrosis in other types of infantile neuronal lesions, are sparse or absent. There is no evidence of vascular occlusion.

The organizing phase of ulegyria was described by Schwartz (1927), although it is not clear whether he referred specifically to the topographic pattern of ulegyria. In two cases studied by the present author the lesions were rather conspicuous, contrary to their vague delineation in the acute phase, due to a massive proliferation of glia and blood vessels and an abundance of macrophages, all affecting the cortex in the depth of the sulci only; the subjacent white matter showed ill defined, ragged patches of partial necrosis without cavitation (Fig. 25).

Residual Lesions. Comprehensive descriptions of the late stages of ulegyria were given by Norman (1944, 1969). There is a characteristic predilection for sulci, with relative sparing of the crowns of the convolutions, to the extent that gross inspection of the uncut cortical surface may not reveal any signs of damage. Slight lesions consist of multifocal, irregular, partly confluent patches of neuronal loss and intense gliosis at the bottom of sulci. The glial scars and adjacent cortex may contain abnormally oriented bundles of fibers staining intensely with myelin stains, giving the lesions a marbled appearance similar to that of status marmoratus of basal ganglia. The term "plaque fibromyelinique" has been used for these cortical lesions; the pathogenetic factors responsible for the abnormal myelin patterns are discussed in Chapter 7.

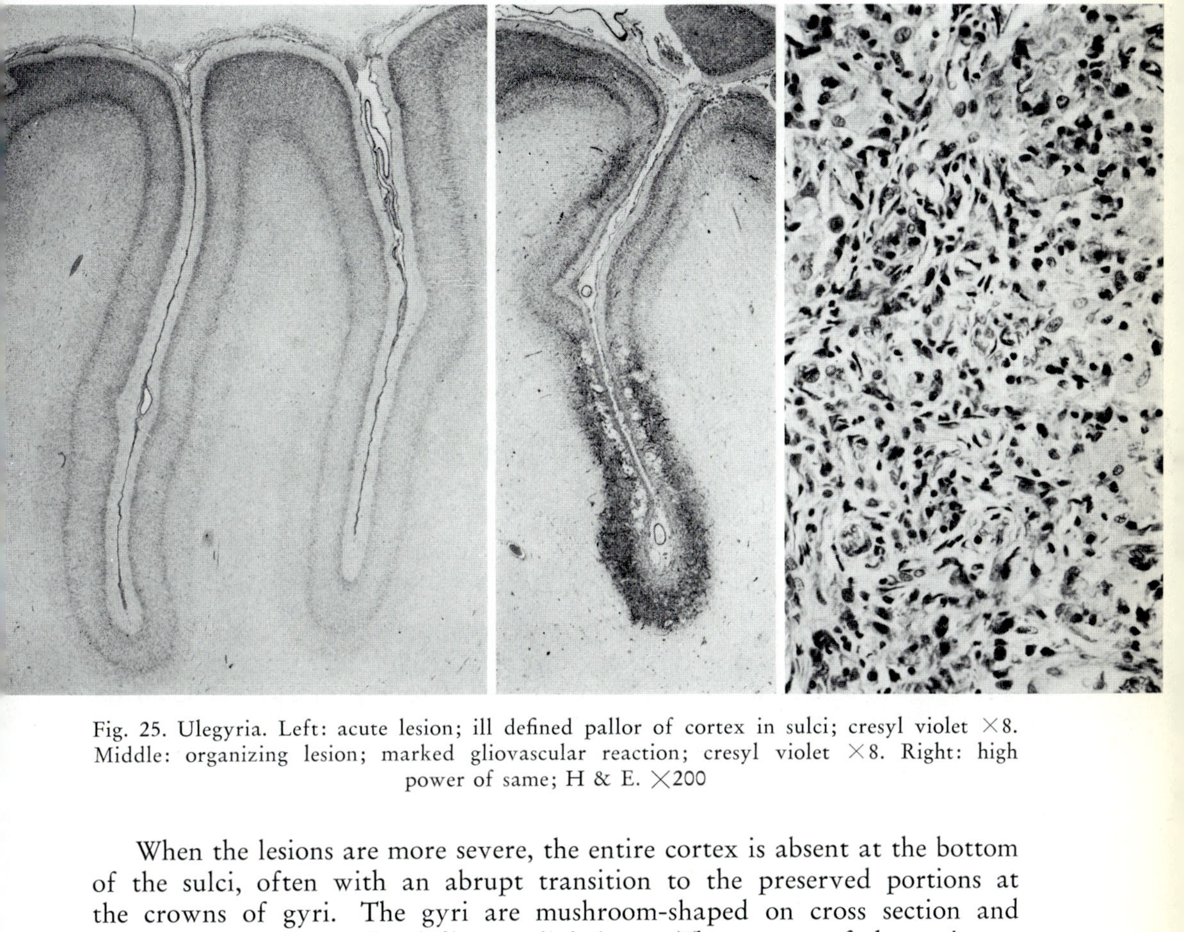

Fig. 25. Ulegyria. Left: acute lesion; ill defined pallor of cortex in sulci; cresyl violet ×8. Middle: organizing lesion; marked gliovascular reaction; cresyl violet ×8. Right: high power of same; H & E. ×200

When the lesions are more severe, the entire cortex is absent at the bottom of the sulci, often with an abrupt transition to the preserved portions at the crowns of gyri. The gyri are mushroom-shaped on cross section and are supported by a stalk of fibrous glial tissue. The crowns of the gyri may consist of islands of cortex between interspaced glial scars, resulting in an irregular granular surface (granular atrophy). Laminar necrosis may occur, most often in the third layer, and there may be areas of cavitation. In the most severe stages the entire cortex is wasted, the greatly shrunken residual gyri consisting mostly of glial scar tissue. Intense gliosis is evident in Holzer stains, particularly in the subcortical white matter in the region of the U fibers. The degree of affectation of underlying white matter varies with the severity of the cortical lesions. Small cortical defects at the depth of sulci may overlie myelinated white matter, although the projection fibers normally entering the cortex are absent. More severe lesions show loss of myelin, glial fibrosis and severe atrophy of white matter with intense gliosis in Holzer stains. Leptomeningeal and cortical arteries may show mineralization of the elastica and diffuse or patchy proliferation of the intima (Chapter 12). These changes are secondary to severe atrophy and are not specific for ulegyria.

Several patterns of distribution of ulegyria are observed. Meyer (1953) found ulegyria distributed in watershed zones in 30 of 153 cases of residual lesions of infantile cerebral damage. Watershed lesions correspond to the

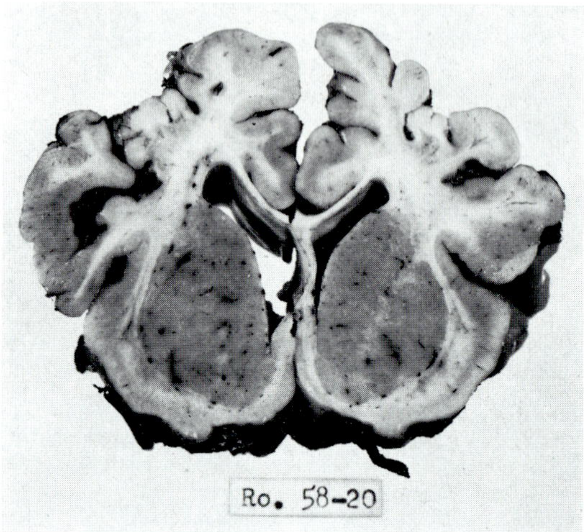

Fig. 26. Bilateral ulegyria in watershed distribution (Walsh and Lindenberg, 1961)

boundaries between the irrigation territories of the main cerebral arteries, and are commonly bilateral in a narrow zone arching parasagittal from the second frontal convolution into the parietal and occipital lobes, or they may occur in small patches along this zone (Fig. 26). There may be variance in the distribution of the zones, probably corresponding to variance in arterial territories. The boundary between the middle and posterior cerebral arteries at the surface of the temporal lobe is less frequently affected. In other instances ulegyria may occur within the territory of one major cerebral artery, such as at the frontal lobes or at the medial surface of the occipital lobes. Ulegyria also may fringe cavitated defects situated within the territories of main cerebral arteries (Norman *et al.*, 1957). A bilateral parasagittal distribution of ulegyria in a pattern suggestive of venous drainage territories is also common. These lesions are often bilateral but may occur unilaterally as well. In the case 1 of Friedman and Courville (1941) ulegyria was confined to the right hemisphere where it coexisted with an encapsulated subdural hematoma; the association may suggest that compression of the cortex by a space-occupying hematoma aggravates cortical ischemia causing ulegyria; on the other hand, hemispheric atrophy may facilitate the formation of the subdural hematoma (Chapter 19). The characteristic features of ulegyria may coexist and show transitions with widespread, diffuse cortical sclerosis with laminar necrosis or diffuse loss of neurons of the type described in Chapter 10.

Pathogenetic Considerations. The relation of ulegyria to disturbed parturition is indicated by its common association with other lesions of known perinatal origin, and from documentations of corresponding perinatal histories. Furthermore, these lesions have been produced experimentally in monkeys by perinatal asphyxia (Myers, 1972). The occurrence of ulegyria in watershed areas is strikingly similar to the watershed lesions in adult brains.

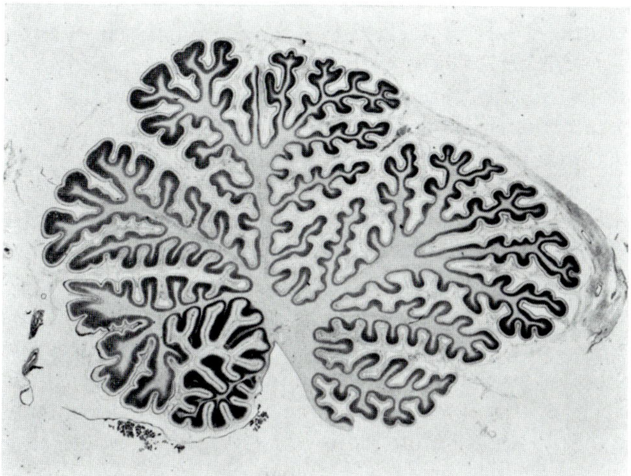

Fig. 27. Centrolobular cerebellar sclerosis; cresyl violet ×6

The latter had been attributed to specific vascular disease processes (thromboangiitis obliterans), but this interpretation is now largely abandoned; these lesions are known to result from insufficient perfusion either from a blockage proximal to the origin of two major arteries or from a generalized drop in blood pressure, such as during shock (Romanul and Abramowicz, 1964). Only the latter disturbance is applicable to the perinatal lesions. Severe hypoxia induces circulatory collapse (Noell and Schneider, 1942), as discussed in Chapter 2. It is most logical to attribute ulegyria, particularly when occurring in watershed distribution, specifically to this phase of circulatory collapse induced by severe hypoxia.

Lesions of the Cerebellar Cortex. Perinatal damage to the cerebellar cortex is less frequent than to the cerebral cortex; it was present in 56 of 153 cases of infantile circulatory cerebral lesions (Myer, 1949). Infantile lesions of cerebellar cortex are known largely from their residual state, when they present as atrophy and sclerosis of cerebellar foliae, a change accompanied miscroscopically by loss of Purkinje cells, loss, or diminution, respectively, of the granular layer and intense glial proliferation. With complete depletion of neuronal elements, the laminar architecture of the cortex is represented only by a layer of proliferated Bergmann glia cells underneath a shrunken molecular layer. Although such sclerosis occurs in the context of cavitated lesions, it manifests more commonly as diffuse shrinkage of the tissue without any tendency to cavitate.

Several patterns of cerebellar cortical sclerosis may be distinguished. Lesions suggestive of watershed distribution are found at the boundaries between the territories of the superior and inferior cerebellar arteries—that is, in a band stretching across the convexity of the cerebellar hemispheres. The lesions are usually bilateral and consist of a zone of patchy or confluent foci of sclerosis extending from the surface into the depth of the hemisphere. This type of cortical lesion is probably the one that is linked most intimately to perinatal damage, but it is relatively uncommon; it was found in only 4 of 153 cases (Meyer, 1953), which is about 8 times less frequent than watershed lesions in the cerebral hemispheres. Cerebellar sclerosis of this type was observed coexistent with ulegyria by Norman *et al.* (1957).

Another regional pattern of cortical sclerosis affects the deeply situated portions of the cortex bordering the central white matter (Fig. 27) while sparing the superficial cortex (Meyer, 1949). This peculiar pattern has been attributed either to the extension into the cortex of white matter edema, or to a specific type of circulatory disturbance; it is not specific for perinatal onset and has been reported for damage originating in adult life, such as for CO intoxication. A reverse pattern, that is sclerosis of superficially situated gyri, also occurs and is considered characteristic of agents acting via the CSF spaces, such as for meningitis, hematomas or superficial compression. Focal necrosis of the crowns of cerebellar gyri with tissue pigmentation are characteristic of superficial siderosis (Chapter 9). Sclerosis of superficially situated gyri can be found in the absence of any clues as to the nature of the pathogenetic agent.

These regional patterns may be compared with focal cortical sclerosis having no characteristic regional distribution or with widespread sclerosis affecting the cortex of the entire cerebellum. Focal or widespread cortical sclerosis in patients with perinatal brain damage frequently develops secondary to convulsive disorder (Chapter 10). Severe postnatal anoxia or local circulatory disturbances during infancy, *e.g.*, from cerebral phlebothrombosis (Chapter 13), may also induce diffuse or focal cerebellar sclerosis on a nonconvulsive basis. The origin of such residual lesions is often difficult to determine in retrospect. Induction of widespread cerebellar sclerosis by perinatal asphyxia appears to be uncommon however. An interesting case was reported by Norman (1940). Status marmoratus of the basal ganglia was associated with bilateral hemispheric cerebellar atrophy, loss of Purkinje cells, diminution of the granular layer and heavy gliosis; there was marked atrophy of the olivary nuclei, probably secondary, but no loss of cells was found in the pontine nuclei. The patient, a 33-year-old idiot, was not known to be epileptic.

The differential diagnosis of widespread cerebellar cortical sclerosis of infantile origin must include scarred endstages of lesions produced by selective damage to the outer granular layer; these lesions typically induce granular layer aplasia and heterotopia of granule cells with persistence of the Purkinje cell population (Chapter 31), but a more severe damage may result in devastation of the entire neuronal population.

Cerebro-Cerebellar Atrophy (Crossed Cerebellar Atrophy). Atrophy of the contralateral cerebellar hemisphere may develop following extensive lesions of one cerebral hemisphere. The literature on this rather capricious type of change has been reviewed by Verhaart and van Wieringen-Rauws (1950). The crossed cerebellar atrophy is transneuronal and may develop antegrade by way of the cerebro-pontine tracts, or retrograde by way of the thalamus and superior cerebellar peduncle. In the first case the atrophy has to progress beyond the pontine nuclei, in the second beyond the dentate nucleus, at which points degenerative changes normally stop. The causes and conditions of the transneuronal extension of the degenerative process are unknown, and their development cannot be predicted from the cerebral lesions. Generally, the cerebral lesions are extensive, develop early in youth, and were present for many years; on the other hand, neither the regional distribution of lesions in the cerebrum nor the resultant changes in the cerebellar cortex are predictable or characteristic, nor does crossed cerebellar atrophy consistently follow large cerebral lesions.

References

Banker, B. Q., Larroche, J. C.: Periventricular leukomalacia of infancy. Arch. Neurol. 7: 386—410, 1962.

— Neuropathological effects of anoxia and hypoglycemia in newborn. Develop. Med. Child. Neurol. 9: 544—550, 1967.

Bresler: Klinische und pathologisch-anatomische Beiträge zur Mikrogyrie. Arch. Psychiat. 31: 566—573, 1899.

Courville, C. B.: Cerebral Palsy. A brief introduction to its history, etiology and pathology, with some notes on the resultant clinical syndromes and their treatment. Los Angeles: San Lucas Press 1954.

Friedman, A. P., Courville, C. B.: Atrophic lobar sclerosis of early childhood. Report of two cases with special reference to asphyxial etiology. Bull. Los Angeles neurol. Soc. 6: 32—45, 1941.

Köppen, M.: Beiträge zum Studium der Hirnrindenerkrankungen. Arch. Psychiat. 28: 931—963, 1896.

Malamud, N., Itabashi, H., Caston, J., Messinger, H.: An etiologic and diagnostic study of cerebral palsy. J. Pediat. 65: 270—293, 1964.

Meyer, J. E.: Zur Ätiologie und Pathogenese des fetalen und frühkindlichen Cerebralschadens. Z. Kinderheilk. 67: 123—136, 1949.

— Über Gefäßveränderungen beim fetalen und frühkindlichen Cerebralschaden. Arch. Psychiat. Z. Neurol. 186: 437—455, 1951.

— Über die Lokalisation frühkindlicher Hirnschäden in arteriellen Grenzgebieten. Arch. Psychiat. Z. Neurol. 190: 328—341, 1953.

Myers, R. E.: Two patterns of perinatal brain damage and their conditions of occurrence. Amer. J. Obstet. Gynecol. 112: 246—276, 1972.

Noell, W., Schneider, M.: Über die Durchblutung und die Sauerstoffversorgung des Gehirns im akuten Sauerstoffmangel. Pflügers Arch. ges. Physiol. 246: 181—249, 1942.

Norman, R. M.: Cerebellar atrophy associated with état marbré of the basal ganglia. J. Neurol. Psychiat. 3: 311—318, 1940.

— Atrophic sclerosis of the cerebral cortex associated with birth injury. Arch. Dis. Child. 19: 111—121, 1944.

— Cerebral birth injury. In: Greenfield's Neuropathology. London: E. Arnold 1969.

Norman, R. M., Ulrich, H., McNemeny, W. H.: Vascular mechanisms of birth injury. Brain 80: 49—58, 1957.

Romanul, F. C. A., Abramowicz, A.: Changes in brain and pial vessels in arterial border zones. Arch. Neurol. 11: 40—65, 1964.

Schwartz, P.: Traumatische Schädigungen des Zentralnervensystems durch die Geburt. Erg. inn. Med. Kinderheilk. 31: 164—372, 1927.

Verhaart, W. J. C., van Wieringen-Rauws, G. A.: On cerebro-cerebellar atrophy. Fol. Psychiat. Neurol. Neurochir. 53: 481—501, 1950.

7. Lesions of Basal Ganglia, Brain Stem and Cord

Status Marmoratus. Marbled state of the basal ganglia was described first by Anton (1893) for a 9-year-old choreo-athetotic boy in whom abnormal whitish areas and interspaced irregular zones of gray matter were found in the posterior halves of both putamina. Microscopic examination showed scar tissue containing myelinated nerve fibers. Anton concluded that the lesions were residual to vascular softenings dating to the first year of life, and were the anatomical substrate of the chorea. Vogt and Vogt (1920, 1926) and their co-workers reported several cases of the disease, which they considered a congenital selective malformation of the striatum; they introduced the terms "état marbré" or "status marmoratus". Their interpretation was not sustained in subsequent clinico-pathological studies in which the relation between marbled state and complicated birth or postnatal disease processes was documented (Norman, 1947; Malamud, 1950). Scholz (1924) had emphasized the correspondence between areas of abnormal myelin staining and zones of glial scarring.

The term marbled state generally denotes abnormally myelinated lesions in the basal ganglia, while the term "plaques fibromyeliniques" has been used to describe abnormally myelinated cortical scars in ulegyria; the latter usually do not show a definite marmorate pattern. Both types of lesions are equivalent (Bielschowsky, 1924), and the discussion of abnormal myelination in this chapter is equally pertinent to the abnormal myelination of cortical lesions (Chapter 6).

Marbled state of the basal ganglia is not very rare; more than 50 cases are found in the literature, but many more are collected unpublished in the files of neuropathologic services. Series of cases were reported by Scholz *et al.* (1938), 7 cases, and Malamud (1950), 15 cases. The statistical data in the following text were extracted from 42 well documented cases in the literature.

Complicated parturition was recorded for 70 percent of cases, the true frequency probably being even higher since many reports lack pertinent data. Typical complications are prolonged birth, severe cyanosis and need of resuscitation, or convulsions, rigidity or other neurologic signs developing soon after birth. Complications from the umbilical cord were specified by Sylvester (1960), one infant having a cord prolapse, the second a firm knot in the cord, and the third the cord wound tightly around the infant's neck. The disease appears to be most common for infants delivered at term, which is specifically mentioned for more than one-half, while prematurity is stated for less than 5 percent, the rest having insufficient data. The relation between marbled state and perinatal distress is corroborated by the frequent coexistence of marbled state with other types of perinatal cerebral lesions as specified below. Marbled state of basal ganglia has been observed coexistent with bilateral ulegyria in a rhesus monkey who suffered from asphyxia shortly before delivery (Myers, 1969).

A small number of cases of marbled state, approximately 10 percent, must be considered of postnatal onset. These have no history of complicated birth and a normal postnatal development. The neurologic disturbances develop upon an acute febrile disease during the first year of life (Scholz, 1924; Vogt and Vogt, 1926; Malamud, 1950; and others).

The most characteristic though not mandatory symptom of marbled state is bilateral choreo-athetosis from early infancy. Malamud (1950) concluded from a review of his cases that hyperkinetic symptoms result only when the caudate nucleus is involved bilaterally and the corticospinal tract intact. Other common symptoms are severely retarded motor and intellectual development, spastic paraplegia and epilepsy. The symptoms are not progressive. Severe debilitation shortens life expectancy, the average age at death being 12 years. Less than 8 percent attain the age of 30 years, but one patient (Christensen and Stubbe Teglbiaerg, 1946) lived to 74. Males predominate by more than 2 to 1.

The morbid anatomy of the acute phase of the lesions that lead later on to marbled state has not been well documented and there are no evident gross changes in the cut brain. Microscopic scrutiny of the basal ganglia of severely asphyxiated newborns occasionally discloses patches of neurons undergoing eosinophilic degeneration in the thalamus or, less often, in the striatum. These foci may well be the early lesions of marbled state. Scholz *et al.* (1938) reported focal neuronal necrosis in the basal ganglia of a 6½-month-old infant with a history of protracted birth; they considered the foci early lesions of status marmoratus, but interpretation of their case is difficult as the lesions were relatively recent and the infant had a thrombosis of the sinus rectus. The abnormal pattern of myelin staining characteristic of marbled state is never found in newborns, evidently because the nuclei are not myelinated at the time when the lesions form. The minimum length of survival required for the development of status marmoratus may be estimated from case 2 of Löwenberg and Malamud (1933), in whom status marmoratus was found at the age of 8 months in an infant with prolonged instrumental delivery, who developed seizures at 3 months.

Marbled state of basal ganglia in survivors is evident on gross inspection of the cut brain, the lesions appearing as spotty or irregular, whitish streaks in the striatum (Fig. 28) or thalamus. The affected nuclei may be of normal size or moderately to severely atrophic, depending on the extent of damage. Microscopic examination discloses 3 characteristic features: Focal loss of neurons; intense glial scarring; and, an abnormal distribution of myelinated fibers. The areas of abnormal myelin staining are composed of a feltwork of thin crisscrossing fibers; some of these have all the features of myelinated nerve fibers while others, particularly the very thin ones, are difficult to identify. The distribution of these fibers is abnormal in that they are not confined to sharply delineated bundles as is characteristic of the normal myeloarchitecture of the striatum. Instead, the fibers are dispersed diffusely, producing a faint patchy staining that forms interlacing networks by confluence; a perivascular accentuation is common. Large lesions consist of dense patches of fibers having irregular outlines and adjacent satellite foci. The

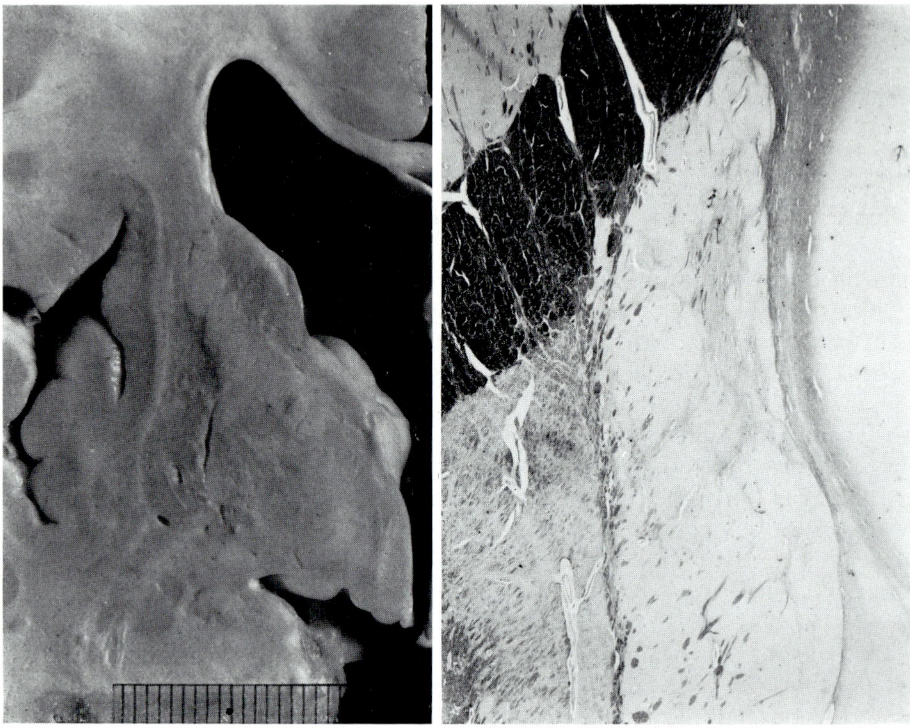

Fig. 28. Status marmoratus; shrinkage and scarring of putamen; right ×9.5

areas of abnormal myelin staining correspond, generally, to areas of intense reactive fibrillary gliosis in Holzer stains. There is, however, no precise congruity of the zones staining with myelin stains and those staining with Holzer stains. Case (1934) emphasized this point on staining the same sections with Holzer and myelin stains but gave no technical data. The present author obtained the best results by counterstaining Holzer preparations with phloxine. The preparations show that the intensity of gliosis in Holzer stain is not proportional to the density of fibers staining with phloxine although both tend to occur in the same general regions; myelinated fibers can be seen traversing, and continuing beyond, areas of gliosis. The areas of gliosis and abnormal myelin staining correspond to patchy loss of the neuronal population; mineralized neurons are often seen in these areas, particularly in the thalamus. Neuronal loss in the striatum affects large and small cells alike, but the latter may be affected to a greater degree. An increase in capillary density in the affected areas may develop as a result of tissue shrinkage.

Status marmoratus affects characteristically the striatum, the putamen being affected most often in its rostral and dorso-lateral portion, the caudate nucleus in its head. The lesions are nearly always bilateral but usually without strict symmetry; unilateral lesions are exceptionally rare (Scholz *et al.*, 1938). Marbling of the striatum is associated with changes in the thalamus in about 80 percent of cases, but this figure needs cautious interpretation since the thalamic lesions may either represent concurrent marbled state of the thalamus or be the result of secondary thalamic degeneration induced by devastation of the cerebral cortex from ulegyria. Also, it is more difficult to assess marbled state in the thalamus than in the striatum because of considerable individual variance in thalamic myeloarchitecture. In some instances the severity of the marbled lesions is greater in the thalamus than in the striatum (Carpenter, 1955) and rare cases show marbling exclusively in the thalamus (Norman, 1949). It is perhaps significant that predominance of thalamic lesions was observed in infants born prematurely, while the majority of infants with typical distribution of status marmoratus in the striatum were term.

Marbled state of the basal ganglia is frequently associated with other cerebral lesions; affectation of the cerebral cortex was present in 60 percent of cases, consisting of ulegyria or laminar or focal necrosis, often with abnormal myelin staining. Residual cavities of periventricular infarcts were the predominant lesions in infants reported by Pfeiffer (1925) and Juba (1937). No lesions were found in the pallidum in approximately 40 percent of cases; the others showed lesions that were less severe than those in the striatum. Affectation of claustrum and subthalamic nucleus is relatively common while substantia nigra, amygdala and mammillary bodies are usually spared. Focal sclerosis may occur in the cerebellum, but its attribution to concurrent primary lesions or to postconvulsive damage is controversial (Malamud, 1950).

The interpretation of marbled state of the basal ganglia has created considerable interest. Most investigators accepted the affinity of the marbled areas for myelin stains as *prima facie* evidence of an abnormal distribution of myelinated fibers; interpretations differed only in terms of whether marbling is produced by regeneration of myelinated fibers, formation of myelin around normally nonmyelinated fibers, redundant myelin formation, or tissue shrinkage with resultant increase in fiber density. These interpretations agree in considering marbling a residual lesion; whereas, Alexander (1942) thought that the abnormal distribution of myelinated fibers was due to a malformation of tracts that normally descend into the pons. The overlap between areas of abnormal myelin staining and of Holzer gliosis inherently creates difficulties in distinguishing glial fibers from thin nerve fibers, and the attribution of abnormal myelin staining to nerve fibers has been challenged. Sylvester (1960) thought that the principal component of marbling was gliosis and not hypermyelination since the marbled areas lost the myelin stain on progressive differentiation before the myelinated fibers lost theirs. Belloni (1952) and Jacob (1968) commented on the affinity of iron hematoxylin stains for glial fibers, particularly in areas of old gliosis. Electron microscopic examination of marbled basal ganglia and plaques fibromyeliniques in the cerebral cortex produced a new point of view in showing that formation of abnormally thick myelin sheaths can occur around what was presumed to be processes of fibrillary astrocytes in glial scars (Bignami and Ralston, 1968; Borit and Herndon, 1970). In conclusion, status marmoratus can be considered characteristic of damage occurring before the onset of myelin formation; the lesions derange subsequent myelination of the affected nuclei either in terms of deviating the course, density, caliber or growth of the fibers that normally enter the damaged areas, or in terms of inducing abnormal deposition of myelin about structures that normally do not become myelinated.

Other Types of Lesions in Basal Ganglia. Not all infantile lesions of thalamus or striatum induce marbled state. Rosales and Riggs (1962) described symmetric thalamic degeneration in 3 infants, 6, 15, and 16 months old, with profound neurogenic dysfunctions from birth. The damage affected mainly the lateral thalamic nuclei and was characterized by gliosis and numerous mineralized neurons. There were no other lesions in the brains, and the distribution of myelinated fibers was apparently not grossly disturbed, although the authors mention an arrangement in brush-like bands in the thalamus.

Predominant or selective lesions of the pallidum in patients with a history of perinatal disturbance have been reported under the name "status dysmyelinisatus"; they are discussed in Chapter 8 as they likely represent early descriptions of posticteric encephalopathy. Not all pallidal lesions can be attributed to kernicterus, however, as shown by 2 exceptional cases reported by Hallervorden (1949) and Jolly and Norman (1965). In the case of Hallervorden an unsuccessful attempt at suicide by carbon monoxide during the 5th month of pregnancy resulted, in the infant, in bilateral cavitation of the globus pallidus, atrophy of the striatum, almost complete loss of nerve cells in the lateral thalamic nuclei, and extensive polymicrogyria in the frontal lobes. The infant described by Jolly and Norman (1965) was the surviving twin of a coexistent extra- and intrauterine pregnancy, with a history of severe maternal shock upon rupture of the tube at the calculated fetal age of 91 days. This infant had extreme atrophy of the pallida associated with extreme and atypical status marmoratus of the thalamus, suggestive of a malformation of the thalamic radiation, and a moderate atrophy of the striatum. In discussing their case, the authors state that they never saw lesions in the globus pallidus of newborns that were not associated with changes in putamen or subthalamic nucleus. The nerve cells of the pallidum and thalamic nuclei mature considerably earlier than those of the striatum and have acquired large cell bodies with substantial cytoplasm when most of the striatal cells are still in the neuroblast stage (Chapter 1). This renders it probable that selective pallidal necrosis, or combined pallidal and thalamic necrosis, may be a pattern characteristic of an earlier developmental period than damage of the pallidum as a component of more severe lesions in the striatum.

Pontosubicular Neuronal Necrosis. Neuronal necrosis limited to the ventral pons was reported in a study on pulmonary hemorrhages in newborns by MacAdams (1967) for 40 infants, representing 17 percent of autopsies. A neuropathologic study of 22 infants, comprising 10 percent of autopsies, showed the pontine changes associated with neuronal necrosis in the subicular

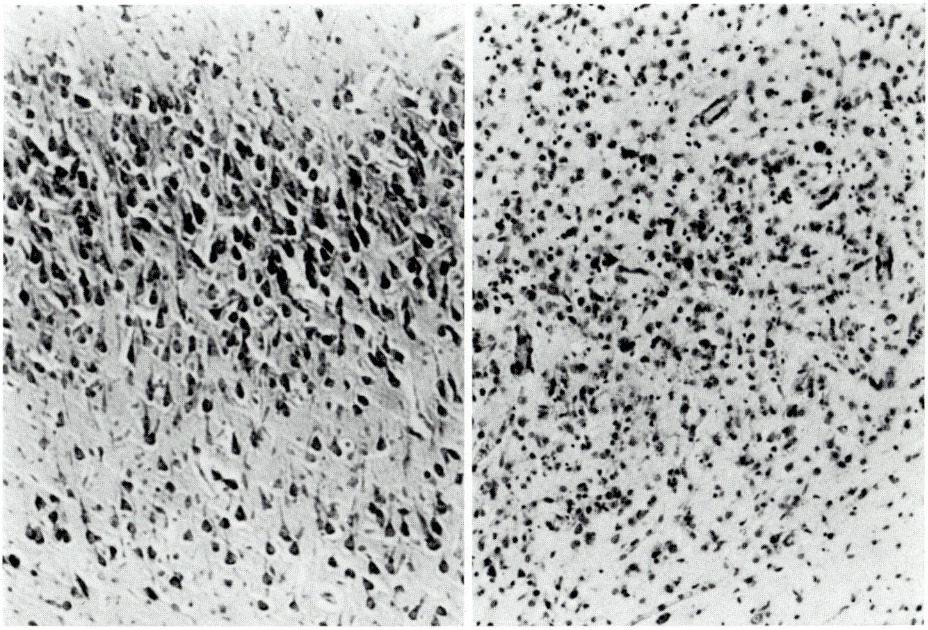

Fig. 29. Neuronal necrosis in subiculum (right) compared with normal architecture (left); cresyl violet ×250

segment of the Ammon's horn (Friede, 1972). These lesions were not observed in prematures less than 30 weeks gestation nor in children older than 2 months, suggesting a rather narrow age range for their occurrence. There was a more than 3 to 1 preference for males, but no sex predilection was noted in the series of MacAdams (1967). The most severe lesions were found in mature newborns with a history of respiratory distress having a high incidence of pulmonary lesions. Pontosubicular neuronal necrosis often coexists with other perinatal lesions, such as subependymal and intraventricular hemorrhages, periventricular infarcts or kernicterus.

The presence of the acute lesions is not obvious on gross inspection of the cut brain. Microscopic findings consist of neuronal necrosis, characterized by karyorrhexis and shrinkage of the cells. Karyorrhexis is identified by loss of definition of the nuclear membrane and disintegration of the nucleus into basophilic granules or into irregular lumps, inducing complete loss of basophilic material from the cells. Eosinophilic staining of the cytoplasm may

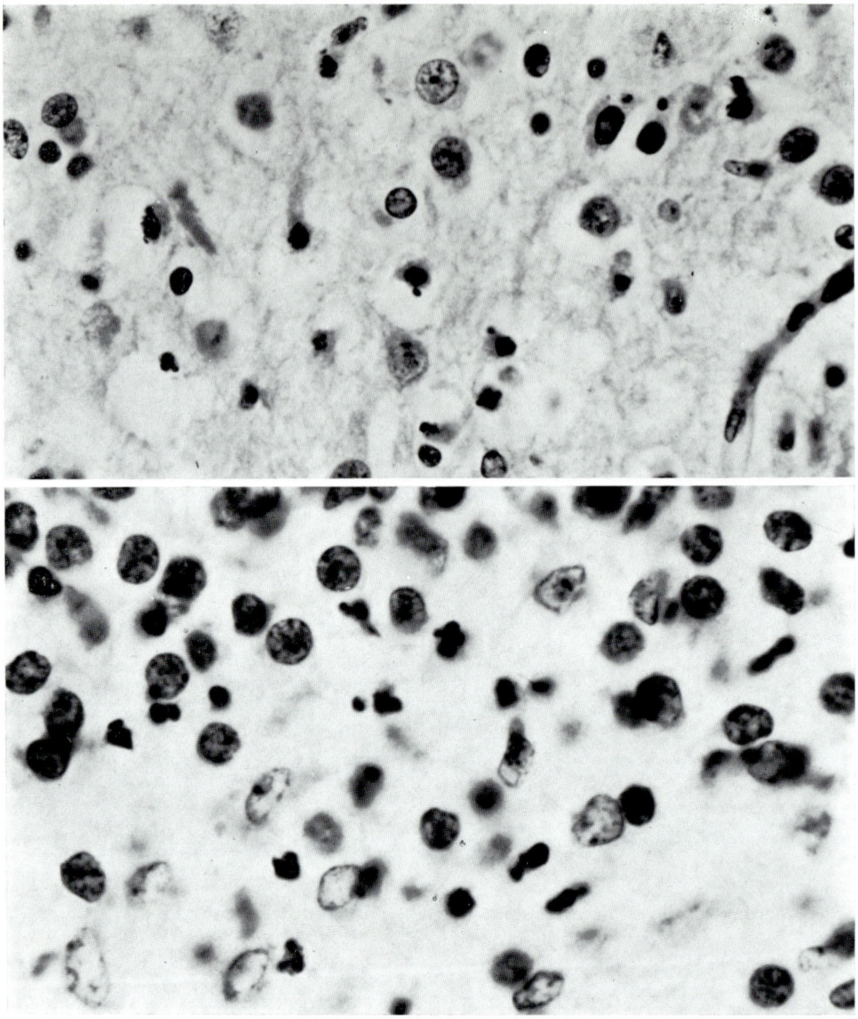

Fig. 30. Karyorrhexis of subicular neurons; H & E ×480. Karyorrhexis in cerebellar granular layer in a case of subtotal hemispheric necrosis; H & E ×1,000

be seen but is not a consistent feature. There is little or no glial response in lesions less than 48 hours old. Lesions 3 to 5 days old show progressive dropping out of neurons, astrocytic proliferation and migrating microglia and macrophages scattered through the tissue; there is no tendency to cavitate (Figs. 29–31).

Neuronal necrosis affects predominantly pons and subiculum. In the pontine gray matter it subsides sharply at the boundary to the tegmentum which is generally spared; the cerebellar Purkinje cells also are usually intact. Pontine changes vary in intensity from a few scattered karyorrhectic cells to subtotal necrosis of the entire pontine gray matter. Neuronal necrosis in

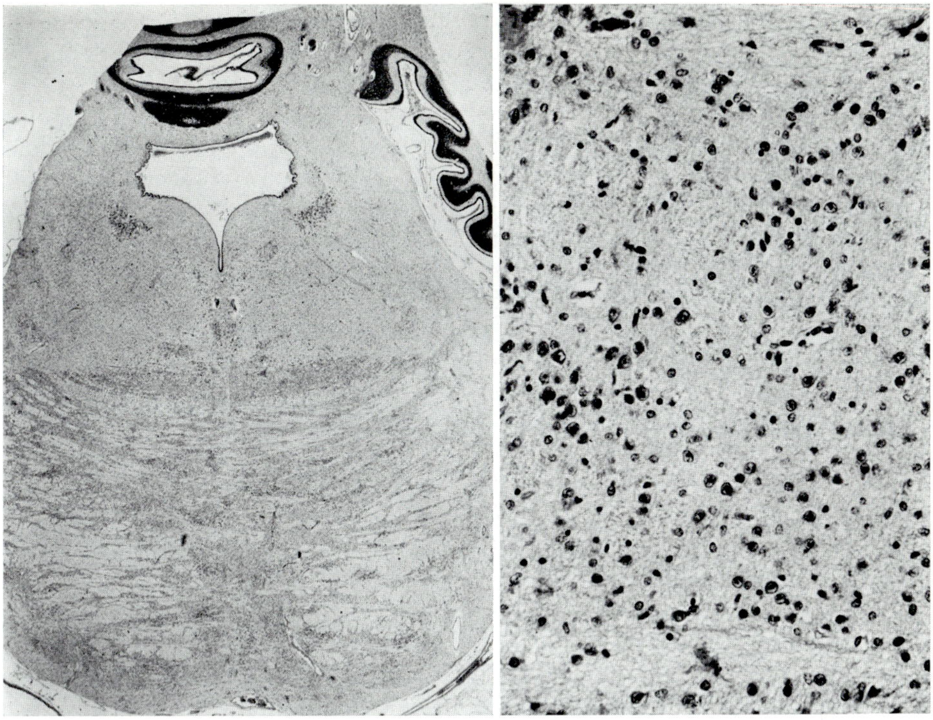

Fig. 31. Pontosubicular neuronal necrosis; subtotal loss of neurons in pontine gray matter; cresyl violet ×6.5; H & E ×200

the subicular segment of the pyramidal layer of the Ammon's horn may extend into the adjacent portion of Sommer's sector and into the entorhinal cortex and, occasionally, into the adjacent temporal cortex; the damage diminishes with distance from the subiculum. The cerebral cortex is spared, but scattered karyorrhectic neurons are often found in the supracallosal gyri, though always fewer than in pons and subiculum. There may be focal neuronal necrosis in the basal ganglia.

Neuronal necrosis of pons and subiculum of the type described above may also present as a component of massive and widespread cerebral damage, as in the 15 infants described under the designation "massive cerebral necrosis in the newborn" by Larroche (1968). These babies, born between 36 and 40 weeks gestation, all had convulsions or status epilepticus, and severe bioelectric anomalies were found for 4 of 5 who had an EEG. The microscopic changes described above were associated with widespread patchy or laminar loss of cells in the neocortex, neuronal loss in basal ganglia, affecting particularly the thalamus, and intense karyorrhexis in the internal cerebellar granule layer. It may be mentioned at this point that another pattern of brain stem lesions in infants—that of hypotensive brain stem necrosis (Chapter 9)— also occurs either as a selective brain stem lesion or as component of widespread anoxic encephalopathy.

The severity and relative selectivity with which perinatal neuronal necrosis may affect the pontine gray matter opens a Pandora box of differential diagnostic problems in regard to the identification of its residual lesions. There is a dichotomy between marbled state of basal ganglia and pontosubicular neuronal necrosis, in that the former is known only from its residual state, the latter almost exclusively from its acute lesions. Subacute stages of pontosubicular necrosis, after several months survival, show marked atrophy of the pons which is readily apparent on gross inspection of the brain stem; there is little or no atrophy in the cerebellar hemispheres. Microscopic examination of the pons discloses reduction in the volume of pontine gray matter with reduction in neuron population and relatively little gliosis. Identification of these lesions as subacute stages of pontosubicular neuronal necrosis is possible by demonstrating the characteristic loss of cells in the subiculum (Friede, 1972). Greater difficulties may be encountered if there are also lesions in other portions of the brain.

Marked pontine atrophy is a characteristic feature of neocerebellar aplasia (Chapter 30), where it is associated with deficiency of the hemispheric cerebellar cortex. For some cases, however, the cerebellar cortex is hypoplastic rather than deficient, having hypoplastic cortical gyri. Brun (1918) referred to these cases as neocerebellar hypoplasia in distinction from aplasia. Representative reports were given by Koster (1926), Krause (1929), and Biemond (1929). These lesions probably were less severe degrees of neocerebellar aplasia rather than perinatally acquired, an interpretation consistent with the presence of anomalies in the architecture of the dentate nucleus as often seen in neocerebellar aplasia (Chapter 30). Other observations are more difficult to interpret. A 14-day-old premature girl described by Scherer (1933) had poor postnatal development and never recovered from a gastroenteritis at the age of 1 month; convulsions developed at 15 months and death came at 18 months. Pontine atrophy was associated with sclerosis of the Ammon's horn and with loss of Purkinje cells, but the latter changes may have been secondary to convulsions. Case 1 of Norman and Urich (1958) was a 5-month-old infant which exhibited thalamic and mammillary necrosis in addition to pontine and cerebellar lesions. The authors concluded that a malformation of one nuclear group induces transneuronal degeneration in others and considered their case as disclosing a bond between malformation and abiotrophy.

Difficulties may also arise from the affectation of the pontine gray matter in the context of more widespread hemispheric cortical lesions as, for example, the lesions described by Larroche (1968) discussed earlier in this chapter which may be considered transitional to those of progressive sclerosing cortical atrophy (Chapter 10). The latter usually does not produce secondary, transneuronal degeneration of the pontine gray matter. Skullerud *et al.* (1973) described 3 siblings having nearly identical histories of progressive neurologic deterioration. Autopsy findings in one disclosed laminar degeneration of the cerebral cortex and near complete absence of neurons in the pontine gray matter, but little or no changes in basal ganglia, brain stem and cerebellum. Near complete loss of pontine neurons was observed by the present author in 2 siblings succumbing to congenital renal disease. There was also subicular and patchy cortical loss of neurons. Cases such as these are still difficult to classify.

Brain Stem Lesions Produced by Experimental Perinatal Asphyxia in Laboratory Animals. The available data on experimental perinatal asphyxia, though quite extensive, often do not permit direct application to the understanding of autopsy findings in human infants. Experimental asphyxia produced by clamping of the umbilical cord of guinea pig fetuses resulted in rather indistinct chromatolytic changes in large interneurons of the reticular formation (Windle *et al.*, 1944; Bailey and Windle, 1959). A more characteristic pattern of damage was produced in rhesus monkeys, who developed symmetric necrosis of inferior colliculi, gracile and medial cuneate nuclei, the roof nuclei of the cerebellum, the ventral posterior thalamic nuclei, the pallidum, putamen and the vestibular nuclei (Ranck and Windle, 1959; Windle, 1963; Myers, 1971). This type of damage is not a recognized feature in human newborns suffering from perinatal asphyxia, but it has obvious similarities to hypotensive brain stem necrosis following cardiac arrest (Chapter 9). Miller and Myers (1972) observed a similar pattern of brain stem damage following circulatory arrest in adult monkeys. One has to surmise, therefore, that the lesions described by Rank and Windle (1959) are not specific for damage during the perinatal period; they may be the equivalent of hypotensive brain stem necrosis, or they may represent a type of damage more readily induced in monkey than in man.

Experimental perinatal anoxia has also been linked to a diffuse loss of neurons in the cerebral cortex affecting cortical thickness as well as cortical neuronal organization (Hicks *et al.*, 1962; Faro and Windle, 1969). The disturbances of cortical architecture in these experiments are of a degree which would almost certainly escape detection in routine examination of human neuropathologic material.

Ischemic Necrosis of Spinal Cord. Ischemic changes in the spinal cord of newborn infants are extremely rare. A case of bilateral paralysis of arms from birth to age 10 days was described by Adams and Cameron (1965). The cervical cord showed bilateral necrosis of the gray matter of ventral horns with cavitation extending from C_2 to C_7. The lesions were attributed to severe impairment of cervical cord circulation. Further reports of similar cases are needed for a definite classification of this type of lesion, since hypotensive brain stem necrosis may also induce lesions in the gray matter of cord.

References

Adams, J. H., Cameron, H. M.: Obstetrical paralysis due to ischaemia of the spinal cord. Arch. Dis. Child. 40: 93—96, 1965.

Alexander, L.: The fundamental types of histopathological changes encountered in cases of athetonis and paralysis agitans. A. Research Nerv. Ment. Dis., Proc. (1940) 21: 334—493, 1942.

Anton, G.: Über die Beteiligung der basalen Gehirnganglien bei Bewegungsstörungen bei der Chorea. Wien. klin. Wschr. 6: 859—861, 1893.

Bailey, L. J., Windle, W. F.: Neurological, psychological and neurohistological defects following asphyxia neonatorum in the guinea pig. Exp. Neurol. 1: 467—482, 1959.

Belloni, G. B.: Sulla istopatologia dello status marmoratus e delle placche fibromieliniche. Proc. 1st Int. Congr. Neuropath. 2: 235—241, 1952.

Bielschowsky, M.: Über den Status marmoratus des Striatums und atypische Markfasergeflechte der Hirnrinde. J. Psychol. Neurol. (Lpz.) 31: 121—151, 1924.

Biemond, A.: Hypoplasia ponto-neocerebellaris with malformation of the dentate nucleus. Fol. Psych. Neurol. Neurochir. Neerl. 58: 2—7, 1955.

Bignami, A., Ralston, H. J., III.: Myelination of fibrillary astroglial processes in long term Wallerian degeneration. The possible relationship to "status marmoratus". Brain Res. 11: 710—713, 1868.

Borit, A., Herndon, R. M.: The fine structure of plaques fibromyeliniques in ulegyria and in status marmoratus. Acta Neuropath. 14: 304—311, 1970.

Brun, R.: Zur Kenntnis der Bildungsfehler des Kleinhirns. Schweiz. Arch. Neurol. Psychiat. 1: 61—123, 1917; 2: 48—105; 3: 13—88, 1918.

Carpenter, M. B.: Status marmoratus of the thalamus and striatum (associated with athetosis and dystonia). Neurology 5: 139—146, 1955.

Case, T. J.: Status marmoratus related to early encephalitis. Arch. Neurol. Psychiat. 31: 817—823, 1934.

Christensen, E., Stubbe Teglbiaerg, H. P.: Double athetosis with status marmoratus. Acta Psychiat. Neurol. 21: 177—194, 1946.

Faro, M. D., Windle, W. F.: Transneuronal degeneration in brains of monkeys asphyxiated at birth. Exp. Neurol. 24: 38—53, 1969.

Friede, R. L.: Ponto-subicular lesions in perinatal anoxia. Arch. Path. 94: 343—354, 1972.

Hallervorden, J.: Über eine Kohlenoxydvergiftung im Fetalleben mit Entwicklungsstörung der Hirnrinde. Allg. Z. Psychiat. 124: 289—298, 1949.

Hicks, S. P., Cavanaugh, M. C., O'Brien, E. D.: Effects of anoxia on the developing cerebral cortex in the rat. Amer. J. Path. 40: 615—635, 1962.

Jacob, H.: Dissociation glio-myélinique und Hämatoxylinaffinität von Gliafasern. Acta neuropath. (Berl.), Suppl. IV: 158—164, 1968.

Jolly, G. F., Norman, R. M.: Co-existing intra- and extra-uterine pregnancy associated with cerebral malformation in the surviving twin. J. Obstet. Gynaec. 72: 125—130, 1965.

Juba, A.: Über eine frühinfantile Großhirnmißbildung (Polyporencephalie und Status marmoratus). Z. Neurol. Psychiat. 157: 622—635, 1937.

Koster, S.: Two cases of hypoplasia pontoneocerebellaris. Acta Psychiat. Neurol. 1: 47—83, 1926.

Krause, F.: Über einen Bildungsfehler des Kleinhirnes und einige faseranatomische Beziehungen des Organs. Z. ges. Neurol. Psychiat. 119: 788—815, 1929.

Larroche, J. C.: Nécrose cérébrale massive chez le nouveau-né. Biol. Neonat. 13: 340—360, 1968.

Löwenberg, K., Malamud, W.: Status marmoratus. Etiology and manner of development. Arch. Neurol. Psychiat. 29: 104—124, 1933.

MacAdams, A. J.: Pulmonary hemorrhage in the newborn. Amer. J. Dis. Child. 113: 255—262, 1967.

Malamud, N.: Status marmoratus. A form of cerebral palsy following either birth injury or inflammation of the central nervous system. J. Pediat. 37: 610—619, 1950.

Miller, J. R., Myers, R. E.: Neuropathology of systemic circulatory arrest in adult monkeys. Neurology 22: 888—904, 1972.

Myers, R. E.: Atrophic cortical sclerosis associated with status marmoratus in a perinatally damaged monkey. Neurology 19: 1177—1188, 1969.

— Brain damage induced by umbilical cord compression at different gestational ages in monkeys. Medical Primatology 1970. Proc. 2nd Conf. exp. Med. Surg. Primates, New York 1969, pp. 394—425. Basel: Karger 1971.

Norman, R. M.: Etat marbré of corpus striatum following birth injury. J. Neurol. Neurosurg. Psychiat. 10: 12—25, 1947.

— Etat marbré of the thalamus following birth injury. Brain 72: 83—89, 1949.

— Urich, H.: Cerebellar hypoplasia associated with systemic degeneration in early life. J. Neurol. Neurosurg. Psychiat. 21: 159—166, 1958.

Pfeiffer, F.: Chorea Athetose bei der Little-Lähmung. Arch. Psychiat. 72: 728—754, 1925.

Randk, J. B., Windle, W. F.: Brain damage in the monkey, Macaca mulatta by asphyxia neonatorum. Exp. Brain Res. 1: 130—154, 1959.
Rosales, R. K., Riggs, H. E.: Symmetrical thalamic degeneration in infants. J. Neuropath. exp. Neurol. 21: 372—376, 1962.
Scherer, H. J.: Beiträge zur pathologischen Anatomie des Kleinhirnes. III. Genuine Kleinhirnatrophien. Z. ges. Neurol. Psychiat. 145: 335—405, 1933.
Scholz, W.: Zur Kenntnis des Status marmoratus. Infantile partielle Striatumsklerose. Z. Neurol. Psychiat. 88: 355—383, 1924.
— Wake, I., Peters, G.: Der Status marmoratus, ein Beispiel systemähnlicher Hirnveränderungen auf der Grundlage von Kreislaufstörungen. Z. Neurol. Psychiat. 163: 193—232, 1938.
Skullerud, K., Torvik, A., Skaare-Botner, L.: Progressive degeneration of the cerebral cortex in infancy. Acta Neuropath. 24: 153—160, 1973.
Sylvester, P.: Marbling and perinatal anoxia. Acta Pediat. 49: 338—344, 1960.
Vogt, C., Vogt, O.: Zur Lehre der Erkrankungen des striären Systems. J. Psychiat. Neurol. 25: 627—846, 1920.
— — Die nosologische Stellung des Status marmoratus des Striatum. Psychiat.-neurol. Wschr. 28: 85—87, 1926.
Windle, W. F.: Neuropathology of certain forms of mental retardation. Science 140: 1186—1189, 1963.
— Becker, R. F., Weil, A.: Alterations in brain structure after asphyxiation at birth. An experimental study in the guinea pig. J. Neuropath. exp. Neurol. 3: 224—238, 1944.

8. Kernicterus (Bilirubin Encephalopathy)

The first report of kernicterus is generally attributed to Orth (1875), although his description is somewhat unclear and emphasizes staining of the superficial portions of brain tissue in the ventricular walls and at the hemispheric surface. The first comprehensive description of the disease was given by Schmorl (1903) who distinguished two types of cerebral lesions in icteric infants. One type consisted of a diffuse staining of the tissue and was found in infants with periventricular infarcts. This type of lesion has rarely been reported in the subsequent literature. The second type, called kernicterus by Schmorl, was observed in six infants who showed selective icteric discoloration of the subthalamic nuclei, Ammon's horn, lentiform nuclei, and dentate and olivary nuclei; the thalamus and cerebral cortex were spared. An intense yellow discoloration of many, though not all, of the nerve cells and a delicate staining of the intervening tissue were observed microscopically in the affected nuclei. The early literature on subsequent case reports was reviewed by Zimmerman and Yannet (1933) and Péhu and Pollet (1939). The term kernicterus is now generally used to designate the pathologic lesions as well as the clinical features of the disease.

Kernicterus was considered a nosologic entity during the first part of the century and many now obsolete hypotheses were proposed on its etiology and pathogenesis. The discovery of the Rh factor by Landsteiner and Wiener (1940) opened the way for the recognition of kernicterus as a cerebral complication of icterus gravis from fetal erythroblastosis caused by iso-immunization of the mother by the Rh antigen of the fetus (Levine *et al.*, 1941). Subsequent investigations made clear that kernicterus is not a complication of a specific hemolytic disease, but rather one of infantile hyperbilirubinemia regardless of its etiology. Accordingly, the terms "bilirubin encephalopathy" (Waters *et al.*, 1954) or "bilirubin toxicosis" (Chen, 1964) have been proposed.

Metabolism of Bilirubin. The bilirubin formed from the breakdown of blood is normally taken up by the liver where it is conjugated with glucuronic acid. Conjugation is accomplished by means of a series of enzymatic reactions leading to the formation of uridine-diphosphate glucuronide which serves as a donor of glucuronyl radicals for the formation of bilirubin diglucuronide. The reaction is mediated by UDP glucuronyl-transferase (Lathe and Walker, 1958). The conjugated bilirubin is water-soluble and is excreted by the kidneys. Conjugated bilirubin is also called "direct reacting bilirubin", in distinction from the "indirect bilirubin" which is unconjugated and in plasma normally is bound to serum albumin.

The significance of bilirubin production and the different steps of its elimination have been the subject of extensive investigations. Most authors agree that the fundamental defect in neonatal hyperbilirubinemia is not hemolysis, but insufficient rates in the hepatic uptake of bilirubin, of bilirubin conjugation, and the excretion of bilirubin conjugates. The rate-limiting factor among the processes of bilirubin elimination appears to be the synthesis of bilirubin conjugates due to low activities of hepatic glucuronyltransferase activity and ancillary enzymes (Lathe and Walker, 1958). Glucuronide formation in the human newborn is 10 percent, or less, of the adult value; a postnatal increase of conjugation to normal adult rates has occurred by the third postnatal month (Vest, 1958). The urinary excretion of conjugates is still lower in premature than in term babies (Brown and Burnett, 1957). No significant amounts of conjugated bilirubin are found in the plasma of children suffering from Rh or ABO incompatibility, or prematurity (Winsnes and Bratlid, 1972). The lack in the enzymatic conjugation process is now widely accepted as the cause of neonatal hyperbilirubinemia. Any condition that induces hemolysis in the newborn adds to the load on the conjugation mechanism already working at capacity, thus increasing the risk of kernicterus. Any factor inducing hepatic damage will further impair conjugation. Hyperbilirubinemia may also result from an inherited defect of hepatic glucuronyltransferase as in familial nonhemolytic anemia, or as in rats of the Gunn strain. Deficient conjugation of bilirubin, therefore, emerges as a key factor in kernicterus, and it stands to reason that kernicterus does not develop in adults having no conjugation defect nor does it develop from congenital atresia of bile ducts in newborns as the sole cause. Various etiologic processes underlying kernicterus are reviewed briefly in the following paragraphs. The pathogenetic mechanisms relating to the exchange of bilirubin between plasma and brain tissue are discussed at the end of this chapter.

Etiologies of Kernicterus. Erythroblastosis fetalis or hemolytic anemias due to iso-immunization are caused in approximately 80 percent of cases by Rh incompatibility and in approximately 20 percent by the ABO system. Fetal erythroblastosis occurs in approximately 5 percent of marriages in which the mother is Rh negative and the father Rh positive and in 1 to 5 percent of marriages with the ABO constellation. Erythroblastosis due to Rh incompatibility is rare in the first pregnancy, because previous sensitization of the mother by a preceding pregnancy or by blood transfusion is required; jaundice develops during the second to fifth day. ABO incompatibility occurs in the first pregnancy in 40 to 50 percent of cases; jaundice develops during the first 24 hours and is associated with mild anemia and few other symptoms (Zuelzer and Cohen, 1957).

The occurrence of kernicterus in erythroblastosis was found to be related to the severity of the hemolytic anemia; it is likely to occur with serum bilirubin levels above 30 mg% and is rare at levels below 20 mg% (Hsia *et al.*, 1952). The neurologic symptoms of kernicterus usually become manifest between the second and fifth day of life, with initial somnolence, apathy and hypotonia; disturbances of motor coordination, rigidity, opisthotonos, trismus, spasms, high pitched cry or excitation lead to cyanosis and coma; convulsions are uncommon. A precipitous decrease in serum bilirubin may occur with the onset of neurologic symptoms (Ackerman *et al.*, 1971). The prognosis is severe after neurologic complications have appeared and the majority of affected infants die within the first or second week. Exchange transfusions may prevent the development of kernicterus.

Another cause of kernicterus is severe hemolytic anemia in the newborn period caused by erythrocyte deficiency of glucose-6-phosphate dehydrogenase, particularly in Mediterranean and Chinese populations in whom this defect is more prevalent. Jaundice and kernicterus may be precipitated by exposure to normally innocuous drugs, such as primaquine, sulfonamide, or naphthalene (Smith and Vella, 1960; Panizon, 1960; Naiman, 1964). An increased incidence of kernicterus with high intake of vitamin K (Schall, 1958) may also depend on increased hemolysis, but other pathogenetic factors may be involved as well.

The frequency of autopsy cases of kernicterus as a complication of erythroblastosis with icterus gravis and high bilirubin levels has diminished greatly with the introduction of exchange transfusions in 1950. Consequently, greater attention has been focused on the occurrence of kernicterus in infants with relatively low bilirubin levels having one or more predisposing factors including prematurity, low birth weight, hypoxia, acidosis or septicemia (Corner, 1955; Brown and Zuelzer, 1957; Stern and Denton, 1965; Gartner *et al.*, 1970). In these infants kernicterus develops at serum bilirubin levels substantially below 20 mg% and often in the absence of typical neurologic manifestations. Males predominate moderately.

Kernicterus may also develop in infantile hyperbilirubinemia due to nonhemolytic familial diseases, as in Crigler-Najjar and Gilbert diseases, both having in common a deficiency of hepatic glucuronyl-transferase activity. In the family described by Crigler and Najjar (1952) jaundice was present from birth; extrapyramidal signs with distorted posture and athetosis developed at 1 to 3 months, progressive deterioration and death within the first year of life. A defect clinically and pathologically analogous to that in the Crigler-Najjar family was found in homozygous rats of the Gunn strain, which also lack hepatic glucuronyl-transferase activity (Johnson *et al.*, 1959). Hyperbilirubinemia of the indirect type usually appears within a few hours after birth; it reaches levels of 10 to 20 mg% during the first weeks of life and falls thereafter to an average of 7 mg% at which it remains. Kernicterus develops spontaneously in 65 percent of rats; its gross and microscopic features are strikingly similar to kernicterus in man (Blanc and Johnson, 1959).

Survival of kernicterus may be followed by posticteric encephalopathy with residual neurologic symptoms referring mainly to the basal ganglia, including choreo-athetoid movements, spasticity, strange postures and muscular rigidity, hypotonus, opisthotonos, ataxia and mental deficiency. The clinical course may vary greatly. Loss of hearing, strabismus and dental anomalies with semi-lunar defects in the enamel of incisors and canines have also been reported in survivors.

Gross and Microscopic Lesions. Among the many descriptions of the lesions of kernicterus, those of Claireaux (1950), Haymaker *et al.* (1961), and Chen (1964) provide the greatest detail. The gross features consist of icteric discoloration of certain nuclear groups in a symmetrical and highly selective pattern and of absent staining in the rest of the brain tissue. The affectation of given nuclei varies somewhat from case to case. The most common sites of staining are the pallidum, subthalamic nucleus and Ammon's horn, while staining of the thalamus and the striatum is less common; the cerebral cortex and white matter are usually spared, unless there are unrelated destructive lesions such as periventricular infarcts. Icteric staining in the brain stem involves mainly the cranial nerve nuclei of the tegmentum, particularly the oculomotor, vestibular and hypoglossal nuclei, as well as the inferior olivary and dentate nuclei and the cerebellar flocculi. Diffuse staining may occur in the reticular formation, the substantia nigra and, on occasion, in the spinal cord. Discoloration is caused by the presence in the tissue of bilirubin in the unconjugated form (Claireaux *et al.*, 1953; Waters *et al.*, 1954).

Efforts to demonstrate the cellular distribution of bilirubin in the tissue may meet with variable success, depending on the period of storage in formalin and the methods of processing of the tissue. Staining fades rapidly upon storing the brains in formalin at room temperature. An intense yellow discoloration of neurons and their processes may be seen in frozen section under favorable conditions. Selective staining of some of the neurons may leave others in their immediate vicinity unstained; the stained neurons may be considered necrobiotic. Deposition of bilirubin crystals is uncommon. Staining is no longer present in paraffin-embedded sections, although some residual pigment, or even crystalline material, is observed on occasion.

The intensity of histologic changes in the various nuclear groups varies considerably in acute cases of kernicterus, and it is often not related to the presence of icteric discoloration in the gross specimen. In many instances only early, nonspecific alterations are seen, such as shrinkage and pyknosis of cells, early eosinophilic degeneration, chromatolysis and vacuolization of cytoplasm, and sponginess of the neuropil. Incrustation of neurons by pericellular basophilic granules is seen on occasion. Alterations of this type are found in the pallidum and red zone of the substantia nigra, the subthalamic nucleus, hippocampus, third and fourth cranial nerve nuclei, tegmental reticular formation and cerebellar roof nuclei with variable involvement of thalamus and other nuclear groups. The cerebral and cerebellar cortex, striatum, amygdala and other nuclear groups are usually free of changes. The presence of early or borderline cellular changes in a majority of autopsy cases of kernicterus implies that the lesions develop in the terminal phase of the disease, attesting to the grave prognosis of neurologic complications. Subacute lesions are seen with longer survival; there is loss of neurons, reactive astrocytic proliferation and the scattering of macrophages in the tissue. A survival of 3 weeks has

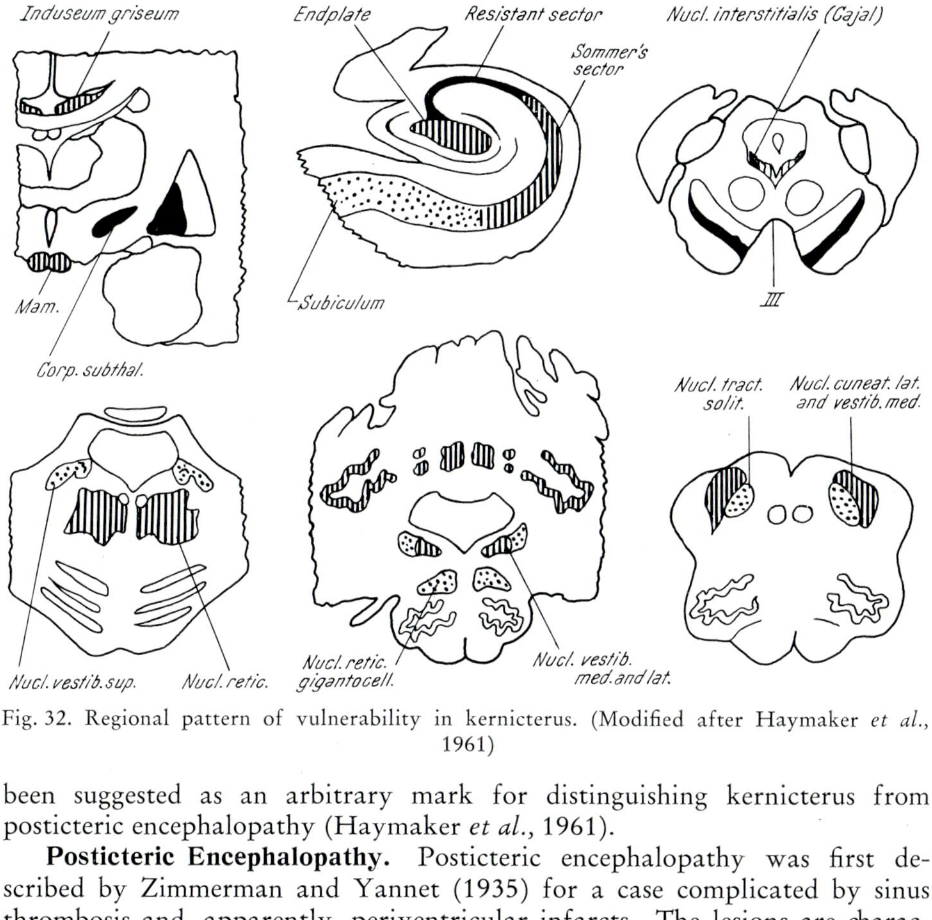

Fig. 32. Regional pattern of vulnerability in kernicterus. (Modified after Haymaker *et al.*, 1961)

been suggested as an arbitrary mark for distinguishing kernicterus from posticteric encephalopathy (Haymaker *et al.*, 1961).

Posticteric Encephalopathy. Posticteric encephalopathy was first described by Zimmerman and Yannet (1935) for a case complicated by sinus thrombosis and, apparently, periventricular infarcts. The lesions are characterized by atrophy of the nuclei with loss of nerve cells and glial scarring in the pallidum, subthalamic nucleus, particularly its lateral portion, the resistant sector of the Ammon's horn, the red portion of the substantia nigra, and the superficial nucleus of Cajal in the midbrain (Fig. 32). Less severe or less consistent changes are seen in the end-plate and Sommer's sector of the Ammon's horn, the mammillary bodies, and induseum griseum, the oculomotor, trochlear, vestibular and cuneate nuclei, the reticular formation of the pons, and the dentate nuclei; occasional damage is observed in subiculum and in other stem nuclei (Haymaker *et al.*, 1961). No residual pigmentation is evident on gross or microscopic inspection. Lesions are uncommon in the cerebral and cerebellar cortex, striatum and pontine gray matter. The most characteristic features of posticteric encephalopathy are the combined affectation of the subthalamic nucleus, pallidum and the resistant sector of the Ammon's horn. Significant damage of the dentate and olivary nuclei is rarely seen, although the staining of these nuclear groups in the acute phase is often prominent.

There are only a few reports on cerebral lesions in familial nonhemolytic jaundice. Autopsy observations on Crigler-Najjar disease, reviewed by Gardner and Konigsmark (1969), showed gross pigmentation or microscopic lesions consistent with kernicterus. A case observed by these authors was unusual in that a progressive neurologic disturbance began at the age of 15$^{1}/_{2}$ years. The lesions in this brain differed from typical posticteric encephalopathy in their preferential affectation of the thalamus, putamen, caudate nucleus, dentate and red nuclei, while the pallidum, subthalamic nucleus and Ammon's horn were either normal or only mildly affected. No pigment was found in the tissue. The authors considered the case kernicterus of late onset. A similar observation by Jellinger *et al.* (1970) shows residual damage consistent with kernicterus superimposed by more recent partial necrosis of cerebral cortex, Ammon's horn and striatum, with marked gross discoloration of these regions. A case of constitutional nonhemolytic hyperbilirubinemia (Gilbert's disease) also showed affectation of the putamen, red nucleus, corpora quadrigemina, the third layer of cerebral cortex and Sommer's sector, in addition to the classic pattern of posticteric encephalopathy (Jervis, 1959).

Kernicterus, Status Dysmyelinisatus and Lesions of Perinatal Anoxia. Status dysmyelinisatus was described by Vogt and Vogt (1920) for two infants with extrapyramidal rigidity. The cerebral lesions were characterized by subtotal or complete loss of neurons in the pallidum and by reduced density of myelinated fibers within the nucleus and the ansa lenticularis. The designation "status dysmyelinisatus" refers to the latter change. Intense gliosis and selective staining of the shrunken nucleus with Holzer stains was also observed. Both of the cases described by Vogt and Vogt had coexistent lesions in the subthalamic nuclei. The significance of this report needs to be assessed in the light of the author's preoccupation with the various tissue patterns of striatal lesions to the point of ignoring the underlying etiologies; for example, atrophy of the striatum caused by Huntington's chorea or by general paresis was classified as état fibreux. Several additional cases of status dysmyelinisatus were published in the subsequent literature, and Hallervorden and Meyer (1956) briefly reviewed a series of 10. Hence, "status dysmyelinisatus" became established as a disease entity *sui generis,* even after posticteric encephalopathy had been recognized. Zimmerman and Yannet (1935) were the first to draw attention to the similarity between status dysmyelinisatus and posticteric encephalopathy. There had been no mention of neonatal icterus in the case reports on status dysmyelinisatus, except for Balthasar (1939); however, the characteristic involvement of pallidum and subthalamic nuclei was observed by Onari (1925), Kreyenberg (1931), de Lange (1939), Inose (1941), and Hallervorden and Meyer (1956). Only in the carefully studied case of Papez *et al.* (1938) were the lesions highly selective to the pallidum. No additional cases of "status dysmyelinisatus" have been reported in the more recent literature. In the light of these observations there is no justification for continued use of the term "status dysmyelinisatus" as the lesions are evidently those of posticteric encephalopathy.

A similar overlap existed in the literature in regard to anoxic and icteric cerebral lesions. Scholz (1941) reported loss of nerve cells and scarring of the pallidum, nucleus subthalamicus and nucleus dentatus in an 18-year-old boy with pulmonary stenosis and atrial and ventricular septal defect as an example of brain damage from chronic hypoxia caused by congenital cardiac disease; the report has been widely quoted. However, the lesions are not consistent with those found in congenital cardiac disease (Chapter 14), and the patient's history discloses that he was born cyanotic and with respiratory distress as the second of twins. Meriwether *et al.* (1955) later attributed neuronal necrosis in the pallidum to neonatal asphyxia and considered jaundice per se of no pathologic significance. There is no question that perinatal asphyxia and kernicterus often coexist; Chen (1964) observed amniotic aspiration in the lungs of 84 percent of his cases of kernicterus. Indeed, anoxia may play a role in triggering kernicterus, as discussed later in this text. Hence, posticteric encephalopathy may coexist with residual lesions characteristic of perinatal asphyxia. Of the 7 cases of posticteric encephalopathy reviewed by Haymaker *et al.* (1961), one showed marbled state of the anterior thalamic nuclei; marbled state of the striatum has been found repeatedly associated with "status dysmyelinisatus" (Onari, 1925; Scharapow and Tschernomordik, 1928; Balthasar, 1939). The residual cavities of periventricular infarcts (Chapter 5) may also coexist with posticteric encephalopathy.

In conclusion, the weight of the available clinical, pathologic and experimental evidence reviewed here and in other pertinent sections of this text strongly indicates that the so-called "status dysmyelinisatus" is identical to posticteric encephalopathy, and that these icteric lesions can be distinguished in type and regional distribution from those caused by perinatal anoxia in the absence of jaundice. Lesions similar to status dysmyelinisatus also occur with other CNS diseases, in particular neuraxonal dystrophy (Chapter 43).

Pathogenetic Considerations. The etiologic factors causing hyperbilirubinemia in the newborn are reviewed at the beginning of this chapter.

The following considerations concern factors affecting the state of bilirubin in the blood stream and its transfer into the tissue. Bilirubin in serum is strongly bound to plasma albumin, one mole of the protein binding two moles of bilirubin. Unbound bilirubin is a highly lipid-soluble molecule and has the capacity for rapidly passing the blood brain barrier. Its failure to do so in the nondamaged brain is obviously the result of its protein binding. Factors affecting the protein binding of bilirubin need to be considered in the pathogenesis of kernicterus. One is the competition for binding sites on the protein molecules between bilirubin and other substances. Salicylic acid or sulfonamides (Odell, 1959) may release free bilirubin by competing for its binding sites, and their medication increases the mortality of kernicterus (Silverman *et al.*, 1956). They also provide a convenient experimental model for the controlled induction of neurologic complications in Gunn rats (Schutta and Johnson, 1971). The protein binding of bilirubin is pH dependent (Odell and Cohen, 1960), so that a decrease in pH or an increase in the bilirubin-albumin ratio at low pH increase the cytotoxicity in tissue cultures (Silberberg *et al.,* 1970). Hypoalbuminemia from insufficient formation of albumin or from loss of plasma proteins also reduces the number of binding sites available for bilirubin. The transfer of bilirubin from the blood stream into the tissue may be facilitated, on the other hand, by the simultaneous passage of albumin, or by an increased concentration of albumin in the cerebrospinal fluid; the bilirubin content of cerebrospinal fluid of infants increases with its protein content (Nasralla *et al.,* 1958).

Disturbances of the albumin-bilirubin equilibrium may facilitate the entrance of bilirubin into brain tissue, but neither the reason for the selective affectation of certain nuclear groups nor the precise nature of the cytotoxic action of bilirubin in the tissue are well understood. The entrance of bilirubin into the brain tissue has been thought to be merely the result of greater permeability of the immature blood brain barrier (Spatz, 1934). This concept, however, is not based on specific observations correlating the regional permeability of the blood brain barrier with the affectation of certain nuclei in kernicterus. It was also proposed that the bilirubin circulating in the blood may enter into the tissue because of its toxic effect on the blood brain barrier (Ernster *et al.,* 1957). In support of this concept Rozdilsky and Olszewski (1960) observed an increased uptake of protein from the blood stream into brain tissue after repeated intravenous injections of a bilirubin-protein complex; they concluded that prolonged high concentrations of bilirubin in the blood stream may facilitate its entrance into the tissue by damaging barrier mechanisms. An alternate postulate is that the entrance of bilirubin into the tissue is secondary to the damage of certain nuclear groups by asphyxia, increasing the permeability of the blood brain barrier in the damaged regions. Kernicterus was readily induced by injection of non-conjugated bilirubin into asphyxiated monkeys but not in normal controls (Lucey *et al.,* 1964), and similar results were obtained in asphyxiated newborn rabbits (Chen *et al.,* 1965). These experiments are particularly relevant to the understanding of kernicterus in asphyxiated prematures.

There is no agreement on the type of cytotoxic effect of bilirubin on brain tissue. Bilirubin has been shown to inhibit oxidative phosphorylation (Ernster *et al.,* 1957). Unconjugated bilirubin causes uncoupling of oxidative phosphorylation in isolated brain mitochondria; protection from this effect is achieved by adding serum albumin in quantities sufficient to bind 100 percent of the added bilirubin (Vogt and Basford, 1968). The experiments by Diamond and Schmid (1967), however, indicate that the pigment concentrations required to initiate uncoupling *in vitro* are much higher than those found in the brains of neurotoxic animals. Electron microscopic studies suggest that the primary event of bilirubin toxicity consists of cytoplasmic disorganization; alterations in the fine structure of mitochondria, which become enlarged and filled with glycogen-containing vesicles, were thought to be secondary changes (Schutta *et al.,* 1970; Schutta and Johnson, 1971).

References

Ackerman, B. D., Dyer, G. Y., Taylor, P. M.: Decline in serum bilirubin concentration coincident with clinical onset of kernicterus. Pediatrics 48: 647—649, 1971.

Balthasar, K.: Über die Beteiligung des Globus pallidus bei Athetose und Paraballismus. Dtsch. Z. Nervenheilk. 148: 243—261, 1939.

Blanc, W. A., Johnson, L.: Studies on kernicterus. J. Neuropath. exp. Neurol. 18: 165—187, 1959.

Brown, A., Burnett, H.: Studies on the neonatal development of the glucuronide conjugating system. Amer. J. Dis. Child. 94: 510—511, 1957.

— Zuelzer, W. W.: Studies in hyperbilirubinemia. I. Hyperbilirubinemia of the newborn unrelated to isoimmunization. Amer. J. Dis. Child. 93: 263—273, 1957.

Chen, H. C.: Kernicterus in the Chinese newborn. J. Neuropath. exp. Neurol. 23: 527—549, 1964.

— Lien, I. N., Lu, T. C.: Kernicterus in newborn rabbits. Amer. J. Path. 46: 331—345, 1965.

Claireaux, A. E.: Hemolytic disease of the newborn. Arch. Dis. Child. 25: 61—80, 1950.

— Cole, P. G., Lathe, G. H.: Icterus of the brain in the newborn. Lancet 2: 1226—1230, 1953.

Corner, B.: Kernicterus and prematurity. Amer. J. Dis. Child. 90: 520—521, 1955.

Crigler, J. F., Najjar, V. A.: Congenital familial nonhemolytic jaundice with kernicterus. Pediatrics 10: 169—179, 1952.

De Lange, C.: Angeborene Systemerkrankung des Zentralnervensystems. Ann. Pediat. 152: 309—315, 1939.

Diamond, I., Schmid, R.: Oxidative phosphorylation in experimental bilirubin encephalopathy. Science 155: 1288—1289, 1967.

Ernster, L., Herlin, L., Zetterstrôm, R.: Experimental studies on the pathogenesis of kernicterus. Pediatrics 20: 647—652, 1957.

Fitz, G. G. M., Greenfield, J. G., Kounine, B.: Neurological sequelae of "kernicterus". Brain 62: 292—310, 1939.

Gardner, W. A., Konigsmark, B.: Familial nonhemolytic jaundice: Bilirubinosis and encephalopathy. Pediatrics 43: 365—376, 1969.

Gartner, L. M., Snyder, R. N., Chabon, R. S., Bernstein, J.: Kernicterus: High incidence in premature infants with low serum bilirubin concentrations. Pediatrics 45: 906—917, 1970.

Hallervorden, J., Meyer, J.-E.: Cerebrale Kinderlähmung. (Früherworbene körperliche und geistige Defektzustände.) Handbuch der Spec. Path. Anat. Histol. XIII/4: 194—282, 1956.

Haymaker, W., Margoles, C., Pentschew, A., Jacob, H., Lindenberg, R., Sáenz Arroyo, L., Stochdorph, O., Stowens, D.: Pathology of kernicterus and posticteric encephalopathy. Presentation of 87 cases, with a consideration of pathogenesis and etiology. In: Kernicterus in Cerebral Palsy, pp. 21—228. Springfield, Ill.: Ch. C Thomas 1961.

Hsia, D. Y. Y., Allen, F. H., Gellis, S. S., Diamond, L. K.: Studies of serum bilirubin in relation to kernicterus. New Engl. J. Med. 247: 668—671, 1952.

Inose, T.: Athetose bei der symmetrischen pallidären Gliose. Abstract in: Zbl. Neurol. 100: 65—65, 1941.

Jellinger, K., Minauf, M., Weißenbacher, G.: Hirnveränderungen bei kongenitalem nicht hämolytischem Ikterus. Acta Neuropath. 16: 141—147, 1970.

Jervis, G. A.: Constitutional nonhemolytic hyperbilirubinemia with findings resembling kernicterus. Arch. Neurol. Psychiat. 81: 55—64, 1959.

Johnson, L., Sarmiento, F., Blanc, W. A., Day, R.: Kernicterus in rats with an inherited deficiency of glucuronyl transferase. Amer. J. Dis. Child. 97: 591—608, 1959.

Kreyenberg, G., Status dysmyelinisatus des Pallidum bei kongenitaler bilateraler Athetose. Z. Neurol. Psychiat. 132: 806—814, 1931.

Landsteiner, K., Wiener, A. S.: Agglutinable factor in human blood recognized by immune sera for rhesus monkey. Proc. Soc. exp. Biol. Med. 43: 223—223, 1940.

Lathe, G. H., Walker, M.: The synthesis of bilirubin glucuronide in animal and human liver. Biochem. J. 70: 705—712, 1958.

Levine, P., Burnham, L., Katzin, E. M., Vogel, P.: Role of iso-immunization in the pathogenesis of erythroblastosis fetalis. Amer. J. Obstet. Gynec. 42: 925—937, 1941.

Lucey, J. F., Hibbard, E., Behrman, R. E., de Gallardo, E., Windle, W. F.: Kernicterus in asphyxiated newborn rhesus monkeys. Exp. Neurol. 9: 43—59, 1964.

Meriwether, L. S., Hager, H., Scholz, W.: Kernicterus. Hypoxemia, significant pathogenic factor. Arch. Neurol. Psychiat. 73: 293—301, 1955.

Naiman, J. L.: Red cell glucose-6-phosphate dehydrogenase deficiency. A newly recognized cause of neonatal jaundice and kernicterus in Canada. Canad. med. Ass. J. 91: 1243—1249, 1964.

Nasralla, M., Gawrowska, E., Hsia, D. Y. Y.: Studies on the relation between serum and spinal fluid bilirubin during early infancy. J. clin. Invest. 37: 1403—1412, 1958.

Odell, G. B.: The dissociation of bilirubin from albumin and its clinical implications. J. Pediat. 55: 268—279, 1959.

— Cohen, S.: The effect of pH on the protein binding of bilirubin. Amer. J. Dis. Child. 105: 525—525, 1960.

Onari, K.: Über zwei klinisch und anatomisch kompliziert liegende Fälle von Status marmoratus des Striatum. Z. Neurol. Psychiat. 98: 457—486, 1925.

Orth, T.: Über das Vorkommen von Bilirubinkrystallen bei neugeborenen Kindern. Virchow Arch. 63: 447—462, 1875.

Panizon, F.: L'ictère grave du nouveau-né associé à une déficience en glucose-6-phosphate déhydrogenase. Biol. Neonat. 2: 167—177, 1960.

Papez, J. W., Hertzman, J., Rundles, R. W.: Athetosis and pallidal deficiency. Arch. Neurol. Psychiat. 40: 789—799, 1938.

Péhu, M., Pollet, M.: L'ictère nucléaire du nouveau-né. Rev. Franc. Pediat. 15: 349—390, 1939.

Rozdilsky, B., Olszewski, J.: Permeability of cerebral vessels to albumin in hyperbilirubinemia. Neurology 10: 631—638, 1960.

Schall, L.: Vit. K und Kernikterus der Frühgeborenen. Münch. med. Wschr. 100: 932—933, 1958.

Scharapow, B. I., Tschernomordik, P. M.: Zur Pathologie der Stammganglien (Ein Fall des Status marmoratus und des Status dysmyelinisatus). J. Psychol. Neurol. 35: 279—282, 1928.

Schmorl, G.: Zur Kenntnis des Icterus neonatorum. Verh. Dtsch. Ges. Path. 6: 109—115, 1903.

Scholz, W.: Über den Einfluß chronischen Sauerstoffmangels auf das menschliche Gehirn. Z. ges. Neurol. Psychiat. 171: 427—450, 1941.

Schutta, H. S., Johnson, L.: Electron microscopic observations on acute bilirubin encephalopathy in Gunn rats induced by sulfadimethoxine. Lab. Invest. 24: 82—89, 1971.

— — Neville, H. E.: Mitochondrial abnormalities in bilirubin encephalopathy. J. Neuropath. exp. Neurol. 29: 296—305, 1970.

Silberberg, D. H., Johnson, L., Ritter, L.: Factors influencing toxicity of bilirubin in cerebellum tissue culture. Pediatrics 77: 386—396, 1970.

Silverman, W. A., Andersen, D. H., Blanc, W. A., Crozier, D. N.: A difference in mortality rate and incidence of kernicterus among premature infants allotted to two prophylactic antibacterial regimes. Pediatrics 18: 614—624, 1956.

Smith, G. D., Vella, F.: Erythrocyte enzyme deficiency in unexplained kernicterus. Lancet 1: 1133—1134, 1960.

Spatz, H.: Die Bedeutung der vitalen Färbung für die Lehre vom Stoffaustausch zwischen dem Zentralnervensystem und dem übrigen Körper. Arch. Psychiat. Nervenkr. 101: 267—358, 1934.

Stern, L., Denton, R. L.: Kernicterus in small premature infants. Pediatrics 35: 483—485, 1965.

Vest, M.: Insufficient glucuronide formation in the newborn and its relationship to the pathogenesis of icterus neonatorum. Arch. Dis. Child. 33: 473—476, 1958.

Vogt, C., Vogt, O.: Zur Lehre der Erkrankungen des striären Systems. J. Psychiat. Neurol. 25: 627—846, 1920.

Vogt, M. T., Basford, R. E.: The effect of bilirubin on the energy metabolism of brain mitochondria. J. Neurochem. 15: 1313—1320, 1968.

Waters, W., Richert, D., Rawson, H.: Bilirubin encephalopathy. Pediatrics 13: 319—325, 1954.

Winsnes, A., Bratlid, D.: Unconjugated and conjugated bilirubin in plasma from patients with erythroblastosis and neonatal hyperbilirubinemia. Acta Paediat. Scand. 61: 405—412, 1972.

Zimmerman, H. M., Yannet, H.: Kernicterus: Jaundice of the nuclear masses of the brain. Amer. J. Dis. Child. 45: 740—759, 1933.

— — Cerebral sequelae of icterus gravis neonatorum and their relation to kernicterus. Amer. J. Dis. Child. 49: 418—430, 1935.

Zuelzer, W. W., Cohen, F.: ABO-hemolytic disease and heterospecific pregnancy. In: Symposium on pediatric hematology. Pediatric Clinics of North America, pp. 405—428. 1957.

9. Various Topographic Patterns of Postnatal Neuron Loss

The subject matter of the present chapter is in many ways related to and continuous with that covered in Chapters 6 and 7, and even some of the etiologic and pathogenetic mechanisms are the same. The lesions are discussed in separate chapters, however, because of differences in the onset of the underlying disease processes in relation to birth. The lesions described earlier (Chapters 6, 7), such as ulegyria, marbled state, or pontosubicular neuronal necrosis, date for most cases to the immediate perinatal period, developing rarely postnatally and hardly ever after the age of 6 months. The types of neuron loss described in the present chapter are usually not related to the stresses and derangements set off by birth; they date only occasionally to the perinatal period, and they are found in children or adults as well. All of these features are equally pertinent to the progressive sclerosing cortical atrophy described in Chapter 10.

Age-Dependent Variation in Anoxic Tissue Damage, General Remarks. Anoxic encephalopathy is caused by general anoxia, severe nonvasculo-occlusive ischemia or systemic circulatory failure. The resultant lesions in adults are commonplace and well known, consisting of "elective parenchymal necrosis" involving all or part of the neuronal populations of various nuclear groups of the brain, most commonly the cerebral cortex, basal ganglia and cerebellar cortex. The principal microscopic feature of the acute lesions consists of eosinophilic degeneration of neurons. Their dropping out later on is associated with reactive proliferation of the gliovascular stroma, particularly the astrocytes forming a glial scar. Ultimately there is atrophy and sclerosis of the affected regions. Cavitation is not typical although it may develop in extreme lesions.

Anoxic encephalopathy in childhood shows the same general features as in adults; in early infancy, however, it differs in its regional distribution as well as its cytopathology. Eosinophilic neuronal degeneration is uncommon in the asphyxiated newborn. The acute lesions of ulegyria, or of massive hemispheric necrosis in newborns (Larroche, 1968), rarely manifest in eosinophilic degeneration of the cortical pyramidal cells; instead, there is cytoplasmic swelling, chromatolysis, nuclear pyknosis, and occasional karyorrhexis

(Chapter 6). Pontosubicular neuronal necrosis, which may be associated with these lesions, is characterized by karyorrhexis, and it only occasionally shows a discernable eosinophilia of the cytoplasm (Chapter 7). On the other hand, patches of neurons undergoing eosinophilic degeneration are seen, on occasion, in the thalamic nuclei of term infants. Such variances in the cytologic expression of neuronal damage may depend on regional or age-related changes in neuronal vulnerability, age-dependent differences in the manifestations of cell necrosis or, perhaps, also differences in the damaging agent or the tissue environment. Any of these changes does not necessarily develop for each given nucleus at the same developmental period. The regional variance in the morphologic expression of tissue damage renders it much more difficult to assess acute lesions in the newborn brain than in the adult.

Hypotensive Brain Stem Necrosis. Neuronal necrosis confined to certain nuclear groups of the brain stem was reported for 4 cases by Gilles (1969), 2 infants 17 and 18 months old, the others 9 and 22 years. All had a history of cardiac arrest, surviving in an unresponsive, decerebrate state for various lengths of time. The lesions were characterized by symmetric loss of neurons and glial scarring in the motor cranial nerve nuclei, including oculomotor, trochlear, trigeminal, abducens, facial and hypoglossal nerve nuclei, as well as bilateral symmetric necrosis in the tegmentum, the superior and inferior colliculi, cuneate and gracilis nuclei and other nuclei (Fig. 33). The lesions were at maximum in the central portion of a given nucleus, sparing the cells at its periphery. Anoxic encephalopathy with diffuse loss of neurons was found in cerebral cortex and basal ganglia in 3 of the cases, but the 4th had only brain stem lesions. The present author's material includes 8 cases of hypotensive brain stem necrosis, 3 adults and 5 infants 1, 2, 12 days, 6 weeks and 2 years old. There was a history of cardiac arrest for all. Lesions of a few days survival presented as bilateral, symmetric eosinophilic degeneration of neurons in the central portions of the cranial nerve motor nuclei, of scattered cells in the tegmentum, the magnocellular part of the reticular formation and the lateral and ventral columns of the spinal cord. Cases of longer survival showed dropping out of neurons and reactive gliosis as described by Gilles. Cerebral and cerebellar cortices were spared for 3 cases: Diffuse eosinophilic changes or neuronal loss were found in the cerebral cortex of 2 adults and 2 infants, and 1 infant had ulegyria in the organizing state. The similarity of these observations with those of Gilles implies that hypotensive brain stem necrosis is relatively more frequent in infants than in adults, particularly when considering the rather large number of anoxic encephalopathies in adults in whom there are no brain stem lesions. Lesions similar to hypotensive brain stem necrosis were produced in monkeys by systemic circulatory arrest (Miller and Myers, 1972; p. 73).

The lesions of congenital hypoplasia of cranial nerve nuclei (Chapter 32) must be considered in the differential diagnosis, but the clinical history will disclose abnormal facies from birth on for congenital hypoplasia, and a history of postnatal cardiac arrest followed by neurologic deficits for hypotensive brain stem necrosis. The problems are illustrated in the report of Richter (1960). The infant became cyanotic 2 hours after birth and remained so thereafter; it was readmitted to the hospital in poor condition and died at the age of 1 month. The left facial nucleus showed patchy loss of neurons, mainly in its central portion, while the right nucleus was nearly completely depleted of neurons; multiple congenital anomalies were present. Although this case probably represents congenital hypoplasia of the facial nucleus, its interpretation is complicated by the history of peri- and postnatal hypoxia. The unilateral lesions described by Norman (1974), on the other hand, are more closely related to hypotensive brain stem necrosis.

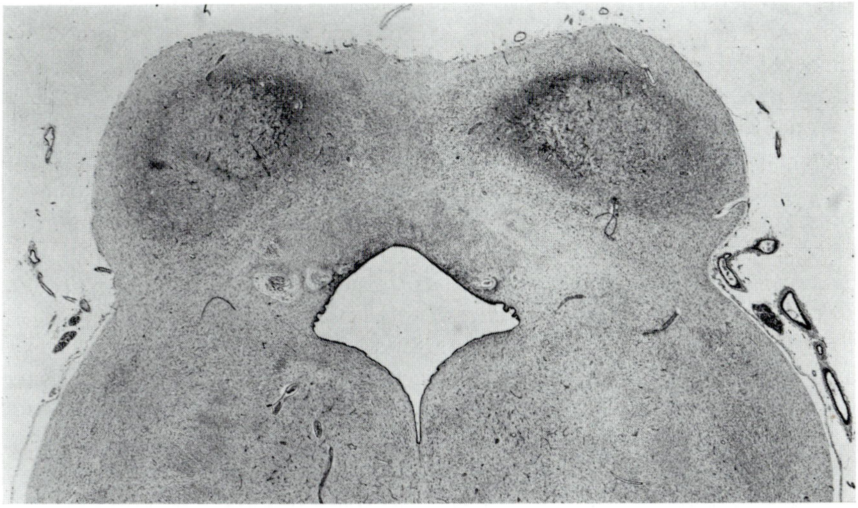

Fig. 33. Hypotensive brain stem necrosis; bilateral necrosis of superior colliculi; cresyl violet ×6.5

Hypoglycemic Lesions. Postnatal hypoglycemia was suggested as a possible cause of neurologic deficits and retarded development (Haworth and McRae, 1965; Cornblath *et al.*, 1964). However, its significance in the production of cerebral lesions is difficult to assess as hypoglycemia often coexists with respiratory difficulties or convulsions which by themselves may cause cerebral lesions. Extremely low or negative values for blood sugar have been observed in newborns, without evident symptoms attributable to hypoglycemia (Haworth and Ford, 1960). A series of 27 infants with seizures associated with hypoglycemia was reviewed by Ethridge and Millichap (1964); they found no correlation between the seizures and the degree of hypoglycemia, and the seizures were not triggered by fasting. They concluded that the seizures were symptoms of pre-existent cerebral damage. Pildes *et al.* (1974; references) in a prospective study of 39 hypoglycemic infants and 41 matched controls found smaller head circumferences for the hypoglycemic group; however, for only 2 of 30 infants could neurologic abnormalities be attributed solely to hypoglycemia. These observations suggest that a transient asymptomatic hypoglycemia in the newborn, even if severe in degree, is an unlikely cause of cerebral lesions. Brain damage may result, however, if hypoglycemia persists for a prolonged period and with neurologic manifestations; however, the type of lesion resulting from such damage is still not clearly defined.

Pronounced microcephaly with cavitated laminar cortical necrosis affecting predominantly the second and third cortical layers were attributed to hypoglycemia by Banker (1967). There were no changes in the cerebellum. These observations agree with the experimental data on insulin-induced hypoglycemia in monkeys (Myers and Kahn, 1971), demonstrating diffuse loss of neurons in the basal ganglia, cerebral cortex and Ammon's horn, and sparing of the cerebellar cortex. A preferential devastation of the upper cortical layers was found for severe lesions. Anderson *et al.* (1967) report different findings for infants succumbing in a state of severe hypoglycemia. There was swelling and chromatolysis of large nerve cells throughout the brain stem and spinal cord, lacking a selective pattern of regional distribution; eosinophilic degeneration was minimal or absent. No lesions were found in 3 infants who had died some time after their hypoglycemia had been treated. The authors suggest that the changes in untreated cases were caused by hypoglycemia. Conversely, one may conclude that the changes in the untreated cases were reversible in nature. Griffiths and Laurence (1974) found no significant histopathologic differences between the brains of 17 hypoxic and 17 hypoxic as well as hypoglycemic infants. Chase *et al.* (1973) in an experimental study of rats rendered hypoglycemic for 18 days after birth detected chemical changes indicative of reduced myelin lipids, protein and cell numbers in the brains whose weights were less than normal.

Retrolental Fibroplasia. Infants afflicted by retrolental fibroplasia due to the toxic effect of high oxygen concentration on the immature retina are often mentally retarded. No definite cerebral lesions have been recorded, and a personal inquiry by Bender and Andermann (1965) failed to produce any relevant observations.

Familial Degeneration of the Pallidonigral System. McCormick and Lemmi (1965) reported two negro sibs, 35 and 21 months, with histories of multiple infections, fever, hepatosplenomegaly and progressive neurologic deterioration with spasticity, hypotonicity, convulsions and death. The cerebral lesions consisted of loss of neurons and a tendency of cavitation in the globus pallidus, subthalamic nucleus and the reticular zone of the substantia nigra. The etiology of the process was unclear.

Infantile Bilateral Striatal Necrosis. This disease process was first described by Marinesco and Draganesco (1929) and became more widely recognized through the publications of 4 cases by Verhaart (1938) and of another by Hawke and Donohue (1950). Several additional cases have been observed since then, but the report of Verhaart is also often quoted in the literature as an early description of Leigh disease (Chapter 45).

Striatal necrosis affects infants or children, usually during the course of a febrile infectious disease upon which drowsiness, coma and anomalies in tone develop; convulsions occur on occasion. The infants described by Verhaart (1938) were between 5 and 8 months old, and all died during the acute phase of the disease; older infants and children were afflicted in the other reports. Late sequela of the disease in survivors are paralysis of trunc and extremities, impaired consciousness, hyper- or hypotonus, and occasional involuntary movements. The initial reports pertain to sporadic cases, but 5 occurrences in 2 sibs were reported by Miyoshi *et al.* (1969), and another familial occurrence by Roessmann and Schwartz (1973).

Sectioning of the brain discloses bilateral necrosis of putamen and caudate nucleus, which are softened and yellowish discolored at the early stages of the disease or shrunken and sunken below the cut surface after some survival. The necrosis affects the entire nuclear territory and tends to stop at its boundaries with the white matter, typically sparing the internal capsule. Microscopic examination shows loss of the entire neuronal population without selectivity for either large or small cells. In the subacute stages there is massive microglial invasion and lipid-laden macrophages; ultimately the nuclear territory is shrunken and the tissue replaced by a loose, spongy webb of glial scar tissue. In addition to the changes in the striatum, there may be less severe, patchy neuronal loss in pallidum, red nuclei, subthalamic nuclei, cerebral cortex, colliculi and periaqueductal tissue. In the case of Mathieson and Olszewski (1960) the lesions in the basal ganglia coexisted with central pontine myelinolysis.

The pathogenesis of infantile striatal necrosis is obscure; familial occurrence may suggest an inherited metabolic defect or a relationship to heredodegenerative disease processes, but there is no evicence to substantiate this assumption.

Superficial Siderosis. The earliest reported instance of superficial siderosis (subpial cerebral siderosis, marginal siderosis, Randzonensiderose) may well be that of Hamill (1908), but the interpretation of his case is uncertain. The disease became widely recognized following the report of two cases by Noetzel (1940). Hughes and Oppenheimer (1969) quote 27 cases reported in the subsequent literature, to which they added a series of 9 of their own. Superficial siderosis was observed, for the most part, for adults, but it is also seen in childhood and infancy; there has been little appreciation of the fact that it occasionally may develop in consequence of neonatal leptomeningeal hemorrhage (Fig. 34). The clinical course in adults is usually marked by a progressive disorder lasting several years, such as unsteadiness of gait, cerebellar signs, diminution of hearing, pyramidal signs and other neurologic deficits, and, in some cases, also, mental deterioration. A hemorrhagic or xanthochromic cerebrospinal fluid was observed for some cases during the early phases of the disease.

The morbid anatomy is characterized by a diffuse, light yellow, rusty to dark brownish discoloration of the surfaces of the central nervous system, occasionally with regional accentuation. The color does not fade upon storage of the tissue in formalin. On the cut surface the discoloration is confined to a narrow band of subpial tissue, a few mm in width, and to the surfaces of the ventricular walls. Microscopic examination discloses fibrosis of the leptomeninges and hemosiderin in macrophages as well as in meningeal fibrocytes. The pattern of tissue damage in the cerebellar cortex is rather characteristic: The crowns of adjacent gyri are scarred or even cavitated while the intrasulcal cortex is spared. There is loss of Purkinje cells and of the granular layer at the crown of gyri and deposition of a dark brown pigment in glial cells and macrophages. The pigment may be concentrated in perivascular distribution, or there may be a heavy deposition in the layer of Bergmann-

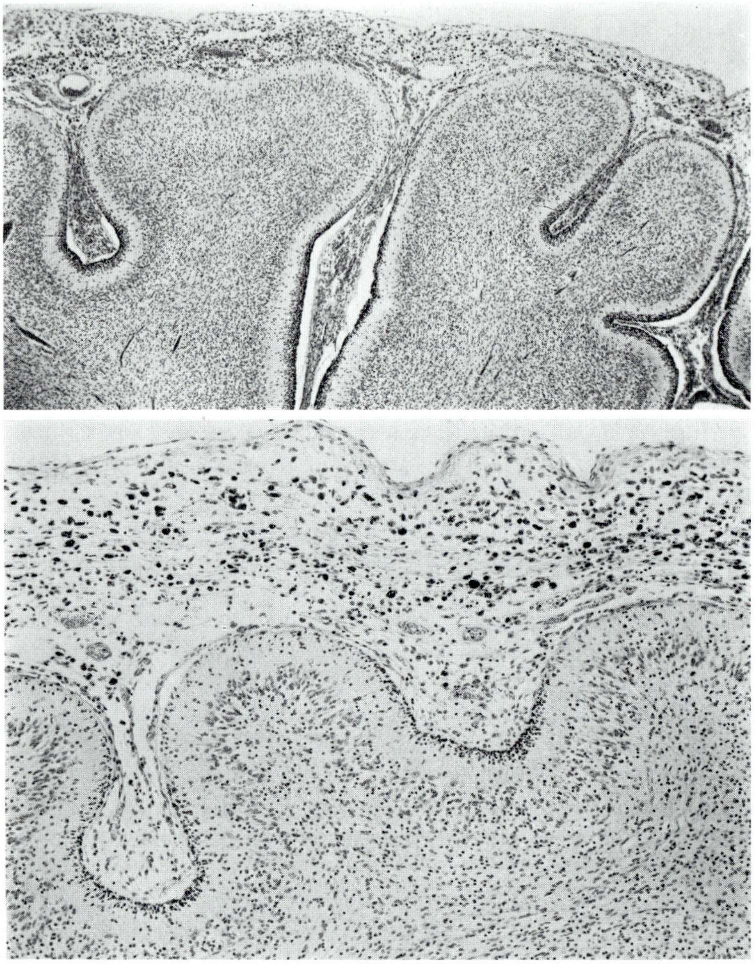

Fig. 34. Superficial siderosis; formative stage in a young infant with organized subarachnoid hemorrhage. Top: H & E ×32; bottom: iron stain ×80

glia cells. These lesions range from focal loss of nervous parenchyma and reactive gliosis to superficial defects at the crowns of the gyri, the latter extending no deeper than the thickness of the cortex.

Deposits of pigment in the cerebral cortex may extend into the upper cell layers, the extent of tissue destruction usually being less than for cerebellar cortex. The spinal cord and brain stem are encompassed by a subpial zone of gliosis and pigmentation, showing pallor in myelin stains from the demyelination or destruction of superficial fibers. Pigmentation in the spinal cord may reach the gray matter and may, on occasion, even affect neuronal perikarya. Cranial nerves and spinal roots show heavy deposition of pigment as well as loss of fibers and atrophy. There is granular ependymitis at the ventricular surfaces with deposition of granular pigment in the proliferated subependymal glia; there is also pigment deposition in the choroid plexus epithelia. The affected regions stain heavily for iron, hemosiderin granules being concentrated in macrophages or dispersed throughout the tissue. There is also a diffuse staining or fine dusting of the neuropil.

The lesions of superficial siderosis often contain scattered brightly eosinophilic, spherical or oval masses staining at variable intensity for iron. Most have a homogeneous or finely granular internal structure, but some may contain a flattened peripheral nucleus. The origin of these eosinophilic bodies has been a matter of debate, but the most probable interpretation is that they are derived from degeneration of astrocytes or macrophages. The eosinophilic bodies are not specific for superficial siderosis and are seen in gliotic scar tissue bordering organized intracerebral hematomas in general.

Many cases of superficial siderosis had sources of presumably repetitive hemorrhage into the CSF spaces from angiomas, metastatic meningeal carcinomas, ependymomas, other tumors or a bleeding disorder. Four of the 9 cases of Hughes and Oppenheimer (1969) had undergone cerebral hemispherectomy in childhood. The absence of detectable sources of intracranial hemorrhage in some instances caused discussion as to whether superficial siderosis invariably results from bleeding into the CSF (Castaigne *et al.*, 1967); yet, this mechanism is strongly implicated by the available evidence.

In some of the early publications superficial siderosis was thought to represent a form of hemochromatosis in which lesions are confined to the central nervous system, but this interpretation has not met with general acceptance. The involvement of the central nervous system in generalized hemochromatosis occurs only for those regions lacking a blood brain barrier—the choroid plexus, area postrema, tuber cinereum and others—(MacDougal and Adams, 1950; Noetzel and Ohlmeier, 1963). The only overlap between the lesions of hemochromatosis and superficial siderosis consists in the involvement of the choroid plexus whose epithelia are capable of uptake of substances from either the blood or the CSF. Superficial siderosis can be produced experimentally by the injection of iron-containing substances into the subarachnoid space (Iwanowski and Olszewski, 1960), but not by their injection into the blood stream (Noetzel and Ohlmeier, 1963). Such experiments, however, require numerous injections, and the lesions tend to be less severe than those in man. It is unlikely, therefore, that a single or a few subarachnoid hemorrhages can cause superficial siderosis without the influence of additional unknown factors (Iwanowski and Olszewski, 1960). Electron microscopic studies of experimental superficial siderosis disclose storage of particles having a subunit structure of ferritin almost exclusively in astrocytes and in actively proliferating microglia, sparing the neurons (Blinzinger, 1968). These data are consistent with the assumption that iron must be dispersed in soluble form to permit its entrance into the nervous parenchyma.

References

Anderson, J. M., Milner, R. D. G., Strich, S. J.: Effects of neonatal hypoglycemia on the nervous system: a pathological study. J. Neurol. Neurosurg. Psychiat. 30: 295—310, 1967.

Banker, B. Q.: Neuropathological effects of anoxia and hypoglycemia in newborn. Develop. Med. Child. Neurol. 9: 544—550, 1967.

Bender, L., Andermann, K.: Brain damage in blind children with retrolental fibroplasia. Arch. Neurol. (Chic.) 12: 644—649, 1965.

Blinzinger, K.: Elektronenmikroskopische Beobachtungen bei experimentell erzeugter Randzonensiderose des Kaninchengehirns. Acta Neuropath., Suppl. IV: 146—157, 1968.

Castaigne, P., Escourolle, R., Laplane, D., Berger, B., Augustin, P.: Etude anatomo-clinique d'un cas de sidérose marginale du système nerveux central. Rev. Neurol. 116: 105—118, 1967.

Chase, H. P., Marlow, R. A., Dabiere, C. S., Welch, N. N.: Hypoglycemia and brain development. Pediatrics 52: 513—521, 1973.

Cornblath, M., Wybregt, S. H., Beans, G. S., Klein, R. I.: Symptomatic neonatal hypoglycemia. Pediatrics 33: 388—402, 1964.

Ethridge, J. E., Millichap, J. G.: Hypoglycemia and seizures in childhood. The etiologic significance of primary cerebral lesions. Neurology (Chic.) 14: 397—404, 1964.

Gilles, F. H.: Hypotensive brain stem necrosis. Selective symmetrical necrosis of tegmental neuronal aggregates following cardiac arrest. Arch. Path. 88: 32—42, 1969.

Griffiths, A. D., Laurence, K. M.: The effect of hypoxia and hypoglycaemia on the brain of the newborn human infant. Develop. Med. Child. Neurol. 16: 308—319, 1974.

Hamill, R. C.: Report of a case of melanosis of the brain, cord and meninges. J. nerv. ment. Dis. 35: 594—594, 1908.

Hawke, Wm. A., Donohue, Wm. L.: Bilateral symmetrical necrosis of the corpora striata. J. nerv. ment. Dis. 113: 20—39, 1950.

Haworth, J. C., Ford, J. P.: Blood-sugar in infants after lactose feeds. Lancet 2: 794—797, 1960.

— McRae, K. N.: The neurological and developmental effects of neonatal hypoglycemia: a follow-up of 22 cases. Canad. med. Ass. J. 92: 861—865, 1965.

Hughes, J. T., Oppenheimer, D. R.: Superficial siderosis of the central nervous system. Acta Neuropath. 13: 56—74, 1969.

Iwanowski, L., Olszewski, J.: The effects of subarachnoid injections of iron-containing substances on the central nervous system. J. Neuropath. exp. Neurol. 19: 433—448, 1960.

Larroche, J. C.: Nécrose cérébrale massive chez le nouveau-né. Ses rapports avec la maturation, son expression clinique et bioeléctrique. Biol. Neonat. 13: 340—360, 1968.

McCormick, W. F., Lemmi, H.: Familial degeneration of the pallidonigral system. Neurology (Minneap.) 15: 141—153, 1965.

McDougal, D. B., Adams, R. D.: The neuropathological changes in hemochromatosis. J. Neuropath. exp. Neurol. 9: 117—118, 1950.

Marinesco, G., Draganesco, S.: Contribution anatomo-clinique à l'étude du syndrome de Foerster. Encéphale 24: 685—699, 1929.

Mathieson, G., Olszewski, J.: Central pontine myelinolysis with other cerebral changes. Neurology (Minneap.) 10: 345—354, 1960.

Miller, J. R., Myers, R. E.: Neuropathology of systemic circulatory arrest in adult monkeys Neurology (Minneap.) 22: 888—904, 1972.

Miyoshi, K., Marsuoka, T., Mizushima, S.: Familial holotopistic striatal necrosis. Acta Neuropath. 13: 240—249, 1969.

Myers, R. E., Kahn, K. J.: Insulin-induced hypoglycemia in the non-human primate. II. Long-term neuropathological consequences. In: Brain Hypoxia (Brierley, J. B., Meldrum, B. S., eds.), Chapter 20. Reprinted from Clinics in Developmental Medicine No. 39/40: 195—206, 1971.

Noetzel, H.: Diffusion von Blutfarbstoff in der inneren Randzone und äußeren Oberfläche des Zentralnervensystems bei Subarachnoidalblutung. Arch. Psychiat. Nervenkrank. 11: 129—138, 1940.

Noetzel, H., Ohlmeier, R.: Zur Frage der Randzonensiderose des Zentralnervensystems. Tierexperimentelle Untersuchung. Acta Neuropath. 3: 164—183, 1963.
Norman, M. G.: Unilateral encephalomalacia in cranial nerve nuclei in neonates: Report of two cases. Neurology (Minneap.) 23: 424—427, 1974.
Pildes, R. S., Cornblath, M., Warren, I., *et al.*: A prospective study of neonatal hypoglycemia. Pediatrics 54: 5—14, 1974.
Richter, R. B.: Unilateral congenital hypoplasia of the facial nucleus. J. Neuropath. exp. Neurol. 19: 33—41, 1960.
Roessmann, U., Schwartz, J. F.: Familial striatal degeneration. Arch. Neurol. (Chic.) 29: 312—317, 1973.
Verhaart, W. C. J.: Symmetrical degeneration of the neostriatum in Chinese infants. Arch. Dis. Child. 13: 225—233, 1938.

10. Progressive Sclerosing Cortical Atrophy: Spongy Glio-Neuronal Dystrophy

The etiologic definition of the disease, or group of diseases, described in this chapter is controversial. Pertinent cases are reported under the names of progressive sclerosing cortical atrophy, progressive cerebral poliodystrophy, "Alpers' disease", or spongy glioneuronal dystrophy, or as hemiatrophy if there is lateralization of the lesions. No satisfactory subclassification can be arrived at on the basis of morphologic examination alone, and there is no generally accepted definition of clear-cut nosologic entities. Much of the pathogenetic discussion has centered on the significance of convulsions: The cerebral lesions may be considered postictal damage, or the convulsions may be a nonobligatory symptom of an acquired or an inborn progressive destructive disease process which affects mainly the cerebral gray matter. A combined description of the histopathology of these lesions is given in the present chapter, including the processes known as hemiatrophy.

The term "progressive sclerosing cortical atrophy" was introduced by Schob (1930) who appears to have been the first investigator to classify it as being different from other types of cortical atrophy. He divided diffuse cortical atrophies of infancy into two groups: 1. Widespread ulegyria, which he used synonymous with "lobar sclerosis". The lesions, described in Chapter 6, are characterized by focal destruction and scarring of the cerebral cortex, predominantly in sulci. Ulegyria commonly results from perinatal asphyctic-circulatory damage. 2. Progressive sclerosing cortical atrophy differs from ulegyria in that there is a diffuse, uniform shrinkage of gyri as well as sulci, involving large portions of one or both cerebral hemispheres, usually without sharp boundaries. The atrophy is due to diffuse loss of neurons in the upper layers or the entire width of the cortex, with survival and reactive proliferation of glia tissue.

Schob's classification was accepted in the review of Hallervorden and Meyer (1956) and, in principle, also by Norman (1969) who designated this group by the name of hemiatrophy which he used synonymous with "lobar atrophy of Schob". A conceptionally clear survey of cases of hemiatrophy was reported by Josephy (1945). The term hemiatrophy, however, is arbitrarily restricted to cases having unilateral lesions. Further, hemiatrophy has not always been used to designate a specific type of lesion: Alpers and Dear (1939) classified a variety of "primary" or "secondary" processes which result in reduction of the volume of one hemisphere as "hemiatrophy".

The designations "Alpers' disease" or "progressive cerebral poliodystrophy" are used mainly for bilateral lesions in younger infants, while hemiatrophy has been applied mostly to cases of unilateral lesions found later in life. Accordingly, the average age of the 38 cases of poliodystrophy reviewed by Greenhouse and Neubuerger (1964) was 71 months and for the cases of hemiatrophy reviewed by Josephy (1945) approximately 36 years. These statistics may result from the arbitrary selection and grouping of cases: Designating a disease entity by the name of hemiatrophy automatically excludes the cases of short clinical course in which there is no atrophy and those having bilateral lesions. The present text follows the lead of the comprehensive survey by Wolf and Cowen (1954) who described all these types of lesions under the name "diffuse progressive cerebral cortical atrophy".

Clinical Features. Most cases of progressive sclerosing cortical atrophy have a normal history of birth and normal development during the first weeks of life. Approximately one-fifth of the reported cases have a history of disturbed parturition, and some of these had neurologic defects from birth; for these it appears that the postnatal disease process had become superimposed on a perinatal lesion. There is no sex predilection. The onset of the disease occurs most often during the first 2 to 4 years of life and is marked by sudden convulsions developing from apparent normalcy or in the course of a febrile disease. The progression of the disease is often stormy, characterized by repeated convulsions and mental and neurologic deterioration accompanied with quadruparesis and spasticity; some patients die in status epilepticus. Other cases run a more protracted course, with continuous or intermittent progression and repeated convulsions, which pertains in particular to many of the cases described as hemiatrophy. In a few instances the disease appears to have become stationary (Töppich, 1935; Josephy, 1945). Although most cases of hemiatrophy have a history of onset during early infancy, there are instances for which the convulsions first occurred during puberty or early adult life (Spielmeyer, 1906; Moore, 1943). The present author had the opportunity to observe a rare instance of extremely late onset. A 42-year-old woman had sudden onset of convulsions, first generalized, then right sided, running an intractable course to death within 38 days. The brain showed the lesions characteristic of hemiatrophy. The left hemisphere, 380 gms, showed laminar loss of nerve cells without cavitation; the right, 454 gms, showed similar though less pronounced changes; no other lesions were found in the brain. Cases of hemiatrophy invariably develop hemiparesis, often progressively, during the course of the disease and aggravating subsequent to convulsions. In other instances the convulsive disorder may become superimposed on hemiparesis existing from early infancy (Siegmund, 1923).

Gross and Microscopic Features. The morbid anatomy of residual lesions is described first as progressive sclerosing atrophy is known best from its late stages. Diffuse atrophy of the cerebral cortex is characterized by reduction in hemispheric volume and in brain weight. There is uniform shrinkage of the cortex, with widely gaping sulci and narrow gyri which are firm to the touch. The gyral pattern is well retained and focal destructive lesions are absent. The overlying meninges are delicate, but moderate to severe fibrosis is present in some cases. The degree of atrophy may vary among portions of the hemisphere, but there is no tendency to focal confinement, and transitions tend to be gradual. The cut surface of the brain shows moderate to marked enlargement of the lateral ventricles and a thin corpus callosum; the cortex is narrowed but usually sharply delineated from white matter. In some instances there is abnormal porosity of the upper cortical layers due to an excessive spongy state, which may be accentuated by an artefactual tearing of the tissue at this level upon slight mechanical stress. The normal pattern of gyri and sulci is preserved even with excessive atrophy, as the lesions do not tend to cavitate. The Ammon's horn may be either spared or involved unilaterally or bilaterally. The basal ganglia are often grossly normal, but there is thalamic atrophy, due to secondary degeneration, and enlargement of the third ventricle. The cerebellar hemispheres are often of normal size and protrude over the hemispheres. In other instances there may be focal or diffuse cerebellar atrophy, or crossed atrophy contralateral to the cerebral hemispheric atrophy.

The microscopic changes consist of a severe and widespread depletion of cortical neurons, mostly in the third or the second to fourth cortical layers, which frequently show a spongy state. The fifth and sixth cortical layers may be intact; in these instances the cases have been described as "hemiparesis with intact corticospinal tract" (Spielmeyer, 1906; Bielschowsky, 1916). The affectation of the cortical layers may vary from one region to the next, and the entire depth of the cortex is involved when the lesions are severe. The large pyramidal cells appear to be more resistant to damage and may be the only survivors. Glial proliferation is marked, to the extent that it led early investigators to the erroneous conclusion that the disease was due to a primary excessive growth of glial tissue. No obstructive lesions are demonstrated in the blood vessels, except for the occasional finding of secondary intimal fibrosis. The subcortical white matter may be myelinated but shrunken. Severe cortical atrophy, with total depletion of the neuronal population, results in atrophy of the underlying white matter which lacks myelinated fibers, the hemisphere being reduced to a thin shrunken shell. Microscopic changes in basal ganglia vary considerably and are, as a rule, less severe than those in the cortex, except for secondary thalamic degeneration. Microscopic changes in the cerebellum vary from normalcy to loss of Purkinje cells, to focal or widespread sclerosis and atrophy of the entire cortex.

There are relatively few reports on cases of diffuse, severe, bilateral cortical atrophy of the type described as "walnut brain" by Courville (1953). Reports on unilateral lesions are comparatively more frequent, as the latter have always commanded greater attention. It is difficult, therefore, to assess the relative frequency of unilateral and bilateral lesions. Unilateral lesions affect left and right hemisphere with equal frequency. The gross appearance of the brain suggests restriction of the process to one hemisphere, but it is common to find microscopic changes of a lesser degree in the contralateral hemisphere as well. If the onset of hemiatrophy dates to infancy, there is corresponding thickening of the bones of the cranial vault due to apposition of bone at the inner table (Fig. 35). There may be asymmetry of face and cranium and enlargement of homolateral nasal sinus, changes readily detected on X-ray examination. The growth of the paralysed extremities is retarded. Hemiatrophy is frequently accompanied by atrophy of the contralateral cerebellar hemisphere; the latter occasionally results in unilateral thickening of the occipital bone. The affected cerebellar hemisphere may appear entirely normal on histologic examination (Mott and Tredgold, 1900; Moore, 1953). An unusual case of combination of hemiatrophy with an organizing subdural hematoma overlying the atrophic hemisphere was described by Stroh (1925). This infant had a single seizure at 6 to 7 months and subsequent hemiparesis and died at 10 months. No changes were found in the contralateral hemisphere.

The acute and subacute lesions have often been described under "progressive cerebral poliodystrophy". The tissue changes are similar to those described above, except that loss of neurons may be less pronounced and cortical atrophy is mild or absent because of the shorter duration of the disease. The infant described by Alpers (1931) is exemplary: A girl developed normally for the first few weeks after a normal birth; severe generalized convulsions occurred at approximately 3 months; a stormy course terminated in stupor and death at 4 months. Microscopic examination disclosed neuronal loss in the upper cortical layers and also in basal ganglia and thalamus. The only clear difference between this case and sclerosing cortical atrophy of Schob is the length of survival and the corresponding state of organization of the cortical lesions. The same applies to many of the cases reported under the eponym "Alpers' disease" such as that of Freedom (1931), that of Levin (1936) who considered the lesions an early phase of lobar sclerosis, and to others reviewed by Greenhouse and Neubuerger (1964). Two of the three cases reported by Ford *et al.* (1951) had more severe lesions in one hemisphere than in the other. The transition from the acute neuronal loss without cortical shrinkage to the diffuse atrophy with longer survival is evident from the series of cases by Wolf and Cowen (1954) and Courville (1960). Progression of the lesions in a given case was demonstrated by Blackwood *et al.* (1963) from findings in biopsies at 25 and 27 months and autopsy findings $1^1/_2$ years later.

A minority of the cases of progressive sclerosing cortical atrophy have a definite history of disturbed parturition, others a history of a neurologic deficit from early infancy preceding the onset of the convulsive disorder. The case described by Crome (1951), for example, was a boy born 5 weeks premature who developed fits at the age of 5 weeks in the course of severe gastroenteritis and died severely debilitated at 2 years $7^1/_2$ months. The brain showed hemiatrophy combining the lesions of lobar ulegyria consistent with perinatal asphyxia with those of Schob's progressive sclerosing cortical atrophy. Weller and Norman (1955) described a twin to a normal sibling

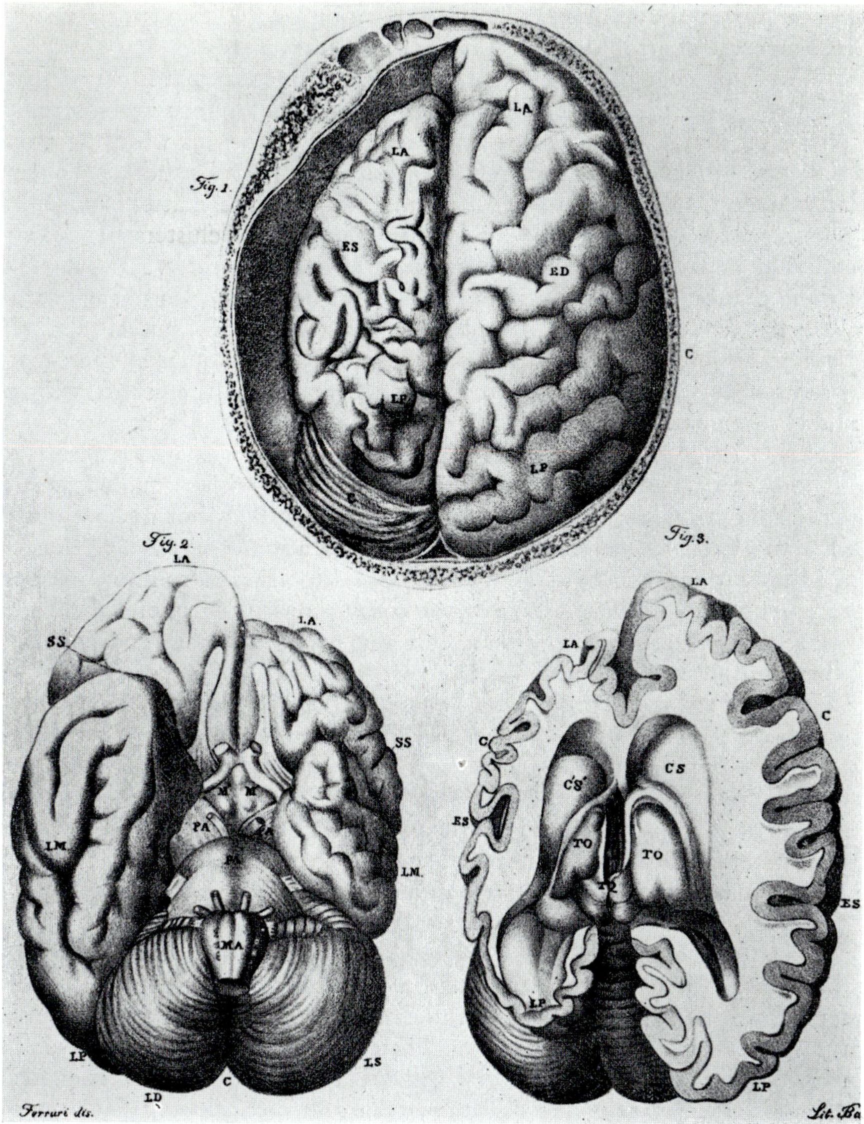

Fig. 35. Cruveilhier's illustration of hemiatrophy

who developed slowly from birth and started convulsions at 16 months followed by a downhill course. There was laminar atrophy in the cortex and focal loss of nerve cells in basal ganglia; the changes were attributed in part to birth injury and in part to superimposed convulsive damage. Periventricular cysts suggestive of subependymal hemorrhages were associated with severe bilateral cortical atrophy in case 5 of Courville (1960). This led the author to conclude that all changes of diffuse cortical atrophy are due to perinatal asphyxia. It is more likely, however, that instances like the ones quoted above represent superimposition of the lesions of progressive sclerosing cortical atrophy on preexisting perinatal damage.

Maldevelopment of the brain is often emphasized as a distinctive feature of "Alpers' disease", although reports on pertinent findings are sparse. The emphasis on maldevelopment stems from Alpers' paper in which he stressed numerous ancillary findings which he considered abnormal, such as periventricular matrix tissue and scattered neurons in the white matter, and a focus of "multinucleated giant cells", which probably were clusters of dislocated ependymal cells characteristic of certain portions of the ventricular wall. All these changes are, at best, minor variations of findings in normal infants. Similar trivial changes were described by Kramer (1953), but he also refers to temporal microgyria of unspecified type and to heterotopias in white matter. Christensen and Krabbe (1949) describe pachygyria of the cortex with profound disorganization of cortical layering and concluded that most of this disorganization was due to maldevelopment.

The case of Christensen and Krabbe (1949) is widely quoted as a key case without convulsions; however, the description does not make clear how much actual cell loss had occurred, and the separation of cortical tissue shown in the illustrations does not seem to correspond to areas of cell loss or extreme status spongiosus. Other cases without convulsions often quoted in the controversy embroiling "Alpers' disease" are reviewed later in this chapter. Many of these differ much more from the case described by Alpers (1931) than the latter differs from progressive lobar sclerosis of Schob. Hence, there is no justification, historically or otherwise, for retaining the eponym of "Alpers' disease" or for separating it from progressive sclerosing cortical atrophy. If historical credit for a detailed description of the disease is to be given, it should go to Kast's (1887) report on two cases: The first, a boy, developed normally to 6 months; the infant then had frequent seizures during which he developed first a hemiparesis, later quadruparesis, and died debilitated at the age of 14 months. The sagittal sinus was filled with liquid blood, excluding the diagnosis of sinus thrombosis which was already well known at that time. There was severe bilateral cortical atrophy with loss of neurons and marked gliosis. The report includes the first microscopic description of status spongiosus, the texture of the tissue being compared to pumice. The second infant, a girl, developed first generalized than right-sided convulsions, with ensuing hemiparesis and death at 3 years 11 months. A typical instance of hemiatrophy was disclosed at autopsy. The author, in his discussion of the cases, anticipates most of the arguments put forward in the later literature.

Pathogenetic Considerations. The difficulties in the interpretation of progressive sclerosing cortical atrophy lie in the absence of identified etiologic factors and in the interpretation of the cause-effect relationship between cerebral damage and convulsions. Scholz (1933, 1951) documented diffuse neuronal loss from repeated, prolonged, closely spaced convulsions and emphasized that the damage tends to be more severe in children than in adults. The severity of cortical devastation following status epilepticus was again stressed by Zimmerman (1938) and Norman (1946). Recent data by Wasterlain and Plum (1973) confirm that convulsive damage is more severe in the immature brain: Determinations of DNA showed that convulsions that leave the brains of adult rats undamaged produce loss of cells in immature ones. The induction of neuronal necrosis by convulsions involves the interaction of several factors, such as local circulatory disturbances in the cerebral tissue, impaired respiration during the seizure, an increase in the metabolic rate of neurons during the convulsive discharge, age-dependent differences in neuronal metabolism, hyperpyrexia from convulsions, or the occurrence of the latter during febrile diseases, fever increasing the metabolic rate in proportion with the increase in body temperature.

The interpretation of progressive cortical atrophy in terms of postictal damage is particularly attractive for the cases of hemiatrophy as it is difficult to explain lateralization of the lesions for inherited metabolic or degenerative disease processes. Cases of hemiatrophy without convulsions are on record (Töppich, 1935; Josephy, 1945), but without reliable information on birth or on infancy, and the process appeared to have become stationary during infancy. The interpretation of the cortical damage as postictal, however, postpones rather than settles etiologic classification. In many instances the lesions may actually be the product of a vicious cycle, in which anoxic cortical damage predisposes to convulsions which, in turn, cause more anoxic damage. The cycle may be triggered by perinatal damage or by postnatal diseases; meningitis has been implicated (Hallervorden and Meyer, 1956). There are also instances for which cerebral damage appears to be component of systemic diseases. Wefring and Lamvik (1967) report two sibs with subtotal hepatic atrophy from cirrhosis who had laminar spongy degeneration of the cerebral cortex; both had had convulsions. Marked spongiform degeneration of the cerebral cortex was also seen in a 14-month-old infant with acute hepatitis who had suffered from recurrent convulsions (Cameron *et al.*, 1968). Further, the identification of slow virus diseases has prompted speculation that progressive sclerosing cortical atrophy may represent an infantile form of Creutzfeldt-Jakob disease (Crompton, 1968).

Many cases do not readily fit the mold of postictal cerebral cortical damage. Indeed, "Alpers' disease" has never been defined in more precise terms than a progressive disorder of gray matter in infancy, and the diagnosis, therefore, was bound to become a repository for infantile gray matter lesions defying further classification. There are, for example, rather heterogeneous reports such as the infant of Jervis (1957) who had marked cerebellar degeneration and deposition of cholesterol in the basal ganglia. De Jong and Bebin (1956) reported a case with widespread demyelination. The general swelling of nerve cells with focal dispersion of Nissl substance in the case of Rusk and Nixon (1927) is suggestive of storage disease. Glia cells of Alzheimer type I were associated with focal lesions in the white matter in the 22-year-old woman described by Löken and Hörsdal (1961). All these cases had coexistent diffuse changes in the gray matter.

Jellinger and Seitelberger (1970) in an attempt at classification distinguish a symptomatic type, an idiopathic type and unclassifyable cases. They consider the symptomatic type secondary to complicated birth or to postnatal disease processes, as described above. The idiopathic type is represented by approximately 30 case reports in the literature, two-thirds familial for whom there was no evidence of exogenous disease. The idiopathic type was considered a nosologic entity called spongy glio-neuronal dystrophy, a term proposed by Klein and Dichgans (1969). These familiar cases, those having an onset of neurologic disturbances before the first seizures, those for whom the seizures were out of proportion to the severity of cerebral damage, or those having an unusual distribution of the cerebral lesions are of particular interest. The two siblings described by Liu and Sylvester (1960) had a progressive encephalopathy from early infancy with fits, blindness, hypertonus and nystagmus, the older dying at 38 months, the younger at 16 months. Widespread changes in gray and white matter were associated with absence or paucity of cells in the substantia nigra, optic atrophy, and cortical and subcortical sclerosis. Laurence and Cavanagh (1968) describe sibs with severe cortical atrophy and consider hypoglycemia as a possible pathogenetic factor in the first two of their cases (Chapter 9). Three sibs (Skullerud *et al.*, 1973) had similar clinical courses; one of them was studied at autopsy and had marked cortical atrophy affecting the third and fifth layers, near depletion of neurons in the pontine gray matter, loss of ventral horn cells in the spinal cord and neurogenic atrophy of muscles. Three siblings (Dekaban, 1973) showed—in addition to widespread spongy degeneration of neocortex, thalamus, and red and dentate nuclei—a severe spongy degeneration of the macula; they had had marked reduction in photic response. The familial occurrence of poliodystrophic disease processes is reinforced by additional reports (Bohnert and Noetzel, 1974).

The interpretation of familial cases needs to consider the inherited metabolic defects (Chapter 45), some of which, *e.g.*, galactosemia, hyperammonemia, or hyperprolinemia may show a preferential damage to the gray matter. Attempts at a submicroscopic identification (Suzuki and Rapin, 1969; Sandbank and Lerman, 1972) disclosed giant mitochondria, but the changes may be secondary rather than causes of the disease.

One has to conclude that the lesions described as progressive sclerosing atrophy in this chapter probably represent a heterogeneous group of conditions causing similar residual lesions. Some are postictal lesions, while others may form on the basis of one or several inherited or acquired progressive cerebral diseases. One may expect that further research on this group will identify specific entities, particularly in regard to the familial cases, but it is doubtful that histopathologic criteria will form the basis of their definite identification.

References

Alpers, B. J.: Diffuse progressive degeneration of the gray matter of the cerebrum. Arch. Neurol. Psychiat. (Chic.) 25: 469—505, 1931.

— Dear, R. B.: Hemiatrophy of the brain. J. nerv. ment. Dis. 89: 653—671, 1939.

Bielschowsky, M.: Über Hemiplegie bei intakter Pyramidenbahn. J. Psychol. 22: 225—266, 1916.

Blackwood, W., Buxton, P. H., Cumings, J. N., *et al.*: Diffuse cerebral degeneration in infancy (Alpers' disease). Arch. Dis. Child. 38: 193—204, 1963.

Bohnert, B., Noetzel, H.: Beitrag zur familiären spongiösen glio-neuralen Dystrophie. Arch. Psychiat. Nervenk. 218: 353—368, 1974.

Cameron, A. H., Jones, E. L., Smith, W. T., Wood, B. S. B.: Combined hepatic and cerebral degeneration in infancy. J. Path. Bact. 96: 227—230, 1968.

Christensen, E., Krabbe, K. H.: Poliodystrophia cerebri progressiva (infantilis). Arch. Neurol. Psychiat. (Chic.) 61: 28—43, 1949.

Courville, C. B.: Contributions to the Study of Cerebral Anoxia. Los Angeles: San Lucas Press 1953.

— Widespread softening of the cerebral gray matter in infancy. Probable etiology in the paranatal circulatory disorder. Bull. Los Angeles neurol. Soc. 25: 72—88, 1960.

Crome, L.: Congenital hemiatrophy of the brain. Arch. Dis. Child. 26: 608—615, 1951.

Crompton, M. R.: Alpers' disease—A variant of Creutzfeldt-Jakob disease and subacute spongiform encephalopathy? Acta Neuropath. (Berl.) 10: 99—104, 1968.

Dekaban, A. S.: Topistic, spongiform degeneration of the cerebral gray matter and retina in three siblings. J. Neuropath. exp. Neurol. 32: 165—165, 1973.

De Jong, R. N., Bebin, J.: Clinical pathologic conference. Neurology (Minneap.) 6: 208—217, 1956.

Ford, F. R., Livingston, S., Pryles, C. V.: Familial degeneration of the cerebral gray matter in childhood. J. Pediat. 39: 33—43, 1951.

Freedom, L.: Cerebral birth palsies: a contribution to their pathology with a report of a hitherto undescribed case. Arch. Neurol. Psychiat. 26: 524—548, 1931.

Greenhouse, A. H., Neubuerger, K. T.: The syndrome of progressive cerebral poliodystrophy. Arch. Neurol. 10: 47—57, 1964.

Hallervorden, J., Meyer, J. E.: Cerebrale Kinderlähmung. In: Handbuch der speziellen pathologischen Anatomie und Histologie. Henke Lubarch, Vol. 13, Part 4, 1956.

Jellinger, K., Seitelberger, F.: Spongy glio-neuronal dystrophy in infancy and childhood. Acta Neuropath. 16: 125—140, 1970.

Jervis, G. A.: Degenerative encephalopathy of childhood. J. Neuropath. exp. Neurol. 16: 308—320, 1957.

Josephy, H.: Cerebral hemiatrophy. J. Neuropath. exp. Neurol. 4: 250—261, 1945.

Kast, A.: Zur Anatomie der cerebralen Kinderlähmung. Arch. Psychiat. 18: 437—448, 1887.

Klein, H., Dichgans, J.: Familiäre juvenile glio-neurale Dystrophie. Akut beginnende progressive Encephalopathie mit rechtsseitigen occipito-parietalen Herdsymptomen und Status epilepticus. Arch. Psychiat. Nervenkr. 212: 400—422, 1969.

Kramer, W.: Poliodysplasia cerebri. Acta psychiat. neurol. scand. 28: 413—427, 1953.

Laurence, K. M., Cavanagh, J. B.: Progressive degeneration of the cerebral cortex in infancy. Brain 91: 261—280, 1968.

Levin, P. M.: Cortical encephalomalacia in infancy. A contribution to the study of infantile paralysis. Arch. Neurol. Psychiat. 36: 264—292, 1936.

Liu, M. C., Sylvester, P. E.: Familial diffuse progressive encephalopathy. Arch. Dis. Child. 35: 345—351, 1960.

Löken, A. C., Hörsdal, O.: Progressive degenerative encephalopathy of unusual type. J. Neuropath. exp. Neurol. 20: 427—439, 1961.

Moore, J.: Hemiatrophy of brain with contralateral cerebellar atrophy. J. nerv. ment. Dis. 98: 31—41, 1943.

Mott, F. W., Tredgold, A. F.: Hemiatrophy of the brain and its results on the cerebellum. Brain 23: 239—263, 1900.

Norman, R. M.: The neuropathology of status epilepticus. Med. Sci. Law 4: 46—51, 1964.

— Malformations of the nervous system. In: Greenfield's Neuropathology. London: Arnold 1969.

Rusk, G. Y., Nixon, C. E.: Diffuse cortical sclerosis. A clinical and pathologic report of two cases. J. Lab. clin. Med. 12: 644—660, 1926/27.

Sandbank, U., Lerman, P.: Progressive cerebral poliodystrophy—Alpers' disease. J. Neurol. Neurosurg. Psychiat. 35: 749—755, 1972.

Schob, F.: Pathologische Anatomie der Idiotie. In: Bumke's Handbuch der Geisteskrankheiten, Vol. 11 (Spezieller Teil VII), p. 779. Berlin: Springer 1930.

Scholz, W.: Über die Entstehung des Hirnbefundes bei der Epilepsie. Z. ges. Neurol. Psychiat. 145: 471—515, 1933.

— Die Krampfschädigungen des Gehirns. Monogr. Neurol. Psychiat. 75: 1—114, 1951.

Siegmund, H.: Die Entstehung von Porencephalien und Sklerosen aus geburtstraumatischen Hirnschädigungen. Virchow Arch. 241: 237—276, 1923.

Skullerud, K., Torvik, A., Skaare-Botner, L.: Progressive degeneration of cerebral cortex in infancy. Acta Neuropath. 24: 153—160, 1973.

Spielmeyer, W.: Hemiplegie bei intakter Pyramidenbahn. Münch. med. Wschr. 53, II; 1404—1407, 1906.

Stroh, H.: Halbseitige Mikrencephalie durch degenerative Atrophie infolge Pachymeningitis haemorrhagica interna bei Müller-Barlowscher Krankheit. Z. Neurol. Psychiat. 99: 1—17, 1925.

Suzuki, K., Rapin, I.: Giant neuronal mitochondria in an infant with microcephaly and seizure disorder. Arch. Neurol. (Chic.) 20: 62—72, 1969.

Töppich, G.: Über die sklerosierende Hemisphärenatrophie. Arch. Psychiat. 103: 335—346, 1935.

Wasterlain, C. G., Plum, F.: Vulnerability of developing brain to electroconvulsive seizures. Arch. Neurol. (Chic.) 29: 38—46, 1973.

Wefring, K. W., Lamvik, J. O.: Familial progressive poliodystrophy with cirrhosis of the liver. Acta Paed. Scand. 56: 295—300, 1967.

Weller, S. D. V., Norman, R. M.: Epilepsy due to birth injury in one of identical twins. Arch. Dis. Child. 30: 453—456, 1955.

Wolf, A., Cowen, D.: Cerebral atrophies and encephalomalacias of infancy and childhood. Res. Publ. Ass. Res. Nerv. Ment. Dis. 34: 199—330, 1954.

Zimmerman, H. M.: The histopathology of convulsive disorders in children. J. Pediat. 13: 859—890, 1938.

11. Porencephaly, Hydranencephaly, Multilocular Cystic Encephalopathy

Reaction of Immature Nervous Tissue to Necrosis. Our understanding of the peculiarities of the reactions of immature nervous tissue to destructive lesions originates from the experimental investigations of Spatz (1921) who compared the histopathology of a double transection of the spinal cord in adult and newborn rabbits. The main conclusions of his 318 page report may be summarized as follows: 1. Liquefaction and dissolution of necrotic tissue develops in newborns with exceptional rapidity. Organization of the lesions is essentially completed after 8 days, and the last phagocytes have disappeared by the 12th day. There is little or no proliferation of "fixed" elements and no gliomesodermal scar develops, as organization is mainly carried out by macrophages which disappear rapidly from the lesions. The residual cavity forms a smooth-walled porus. Etiologically different lesions may produce similar residual pori. 2. The reactivity of glial tissue is very limited, in that there is no fibrillary gliosis and development of hypertrophic glial forms is rare. The changes in glial tissue may be interpreted, essentially, as an arrest in its development, particularly in regard to the abrogation of myelination gliosis. The walls of the porus are formed by a thin layer of glial tissue deficient in neurons, but there is no evidence of actual glial scarring. In the subpial zones of the cord there may be persistence of glial tissue at the leptomeninges, resulting in the formation of thin gliomesodermal membranes; glial tissue may become deficient in the latter, with wide surface communication of the defect. 3. The profile of the cord is altered by a failure in growth of the destroyed tracts which may become displaced secondarily by the growth and myelination of those fiber systems whose development is not abrogated by the lesion. No comparable displacement occurs at higher ages, when the tracts become atrophic without change in their relative position. Development of gray matter may also be retarded, and formation of an abnormal lateral sulcus in the cord is a fairly consistent secondary change.

Spatz stressed the significance of his observations for the understanding of porencephaly: that the smoothness of the defects and the absence of scarring are peculiarities of fetal lesions which should not be considered evidence of malformation. He proposed that the myelination period is the critical determinator, after which the formation of pori no longer occurs. It seems likely, however, that other aspects of tissue maturation antedating myelination are even more important: The characteristic smoothness of the walls and the absence of glial scarring of porencephalic defects dating to fetal life may be contrasted with the dull, irregular, shaggy surface of the walls of encephaloclastic lesions occurring near the end of gestation, such as those of multilocular cystic encephalopathy; both lesions antedate myelination of the hemispheric white matter.

Several factors may contribute to the peculiarities of the response of immature nervous tissue to injury: Its water content is higher than for adults and its texture much looser; its metabolism differs from the adult, and the maturation of the various metabolic pathways is not concurrent; finally, the capacity of certain cell types to develop characteristic tissue responses appears to develop at different periods. The relative significance of each of these factors cannot be assessed precisely at present, but the differences in cellular maturation are of particular interest to the morphologist. The microglia-monocyte-macrophage system appears to mature much earlier than the astroglia. Resorption of the necrotic tissue by macrophages can be seen in the fetal brain when astrocytic response is still minimal, and its speed appears to be even greater than in the adult. Monocytes have been found in the circulating fetal blood as early as the 4th week of gestation; their number varies initially, but values approximating those in term infants are present from approximately the 20th week on (Playfair *et al.,* 1963). The studies of Konigsmark and Sidman (1963), confirmed by subsequent investigators, have shown that circulating monocytes are a source of the macrophage response in cerebral lesions. While the early appearance of circulating monocytes in the fetal blood does not prove that the phagocytic capacities are fully developed at this period, it is certainly consistent with histopathologic observations indicating that the macrophage response matures much earlier than that of astroglia.

Reactive gliosis consisting of proliferation of astrocytes in response to nonspecific tissue damage is one of the most elementary components of neuropathologic lesions. Its features in adults are well established. Astrocytes are known to react to subtotal damage with proliferation, followed within 3 to 5 days, by the development of cytoplasmic hypertrophy. A massive enlargement of the cell body produces pools of translucent, homogeneous, slightly eosinophilic cytoplasm. The enlarged nucleus is often eccentric, but nuclear enlargement usually does not reach the excessive degree seen in metabolic astrocytosis (Chapter 45). Silver impregnations demonstrate that the increase in the size of the cell body is accompanied with a progressive reduction of the number of cell processes, the remaining ones being hypertrophic. Reactive hypertrophy is accompanied with an increase in the activity of various oxydative enzymes in the cytoplasm of astrocytes (Rubinstein *et al.*, 1962; Friede, 1965). There is also a characteristic increase in glycogen in the astrocytic cytoplasm, as may be shown with the electron microscope; contrary to metabolic astrocytosis, there is no intranuclear accumulation of glycogen. The glycogen may be seen with the light microscope in the form of a diffuse dusting of the neuropil with glycogen granules or in the form of local condensations around astrocytic nuclei or in chains of granules outlining astrocytic processes; perivascular accumulation of glycogen results from an increase in glycogen in the glial footplates. The increase in glycogen develops quite rapidly upon damage and antedates the increase in oxydative enzymes. Reactive astrocytosis persists for weeks or months but gives way, eventually, to fibrillary gliosis with minimal or absent hypertrophy of the remaining astrocytes.

The extent of astrocytic hypertrophy in fetal or infantile nervous system varies with maturation. Practically no residual gliosis is seen, even upon massive destructive lesions, during the first half of gestation. The capacity of astrocytes to react with proliferation and hypertrophy appears to develop during the last trimester of gestation and is already evident in the mature newborn, *e.g.*, for ulegyria or for periventricular infarcts. Astrocytic hypertrophy, however, may not reach the extent seen in adult brain; reactive astrocytes in the newborn brain have a medium density of nuclear chromatin, and the nuclei are rarely as vesicular as those of hypertrophic astrocytes in adults. There is also less cytoplasmic hypertrophy, and the volume of cytoplasm seen with the light microscope may be only once or twice that of the nucleus, in distinction to the large lakes of cytoplasm seen in reactive astrocytes in adults.

Experimental studies in rat cerebral cortex indicate that the capacity of astrocytes to respond to injury develops approximately by the second postnatal week. Electron microscopic studies of acute cortical lesions in newborn rats reveal an enlargement of the extracellular space rather than swelling and hypertrophy of astrocytes, and no glial scar formation is seen in residual lesions; the microglial response is very rapid (Sumi and Hager, 1968). The increase in oxydative enzyme activity in reactive astrocytes also does not develop in rats prior to the 10th day of life (Osterberg and Wattenberg, 1963). An increase in cerebral glycogen content near stab wounds of rat cortex was absent at the ages of 4 and 13 days, but it was present at 28 days (Farkas-Bargeton, 1972). An increase in cerebral glycogen was seen in asphyxiated macacus monkeys (Rivera *et al.*, 1970) which are more mature at birth than are rats. The degree of astrocytic maturation of the human newborn is probably more similar to the monkey than to the rat, and an increase in glycogen about astrocytic nuclei may be seen near lesions in newborn brains. The capacity for this type of response appears to develop earlier than that for metabolic astrocytosis (Chapter 45).

Developmental changes associated with the normal maturation of astrocytes and oligodendroglia need to be considered in the assessment of reactive gliosis in the newborn brain. The so-called "myelination glia" consists of precursors of oligodendroglia which form during the myelination gliosis of myelinating tracts (Chapter 1). They have large nuclei of a chromatin content intermediate between oligodendroglia and astrocytes and enlarged, faintly basophilic cell bodies; they may easily be mistaken for reactive astrocytes because the density of nuclear chromatin and the texture of the cytoplasm are similar.

The early phase of differentiation of the matrix tissue is characterized by relatively large, pale, vesicular nuclei having no discernible cytoplasm. Some authors consider these neuronal rather then glial. These maturing nuclei may be paler and more vesicular than those of reactive astrocytes near well defined lesions, and their regional density may vary considerably. Similar enlarged, immature glia nuclei may be seen in the cortex and basal ganglia where they present sources of error in the identification of metabolic astrocytosis in the infantile brain (Chapter 45) or of an early stage of nonspecific, reactive glial proliferation.

Difficulties may be encountered in assessing an increase in glial fibrils in Holzer stains in the brain stem of infants where areas of "fibrillary gliosis" may be seen in the absence of underlying disease processes (Martin *et al.*, 1969). Because of this overlap between the features of normal glial maturation and age-dependent variations in glial response to injury, an extremely cautious approach is indicated in assessing gliosis in the late fetal and early postnatal periods; this is particularly true if the changes are diffusely distributed and unrelated to well defined focal lesions.

Classification of Large Cavities in Infantile Brains. Knowledge of the lesions described in this chapter has been gained almost entirely from examination of residual defects; little verified information is available on their etiology or on the acute stages of the diseases. Etiologic classification, therefore, must remain tentative, and more than one process may be involved in their formation. During the late nineteenth century it was customary to call most or all large hemispheric defects porencephaly. Subsequently, several types of cavitation were subclassified as porencephaly, hydranencephaly and multilocular cystic encephalopathy. There is no consensus in the literature on the usage of these terms; some authors use only one or two of them, and most agree to the existence of transitions. Some of the published cases were ascribed to different categories by different authors. Notwithstanding these differences, the lesions of porencephaly, hydranencephaly and multilocular cystic encephalopathy are sufficiently characteristic to justify their being distinguished as separate types. A summary discussion of pathogenetic factors is given at the end of this chapter.

Porencephaly. The term "porencephaly" was introduced by Heschl (1859) of Krakow, who described a 26-year-old beggar whom he had known and whose clumsy gestures he had thought to be simulated. The autopsy disclosed an asymmetric skull, thicker on the left side; the region of the Sylvian fissure of the left hemisphere showed a large defect with broad communication between the ventricle and the surface of the brain. His report includes brief descriptions of three similar cases. In a second report (1861) Heschl described a 17-year-old hemiparetic girl who had a finger-wide canal in the central region of the left hemisphere penetrating into the lateral ventricle, with a radial arrangement of gyri around the outer opening of the canal. The corresponding region in the contralateral hemisphere showed an indentation with radial arrangement of gyri, but no complete defect. Heschl (1859) considered the lesions connatal defects; he considered and rejected their attribution to a local aplasia of the hemispheric wall and attributed the defects to destruction of the fetal brain. He compared porencephaly with hydranencephaly described by Cruveilhier (1835) and thought that these lesions differ only in the extent of brain destruction; he discussed and rejected the origin of hydranencephaly from fetal hydrocephalus. Hence, most of the discussion that was to ensue about these lesions in the later literature is found here in capsule and is essentially preempted.

In comparing his cases with others in the literature, Heschl (1859) distinguished several types of hemispheric defects: 1. A cavity filled with spongy residual tissue, having no communication with the ventricle or with the subarachnoid space; 2. a cavity communicating with the ventricle only; 3. a cavity communicating with the ventricle as well as with subarachnoid space. This classification evidently accepts a variety of heterogeneous lesions as "porencephalies", and it opened the door for the subsequent indiscriminate application of the term "porencephaly" to a great variety of large hemispheric defects irrespective of their morphologic features, etiology, or time of onset. The series of cases reported by von Kahlden (1895) and the 132 titles reviewed by Schütte (1902) are quite heterogeneous. Most of these authors refer to gross features only, and their reports antedate the recognition of peculiarities of tissue reaction of the immature brain. Approximately three-fourth of the cases published as porencephalies near the turn of the century can be reclassified, at least tentatively, to the categories of hydranencephaly, infarcts from occlusion of major cerebral arteries, traumatic birth hemorrhages, cerebral lesions associated with growing skull fractures, cerebral hemorrhages in adults, or cystic end-stages of lacerations acquired during adult life. The term porencephaly, thus, has been used by some authors for any cavity large enough to expose the ventricular lumen, while others emphasize origin during the developmental period. Yakovlev and Wadsworth (1946) proposed the term "schizencephaly" for congenital hemispheric defects resulting from focal aplasia of the hemispheric walls, in contrast to encephaloclastic porencephalies that result from destruction of the hemispheric walls by perinatal trauma or circulatory disturbance.

The usage of the term "porencephaly" in the present text is restricted to circumscribed hemispheric defects that had occurred *in utero* or before the adult features of the hemisphere were fully developed. The developmental origin of the lesions is evident from smooth walls with minimal scarring, and from developmental disturbances in the architecture of the adjoining cortex, features described at the beginning of this chapter for the experimental lesions produced by Spatz (1921). Encephaloclastic lesions which have an onset during the terminal phase of pregnancy or postnatal life differ from porencephalies in destroying existing cortical tissue without altering cortical architecture, except in terms of atrophy or scarring, and in forming irregular defects with shaggy, rough walls. This restriction of the term porencephaly corresponds to Heschl's (1859) lesions and is justified in that these lesions always were at the core of the cases described as porencephaly. It eliminates from consideration the encephaloclastic lesions described in other chapters as ulegyria (Chapter 6), periventricular infarcts (Chapter 4), infarcts from vasculo-occlusive disease in infancy (Chapters 12, 13) or cystic lesions from peri- or postnatal hematomas (Chapters 2, 3) regardless of the type of communication of these lesions with cerebrospinal fluid spaces. This definition of the term porencephaly is practically synonymous with the "schizencephaly" of Yakovlev and Wadsworth (1946). The latter term is not used, however, as it was coined expressly to emphasize a hypothetical, unproven concept of formal pathogenesis for lesions that have traditionally been described under the term hydranencephaly or porencephaly.

A review of clinical histories of cases of porencephaly gives inconclusive data on pregnancy; however, in Dekaban's (1965) series 4 of 11 patients were illegitimate, with attempted abortion for at least one of them. Neurological symptoms vary with the extent of the lesions, but most patients show severe mental and neurologic defects, cerebral diplegia, blindness, and do not learn to speak or walk. Epilepsy is common but not consistent. Frequent respiratory infections result from aspiration. Life expectancy is shortened by the degree of debilitation and inaniation, although patients may survive to advanced age.

Porencephalic lesions are much more often bilateral than unilateral. The most characteristic location is in the central region involving pre- and postcentral gyri and adjacent frontal convolutions as well as the insula. There is considerable variance in the size of the defects. They present as large cysts filled with clear cerebrospinal fluid and covered with a thin membrane of arachnoid tissue; rupturing of the latter affords a view of the exposed ventricular walls. Smaller lesions present as narrow clefts, either communicating with the ventricle or separated from it by a thin layer of brain tissue; still less extensive lesions present as clefts or cortical indentations of variable depths. Unilateral lesions are often associated with a similar minor lesion in the corresponding portion of the contralateral hemisphere. Beside the typical occurrence in the central region, similar clefts were described in isolated instances in parasagittal distribution or at the orbital surface of the frontal lobe.

Two types of porencephalies may be distinguished based on changes in the adjoining cortex. The first type is characterized by polymicrogyria which may involve the cortex bordering the defect or extend over much of the convexity of the hemisphere; patches of polymicrogyria may be found at distance from the defects. There may be a focus of polymicrogyria in the cortex contralateral to a unilateral cleft surrounded by polymicrogyria. This type of porencephaly was reported by Binswanger (1882) and Otto (1885); Schütte (1902) quoted several later authors. More recently a series of 11 cases was reviewed by Dekaban (1965).

The second type of porencephaly does not show polymicrogyria, but the arrangement of adjacent cortical gyri is abnormal in that some or all of the gyri radiate toward the defect (Fig. 36), often descending into its depth (Heschl, 1861). A similar distortion of gyri may be produced in cortical defects of postnatal traumatic origin from the traction caused by extensive connective tissue scarring. The rearranged gyri near porencephalic defects, however, exhibit little if any glial scarring, and the cortex often shows loss of laminar architecture forming irregular, at times heterotopic, masses of gray matter near the porus. Cortex and heterotopias may be displaced downward

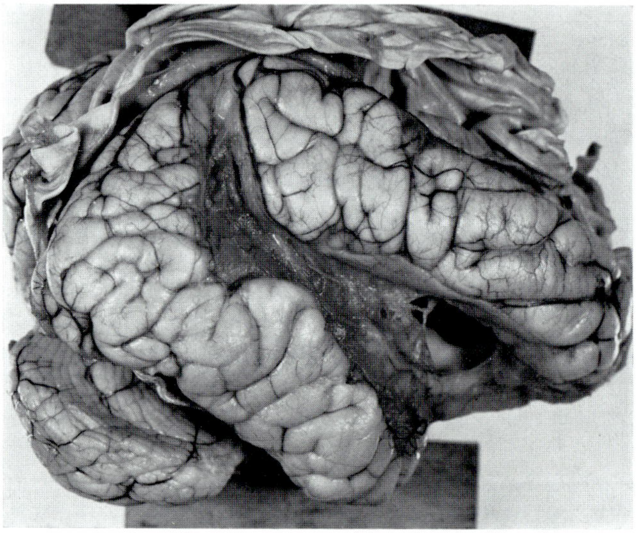

Fig. 36. Porencephaly; anomalous arrangement of gyri toward the defect

while the ventricular wall is displaced upward, resulting in a seam where ependyma and malformed gray matter become approximated.

It is not clear whether the two types of changes in the adjacent cortex are only different in degree, or whether they depend on disturbances originating at different stages of development. Lyon and Robain (1967) suggested that polymicrogyria is the result of subtotal damage due to incomplete ischemia in the tissue adjacent to the defect. The first type of porencephaly may be dated on the basis of the polymicrogyria which can be attributed with reasonable confidence to lesions occurring near the 5th or before the 6th fetal month, as discussed in Chapter 29. Typical instances of porencephalies with polymicrogyria in the formative stage were observed as early as the 24th week of gestation (Fig. 37). No descriptions of still earlier lesions are available, but Solcher (1968) observed large hemorrhagic infarcts in 3 fetuses of less than 25 weeks, without reaching definite conclusion as to pathogenesis. Whether porencephalies of the second type date to a later developmental period, or result from less severe disturbances, or from different types of disturbances, cannot be determined at the present time.

The basal ganglia, cerebellum and brain stem of most cases of porencephaly are free of focal lesions, but the thalamus is often small because of atrophy of thalamic projection nuclei. Scarring or mineralization in the basal ganglia is found for other cases. Atrophy or agenesis of corticospinal tracts depends on the extent of the lesion; the motor cortex is not always affected, as Betz cells were demonstrated in some instances in the cortex next to the defect.

Hydranencephaly. The first comprehensive description of hydranencephaly is generally attributed to Cruveilhier (1835) who reported 3 cases,

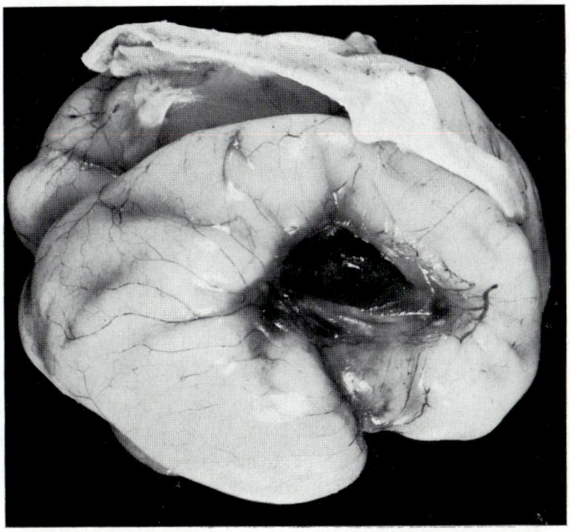

Fig. 37. Porencephaly in a fetus of 24 weeks gestation

2 of which were microcephalic, the 3rd hydrocephalic. He specified 2 types of anencephaly: "anencéphalie hydrocéphalique" or "hydro-anencéphalie" and "anencéphalie avec l'absence de la vue cranienne". Kluge (1902) condensed hydro-anencephaly to "hydranencephaly" which is now widely accepted. The term was criticized by Crome and Sylvester (1958), but without convincing justification as hydranencephaly is no longer used to imply a generic relationship to anencephaly. Their proposed alternate term "hydrencephaly" offers no advantage and is misleading in its allusion to hydrocephalus and to the presence of an encephalon. The descriptive term "bubble brain", derived from German "Blasenhirn", failed to gain acceptance as did the term "hydroencephalodysplasia" or the misnomer "hydro-microcephaly". Lange-Cosack (1944) reviewed 30 case reports of hydranencephaly and added 2 of their own. Muir (1959) studied 6 cases of hydranencephaly and 4 of porencephaly (his 5th "porencephaly" was actually an arhinencephaly). Halsey *et al.* (1971) recently reported 8 cases and reviewed the literature.

The reports on hydranencephaly can readily be divided into two groups. The first group pertains to lesions resulting from intrauterine disturbances:

Arrested, residual defects are found at or shortly after birth. These cases conform to the traditional descriptions of hydranencephaly. The second group has been described under the name "complete hemispheric necrosis" or "hydranencephaly of postnatal onset". This group pertains to infants having a normal history of birth and normal early postnatal development; the cerebral lesions originate during an acute postnatal disease process during the first 18 months of life. Judging from the published cases, hydranencephaly of postnatal onset is approximately 5 times less frequent than that of prenatal onset. The postnatal lesions are described in the following together with multilocular cystic encephalopathy because these two types of lesions cannot always be clearly distinguished. The subsequent text pertains only to hydranencephaly of prenatal onset.

The majority of cases of hydranencephaly of prenatal onset has an inconclusive history of pregnancy. Blunt trauma to the abdomen was recorded for isolated instances (Seitz, 1907; Lange-Cosack, case 2, 1944). Precise definition of the force of the trauma was obtained for an accident at the 22nd week of pregnancy, involving the crash of a glider with impact at an air speed of 70 mph (Fowler *et al.*, 1971). Lange-Cosack (1944) considered the probability of attempted abortion because of a high frequency of illegitimate births and abandoned infants. A case of hydranencephaly with polymicrogyria in the residual cortex was observed following accidental intoxication with household gas at the 24th week of pregnancy (Bankl and Jellinger, 1967).

The symptoms and life expectancy of hydranencephalic infants depend on the extent of cerebral destruction. Infants with destruction of basal ganglia and hypothalamus suffer from disturbances of thermoregulation, sleep and wake pattern, suck and swallowing, and abnormal cry, and frequently die at birth or within the first month. Infants with preserved basal ganglia may appear normal at birth but show persistence of neonatal automatisms, hyperirritability, absence of motor development, spasticity and convulsions during the ensuing months (Halsey *et al.*, 1968). Transillumination of the head is suggestive but not diagnostic of hydranencephaly. Cranial size at birth may be normal or microcephalic, rarely enlarged. Enlargement of the head usually begins during the first weeks of life, up to the third month (Lange-Cosack, 1944). There is no evidence of significant sex predilection.

Postmortem examination shows the cerebral hemispheres replaced by fluid-filled bubbles easily ruptured upon opening the skull. The walls of the bubbles are apposed to the dura mater when fixed *in situ.* The lesions are bilateral and the intact falx separates the two cystic hemispheres. Unilateral occurrence has been observed in few instances. A case reported by Ilberg (1901) had a single, unpaired hemispheric bubble and no falx. The surface of the bubble lacks a residual pattern of convolutions (Fig. 38). The membrane forming its wall is thin and translucent and contains attenuated blood vessels. Its inner surface is smooth, with an opaque layer of nervous tissue arranged in patches, trabecules, or in a thin continous film. No other remnant of the hemispheric wall is seen, in particular there is no tissue layer corresponding to the ventricular walls. The cavity is filled with clear cerebrospinal fluid, but the latter may be opaque, yellowish or hemorrhagic on occasion.

Its evacuation exposes the base of the skull where the remnants of basal ganglia form a characteristic small hump over and anterior to the tentorial hiatus. The membrane replacing the hemispheric wall is continous with the molecular layer of the adjacent cortex. It has an outer layer of connective tissue in continuity with the leptomeninges, which may show pigmentation, hemosiderin-laden macrophages or collagen fibrosis. The inner portion of the membrane consists of sheaths or islands of glial tissue, mostly astrocytes and,

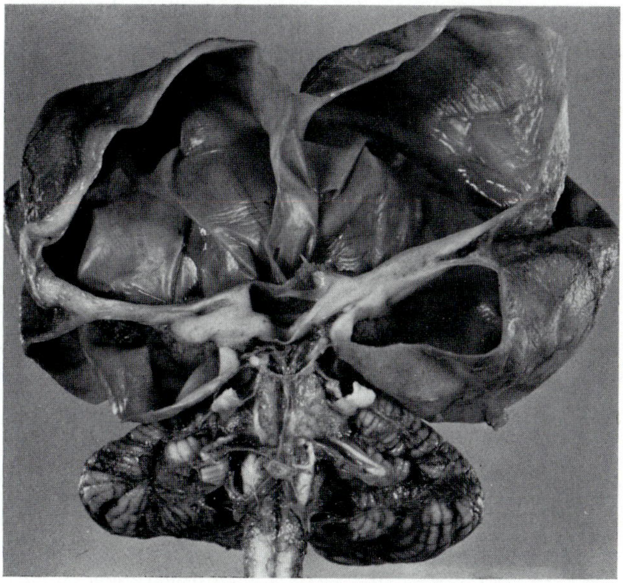

Fig. 38. Hydranencephaly

occasionally, mineralization or a few residual neurons; ependyma is usually absent.

The defect of the hemispheric walls typically corresponds to the territories supplied by the carotid arteries, or the anterior-middle cerebral arteries, respectively. Relative preservation of the temporal lobes and of the tentorial portions of the occipital lobes is characteristic. The cortical remnants may show a normal gyral pattern, the hemispheric wall narrowing abruptly toward the defect; polymicrogyria of the cortex is found in some cases. There is considerable variation in the extent of preservation of occipital and temporal lobes; the Ammon's horn, with an attached segment of choroid plexus, is most resistant and may form the only residuum of the hemispheres at the base of the skull. Still more severe lesions may show absence of the entire hemispheric walls, and the olfactory tracts and bulbs may be absent as well; this does not validate the diagnosis of arhinencephaly (Johnson *et al.*, 1951), even though the lamina cribrosa may be nonperforate.

The extent of preservation of basal ganglia varies. The striatum and thalamus are often intact but commonly rotated outwards so that the internal capsule runs horizontal. The thalamus is always atrophic because of degeneration of its cortical projection nuclei as well as absence of the pulvinar (Halsey *et al.*, 1971). The histologic structure of the basal ganglia may be normal, or there may be disorganization into heterotopic masses of gray matter or focal scarring and mineralization. Absence of the striatum may be associated with absence of substantia nigra. The optic nerve may be atrophic but connected to the lateral geniculate body; with severe lesions only the intraorbital portion of the nerve is preserved; microphthalmia is common. The major cranial arteries, although sometimes attenuated or disproportionate in size, can be identified and show no obstructive lesions. Absence of arteries occurs only in extreme cases in which the diencephalon is destroyed (Környey, 1925; Johnson *et al.*, 1951). An instance of a vasculo-occlusive process causing unilateral hydranencephaly was observed by Meyer (1949) who described an organizing thrombus with triple recanalization in the homolateral middle cerebral artery. Except for absence of the cerebral peduncles and medullary pyramids, there are, typically, no lesions below the level of the oculomotor nucleus (Fig. 39). The cerebellum is grossly normal, but microscopic changes, or even cystic lesions, occur in some cases.

Relatively little attention has been paid to the causes of cranial enlargement developing postnatally in hydranencephalic children. Stenosis of the aqueduct was described for 2 infants by Elo and Otila (1939), but their interpretations are difficult to accept. Other cases showed stenosis (Watson, 1944) or glial obliteration of the aqueduct (Crome and Sylvester, 1958) or of the foramina of Monro (Lange-Cosack, 1944). Obstruction of cerebrospinal fluid circulation in the subarachnoid space must be assumed for cases showing a patent and enlarged aqueduct and fourth ventricle.

The changes in the spinal cord offer an interesting potential for tentative dating of the lesions (Halsey *et al.*, 1971). Complete agenesis of lateral tracts with outward rotation of the dorsal horns and overgrowth of the dorsal tracts may be attributed to lesions occurring before the 5th fetal month. Relatively small lateral tracts may be the result of lesions occurring during the 5th or 6th fetal month, while still later onset may be assumed if the spinal cord shows normal configuration, the cortical tracts presenting as pale, nonmyelinated zones in the lateral columns (Chapter 32).

Basket Brains. Basket brains are lesions intermediate in extent between porencephaly and hydranencephaly. The term basket brain derives from Obersteiner's (1902) description of a case: "the shape of the brain compares best with a small basket having a high handle". There are very large, bilateral hemispheric defects; the cingular gyri and variable amounts of adjoining tissue are spared and form median-sagittal arches of tissue connecting the occipital and the frontal portions of the brain. Polymicrogyria was observed in the residual cortex in several instances. Obersteiner reported his case as porencephaly and considered it the most extensive lesion on record. Similar cases were reported by Cohn and Neumann (1946), Yakovlev and Wadsworth (1946), and Norman *et al.* (1958). Yakovlev and Wadsworth considered the lesions malformations with reactive hyperplasia of the cingular gyri, but Norman *et al.* found evidence of destructive processes in terms of gliosis and calcification of the claustrum. Myers (1969) observed a lesion closely resembling a basket brain subsequent to fetal carotid ligation in a monkey and considered it a forme fruste of hydranencephaly. The existence of basket brains as "intermediate" lesions supports the assumption that porencephaly and hydranencephaly are varying degrees of the same pathologic process (Muir, 1959).

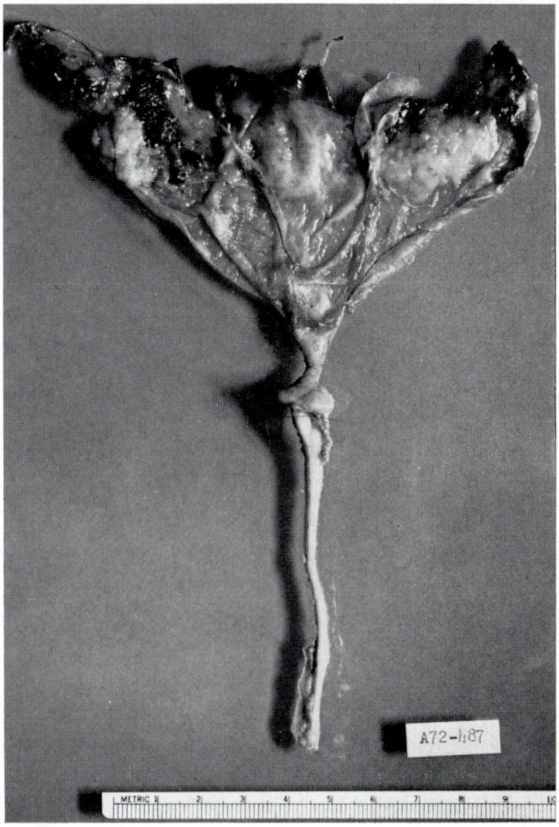

Fig. 39. Hydranencephaly with an extreme degree of destruction of cerebral hemispheres, diencephalon and upper brain stem in a fetus of 39 weeks gestation

Hydranencephaly or Porencephaly and Fetal Infection. A case of hydranencephaly described by Crome and Sylvester (1958) showed asymmetry of lesions and a gradual thinning of the cortex with extensive polymicrogyria. There was calcification of basal ganglia, cerebellar microgyria, and the eyes showed scarring of the macula and retinal pigmentation. Two of the cases described by Halsey *et al.* (1971) had similar features. Crome and Sylvester considered their case suggestive of toxoplasmosis. A more definite relation to infection was demonstrated by Lykke (1957) and Altshuler (1973) who found toxoplasma organisms or cysts in hydranencephalic brains. Navin and Angevine (1968) observed porencephaly with microgyria in an infant with disseminated cytomegalic inclusion disease; the brain tissue adjacent to the defect showed granulomatous encephalitis and inclusion bodies. A case of hydranencephaly in an infant with generalized cytomegalic inclusion disease was described by McElfresh and Arey (1957).

Very unusual lesions were observed by Fowler *et al.* (1972) in 2 autopsied hydranencephalic sibs of a sibship in which 5 hydrocephalic girls were born following hydramnios. The cerebral lesions were characterized by nodular or reticular vascular proliferations with a well developed reticulin network which were called glomeruloids by the authors; these were present in brain and retina. Within the cytoplasm of the cells were ovoid hyaline inclusions,

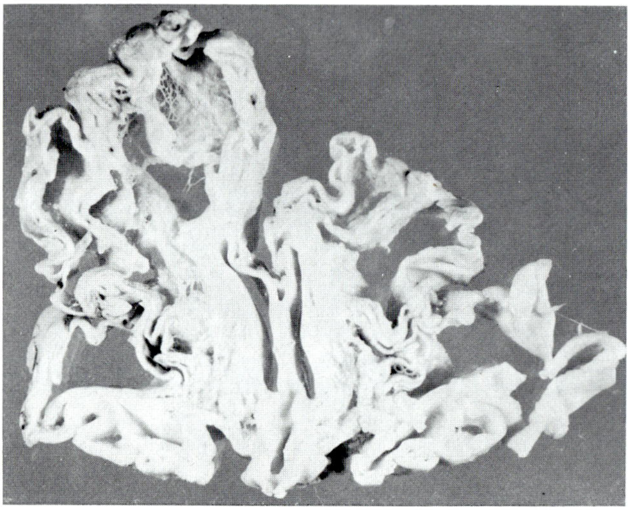

Fig. 40. Multilocular cystic encephalopathy

eosinophilic and PAS-positive, having a filamentous structure in electron micrographs. These cases defy classification at present.

Cavitated Cerebral Lesions in Twins. There appears to be an increased frequency of cerebral lesions in twins (Aicardi *et al.*, 1972). Pertinent cases are listed here for convenience without necessarily implying generic similarity. The only reported instance of hydranencephaly in twins occurred for biamnionic bichorionic twins of equal weights, who survived for 2 and 7 days respectively (Spielmeyer, 1905). The history of pregnancy was inconclusive. All other lesions observed in twins had the features of multilocular cystic encephalopathy. Case 2 of Stevenson and McGowan (1942) is without details on the lesions or the type of twinning. Brocher (1932) described the twin to a macerated fetus, showing poor development from birth with death at the age of 11 months. Multiple large septated cystic cavities were distributed throughout the cortex and white matter of both hemispheres. Manterola *et al.* (1966) report extensive infarction of the hemispheres, sparing the central portions, in a stillborn monochorionic diamnionic infant, about half the size of the surviving twin; the lesions had occurred *in utero*. Bilateral cystic cavities in cortex and white matter were observed in the 7-day-old twin of a macerated monochorionic monoamnionic fetus; cavitated cerebral lesions demonstrated by encephalography were reported for 2 other twins, 1 of which was twin to a macerated fetus having numerous placental anastomoses (Aicardi *et al.,* 1972).

It seems justified to assume a causal relation between twinning and at least some instances of cerebral lesions. The perinatal risk of twins is known to be approximately 4 times greater than for singletons, approximately one-third of the deaths occurring prenatal, the rest peri- and postnatal. By far the most critical factor for survival appears to be a birth weight above

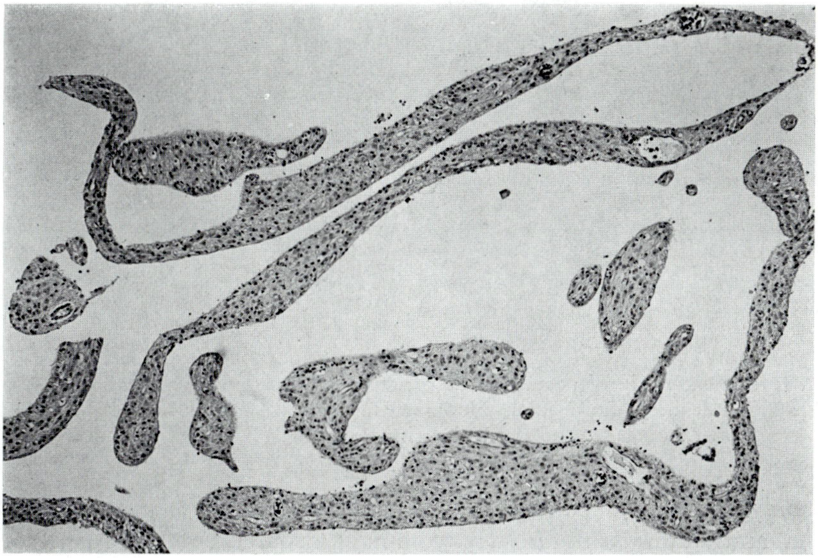

Fig. 41. Glial septa separating the cavities of multilocular cystic encephalopathy; H & E ×52

2,000 gms (Guttmacher and Kohl, 1958; Ferguson, 1964). Monoamnionic twins have a much higher death risk, at 41 percent (Timmons and de Alvarez, 1963), mainly due to cord complications. Also, in some instances of monochorionic twins one fetus preempts the placental blood supply with consequent unequal growth, a mechanism that seems responsible in several of the cases described above.

Multilocular Cystic Encephalopathy and Hydranencephaly of Postnatal Onset. The description of these lesions is combined provisionally because of certain overlaps in clinical histories and in features of the lesions.

Multilocular cystic encephalopathy (Crome, 1958) has been described under different names by almost every author concerned with the subject, such as multicystic encephalomalacia, polyporencephaly, progressive degenerative encephalopathy, multiple encephalomalacia of infancy, encephalomalacia with cavity formation, etc. The brains of these infants are usually smaller than normal and show multiple cavities in the greater part of both hemispheres (Fig. 40). The distribution of the lesions varies, but most are situated in the outer portion of the white matter or in the inner layers of cortex, and they may involve the entire substance of the brain. The cavities are separated from each other by glious tissue of varying thickness and many of the cysts are traversed by fine trabeculae (Fig. 41). Some cases show random disposition of the cavities throughout the hemispheres, but most show the lesions distributed in the territories supplied by anterior and middle cerebral arteries,

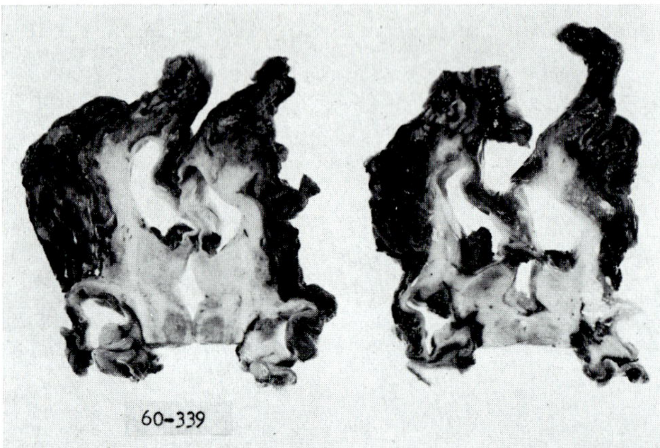

Fig. 42. Hydranencephaly of postnatal onset; note persistence of ventricular walls (Courtesy Walsh and Lindenberg, Bull. Johns Hopkins Univ. 106, 100, 1961, The Johns Hopkins University Press)

commonly sparing the temporal lobes below the superior temporal gyri. Basal ganglia and brain stem also are commonly spared, except for secondary degeneration of corticospinal tracts. The microscopic appearance of these lesions conforms to infarction with organization or incomplete necrosis of brain parenchyma. Organizing cavities are filled with fat-laden macrophages which also scatter through the adjacent glial scar tissue which contains reactive protoplasmatic astrocytes. The extent of organization may vary among lesions, which has been interpreted as a sign of progression of the disease process; more likely, however, such variance depends on the size of the lesions, they all dating to a single damaging event.

The lesions of hydranencephaly of postnatal onset (or extensive bilateral necrosis of cerebral hemispheres) are more massive than those of multilocular cystic encephalopathy. Several instances are described in the older literature, and a series of cases was reported by Lindenberg and Swanson (1967). These lesions differ from hydranencephaly of prenatal onset in that the residual pattern of cortical convolutions is discernable on gross inspection of the hemispheric surface. The cut brain shows necrosis of cortex and white matter, but the ventricular walls persist as intact layers of tissue (Fig. 42). The walls of the defects are shaggy, and strands or trabeculae of glial tissue traverse the cavities. The amount and distribution of the remaining tissue determine whether a given case is classified as postnatal hydranencephaly or as multilocular cystic encephalopathy. The basal ganglia are intact on gross inspection but may show microscopic damage. The lesions present in the initial stage as massive ischemic infarcts without evidence of inflammation. If the acute phase is survived, there is transformation of the hemispheres into a semiliquid, yellowish, succulent mass containing abundant lipid-laden macrophages (Fig. 43). No occlusive lesions have been found in the major cerebral

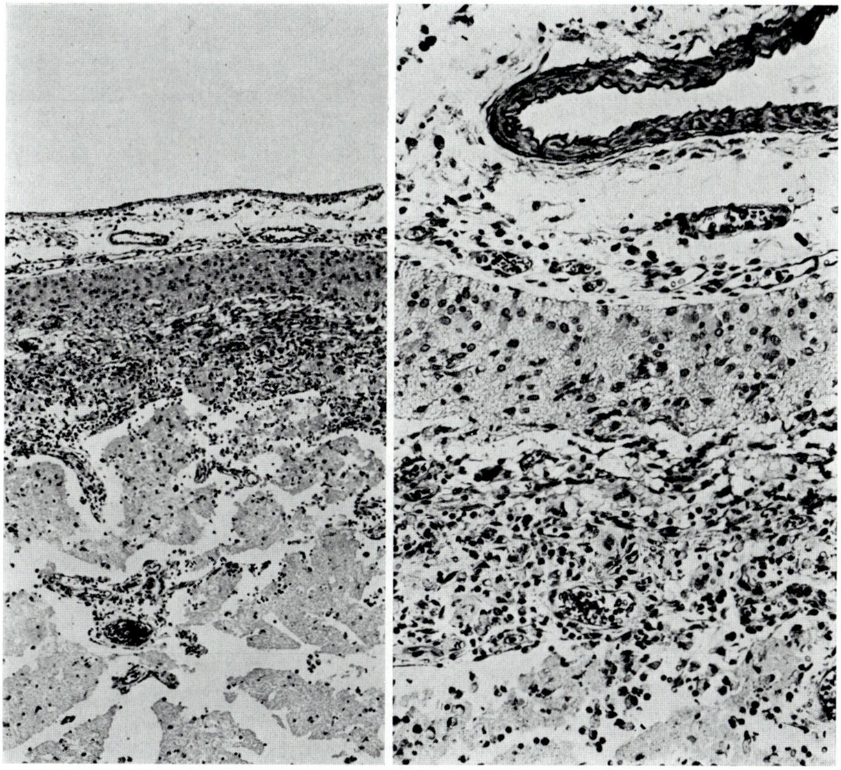

Fig. 43. Organizing stage of postnatal hydranencephaly in a 22-day-old infant. Persistence of the meninges and of the uppermost portion of the molecular layer; complete necrosis and early organization of hemispheric tissue; H & E ×60, ×135

arteries or in carotid arteries. The postnatal development of hemispheric atrophy has been demonstrated by repeat ventriculography (Weiss *et al.*, 1970).

Certain common traits are noted when comparing clinical histories for these two types of lesions. Many of the cases of multilocular cystic encephalopathy were twins or infants with a history of disturbed parturition with prolonged labor, cyanosis at birth, resuscitation, or seizures or neurologic symptoms occurring within a few days after birth. Such clinical histories were reported by Winkelman and Moore (1942), who considered their case a progressive degenerative disorder, by Cohen and Kristiansen (1954, case 1; case

2 had periventricular infarcts), by Kramer (1956, case 1; case 2 was ulegyric) and by Crome (1958). The familial occurrence of multilocular cystic encephalopathy described by Crome and Williams (1960) refers to 2 siblings; one was born after 68 hours initial labor during which meconium was passed, the other was asphyctic at birth and in poor condition thereafter. There is no reason to consider a hereditary factor. The case reported by Neuburger (1935) deserves attention: Birth occurred 5 weeks after attempted suicide with 5 hours exposure to household gas. The infant weighed 3,280 gms and lived for 6 days; abundant cavities occupied most of the white matter and the adjoining cortex, particularly at the depth of the sulci, as is typical for ulegyria. One may speculate, therefore, whether multilocular cystic encephalopathy represents merely severe combined lesions of periventricular infarcts and ulegyria; however, neither of these constituent patterns is apparent for most cases.

The clinical histories of cases of hydranencephaly of postnatal onset report a cerebral disorder of sudden onset between the first days after birth and approximately 18 months. The type of disorder is unclear, but it was identified as hemophilus meningitis for one case and as "meningitis" for another (Lindenberg and Swanson, 1967). Sudden loss of consciousness, coma, convulsions, and a bulging fontanel induced a state of decerebration but was survived for days to several years. Similar histories are reported for cases of extensive hemispheric necrosis (Dahlmann, 1910; Meier, 1912; Schob, 1930; and, probably, Cseh, 1937). Another infant (Jakob, 1931) had normal birth, with onset of symptoms when an umbilical infection became manifest by the 6th day. The lesions, at 3 months of age, were exceptionally severe, resembling hydranencephaly of prenatal onset except for preservation of the ventricular walls. Several other cases had less severe lesions and were described as multilocular cystic encephalopathy (Lumsden, 1950; Negrin *et al.*, 1952; Ford, 1952), but these also had a history of acute postnatal onset. Cerebral phlebothrombosis (as in case 7 of Stevenson and McGowan, 1942) must be considered in the differential diagnosis; its lesions are usually less extensive and differ in regional distribution (Chapter 13). In conclusion, there is overlap in the lesions as well as in clinical histories for cases of multilocular cystic encephalopathy and hydranencephaly of postnatal onset. Both types of lesions seem to derive from severe asphyxia or circulatory disturbances during the pre-, intra- or postnatal period.

Pathogenetic Considerations. Few definite facts are known concerning the pathogenesis of the lesions described in this chapter. The speculative interpretations have been along three lines: First, a primary malformation; second, an infectious process; and, third, a circulatory disturbance.

The concept of a primary malformation clearly is not pertinent to the encephaloclastic lesions of multilocular cystic encephalopathy and hydranencephaly of postnatal onset. Porencephaly as defined in this chapter was considered a primary malformation by Yakovlev and Wadsworth (1946) who proposed the term "schizencephaly", attributing the lesions to focal agenesis of portions of the hemispheric walls. Their interpretation hinges essentially on their interpretation of the membrane bridging the clefts in some instances;

the concept is inconsistent with the transitions between porencephaly and hydranencephaly and with what has been learned from the experimental production of these lesions.

An infective origin of porencephalic and hydranencephalic lesions is suggested by the few cases quoted earlier, but it is difficult to generalize from these observations. Osburn *et al.* (1971) reported hydranencephaly and porencephaly in fetal lambs infected with bluetongue vaccine virus, the type of lesion depending on the period of inoculation. However, their early lesions differed from those in humans in showing extensive destruction of the entire neuraxis including spinal cord. The lesions of later inoculation also differed from those in humans in showing predominantly necrosis in the outer portion of white matter. The similarity between this experimental model and human disease processes is only superficial.

A circulatory origin of porencephalic and hydranencephalic lesions is consistent with their predilection for the territories of carotid arteries and anterior and middle cerebral arteries respectively, which has been emphasized for porencephaly (Dekaban, 1965) as well as for hydranencephaly (Lange-Cosack, 1944; Muir, 1959). Lesions strikingly similar to hydranencephaly were produced experimentally in puppies by injecting into their carotid arteries a mixture of paraffin-oil hardening at body temperature (Becker, 1949). Hydranencephalic lesions showed transitions to less severe cystic lesions comparable to those of multilocular cystic encephalopathy. Bilateral ligation of carotid arteries of fetal monkeys between 70 and 100 days of pregnancy produced hydranencephalic lesions (Myers, 1969); these experiments are of particular interest in demonstrating that ligation before the 70th day failed to induce cavitated lesions but resulted in abnormal gyral patterns of the brain.

It is not known what processes may produce compression or occlusion of carotid arteries in the human fetus. Strangulation by the umbilical cord (Lange-Cosack, 1944) appears to be an exception rather than the rule. Lindenberg and Swanson (1967) considered kinking of intracerebral arteries caused by swelling of the brain. Kinking of the supraclinoid segments of the internal carotid artery has been demonstrated angiographically in adults having space-occupying lesions (Stovring, 1968). This process may have severe consequences in the newborn infant because of its soft, pliable vessels, but the mechanism, nonetheless, remains hypothetical. An additional etiologic factor was disclosed recently in the experiments of Hartley *et al.* (1974) who produced subcortical cavities in sheep by elevating the ewe's temperature to 44 °C for 9 hours daily during the last third of gestation.

On summary, the most logical interpretation of the origin of the cystic lesions described in this chapter is their attribution to fetal circulatory disturbances. However, other etiologic factors may also be responsible for the same—or extremely similar—lesions, as shown by the few cases of documented fetal infections. The possible interrelations between infection, necrosis of brain tissue and disturbances of fetal cerebral circulation remain a matter of conjecture.

References

Aicardi, J., Goutières, F., de Verbois, A. H.: Multicystic encephalomalacia of infants and its relation to abnormal gestation and hydranencephaly. J. Neurol. Sci. 15: 357—373, 1972.

Altshuler, G.: Toxoplasmosis as a cause of hydranencephaly. Amer. J. Dis. Child. 125: 251—252, 1973.

Bankl, H., Jellinger, K.: Zentralnervöse Schäden nach fetaler Kohlenoxydvergiftung. Beitr. path. Anat. 135: 350—376, 1967.

Becker, H.: Über Hirngefäßausschaltung. II. Intracranielle Gefäßverschlüsse. Über experimentelle Hydranencephalie (Blasenhirn). Dtsch. Z. Nervenheilk. 161: 446—505, 1949.

Binswanger, O.: Über eine Mißbildung des Gehirns. Virchow Arch. 87: 427—476, 1882.

Brocher, J. E. W.: Polyporencephalie. Z. ges. Neurol. Psychiat. 142: 107—119, 1932.

Cohen, M., Kristiansen, K.: Multiple encephalomalacia of infancy. Acta psychiat. neurol. scand. 29: 129—138, 1954.

Cohn, R., Neumann, M. A.: Porencephaly. J. Neuropath. exp. Neurol. 5: 257—270, 1946.

Crome, L.: Multilocular cystic encephalopathy of infancy. J. Neurol. Neurosurg. Psychiat. 21: 146—152, 1958.

— Sylvester, P. E.: Hydranencephaly (hydrencephaly). Arch. Dis. Child. 33: 235—245, 1958.

— Williams, C.: The problem of familial multilocular encephalomalacia. Acta Paediat. 49: 175—184, 1960.

Cruveilhier, I.: Anatomic Pathologique du Corps Humain. Paris: Baillière 1829—1835.

Cseh, I.: Multiple Cystenbildung im Gehirn. Frankfurt. Z. Path. 50: 334—546, 1937.

Dahlmann, A.: Beitrag zur Kenntnis der symmetrischen Höhlen im Großhirn des Säuglings. Z. ges. Neurol. Psychiat. 3: 223—248, 1910.

Dekaban, A.: Large defects in cerebral hemispheres associated with cortical dysgenesis. J. Neuropath. exp. Neurol. 24: 512—530, 1965.

Elo, O., Otila, E.: Zum Entstehungsmechanismus der früherworbenen Hydrocephalie. Acta Paediat. 23: 503—547, 1939.

Farkas-Bargeton, E., Olsson, Y., Guth, L., Klatzo, I.: Glycogen reaction to cerebral stab wound during maturation of rat brain. Acta Neuropath. (Berl.) 22: 158—169, 1972.

Ferguson, W. F.: Perinatal mortality in multiple gestations. Obstet. Gynec. 23: 861—870, 1964.

Ford, F. R.: Disseminated encephalomalacia with cavity formation. In: Diseases of the Nervous System in Infancy, Childhood and Adolescence, Third Edition, pp. 363—366. Springfield, Ill.: C. C Thomas 1952.

Fowler, M., Brown, C., Cabrera, K. F.: Hydrencephaly in a baby after an aircraft accident to the mother: Case report and autopsy. Pathology 3: 21—30, 1971.

— Dow, R., White, T. A., Greer, C. H.: Congenital hydrocephalus-hydrencephaly in five siblings, with autopsy studies: a new disease. Develop. Med. Child. Neurol. 14: 173—188, 1972.

Friede, R. L.: Enzyme histochemistry of neuroglia. Progr. Brain Res. 35—47, 1965.

Guttmacher, A. F., Kohl, S. G.: The fetus in multiple gestations. Obstet. Gynec. 12: 528—541, 1958.

Halsey, J. H., Jr., Allen, N., Chamberlin, H. R.: Chronic decerebrate state of infancy. Arch. Neurol. (Chic.) 19: 339—346, 1968.

— — — The morphogenesis of hydranencephaly. J. Neurol. Sci. 12: 187—218, 1971.

Hartley, W. J., Alexander, G., Edwards, M. J.: Brain cavitation and micrencephaly in lambs exposed to prenatal hyperthermia. Teratology 9: 299—304, 1974.

Heschl, R.: Gehirndefect und Hydrocephalus. Vjschr. f. d. prakt. Heilkunde 61: 59—74, 1859.

— Ein neuer Fall von Porencephalie. Vjschr. f. d. prakt. Heilkunde 72: 102—104, 1861.

Ilberg, G.: Beschreibung des Centralnervensystems eines 6tägigen, syphilitischen Kindes mit unentwickeltem Großhirn. Arch. Psychiat. 34: 140—170, 1901.

Jakob, A.: Über ein dreieinhalb Monate altes Kind mit totaler Erweichung beider Großhirnhemisphären („Kind ohne Großhirn"). Dtsch. Z. Nervenheilk. 117—119; 240—265, 1931.

Johnson, E. E., Warner, M., Simonds, J. P.: Total absence of the cerebral hemispheres. J. Pediat. 38: 69—79, 1951.

Kluge, H.: Untersuchungen über Hydranencephalie (Cruveilhier). Z. Heilk. 23: 208—255, 1902.

Konigsmark, B. W., Sidman, R. L.: Origin of brain macrophages in the mouse. J. Neuropath. exp. Neurol. 22: 643—676, 1963.

Környey, S.: Beiträge zur Entwicklungsmechanik und Pathologie des fötalen Zentralnervensystems. Arch. Psychiat. 72: 755—787, 1925.

Kramer, W.: Multilocular encephalomalacia. J. Neurol. Neurosurg. Psychiat. 19: 209—216, 1956.

Lange-Cosack, H.: Die Hydranencephalie (Blasenhirn) als Sonderform der Großhirnlosigkeit. Arch. Psychiat. Nervenkr. 117: 1—51; 595—640, 1944.

Lindenberg, R., Swanson, P. D.: "Infantile hydranencephaly"—A report of five cases of infarction of both cerebral hemispheres in infancy. Brain 90: 839—850, 1967.

Lumsden, E. E.: Multiple cystic softening of the brain in the newborn. J. Neuropath. exp. Neurol. 9: 119—138, 1950.

Lykke, A.: A case of congenital toxoplasmosis. Clin. Reports of the Adelaide Children Hospital 3: 62—66, 1956/57.

Lyon, G., Robain, O.: Etude comparative des encéphalopathies circulatoires prénatales et para-natales (hydranencéphalies, porencéphalies et encéphalomalacies dystiques de la substance blanche). Acta Neuropath. (Berl.) 9: 79—98, 1967.

McElfresh, A. E., Arey, J. B.: Generalized cytomegalic inclusion disease. J. Pediat. 51: 146—156, 1957.

Manterola, A., Towbin, A., Yakovlev, P. I.: Cerebral infarction in the human fetus near term. J. Neuropath. exp. Neurol. 25: 479—488, 1966.

Martin, J.-J., Guazzi, G. C., de Barsy, T.: Sur l'indidence et la signification de certaines glioses fibrillaires du tronc cérébral chez les très jeunes enfants. Z. Hirnforsch. 11: 7—12, 1969.

Meier, E.: Über einen Fall von totaler Erweichung beider Großhirnhemisphären bei einem 5 Monate alten Kinde. Jb. Kinderheilk. 76: 552—567, 1912.

Meyer, J. E.: Zur Ätiologie und Pathogenese des fetalen und frühkindlichen Cerebralschadens. Anatomisch-statistische Untersuchungen. Z. Kinderheilk. 67: 123—136, 1949.

Muir, C. S.: Hydranencephaly and allied disorders: a study of cerebral defects in Chinese children. Arch. Dis. Child. 34: 231—246, 1959.

Myers, R. E.: Brain pathology following fetal vascular occlusion: An experimental study. Invest. Ophthal. 8: 41—50, 1969.

— Cystic brain alterations after incomplete placental abruption in monkey. Arch. Neurol. (Chic.) 21: 133—141, 1969.

Navin, J. J., Angevine, J. M.: Congenital cytomegalic inclusion disease with porencephaly. Neurology (Minneap.) 18: 470—472, 1968.

Negrin, J., Lepow, H., Miller, B.: Multilocular encephalomalacia. J. Neuropath. exp. Neurol. 11: 62—68, 1952.

Neuburger, F.: Fall einer intrauterinen Hirnschädigung nach Leuchtgasvergiftung der Mutter. Ber. gerichtl. Med. 13: 85—95, 1935.

Norman, R. M., Urich, H., Woods, G. E.: The relationship between prenatal porencephaly and the encephalomalacias of early life. J. ment. Sci. 104: 758—771, 1958.

Obersteiner, H.: Ein porencephalisches Gehirn. Arb. Neurol. Inst. Wien. Univ. 8: 1—66, 1902.

Osburn, B. I., Johnson, R. T., Silverstein, A. M., Predergast, R. A., Jochim, M. M., Levy, A. B.: Experimental viral-induced congenital encephalopathies. II. The pathogenesis of bluetongue vaccine virus infection in fetal lambs. Lab. Invest. 25: 206—210, 1971.

— Silverstein, A. M., Predergast, R. A., Johnson, R. T., Parshall, C. J., Jr.: Experimental viral-induced congenital encephalopathies. I. Pathology of hydranencephaly and porencephaly caused by bluetongue vaccine virus. Lab. Invest. 25: 197—205, 1971.

Osterberg, K. A., Wattenberg, L. W.: The age dependency of enzymes in reactive glia. Proc. Soc. exp. Biol. Med. 113: 145—148, 1963.

Otto, R.: Ein Fall von Porencephalie mit Idiotie und angeborener spastischer Gliederstarre. Arch. Psychiat. 16: 215—239, 1885.

Playfair, J. H. L., Wolfendale, M. R., Kay, H. E. M.: The leucocytes of peripheral blood in the human fetus. Brit. J. Haemat. 9: 336—344, 1963.

Rivera, A., Jr., Brann, A. W., Jr., Myers, R. E.: Brain glycogen of the recovering asphyxiated monkey newborn. Exp. Neurol. 309—315, 1970.

Rubinstein, L. J., Klatzo, I., Miquel, J.: Histochemical observations on oxidative enzyme activity of glial cells in a local brain injury. J. Neuropath. exp. Neurol. 21: 116—136, 1962.

Schob, F.: Totale Erweichung beider Großhirnhemisphären bei einem zwei Monate alten Säugling. J. Psychol. Neurol. 40: 365—381, 1930.

Schütte, E.: Die pathologische Anatomie der Porencephalie; zusammenfassendes Referat. Centralbl. Allg. Path. 13: 633—662, 1902.

Seitz, L.: Über die durch intrauterine Gehirnhemorrhagien entstandenen Gehirndefecte und die Encephalitis congenita. Arch. Gynaek. 83: 701—720, 1907.

Solcher, H.: Zur Neuroanatomie und Neuropathologie der Frühfetalzeit. Monogr. Neurol. Psychiat. (Berl.) 127: 1—78, 1968.

Spatz, H.: Über die Vorgänge nach experimenteller Rückenmarksdurchtrennung mit besonderer Berücksichtigung der Unterschiede der Reaktionsweise des reifen und des unreifen Gewebes nebst Beziehungen zur menschlichen Pathologie. (Porencephalie und Syringomyelie.) Nissl-Alzheimer Histolog. Histopathol. Arb., EB: 49—367, 1921.

Spielmeyer, W.: Ein hydranencephales Zwillingspaar. Arch. Psychiat. 39: 807—819, 1905.

Stevenson, L. D., McGowan, L. E.: Encephalomalacia with cavity formation in infants. Arch. Path. 34: 286—330, 1942.

Stovring, J.: Kinking of the supraclinoid segment of the internal carotid artery over neighboring anatomic structures in acute and subacute intracranial mass lesions. Amer. J. Roentgenol. 104: 75—82, 1968.

Sumi, S. M., Hager, H.: Electron microscopic study of the reaction of the newborn rat brain to injury. Acta Neuropath. (Berl.) 10: 324—335, 1968.

Timmons, J. D., de Alvarez, R. R.: Monoamniotic twin pregnancies. Amer. J. Obstet. Gynec. 86: 875—881, 1963.

von Kahlden, L. C.: Über Porencephalie. Beitr. Path. Anat. 18: 231—404, 1895.

Watson, E. H.: Hydranencephaly. Amer. J. Dis. Child. 67: 282—287, 1944.

Weiss, M. H., Young, H. F., McFarland, D. E.: Hydranencephaly of postnatal origin. J. Neurosurg. 32: 715—720, 1970.

Winkelman, N. W., Moore, M. T.: Progressive degenerative encephalopathy. Occurrence in infancy, with antenatal onset simulating "swayback" of lambs; report of a case. Arch. Neurol. Psychiat. 48: 54—71, 1942.

Yakovlev, P. I., Wadsworth, R. D.: Schizencephalies. A study of the congenital clefts in the cerebral mantle. I. Clefts with fused lips. J. Neuropath. exp. Neurol. 5: 116—130, 1946.

— — Schizencephalies. A study of the congenital clefts in the cerebral mantle. II. Clefts with hydrocephalus and lips separated. J. Neuropath. exp. Neurol. 5: 169—206, 1946.

12. Arterial Occlusive Disease in Infancy

The present chapter pertains to the lesions resulting from arterial disease or from the occlusion of otherwise normal arteries in infancy or childhood. Cerebral infarction from these causes is superficially similar to that in porencephaly, hydranencephaly or multilocular cystic encephalopathy (Chapter 11), but there are certain distinctive differences. The latter types of lesions usually develop during fetal life, are often bilateral, and a search of the arteries supplying the destroyed portions of the brain usually yields no evidence of anatomic obstruction or of vascular disease; hence, a systemic disturbance or a transitory occlusive process may be postulated. The vasculo-occlusive processes described in the present chapter are more similar to those in the adult brain in that infarction of a portion of the brain, often unilateral or asymmetric can be traced to an anatomically demonstrable occlusive process in the vascular tree. Also, they typically develop during the postnatal period.

Occlusion of Major Cerebral Arteries in the Newborn. A tabulation of 47 cases of thrombotic or embolic gangrene of extremities in infants (Gross,

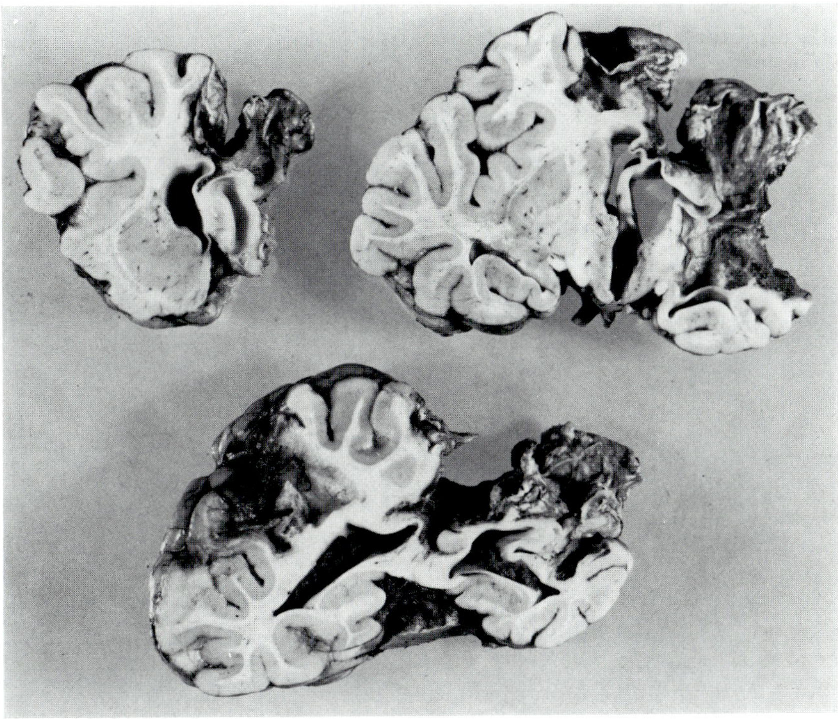

Fig. 44. Residual cavities of perinatal infarcts due to thrombotic or thromboembolic occlusion of internal carotid and stems of anterior and middle cerebral arteries

1945) includes two in whom massive cerebral infarction had occurred as well. One of these (case 5) was attributed to thromboemboli from a recent thrombus of the ductus arteriosus. The other one (case 6) had congenital cardiac disease and had developed—as a characteristic complication of the latter (Chapter 13)—cerebral infarction from thrombosis of the superior sagittal sinus; this infant, in addition, had suffered from thrombosis of the ductus arteriosus and aortic embolization. Clark and Linell (1954) described recent infarcts in the territory of the middle cerebral artery in an infant with erythroblastosis fetalis who died $1^1/_2$ hours after birth. The carotid artery was occluded at its bifurcation by necrotic material which was thought to be an embolus of placental tissue. The placenta contained a few small focal infarcts; a small recent infarct was also found in the spleen. The lesions had presumably occurred during the last days of pregnancy. A child who lived

36 hours (Banker, 1961, case 4) had a recent cerebral infarct and an organized thrombus, estimated to be 2 days old, in the internal carotid and middle cerebral arteries. Two infants, 4 and 11 weeks old, with organizing infarcts in the middle cerebral artery territories were described by Cocker *et al.* (1965). The first showed eccentric proliferation of intima containing hemophages, the second a mineralized organized thrombus. Both lesions were located near the bifurcation of the middle cerebral artery and were thought to be embolic, probably from fetal veins of the placenta. Eggers *et al.* (1973) report a middle cerebral artery infarct complicating leukemia in a 3-month-old child.

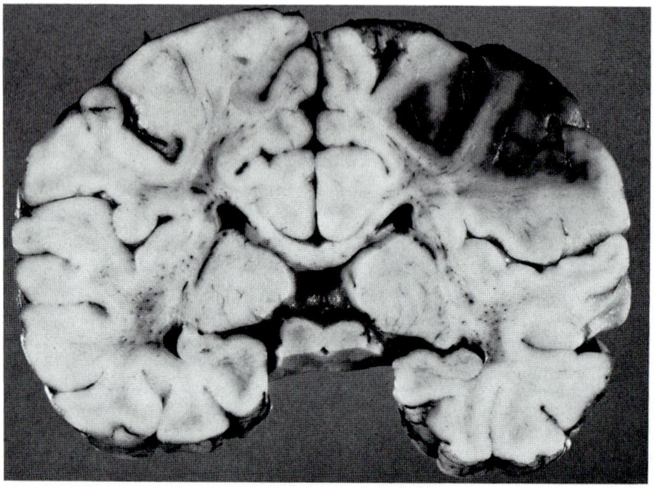

Fig. 45. Acute, mostly ischemic infarct in a newborn

Yates (1959) reported a thrombus of the left vertebral artery in a newborn without corresponding cerebral lesions. A late organizing infarct in the middle cerebral artery territory of a 2-month-old infant (Harvey and Alvord, 1972, case 4) was associated with focal intimal proliferation and hemophages in the middle cerebral artery, indicating a thromboembolic process. A similar case is illustrated in Fig. 44. One may assume that large cavitated hemispheric lesions observed in survivors having a history of neurologic deficits from birth (Hallervorden, 1937; Benda, 1945, 1952; and others) are the endstages of vasculo-occlusive infarcts of early infancy. Case 2 of Norman *et al.* (1957) showed a large cavity in the territory of the left middle cerebral artery in association with ulegyria, marbled state of the thalamus and periventricular infarcts, suggestive of the association of vasculo-occlusive lesions and diffuse perinatal anoxia.

The infarcts described above were large, being caused by occlusion of the carotid artery or of the stems of the cerebral arteries. Very little information is available on smaller infarcts in neonates caused by occlusion of branches of the main cerebral arteries. Siegmund (1923) mentioned the rare occurrence of superficial, wedge-shaped, hemorrhagic infarcts of the cerebral cortex, which he compared in shape with the contusions of the adult brain. Wedge-shaped, subcortical hemorrhagic lesions were seen only twice among more than 300 infants with cerebral damage by Schwartz and Fink (1926), and this type is not mentioned at all in many reviews on the subject. There is reason to believe, however, that small to medium-sized infarcts in the newborn brain, rather than being truly rare, are often neglected, or are misinterpreted as traumatic hemorrhages if the infarcts are hemorrhagic. The present author collected 5 cases of small to medium-sized cerebral infarcts in newborns, 3 hemorrhagic and 2 ischemic, over a 9-year period (Figs. 45, 46). Wedge-shaped, hemorrhagic lesions extending into the subcortical white matter were

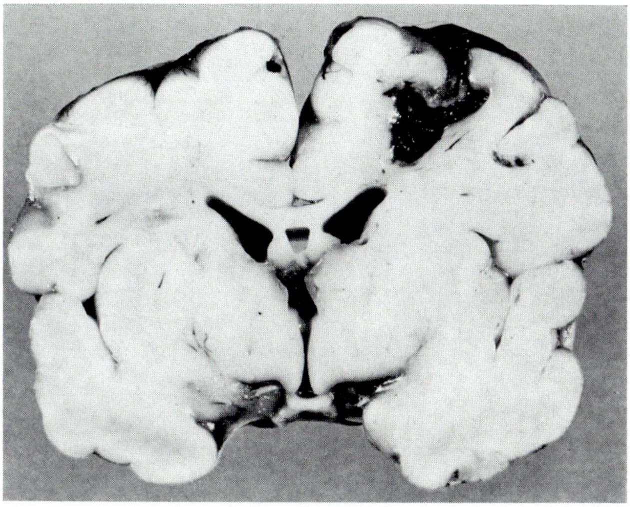

Fig. 46. Massively hemorrhagic infarct in a newborn, simulating primary intracerebral hemorrhage

thought to be cerebral hemorrhages or lacerations from birth trauma on gross inspection, but were identified with hemorrhagic infarcts microscopically. In the first case, a 4-day-old premature, there were wedge-shaped, massively hemorrhagic, liquefying lesions right frontal and parietal caused by embolization of arteries in the subarachnoid space with a villous, epithelium-lined tissue interpreted as placental fragments; the placenta was unfortunately not available for study. The second case, 12 days old, had died from necrotizing enterocolitis; it had a large, mostly liquefying, hemorrhagic infarct in the left parietal lobe; no occluded vessels were found. A third infant, 1 day old, had bilateral, wedge-shaped, recent hemorrhagic infarcts in the parietal lobes. Multiple recent thromboemboli were found in the meningeal arteries. The infant had also suffered from pulmonary and gastrointestinal hemorrhages and consumptive coagulopathy. The fourth case had ischemic infarcts presenting as sharply delineated, grayish discolored areas in the parietal lobe, the occipital pole and the calcarine region, all on the right side. The cerebral arteries with as much as possible of their distal ramifications were dissected before cutting the brain. Many recent thromboemboli were found upon serial sectioning of the coiled up vascular tree (Fig. 47), they had probably arisen from a recent thrombus of the ductus arteriosus. A large discolored area in the right posterior parietal lobe in the fifth case, 1 day old, was traced to a recent arterial thromboembolus of undisclosed origin. This infant had also suffered from left ventricular hypoplasia, mitral and aortic atresia, and atresia of the ascending aortic arch.

One may conclude that vasculo-occlusive disease of major cerebral arteries leading to cerebral infarction is not extremely rare in the newborn. It occurs

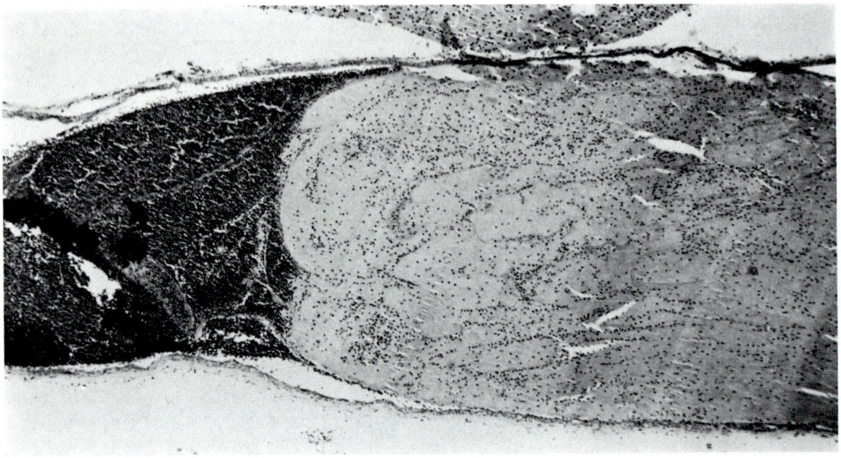

Fig. 47. Recent thromboembolus occluding an artery overlying a recent infarct; H & E ×45

most often unilateral and in the territories of the carotid or middle cerebral arteries; the most common cause appears to be embolization, either from thromboemboli originating from thrombi developing in the course of the involution of the fetal umbilical arteries or the ductus arteriosus (Gross, 1945), or from placental tissue. There has also been speculation as to the possible role of compression or traumatization of major arteries in the neck or cranium during parturition, but no factual evidence has been presented to verify this mechanism.

Arterial Calcification in Infancy. Arterial calcification in young infants is known to occur in: 1. advanced renal disease; 2. in conjuction with anomalies of the heart and great vessels, 3. in vitamin D hypervitaminosis and 4. as an idiopathic disease. Moran and Becker's (1959) review tabulates 44 cases of idiopathic arterial calcification in infancy, nearly all of them less than 1 year old, the average age at death being 3.8 months. The vascular pathology of idiopathic calcification is essentially the same as that of the symptomatic forms, but ancillary findings differ. The idiopathic form nearly always affects the coronary arteries, leading to sudden death in early infancy. Idiopathic mineralization has also been observed in stillborn infants in association with hydramnios (Ivemark *et al.*, 1962), or running a protracted course, leading to death during the 3rd (Holm, 1967) or the 5th year of life (Moran and Steiner, 1962).

The pathologic aspects of infantile arterial mineralization differ from those of adult arteriosclerosis in that there is absence of cholesterol precipitation and of atheroma formation in the intima. The vascular lumen is narrowed from marked fibrous thickening of the intima in association with focal, segmental calcification of the elastic membrane and the media, which may undergo fibrous replacement (Fig. 48). Some authors stress a primary defect of the intercellular substance of the media (Field, 1946), but most consider initial mineralization of the internal elastic membrane to be the critical feature

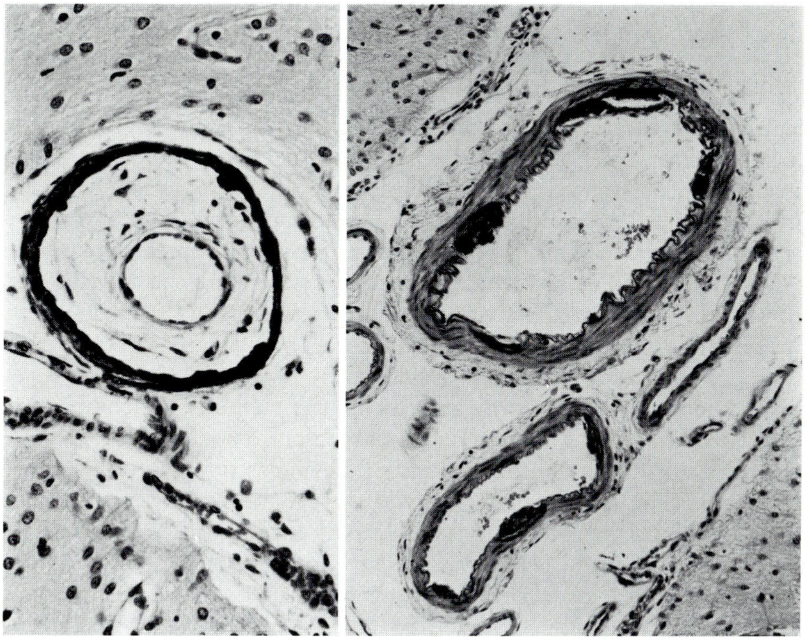

Fig. 48. Mineralization of elastic membrane associated with fibrosis of intima (left) in an infant with congenital renal disease; H & E ×115, ×200

(Stryker, 1946; Cochrane and Bowden, 1954; Moran and Becker, 1959). Moran and Steiner (1962) thought that the primary defect was a disorder of elastic tissue akin to pseudoxanthoma elasticum or osteogenesis imperfecta. However, mineralization of the elastic membranes may also be seen as a presumably secondary change in arteries near residual cerebral lesions.

Infantile vascular mineralization involves, in order of frequency, the coronary arteries, the arteries of kidneys, adrenals, periadrenal tissue, pancreas, spleen, lung, mesentery and thyroid. Cerebral vessels remain unaffected for the majority of cases, but they may become involved on occasion without associated lesions of the cerebral parenchyma (Prior and Bergström, 1948; Cochrane and Bowden, 1954). Extensive mineralization of cerebral arteries may be seen as a symptomatic feature in chronic renal disease of infancy.

Disseminated Vascular Disease in the Congenital Rubella Syndrome. A new note was injected into the problem of disseminated vascular disease in early infancy with Campbell's (1965) report on the vascular pathology of a 4-month-old infant with pulmonary stenosis, whose mother had developed rubella in the 3rd week of gestation. Pulmonary as well as systemic arteries showed focal partial defects of their internal elastic membrane and cushions of intima proliferation. These lesions were attributed to an interference of the rubella virus with elastic tissue formation, a factor to be considered apart from the production of cardiovascular malformation in the congenital rubella syndrome (Chapter 16). Similar vascular changes were recorded by others (Menser *et al.*, 1966), especially by Esterly and Oppenheimer (1967) who stressed the intimal fibromuscular proliferation and the absence of mineralization in 13 cases. Such lesions may lead to stenosis or to aneurysmatic dilation of arteries, and they may also include affectation of cardiac valves by nodular sclerosis (Singer *et al.*, 1967) or thrombotic aortic occlusion associated with systemic arterial hypoplasia (Fortuin *et al.*, 1971). There is still confusion in regard to the differentiation of the rubella lesions from idiopathic mineralization of infancy. Reports diagnosed as the latter (Witzleben, 1970) have been criticised as showing the rubella syndrome (Fortuin *et al.*, 1971), while Esterly and Oppenheimer (1967) quote an early description of idiopathic mineralization as a potential first report of rubella lesions.

Involvement of the cerebral arteries in the rubella syndrome may occur in the form of vasculitis and perivascular calcification (Singer *et al.*, 1967). Endothelial proliferation and deposits of PAS positive material, along with partial destruction of the arterial wall, were observed in small cerebral arterioles and veins in association with small foci of ischemic necrosis of the brain (Rorke and Spiro, 1967). There are no records of occlusion of major arteries or larger infarcts as complications of vascular disease in the congenital rubella syndrome.

Presumed Secondary Vascular Changes Found in Atrophic Arteries Near Residual Perinatal Lesions. Many authors have searched the cerebral vasculature in instances of residual cerebral lesions dating to the perinatal period, but more often than not no distinct lesions were found in the vascular tree. Some studies, however, disclosed narrowing of the vascular lumen from fibrosis and proliferation of the intima, variously associated with mineralization of the elastic membrane. Intimal fibrosis occurs in the form of lacy, spongy intimal tissue composed of loosely woven fibroblasts in the absence of focal collagenous scarring or deposition of hemophages. Considerable narrowing, or even complete obliteration, of the lumen may ensue. These changes extend over considerable distances along the atrophic vessels which appear firm, white and stringy on gross inspection. These alterations need to be distinguished from the musculoelastic cushions normally found at the bifurcations of arteries in infants (Wright, 1963). Intimal thickening may be associated with proliferation, reduplication or mineralization of the internal elastic membrane; there are usually no changes in the media and adventitia. Mineralization of the internal elastic membrane consists of deposition of intensely basophilic material in a segment or throughout the elastic membrane, or of small basophilic granules attached to its surface; there may also be fragmentation of the elastic membrane (Meyer, 1951). Such changes tend to occur locally in areas of old sclerotic lesions in the absence of corresponding arterial changes in the rest of the body and were reported by Juba (1936) in areas of old occipital cavitation and ulegyric scars. Meyer (1951), who searched for them systematically, found them in 28 of 153 cases of infantile circulatory brain damage. Intima fibrosis with or without associated mineralization of the elastic membrane was also recorded for multilocular cystic encephalopathy (Cseh, 1937; Crome, 1958), for hydranencephaly (Lange-Cosack, 1944) or for lesions of phlebothrombotic origin.

The interpretation of these vascular changes has been problematic; they were considered indicative of past thrombosis (Meyer, 1951), of post-meningitic lesions (Eicke, 1947) or of either of these processes (Bertrand and Bargeton, 1955). It is likely, however, that intimal fibrosis develops secondary to a reduced flow of blood through the damaged portions of the brain tissue. Such involutionary vascular changes have been documented in the classic studies of Thoma (1883–84) on the postnatal involution of certain arteries, or on the involution of arterial stumps following limb amputation. He concluded from his measurements that the first response of an artery to reduced blood flow is contracture of the media; this is followed, as a secondary change, by fibrosis of the intima which adjusts the vascular lumen permanently to the reduced flow of blood. Reactive intimal proliferation was produced experimentally by double ligation of arteries (Sokoloff, 1893; Mehrotra, 1953; Williams, 1956). Intimal proliferation also is a common feature in arteries feeding territories affected by watershed type infarcts in the adult brain (Romanul and Abramowicz, 1964) where it may develop either from secondary atrophy or from the organization of platelet thrombi.

Vasculo-Occlusive Processes in Childhood. The diseases described in the preceding portion of this chapter characteristically manifest in early infancy. Others, which typically affect adults, may occur, on occasion, in childhood or early infancy; these are mentioned here only briefly. Premature atherosclerosis differing from the infantile mineralization of arteries may develop as a manifestation of progeria (Rosenthal *et al.*, 1956), or as an idiopathic disease. Atheroma formation, however, generally does not occur before the age of 8 to 12 years, although intimal fibrosis may develop at an earlier age (Janssen, 1957). Strokes of the adult type are almost nonexistent below the age of 10, save for extremely rare exceptions such as the boy, aged 3 years and 11 months, reported by Ford and Schaffer (1927) and the 8-year-old child reported by Harvey and Alvord (1972, case 1).

There are also instances of so-called spontaneous occlusive lesions of carotid or cerebral arteries in children. Wisoff and Rothballer (1961) give a review of 29 cases in this category, 19 of whom survived. They occurred between infancy and 16 years, without specific predilection for a given age group; there was predominance of males (18 of the 23 for which sex was indicated), and the left carotid artery was nearly twice as often involved as the right one. Thrombotic occlusions occurred at the carotid syphon or in the supraclinoid segment and extended into the major cerebral arteries. No underlying anatomic lesions of the arterial wall were detected in some cases (Goldstein and Burgess, 1958; Banker, 1961). The presence of an underlying congenital vascular anomaly was inferred for a 16-month-old boy (Duffy *et al.*, 1957) because the infant also had a thrombosed aneurysm of the right brachial artery and hypoplasia of the right external iliac artery. Ford and Schaffer (1927), in the case quoted earlier described numerous foci of necrosis of the media of the thrombosed vessels, and, to a lesser degree, in other cerebral arteries, in addition to fatty intimal plaques.

Embolization of cerebral arteries in infants or children may result from rheumatic heart disease, subacute bacterial endocarditis, or pulmonary infections. Thrombosis may be induced by adjacent neoplastic disease, or by inflammation such as retropharyngeal infections, granulomatous processes near the artery, and, particularly, by mucor mycosis (Martin *et al.*, 1954; Banker, 1961) because of a tendency of this fungus to invade the wall and lumina of large vessels. Trauma of the carotid artery, particularly to the soft palate, has also been shown to cause carotid artery thrombosis, as documented in the autopsy case of Fairburn (1957) and in numerous clinical studies. The development of arterial occlusion in association with tuberous sclerosis has been recorded (Hilal *et al.*, 1971; Harvey and Alvord, 1972, case 6), presumably as a complication of the vascular anomalies associating with neurocutaneous syndromes. Etiologic factors of arterial vasculo-occlusive disease in infancy were reviewed by Davie and Coxe (1967) and Harvey and Alvord (1972).

Polyarteritis nodosa occasionally develops in childhood or infancy. In the review of the English literature by Fager *et al.* (1951) there were 52 occurrences in children and infants, 8 before the age of 2 years; Benyo and Perrin (1968) found 23 cases before the first year of life. Central nervous system involvement, however, is exceptionally rare at this age, and the 15-month-old infant with necrotizing arteritis reported by Harvey and Alvord (1972, case 5) appears to be unique.

The increasing usage of cerebral angiography has resulted in the radiologic definition of syndromes which are not yet clearly identified in terms of their pathology, such as carotid arteritis (Shillito, 1964) and moya moya disease (Suzuki and Takaku, 1969; Solomon *et al.*, 1970; Hilal *et al.*, 1971). In the latter occlusion of the supraclinoid carotid artery or the stems of cerebral arteries is associated with telangiectasia of the basal ganglia. The pathology of this syndrome appears to vary (Harvey and Alvord, 1972).

Vasculo-Occlusive Disease in Homocystinuria. Homocystinuria, an inborn defect of amino acid metabolism, is known to cause generalized vascular disease in infancy and childhood, in addition to its manifestations in the nervous parenchyma (Chapter 45). Cerebral vasculo-occlusive disease has been observed for more than one-half of cases afflicted with homocystinuria. Cerebral lesions present in the form of single or multiple infarcts of various ages and distribution. Heterogeneous pathogenetic factors were implicated in the few available pathologic studies. White *et al.* (1965) described occlusion of leptomeningeal arteries with organized thrombi in the absence of evidence of preexisting changes in the vascular wall. Cavitated hemorrhagic infarcts secondary to thrombosis of the superior sagittal sinus and cerebral veins were observed by Gibson *et al.* (1964) and Carson *et al.* (1965). Specific vascular alterations present in various organs, but not in the brain, consisting of intimal fibrosis, splitting, irregularity and focal discontinuity of the internal elastic membrane and adventitial proliferation. These changes are probably the result of elevated serum concentration of homocysteine, since they occur in homocysteinemia caused by a deficiency of cystathione synthetase, as well as with elevated serum levels of sulfated amino acids from other causes, such as anomalies of cobalamine metabolism (McCully, 1969).

Dissecting Aneurysms of Cerebral Arteries. Dissecting aneurysms originate at or near the main bifurcation of the internal carotid artery and present either as false luminae extending for considerable distances along the stems of the vessels or as recent thrombi between the elastica and the media. The patient described by Norman and Urich (1957) survived a dissecting aneurysm which had formed at the age of 6 months to the age of 15 years. False luminae extended into the branches of the right middle cerebral artery, and an old infarct was present in the corresponding territory. Wolman (1959) described the origin of a dissecting aneurysm in a 16-year-old youth from a small congenital anomaly of the vascular wall forming an intramural aneurysm lined by elastic membrane. His report contains a review of dissecting aneurysm in cerebral arteries of 17 adults; another review of 24 cases was published by Spudis *et al.* (1962). A thrombosed dissecting aneurysm in an 11-year-old boy was associated with focal areas of necrosis of media (Wisoff and Rothballer, 1961). Jacob *et al.* (1970) report a dissecting aneurysm in the left middle cerebral artery of a 7-year-old girl without further elaboration. This group of cases is still too small to decide whether they belong into one nosologic entity, or whether they present a conglomerate of different types of lesions. The occurrence of arterial fibromuscular dysplasia as a generalized disease in infants and children has recently been reported (Price and Vawter, 1972) and involves anomalies in the arrangement and relationship of elastic, collagen and muscular tissues in arterial walls; such changes may play a role in the production of cerebral vascular thrombotic or aneurysmatic lesions.

Congential Aneurysms of Cerebral Arteries. The frequency of congenital, or berry, aneurysms of cerebral arteries increases strikingly with age. Pathologic observations on congenital aneurysms in newborns are rare. Ferry *et al.* (1974) tabulate 22 verified observations in infants 2 years or less, most localized at the middle cerebral and the basilar arteries. Matson (1965) collected 14 cases of congenital aneurysms in the 1 to 17 year age group, while Patel and Richardson (1971) found only 4 of 58 in the 8 to 10 year age group and none below 7 years. Only 41 of 6,368 aneurysms had ruptured at the ages of 1 to 19 years in the "comparative study" (Nishioka, 1966). Arai *et al.* (1972) collected 20 cases of aneurysms in children less than 5 years and added an exceptional case with multiple aneurysms. The 3-month-old boy reported by Ferry *et al.* (1974) had widespread arteriectasis and aneurysm formation in cerebral, thoracic and abdominal vasculature.

The reported cases of congenital aneurysms in children and juveniles show a relatively high frequency of association with coarctation of the aorta (Chapter 14). Even more common is the association with polycystic kidney disease, although most observed instances in this category had occurred during young adult life (Peebles Brown, 1951; Bigelow, 1953). Forster and Alpers (1943) observed an unruptured aneurysm of the circle of Willis of a 13-week-old boy with polycystic kidney disease.

Aneurysms are found sporadically in association with cerebral malformations, as in the 7-week-old girl with agenesis of the corpus callosum reported by Garcia-Chavez and Mossy (1965). An acquired aneurysm in a 5-year-old boy was observed by Harvey and Alvord (1972, case 3); it had been caused by embolization with a spiklet of grass.

References

Arai, H., Sugiyama, Y., Kawakami, S., Miyazawa, N.: Multiple intracranial aneurysms and vascular malformations in an infant. Case report. J. Neurosurg. 37: 357—360, 1972.

Banker, B. Q.: Cerebral vascular disease in infancy and childhood. J. Neuropath. exp. Neurol. 20: 127—140, 1961.

Benda, C. E.: The late effects of cerebral birth injuries. Medicine 24: 71—110, 1945.

— Structural cerebral histopathology of mental deficiencies. Proc. Int. Congr. Neuropath., Rome, 1952, Vol. 2, pp. 7—50. Turin: Rosenberg and Sellier 1952.

Benyo, R. B., Perrin, E. V.: Periarteritis nodosa in infancy. Amer. J. Dis. Child. 116: 539—544, 1968.

Bertrand, I., Bargeton, E.: Lésions vasculaires dans l'hémiplégie cérébrale infantile. Proc. 2nd Int. Congr. Neuropath., Amsterdam. Excerpta Med. Foundation 2: 519—522, 1955.

Bigelow, N. H.: The association of polycystic kidneys with intracranial aneurysms and other related disorders. Amer. J. med. Sci. 225: 485—494, 1953.

Campbell, P. E.: Vascular abnormalities following maternal rubella. Brit. Heart J. 27: 134—138, 1965.

Carson, N. A. J., Dent, C. E., Field, C. M. B., Gaull, G. E.: Homocystinuria. J. Pediat. 66: 565—583, 1965.

Clark, R. M., Linell, E. A.: Case report: prenatal occlusion of the internal carotid artery. J. Neurol. Neurosurg. Psychiat. 17: 295—297, 1954.

Cochrane, W. A., Bowden, D. H.: Calcification of the arteries in infancy and childhood. Pediatrics 14: 222—231, 1954.

Cocker, J., George, S. W., Yates, P. O.: Perinatal occlusion of the middle cerebral artery. Develop. Med. Child Neurol. 7: 235—243, 1965.

Crome, L.: Multilocular cystic encephalopathy of infancy. J. Neurol. Neurosurg. Psychiat. 21: 146—152, 1958.

Cseh, I.: Multiple Cystenbildung im Gehirn. Frankf. Z. Path. 50: 334—546, 1937.

Davie, J. C., Coxe, W.: Occlusive disease of the carotid artery in children; carotid thrombectomy with recovery in a two-year-old boy. Arch. Neurol. (Chic.) 17: 313—323, 1967.

Duffy, R. E., Portnoy, B., Mauro, J., Wehrle, P. F.: Acute infantile hemiplegia secondary to spontaneous carotid thrombosis. Neurology (Minneap.) 7: 664—666, 1957.

Eggers, Ch., Schmitt, H. P., Fahr, K.: Cerebrale Manifestationen der Leukämie im Säuglingsalter. Neuropädiatrie 4: 458—472, 1973.

Eicke, W. J.: Gefäßveränderungen bei Meningitis und ihre Bedeutung für die Pathogenese frühkindlicher Hirnschäden. Virchow Arch. 314: 88—124, 1947.

Esterly, J. R., Oppenheimer, E. H.: Vascular lesions in infants with congenital rubella. Circulation 36: 544—554, 1967.

Fager, D. B., Bigler, J. A., Simonds, J. P.: Polyarteriitis nodosa in infancy and childhood. J. Pediat. 39: 65—79, 1951.

Fairburn, B.: Thrombosis of internal carotid artery after soft palate injury. Brit. med. J. 1957/II: 750—751, 1957.

Ferry, P. C., Kerber, C., Peterson, D., Gallo, A. A., Jr.: Arteriectasis, Subarachnoid hemorrhage in a three-month-old infant. Neurology (Minneap.) 24: 494—500, 1974.

Field, M.: Medial calcification of arteries in infants. Arch. Path. (Chic.) 42: 607—618, 1946.

Ford, F. R., Schaffer, A. J.: The etiology of infantile acquired hemiplegia. Arch. Neurol. Psychiat. 18: 323—347, 1927.

Fortuin, N. J., Morrow, A. G., Roberts, W. C.: Late vascular manifestations of the rubella syndrome: A roentgenographic-pathologic study. Amer. J. Med. 51: 134—140, 1971.

Forster, F. M., Alpers, B. J.: Aneurysm of circle of Willis associated with congenital polycystic disease of the kidney. Arch. Neurol. Psychiat. 50: 669—676, 1943.

Garcia-Chavez, C., Moossy, J.: Cerebral artery aneurysm in infancy: Association with agenesis of the corpus callosum. J. Neuropath. exp. Neurol. 24: 492—501, 1965.

Gibson, J. B., Carson, N. A. J., Neill, D. W.: Pathological findings in homocystinuria. J. clin. Path. 17: 427—437, 1964.

Goldstein, S. L., Burgess, J. P.: Spontaneous thrombosis of the internal carotid artery in a seven-year-old child. Amer. J. Dis. Child. 95: 538—540, 1958.

Gross, R. E.: Arterial embolism and thrombosis in infancy. Amer. J. Dis. Child. 70: 61—73, 1945.

Hallervorden, J.: Das Geburtstrauma als Ursache der Entwicklungshemmung im Kindesalter. Med. Klinik. 33: 1224—1229, 1937.

Harvey, F. H., Alvord, E. C., Jr.: Juvenile cerebral arteriosclerosis and other cerebral arteriopathies of childhood—Six autopsied cases. Acta Neurol. Scand. 48: 479—509, 1972.

Hilal, S. K., Solomon, G. E., Gold, A. P., Carter, S.: Primary cerebral arterial occlusive disease in children. Part I: Acute acquired hemiplegia. Radiology 99: 71—86, 1971.

— — — — Primary cerebral arterial disease in children. Part II: Neurocutaneous syndrome. Radiology 99: 87—94, 1971.

Holm, V.: Arteriopathia calcificans infantum. Acta Paediat. Scand. 56: 537—540, 1967.

Ivemark, B. I., Lagegren, C., Ljungquist, A.: Generalized arterial calcification association with hydramnios in two stillborn infants. Acta Paediat. 51, Suppl. 135: 103—110, 1962.

Jacob, J., Maroun, F., Heneghan, W., House, A.: Uncommon cerebrovascular lesions in children. Develop. Med. Child. Neurol. 12: 446—453, 1970.

Janssen, W.: Zur Frage der kindlichen Arteriosklerose, besonders der Herzgefäße. Mschr. Kinderheilk. 105: 361—365, 1957.

Juba, A.: Über einen zellig-fibrösen nicht entzündlichen Obliterationsvorgang der meningealen Arterien im Säuglingsalter. Arch. Psychiat. Nervenk. 104: 663—667, 1936.

Lange-Cosack, H.: Die Hydranencephalie (Blasenhirn) als Sonderform der Großhirnlosigkeit. Arch. Psychiat. Nervenkr. 117: 1—51; 595—640, 1944.

McCully, K. S.: Vascular pathology of homocysteinemia: Implications for the pathogenesis of arteriosclerosis. Amer. J. Path. 56: 111—128, 1969.

Martin, F. P., Lukeman, J. M., Ranson, R. F., Geppert, L. J.: Mucormycosis of the central nervous system associated with thrombosis of the internal carotid artery. J. Pediat. 44: 437—442, 1954.

Matson, D. D.: Intracranial arterial aneurysms in childhood. J. Neurosurg. 23: 578—583, 1965.

Mehrotra, R. M.: Experimental studies of changes which occur in ligated arteries and veins. J. Path. Bact. 65: 307—313, 1953.

Menser, M. A., Dorman, D. C., Reye, R. D., Reid, R. R.: Renal artery stenosis in the rubella syndrome. Lancet 1: 790—792, 1966.

Meyer, J. E.: Über Gefäßveränderung beim fetalen und frühkindlichen Cerebralschaden. Arch. Psychiat. Nervenkr. 186: 437—455, 1951.

Moran, J. J., Becker, S. M.: Idiopathic arterial calcification of infancy. Amer. J. clin. Path. 31: 517—529, 1959.

— Steiner, G. C.: Idiopathic arterial calcification in a 5-year-old child. Amer. J. clin. Path. 73: 521—526, 1962.

Nishioka, H.: Report of the cooperative study of intracranial aneurysms and subarachnoid hemorrhage. Section VII, part 1. Evaluation of the conservative management of ruptured intracranial aneurysms. J. Neurosurg. 25: 574—592, 1966.

Norman, R. M., Urich, H.: Dissecting aneurysm of the middle cerebral artery as a cause of acute infantile hemiplegia. J. Path. Bact. 73: 580—582, 1957.

— — McNemeny, W. H.: Vascular mechanisms of birth injury. Brain 80: 49—58, 1957.

Patel, A. N., Richardson, A.: Ruptured intracranial aneurysms in the first two decades of life. A study of 58 patients. J. Neurosurg. 35: 571—576, 1971.

Peebles Brown, R. A.: Polycystic disease of the kidneys and intracranial aneurysms. The etiology and interrelationship of these conditions; review of recent literature and report of 7 cases in which both conditions coexisted. Glasg. med. J. 32: 33—348, 1951.

Price, R. A., Vawter, G. F.: Arterial fibromuscular dysplasia in infancy and childhood. Arch. Path. (Chic.) 93: 419—426, 1972.

Prior, J., Bergström, V.: Generalized arterial calcification in infants. Amer. J. Dis. Child. 76: 91—101, 1948.

Romanul, F. C. A., Abramowicz, A.: Changes in brain and pial vessels in arterial border zones. Arch. Neurol. (Chic.) 11: 40—65, 1964.

Rorke, L. B., Spiro, A. J.: Cerebral lesions in congenital rubella. J. Pediat. 70: 243—255, 1967.

Rosenthal, I. M., Bronstein, I. P., Dallenbach, F. D., *et al.*: Progeria. Pediatrics 18: 565—577, 1956.

Schwartz, P., Fink, L.: Morphologie und Entstehung der geburtstraumatischen Blutungen im Gehirn und Schädel des Neugeborenen. Z. Kinderheilk. 40: 427—474, 1926.

Shillito, J. R.: Carotid arteriitis: a cause of hemiplegia in childhood. J. Neurosurg. 21: 540—551, 1964.

Siegmund, H.: Geburtsschädigungen des kindlichen Gehirns und ihre Folgen. Münch. med. Wschr. 70: 137—139, 1923.

Singer, D. B., Rudolph, A. J., Rosenberg, H. S., *et al.*: Pathology of the congenital rubella syndrome. J. Pediat. 71: 665—675, 1967.

Sokoloff, A.: Über die Bedingungen der Bindegewebsneubildung in der Intima doppelt unterbundener Arterien. Beitr. path. Anat. 14: 11—31, 1893.

Solomon, G. E., Hilal, S. K., Gold, A. P., Carter, S.: Natural history of acute hemiplegia of childhood. Brain 93: 107—120, 1970.

Spudis, E. V., Scharyi, M., Alexander, E., Martin, F.: Dissecting aneurysms in the neck and head. Neurology (Minneap.) 12: 867—875, 1962.

Stryker, W. A.: Arterial calcification in infancy with special reference to the coronary arteries. Amer. J. Path. 22: 1007—1031, 1946.

Suzuki, J., Takaku, A.: Cerebrovascular "moya moya" disease. Arch. Neurol. (Chic.) 20: 288—299, 1969.

Thoma, R.: Über die Abhängigkeit der Bindegewebsbildung in der Arterienintima von den mechanischen Bedingungen des Blutkreislaufs. Virchow Arch. 93: 443—505, 1883; 95: 294—336, 1884.

White, H. H., Rowland, L. P., Araki, S., *et al.*: Homocystinuria. Arch. Neurol. (Chic.) 13: 455—470, 1965.

Williams, G.: Experimental studies in arterial ligation. J. Path. Bact. 72: 569—574, 1956.

Wisoff, H. S., Rothballer, A. B.: Cerebral arterial thrombosis in children. Arch. Neurol. (Chic.) 4: 258—267, 1961.

Witzleben, C. L.: Idiopathic infantile arterial calcification—a misnomer. Amer. J. Cardiol. 26: 305—309, 1970.

Wolman, L.: Cerebral dissecting aneurysm. Brain 82: 276—291, 1959.

Wright, I.: The microscopical appearances of human peripheral arteries during growth and ageing. J. clin. Path. 16: 499—522, 1963.

Yates, P. O.: Birth trauma to the vertebral arteries. Arch. Dis. Child. 34: 436—441, 1959.

13. Thrombosis of Intracranial Sinus and Veins

There are many clinical and pathologic reports on thrombosis of intracranial sinus and veins in infants in the medical literature of the nineteenth and early twentieth centuries. One of the earliest appears to be that of Gerhardt (1857, 1881) for 7 infants developing venous thrombosis during the first months of life in the course of persistent diarrhea, dehydration and cardiac failure. Parrot (1873) described the pathologic findings in several cases and distinguished clearly the "red softenings" produced by venous thrombosis from the "pale softenings" of periventricular infarcts. Bouchut (1884) reviewed 30 cases and Bertier (1907) found 140 in the literature. Series from 26 to 46 cases reported by Hamburger (1920), Zischinsky (1929); Simpson (1932) and Ebbs (1937) further elaborated on the clinico-pathologic features of the disease. The series of 50 cases reviewed by Byers and Hass (1933) was subsequently enlarged to 80 cases by Bailey and Hass (1937). Since the frequency of the disease has decreased in recent years, these older reports still remain the most comprehensive sources of information. Various classifications of the lesions have been used in these studies; many older reports distinguish only venous thrombosis of noninfectious origin from thrombosis occurring in the course of infectious diseases.

A better distinction of etiologic factors and of clinico-pathologic correlations is provided by the classification of Bernheim and Larbre (1956): 1. Thrombosis from the local propagation of infections. 2. Thrombosis complicating meningitis. 3. Thrombosis in the course of general disease processes. 4. Occasional occurrences of unknown origin. The first two of these categories may be classified as thrombophlebitis, the others as phlebothrombosis. However, the distinction between thrombophlebitis and phlebothrombosis in infantile cerebral diseases is not always clear-cut and is often based on the application of a principle of thought rather than on the actual visualization of tissue changes: The walls of infantile cerebral veins are usually too thin to allow demonstration of phlebitic changes, and the presence of thrombi may not correlate with the extent of perivenous infiltrates, particularly in neonatal leptomeningitis. The present chapter deals mainly with the lesions in the third category, that is phlebothrombosis developing in the course of general disease processes. Thrombophlebitis from propagated infections is reviewed briefly at the end of the chapter, and thrombophlebitis complicating leptomeningitis is described in Chapter 17.

Phlebothrombosis Complicating General Disease Processes. Bernheim and Larbre (1956) distinguished within this category: 1. Noninfectious diseases resulting in dehydration, 2. sepsis or general infective disease, 3. congenital cardiac disease. Cerebral phlebothrombosis in noninfective diseases is most frequent in infants 6 to 18 months of age, the majority being less than 1 year, diminishing sharply after the second year. Dehydration results most often from nutritional disorders with vomiting or diarrhea. The term "marantic" thrombosis is frequently used for such cases, but it is not appropriate as marasmus is actually absent for the majority. Phlebothrombosis developing in the course of general infectious diseases such as sepsis and pulmonary infection afflicts slightly older infants and children. It has been observed in children with diphtheria, scarlet fever, dysentery and measles (Zischinsky, 1926). General disease processes were also present if cerebral phlebothrombosis developed after surgery (Evans, 1935). The occurrence of phlebothrombosis as a complication of congenital cardiac disease in young infants was not noted in the older literature and was recognized through the publications of Lhermitte *et al.* (1936), Berthrong and Sabiston (1951), Graser and Burkhard (1953), Weber (1957) and others.

Cerebral phlebothrombosis during the course of general disease processes usually develops after the underlying disease has been present for a few days, most often during its second week. There is no sex preference. An extremely high frequency of 9 percent of autopsies was found in the series of Byers and Hass (1933), who also noted a seasonal increase from dehydrating diseases during the summer months. The frequency has since been greatly reduced by therapeutic measures for correcting electrolyte imbalance and by antibiotic treatment. Accordingly, phlebothrombosis complicating diarrhea or general infections has become less common in most institutions than its occurrence with congenital heart disease, found, for example, in 9 of the 19 cases reported by Banker (1961).

Cerebral phlebothrombosis may be asymptomatic, found incidentally at autopsy, or its symptoms may have been overshadowed by the general disease process. Symptoms of massive cerebral lesions consist of convulsions of sudden onset, paresis, increased intracranial pressure and impairment of consciousness which may be fluctuating with a progressive downhill course.

Gross and Microscopic Features. It is convenient to distinguish phlebothrombosis of the sagittal sinus and external cerebral veins from phlebothrombosis of the internal cerebral veins; there is no intrinsic difference between these lesions and they often overlap. Phlebothrombosis may originate multifocal in different portions of the cerebral venous system, with multiple sites of primary thrombus formation (Fisher, 1901; Friede, 1972).

The superior sagittal sinus is most frequently affected. Firm, friable, grayish-red and adherent thrombi, several cm in length, are most common in the middle third of the sinus, filling it completely; mural thrombi are less frequent. Large thrombi may fill the entire length of the sinus; microscopic examination may show organization by fibroblasts and sprouting capillaries only in the middle portion of the thrombus, indicating that its anterior and posterior extensions are of more recent date. Thrombi may extend from the sagittal into the lateral and straight sinus.

Thrombosis of superficial cortical veins develops secondary to sinus thrombosis, and the latter is always present when the veins are affected. The veins terminating in the middle portion of the sinus are most frequently involved; they are distended, dark blue, firm and protruding; upon organization of the thrombi they turn yellowish-white.

Cerebral lesions form upon extension of a thrombus into the cortical veins. Extreme congestion may be the only change present for a brief interval after the onset of cortical vein thrombosis. Subarachnoid hemorrhage develops almost always in the affected area and may obscure the thrombosed vessels.

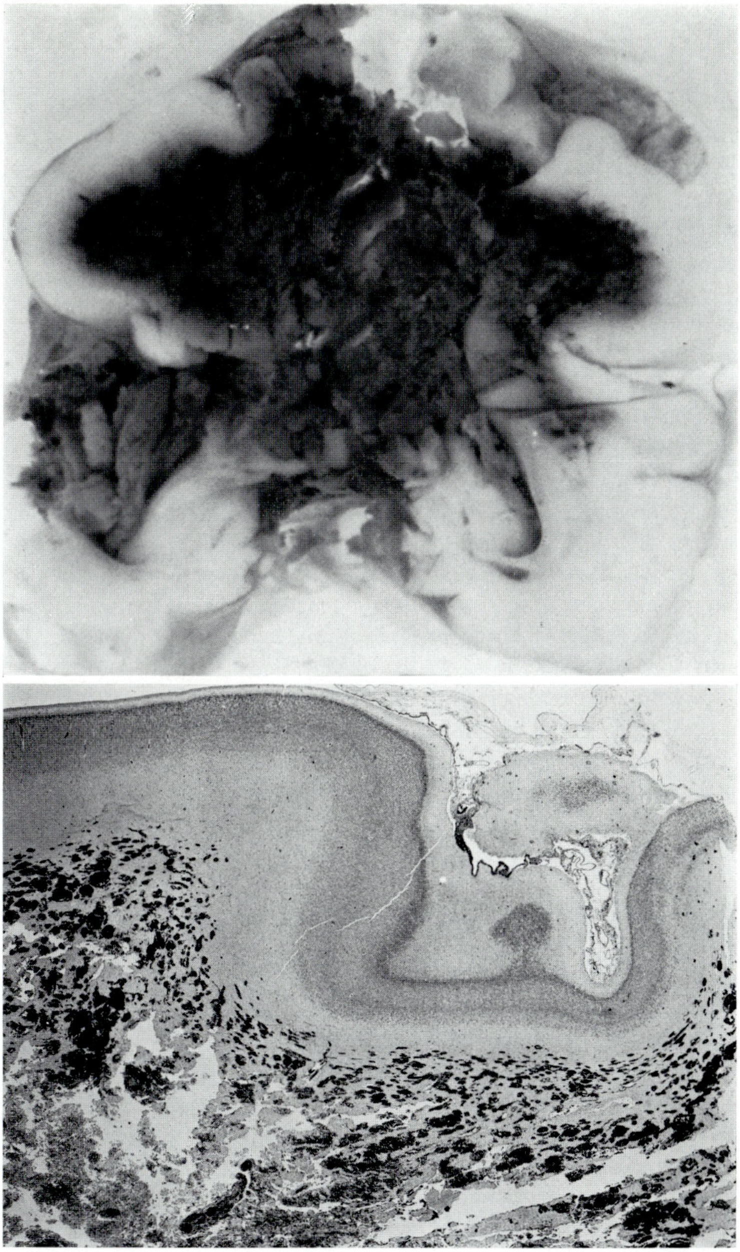

Fig. 49. Massive hemorrhagic infarction of white matter in a newborn with internal cerebral vein phlebothrombosis. Bottom: H & E ×7; numerous fibrinous thrombi were present in veins in the necrotic white matter

It originates either from leakage of excessively congested leptomeningeal veins or from the penetration of parenchymal hemorrhages into the subarachnoid space. Structural damage to the brain varies in extent and localization, consisting of hemorrhagic infarcts with numerous petechiae which tend to become confluent with considerable tissue destruction. Large hematomas may form. The infarcts occur most often at the upper convexity of the hemispheres, involving the cerebral cortex as well as substantial portions of subcortical white matter. Increase in the volume of infarcted tissue and collateral edema may be marked.

Lesions from thrombosis of internal cerebral veins are similar except for distribution. Judging from overall published frequencies, they seem to be somewhat less frequent than thrombosis of external cerebral veins. Ehlers and Courville (1936) surveyed 26 cases of phlebothrombosis of internal cerebral veins, including 5 cases of their own. Scattered reports are found in the later literature. Thrombosis may affect primarily the great vein of Galen—6 of 26 cases reviewed by Ehlers and Courville—or may be associated with thrombosis of other dural sinus including superior sagittal and lateral sinus. Thrombosis of the straight sinus or of the great vein of Galen produces massive bilateral hemorrhagic softening of the entire centrum semiovale (Fig. 49). More restricted hemorrhagic infarctions of the ventricular walls, usually bilateral, may result from thrombosis of tributary veins. The caudate nucleus and thalamus are frequently involved—in 10 of 26 cases (Ehlers and Courville (1936)—which is significant when compared with the constant sparing of basal ganglia by periventricular infarcts from perinatal asphyxia (Chapter 4). Thrombosis of choroid plexus veins may occur, and marked intraventricular hemorrhage is frequent; there may be acute dilation of the ventricles. Hemorrhagic infarction of cerebellum from thrombi in the superior cerebellar veins terminating in the straight sinus is less common. Lesions of brain stem have not been reported.

Residual Lesions. Cerebral phlebothrombosis is fatal for the majority of cases, but residual lesions have been reported in survivors (Norman, 1936; Bailey and Hass, 1937; Courville, 1958; Bailey, 1959). Only 13 cases of residual lesions of verified phlebothrombotic origin were found in a survey of the literature (Friede, 1972). The scarcity of survivals may be overestimated, however, because the sinus are often not available for study and attribution of the lesion to sinus thrombosis must remain tentative, such as for the 3 cases of Woolf (1955). Also, some patients with sinus thrombosis may survive with minimal or without cerebral lesions, or lesions may be mistaken for birth injuries. The possibility of recanalization of thrombi also needs to be considered; however, Norman (1936) demonstrated an organized thrombus after 4 years survival and Dekaban and Norman (1958) after 25 years survival. Hence, it is unlikely that a thrombosed sinus can heal completely without any residual lesion. The sinus may differ, in this regard, from cerebral veins: Experimental obliteration of veins results in rapid endothelial and fibroblast proliferation inducing the formation of new veins which connect to others and soon become filled with circulating blood (Mehrotra, 1953).

Organized thrombi of the sinus consist of a loose mesh of fibrous tissue with scattered capillaries or larger blood channels lined with a single endothelial layer; these are often interpreted as recanalization, although their actual continuity throughout the thrombosed segment is a matter of conjecture. The tissue contains deposits of hemosiderin, and focal mineralization may occur (Fig. 50).

The extent and distribution of residual lesions in the cerebral hemispheres varies considerably. Russell (1954) described organized thrombi in the sagittal

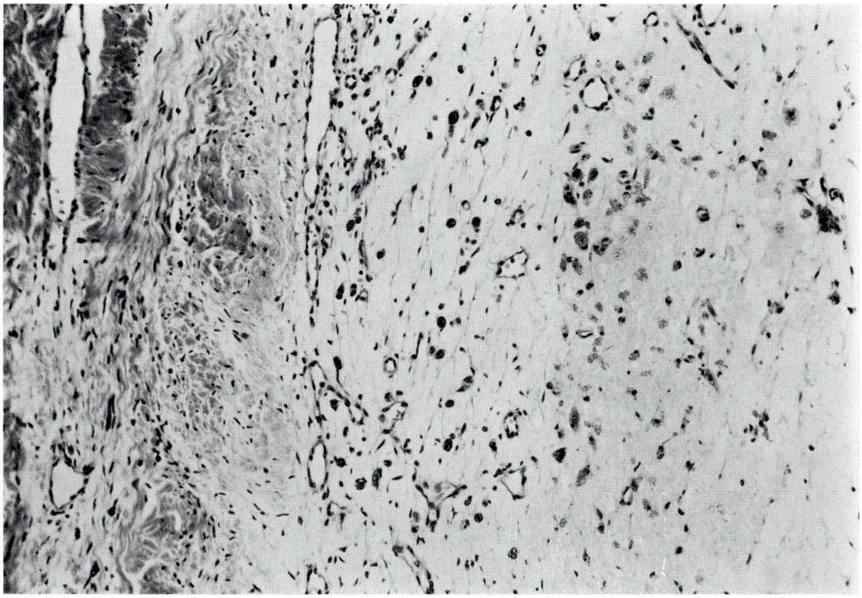

Fig. 50. Old organized thrombus in the superior sagittal sinus; H & E ×110

sinus in the absence of cortical lesions. Lesions range from disseminated small cortical scars, to cavitated defects, to lobar sclerosis and are often bilateral, but without strict symmetry, preferentially located in parasagittal distribution. Cavitated cerebellar lesions are less frequent. Old subarachnoid hemorrhage is noted in the form of arachnoid fibrosis over the affected regions and deposits of hemosiderin in the leptomeninges. Neomembranes of dura mater or hygromas have been found in several cases. Large cavities in cortex and subcortical white matter show the features characteristic of cavitated infarcts, often covered by a persisting upper portion of the molecular layer. The walls of the cavities exhibit marked gliosis, often with perivascular proliferation of reticulum fibers, focal deposits of hematoidin or hemosiderin, hemosiderin-laden macrophages, amorphous mineral deposits, or mineralized neurons. Laminar cortical necrosis adjacent to cavitated lesions may be interpreted as a secondary anoxic change. Hypervascularization may occur in the leptomeninges overlying the cavities or focally in their walls. Widespread phlebectasia and telangiectasia may encompass the lesions and apparently represents collateral circulation from an adaptive enlargement of the still growing vascular system (Fig. 51).

The residual cortical lesions of phlebothrombosis may be distinguished from perinatal anoxic lesions by the pigmentation in the leptomeninges and of the walls of the cavities; the bilateral disposition of the lesions, parasagittal at the convexity of the hemispheres; the random destruction of gyri as well

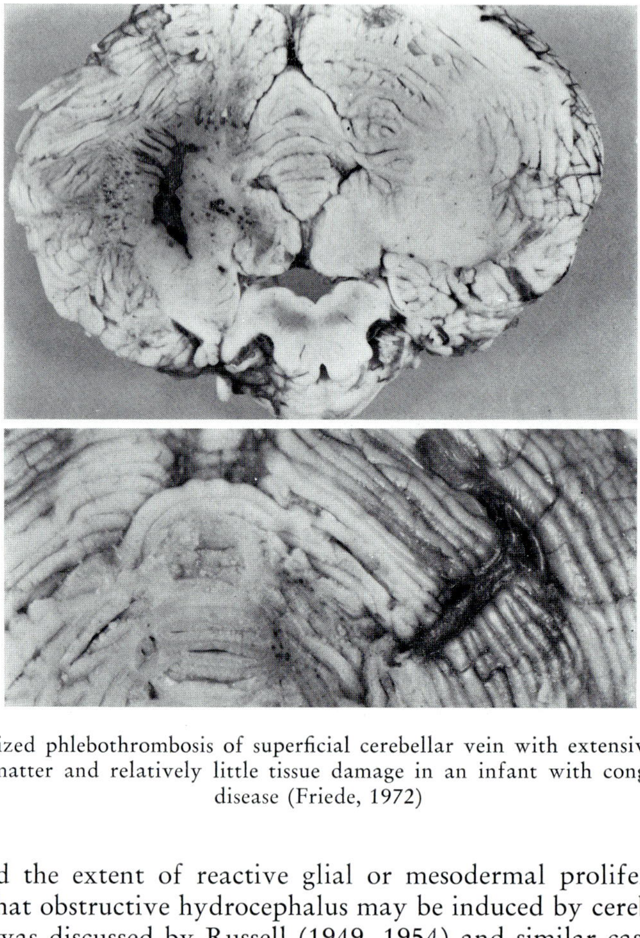

Fig. 51. Organized phlebothrombosis of superficial cerebellar vein with extensive phlebectasia of the white matter and relatively little tissue damage in an infant with congenital cardiac disease (Friede, 1972)

as sulci; and the extent of reactive glial or mesodermal proliferation. The possibility that obstructive hydrocephalus may be induced by cerebral phlebothrombosis was discussed by Russell (1949, 1954) and similar cases are being reported sporadically (Haar and Miller, 1975). The occurrence of this complication is unusual, however, in view of the great difficulty encountered in attempts at inducing hydrocephalus experimentally by obstruction of venous drainage (Chapter 22).

Although one may expect that extensive cavitation of white matter and basal ganglia results from thrombosis of the internal cerebral veins, there are no instances where this has been verified. Dahlmann (1910) described an infant which, after a normal birth and postnatal course, developed persistent convulsions on the 7th day with a rapid increase in head circumference. The autopsy 7 weeks later showed bilateral cavities, up to 8 cm in diameter, in the hemispheric white matter, sparing the cortex. The cavities had brownish walls, were filled with turbid fluid, and there was pigmentation of the ependyma. The clinical history of this case and the type of lesions suggest phlebothrombosis of internal cerebral veins. The differential diagnosis includes periventricular infarcts, which are nonhemorrhagic for the vast majority of cases (Chapter 4) and subependymal hemorrhages, which are usually not extensively destructive to white matter (Chapter 2). The features of these residual lesions are usually sufficiently characteristic to permit their identification, but atypical lesions may pose diagnostic problems.

Pathogenetic Considerations. The induction of cerebral lesions by sinus thrombosis and their extent is dependent on the size and location of the thrombus. The superior sagittal sinus is the main drainage for the convexity of the hemispheres, subject to considerable individual variation in the degree of anastomosis with the middle cerebral and Sylvian veins which drain into the cavernous sinus, superior petrosal sinus and transverse sinus. The frontal third of the superior sagittal sinus may be ligated in man anterior to the Rolandic inflow without disturbances (Jaeger, 1942). Portions of the sinus posterior to the Rolandic inflow may also be resected if the blood flow has been reduced previously by a slowly growing neoplasm (Dandy, 1940; Jaeger, 1951). Dogs and cats tolerate complete and sudden obstruction of the superior sagittal sinus without adverse effect (Beck and Russell, 1946). Becker (1949) injected a paraffin mixture that hardens at body temperature into the sagittal sinus of puppies. Cerebral lesions resulted only when the injected material extended into the superficial cortical veins; then, however, the lesions were massive and fatal.

The preferential origin of thrombi in the middle third of the sagittal sinus may be understood by reference to, among other factors, the entrance of cortical veins. Veins from the frontal lobes enter the sinus at right angle whereas the large posterior veins approach the sinus at an oblique angle and continue within its wall for some distance in a frontal direction. Accordingly, the blood is discharged into the sinus in a direction opposite to its flow in the sinus, which may represent a local factor facilitating thrombus formation.

General factors inducing thrombus formation are changes in the composition of the blood, its rate of flow, and the integrity of the wall of the blood vessels. Phlebothrombosis in infants with general disease processes evidently depends to a large extent on changes in blood composition. Dehydration from diarrhea and vomiting affects blood viscosity, as does the increase in hematocrit that occurs in congenital cardiac disease. Disorders in clotting appear to be less important, as they rarely cause infantile phlebothrombosis; an exceptional case of sinus thrombosis in a newborn with disseminated intravascular coagulation was reported by Leissring and Vorlicky (1966). Mechanical damage to the walls of the sinus does not appear to be a significant factor in thrombus formation. Simpson (1932) postulated that thrombosis may be induced by therapeutic puncture of the sinus, but this was not confirmed in later studies (Ebbs, 1937; Byers and Hass, 1933). Indeed, Beck and Russell (1946) emphasized the difficulty in inducing thrombus formation in the sinus of animals, even with the use of irritant coagulants which consistently induce thrombus formation in peripheral veins.

Sinus thrombosis had been classified as a birth injury on the assumption that the thrombi form at microscopic tears in the wall of the sagittal sinus produced by the deformation of the head during birth (Messen and Stochdorph, 1957). A massive organized thrombus was found in the superior sagittal sinus of an infant with a definite history of severe distress upon birth (Norman, 1937). This case, however, is exceptional. Two cases reported as sinus thrombosis due to birth injury by Schwartz and Fink (1925) were 12 and 16 days old, without clinical histories. The much quoted reports on phlebothrombosis by Marburg and Casamajor (1944) and Marburg *et al.* (1944) include a variety of lesions for which neither the relation to birth injury nor the derivation from phlebothrombosis was convincingly documented. One must conclude, therefore, that cerebral phlebothrombosis is a postnatal disease process unrelated to perinatal trauma for the vast majority of cases.

Thrombophlebitis from Local Propagation of Infections. These lesions result most often from otitis media and mastoiditis. There is no specific predilection for very young infants and the average age is higher than that for phlebothrombosis complicating general disease processes. Thrombosis may develop as a local component of active inflammation, or in the proximity of a focus of infection. Thrombosis of the lateral sinus in cases of otitis or mastoiditis is usually unilateral, most frequently at the sigmoid curvature (Courville and Nielsen, 1935). Less frequent sources of phlebothrombosis from local propagation of infections are dental infections, propagation of infections from the orbit or the cranial bones, rhinopharyngeal infections including sinusitis and tonsillitis, or superficial infective processes of face and scalp. The cavernous sinus or other sinus may be involved depending on the primary localization of the infective process.

Otogenic sinus thrombosis may lead to increased intracranial pressure, especially when the thrombus extends to the confluence sinuum and to the sagittal sinus. Klestadt (1924) recognized this pathogenetic mechanism and referred to it as "otogenic pseudo abscess"; he emphasized the extension of the thrombi beyond the torcular and the difficulty in differential diagnosis with cerebral abscess. Symonds (1931) proposed the term "otitic hydrocephalus", which was modified by McAlpine (1937) to "toxic hydrocephalus". Both terms are unfortunate choices as they equate hydrocephalus with increased intracranial pressure; moreso, both authors used the terms clinically and stated that the underlying pathologic changes were obscure. Otogenic sinus thrombosis, thus, accounts for some of the cases referred to clinically as "pseudotumor cerebri".

Thrombosis of the lateral sinus has a high rate of recovery and does not cause parenchymal lesions in the brain unless the thrombus extends into other sinus, particularly in the superior sagittal sinus. The frequency of this disease has been greatly reduced by antibiotic therapy.

References

Bailey, O. T.: Results of long survival after thrombosis of the superior sagittal sinus. Neurology (Minneap.) 9: 741—746, 1959.

— Hass, G. M.: Dural sinus thrombosis in early life: Recovery from acute thrombosis of the superior longitudinal sinus and its relation to certain acquired cerebral lesions in childhood. Brain 60: 293—314, 1937.

— — Dural sinus thrombosis in early life. The clinical manifestations and extent of brain injury in acute sinus thrombosis. J. Pediat. 11: 755—771, 1937.

Banker, B. Q.: Cerebral vascular disease in infancy and childhood. J. Neuropath. exp. Neurol. 20: 127—140, 1961.

Beck, D. J. K., Russell, D. S.: Experiments on thrombosis of the superior longitudinal sinus. J. Neurosurg. 3: 337—347, 1946.

Becker, H.: Hirngefäßausschaltung II. Intracranielle Gefäßverschlüsse. Über experimentelle Hydranencephalie (Blasenhirn). Dtsch. Z. Nervenheilk. 161: 446—505, 1949.

Bernheim, M.: L'importance des thrombophlébites cérébrales dans la pathologie nerveuse de l'enfant. Ann. Pediat. 187: 153—160, 1956.

— Larbre, F.: Les formes pseudoencéphalitiques des thrombophlébites cérébrales chez l'enfant. Rev. Prat. (Paris) 6: 2965—2973, 1956.

Berthrong, M., Sabiston, D. C., Jr.: Cerebral lesions in congenital heart disease. Bull. Johns Hopk. Hosp. 89: 384—406, 1951.

Bertier, J.: La thrombose médicale des sinus de la dure-mère. Arch. gen. Méd. 84: 313—337, 1907.

Bouchut, J. E.: Clinique de l'hôpital des enfants malades, p. 137. Paris: J. B. Baillière et fils 1884.

Byers, R. K., Hass, G. B.: Thrombosis of the dural venous sinus in infancy and childhood. Amer. J. Dis. Child. 45: 1161—1183, 1933.

Courville, C. B.: Residual cerebral lesions after thrombosis of the superior longitudinal sinus. Review of the literature and report of case. Bull. Los Angeles Neurol. Soc. 23: 160—170, 1958.

— Nielsen, I. M.: Cerebral manifestation following acute otitis media in infancy and in early childhood with particular reference to occurrence of Jacksonian convulsions, conjugate deviation of head and eyes and hemiplegia. Amer. J. Dis. Child. 49: 1—27, 1935.

Dahlmann, A.: Beitrag zur Kenntnis der symmetrischen Höhlen im Großhirnmark des Säuglings mit Bemerkungen über Entstehung von Hirnhöhlen im allgemeinen. Z. Neurol. Psychiat. 3: 223—248, 1910.

Dandy, W. E.: Removal of longitudinal sinus involved in tumors. Arch. Surg. 41: 244—256, 1940.

Dekaban, A. S., Norman, R. M.: Hemiplegia in early life associated with thrombosis of the sagittal sinus and its tributary veins in one hemisphere. J. Neuropath. exp. Neurol. 17: 461—470, 1958.

Dellille, A., Lhermitte, I., Lesobre, R.: Ramollissement hémorrhagique d'origine veineuse chez un enfant atteint de malformation cardiaque. Rev. Neurol. 66: 754—759, 1936.

Ebbs, J. H.: Cerebral sinus thrombosis in children. Arch. Dis. Child. 12: 131—152, 1937.

Ehlers, H., Courville, C. B.: Thrombosis of internal cerebral veins in infancy and childhood. J. Pediat. 8: 600—623, 1936.

Evans, P. R.: Postoperative Sinusthrombose bei Kindern. Lancet II: 12—15, 1935.

Fisher, T.: Four cases of primary thrombosis of cerebral veins and sinuses in children. Brit. med. J. II: 9—12, 1901.

Friede, R. L.: Residual lesions of infantile cerebral phlebothrombosis. Acta Neuropath. 22: 319—332, 1972.

Gerhardt, C., 1857: Quoted in: Gerhardt, C., Lehrbuch der Kinderkrankheiten, 4th Ed., pp. 591—595. Tübingen: Laupp 1881.

Graser, F., Burkhard, I.: Die marantische Sinusthrombose als Komplikation des Morbus caeruleus im Säuglingsalter. Medizinische (Stuttgart) 37: 1194—1195, 1953.

Haar, F. L., Miller, C. A.: Hydrocephalus resulting from superior vena cava thrombosis in an infant. J. Neurosurg. 42: 597—601, 1975.

Hamburger, G.: Über Gefäßthrombosen junger Kinder. Jb. Kinderheilk. 91: 439—454, 1920.
Jaeger, J. R.: Ligation and resection of the superior longitudinal sinus. Arch. Neurol. Psychiat. (Chic.) 48: 977—987, 1942.
— Observations on resection of the superior longitudinal sinus anterior and posterior of the Rolandic venous inflow. J. Neurosurg. 8: 103—109, 1951.
Klestadt, W.: Zerebrale Symptomenkomplexe bei otogener Sinusphlebitis. Z. Laryngol. Rhinol. 13: 83—105, 1924.
Leissring, J. C., Vorlicky, N.: Disseminated intravascular coagulation in a neonate. Amer. J. Dis. Child. 115: 100—106, 1966.
Lhermitte, J., Lerebouillet, J., Kaplan, B.: Ramollissment hémorrhagique d'origine veineuse chez un enfant atteint de malformation cardiaque. Rev. Neurol. 65: 305—312, 1936.
McAlpine, D.: Toxic hydrocephalus. Brain 60: 180—203, 1937.
Marburg, O., Casamajor, L.: Phlebostasis and phlebothrombosis of the brain in the newborn and in early childhood Arch. Neurol. Psychiat. (Chic.) 52: 170—188, 1944.
— Rezek, R. R., Marks, M. B.: Porencephaly. II. Studies in phlebothrombosis and phlebostasis. J. Neuropath. exp. Neurol. 4: 43—58, 1945.
Mehrotra, R. M.: Experimental studies of changes which occur in ligated arteries and veins. J. Path. Bact. 65: 307—313, 1953.
Messen, H., Stochdorph, O.: Die venöse Thrombose. In: Hdb. spec. path. Anat. 13/1 B, pp. 1452—1464. Berlin-Göttingen-Heidelberg: Springer 1957.
Norman, R. M.: Bilateral atrophic lobar sclerosis following thrombosis of the superior longitudinal sinus. J. Neurol. Psychiat. 17: 135—152, 1936.
Parrot, M. J.: Etude sur le ramollissement de l'encéphale chez le nouveau-né. Arch. Physiol. Norm. Path. (Paris) 5: 59—73; 176—195; 283—303, 1873.
Russell, D. S.: Observations on the Pathology of Hydrocephalus. Med. Res. Council Special Rep. Series No. 265. London: Her Majesty's Stat. Off. 1949.
— Hydrocephalus. A. Res. Nerv. Ment. Dis. Proc. 34: 160—175, 1954.
Schwartz, P., Fink, L.: Morphologie und Entstehung der geburtstraumatischen Blutungen im Gehirn und Schädel des Neugeborenen. Z. Kinderheilk. 40: 427—474, 1925.
Simpson, R.: Thrombosis of cerebral vessels in infants. Canad. M.A.J. 26: 317—319, 1932.
Symonds, C. P.: Otitic hydrocephalus. Brain 54: 55—71, 1931.
Weber, G.: Hirnabszesse und zerebrale venöse Thrombosen bei kongenitalen Herzfehlern. Schweiz. med. Wschr. 87: 159—162, 1957.
Woolf, A. L.: The pathology of acute infantile cerebral diplegia. J. ment. Sci. 101: 610—628, 1955.
Zischinsky, H.: Über Vorkommen und Klinik von Thrombosen, insbesondere von Sinusthrombosen und Blutungen des Gehirns und seiner Häute und Embolien am akut Infektionskranken. Kind. Jb. Kinderheilk. 124: 35—71, 1929.

14. Cerebral Lesions in Congenital Cardiac Disease

Congenital cardiac disease is frequently complicated by cerebral lesions. Berthrong and Sabiston (1951) reviewed findings in the central nervous system of 162 cases older than one year, 135 of which were cyanotic, 27 acyanotic. In the cyanotic group there were 25 cases of cerebral infarcts and 8 with hemorrhages, mostly petechiae; five had thrombosis of intracranial sinus or veins, and five had abscesses. Various lesions were found in 8 of the 27 acyanotic cases. A series of 500 cases was published by Terplan (1973).

Of the cerebral lesions associated with congenital cardiac disease, cerebral abscesses have attracted greatest attention, particularly since antibiotics and improved diagnostic and surgical techniques have made them amenable to treatment (Matson and Salam, 1961).

Abscesses. The first observation of a cerebral abscess associated with congenital cardiac disease was made by Farre (1814), but the causal relationship between the two diseases was recognized by Ballet (1880). The reports by Hanna (1941), Marone (1950), Sancetta and Zimmermann (1950), Clark and Clarke (1952), Gluck *et al.* (1952), Newton (1956) and Weber (1957) review the casuistic literature, which increased during this period from 29 to 79 cases.

Cerebral abscesses are found in approximately 4 to 7 percent of patients with congenital cardiac disease (Clark and Clarke, 1952). Two-thirds occurred between the ages of 5 and 20; a preference for the teens is still more striking if only the cases of tetralogy of Fallot are considered. Cerebral abscesses are exceedingly rare below the age of five years, and none have been reported below the age of three (Marone, 1950). There is no striking sex predilection, but males are slightly more frequent.

The vast majority of abscesses occur in association with cyanotic cardiac disease, most frequently with tetralogy of Fallot which accounts for approximately 50 percent. Next in frequency are interventricular septal defects and a wide open foramen ovale. Other types of congenital cardiac anomalies account for only a few cases each. The common denominator of these lesions is a defect permitting the mixture of arterial and venous blood; this is further substantiated by the occurrence of cerebral abscesses with arteriovenous pulmonary fistulas. Le Roux (1959) found 10 examples of pulmonary arteriovenous fistula complicated by cerebral abscess.

The source of infection is usually obscure. Previous infective processes were detected in approximately one-fourth of the cases and include infections of the respiratory tract, teeth, oral cavity or pharynx. Clinical symptoms attributable to the abscess may be vague—headache, lethargy and vomiting being most frequent. Subacute bacterial endocarditis is not a typical source of abscess formation and has been found in only a few cases. Cerebral abscesses complicating congenital cardiac disease need to be distinguished from the local propagation of infectious disease processes such as otitis which may occur independently (Marone, 1950).

The vast majority of abscesses complicating congenital cardiac disease are solitary and only 10 to 20 percent are multiple. Abscesses are distributed with uniform frequency in frontal (Fig. 52), parietal, occipital, or temporal lobes. Hanna (1941) emphasized a predilection for the right hemisphere, but Clark and Clarke (1952) described a two to one preference for the left; no trend of lateralization is evident in later reports. Most abscesses occupy the subcortical white matter of the respective lobes. Few are found in the thalamus or cerebellum. Streptococcus and mixed infections are the most frequent causative organisms, but a variety of others, including actinomyces, have also been observed. Abscesses may rupture into the ventricles or subarachnoid space, with ensuing acute massive purulent meningitis running a rapid, fatal course.

The most significant factor in the formation of these abscesses is evidently the mingling of venous with arterial blood, escaping filtration through the pulmonary capillaries. It is not clear whether local colonization from persistent or intermittent bacteremia, septic microemboli, or superinfection of bland vasculo-occlusive lesions are the mechanisms inducing abscess formation. It is unlikely, however, that abscesses are merely septic complications of phlebothrombotic or arterial occlusive infarcts; they differ from the former in age distribution and from the latter in type and localization. Hanna (1941) observed early abscess formation in a large cerebral infarct, but this appears to be an exception. The most probable sources of abscess formation are septic microemboli derived from minor foci of infection.

Phlebothrombosis. The clinical and pathologic features of phlebothrombosis complicating congenital cardiac disease are the same as those of phlebothrombosis complicating other general diseases in infants (Chapter 13). The reports of Dellille *et al.* (1936), Lhermitte *et al.* (1936), Graser and Burkhard (1953), Berthrong and Sabiston (1951) and Weber (1951) show that this complication occurs mainly in infants under 2 years of age. Among 25 autopsy cases of cerebral infarcts with congenital cardiac disease, only 3 had arterial occlusion; 22 had venous occlusion, 18 of them in the superior sagittal sinus (Cottrill and Kaplan, 1973). Terplan (1973), conversely, considers phlebothrombosis rare.

Infarcts. The frequency of cerebral infarcts as a complication of congenital cardiac disease is difficult to estimate as larger series of cases can only be collected in institutions having facilities for their surgical treatment, which in itself may alter the frequency of embolic infarcts. In the series of Berthrong and Sabiston (1951) 15 of 19 recent cerebral infarcts were postoperative, 6 hours to 20 days after surgery. Old infarcts, antedating surgery, or in cases without surgery, were found in 15 cases. Cohen (1960) reports old encephalomalacia in 9 of 100 cases and Gluck *et al.* (1952) in 5 of 39, which approximates a frequency of 10 percent. In Terplan's series (1973) more than 17 percent of 500 patients had cerebral infarcts, and these were 4 to 5 times more frequent for patients having had surgery or cardiac catheterization.

The size of the lesions varies. Large cerebral infarcts—ischemic or hemorrhagic—occur most often in the territory of the middle cerebral artery, which may be occluded by an organized thrombus. Thrombi or thromboemboli are also demonstrated in the carotid arteries or in small cortical arterial branches (Terplan, 1973). Small lesions range from minor cortical infarcts to old microscopic scars. Multiple, small foci of necrosis and myelin loss in white matter were reported by Bodechtel (1932) and Cohen (1960) but are not common findings in other studies; their presence was reemphasized by Terplan (1973).

The large infarcts are most likely the result of thromboemboli, some paradoxic from the peripheral circulation, others from endocardial thrombi; infarcts in lung, heart, kidney and spleen are more frequent in patients having cerebral lesions than in those having none (Berthrong and Sabiston, 1951). Polycytemia with increased tendency of local thrombus formation has to be considered as an alternate cause of vascular occlusion. Occurrence of carotid thrombosis is rare; findings in a girl with congenital cardiac disease and bilateral carotid artery thrombosis were described by Mymin (1960).

Clarkson *et al.* (1967) drew attention to a cerebral complication induced

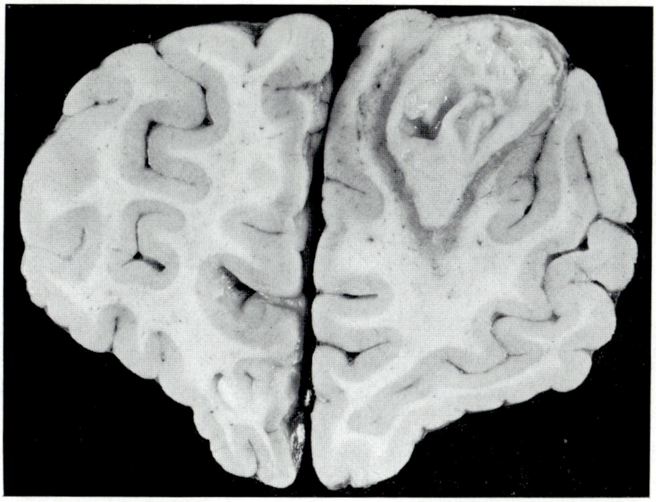

Fig. 52. Frontal abscess complicating congenital cardiac disease

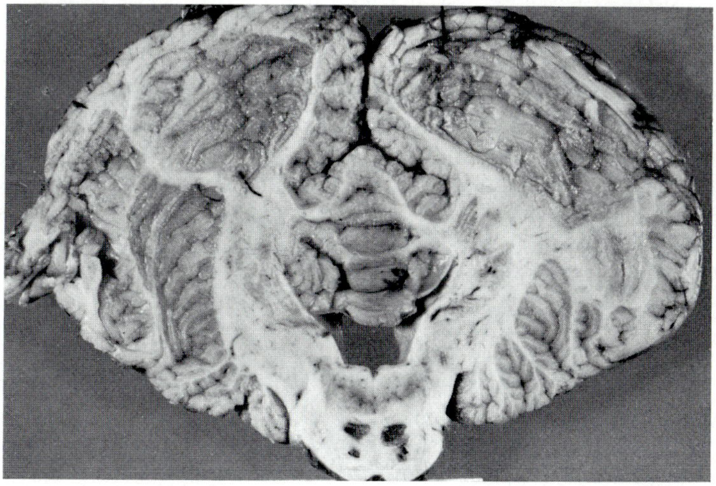

Fig. 53. Bilateral pontine infarcts in an infant with congenital cardiac disease (see text)

by Blalock-Toussig operation for the correction of tetralogy of Fallot. The surgical shunting of the subclavian and pulmonary arteries entails the risk of reduced perfusion in the vertebro-basilar system, and clinical histories of hemiplegia following surgery have been reported. Anatomic description of corresponding lesions are still extant. Terplan (1973) reported a case of cavitated infarcts in the basis pontis in an infant with Blalock-Toussig operation, but there was a thromboembolus in the basilar artery. Similar infarcts in a 3-year-old girl with transposition of great vessels, who had previously undergone balloon septostomy and atrial septectomy, are shown in Fig. 53. There were also multiple recent and old infarcts in the cerebral hemispheres.

This particular pattern of pontine infarction appears to be rare, apparently relating to congenital cardiac disease, but its pathogenesis is not clear.

Aneurysms. Cerebral aneurysms in association with congenital cardiovascular disease occur specifically in aortic stenosis. A first description was given by Eppinger (1871) for a 15-year-old boy with isthmus stenosis and bilateral aneurysms of the anterior cerebral arteries. Aneurysms are found in the distribution typical of berry aneurysms in the circle of Willis and are often multiple. Death occurs most frequently between 23 and 35 years from rupture of the aneurysm with fatal subarachnoid hemorrhage, but patients have been known to survive to advanced age (Wolfman and Shelden, 1927).

Other Lesions. The severe anoxia caused by congenital cardiac disease typically does not produce diffuse neuronal changes. No case of anoxic encephalopathy was found among the 162 cases of Berthrong and Sabiston (1951). One case of diffuse cortical change among 100 was reported by Cohen (1960). Courville (1955) described slight sponginess in the upper cortical layers in a 24-day-old infant with congenital cardiac disease, arhinencephaly, and numerous other malformations; the infant had to be resuscitated and had convulsions since birth, both events being the most probable cause of the diffuse cortical changes. Numerous cases of diffuse cortical necrosis were found in Terplan's (1973) series, but they were related to severe intra- or post-surgical hypotension.

Considerable attention has been paid in the German literature to the extensive congestion of leptomeningeal veins, which is observed in some patients with congential cardiac disease but is absent in the majority. The pertinent observations were reviewed by Erbslöh (1958). Congestion of dilated vessels may also be seen within the nervous tissue (Meessen and Storchdorph, 1952) and was mistaken for an increased incidence of telangiectesia (Cohen, 1960). These alterations are evidently without clinical consequence. Meessen and Storchdorph (1952) attributed an apparently increased vascularity in brain tissue to vascular dilation and denied the presence of a true increase in the number of vessels. Quantitative studies of leptomeningeal vascular density gave inconclusive results (Pollter, 1956).

Terplan (1973) drew attention to the occasional occurrence of nodular encephalitic changes in patients with congenital cardiac disease.

Subendocardial Fibroelastosis. Thrombotic occlusions of middle cerebral arteries with corresponding cerebral infarcts were found in two children, 2 years and 14 months old, suffering from subendocardial fibroelastosis (Stevens, 1959; Castroviejo and Larrauri, 1971); no sources of thromboembolus formation were found in the heart or elsewhere, and the significance of the association of these lesions is still not clear.

References

Ballet, G.: Des abscès du cerveau consécutifs à certaines malformations cardiaques. Arch. gén. Méd. 5: 659—667, 1880.

Berthrong, M., Sabiston, D. C., Jr.: Cerebral lesions in congenital heart disease. Bull. Johns Hopk. Hosp. 89: 384—406, 1951.

Bodechtel, G.: Gehirnveränderungen bei Herzkrankheiten. Z. Neurol. 140: 657—709, 1932.

Castroviejo, I. P., Larrauri, J.: Bilateral thrombosis of the middle cerebral artery in a child aged 14 months. Develop. Med. Child. Neurol. 13: 613—624, 1971.

Clark, D. B., Clarke, E. S.: Brain abscess as a complication of congenital cardiac malformation. Trans. Amer. neurol. Ass. 77: 73—76, 1952.

Clarkson, P., Gomez, M., Wallace, R., Weidman, W.: CNS complications following Blalock Toussig operation. Pediatrics 39: 18—23, 1967.

Cohen, M. M.: The central nervous system in congenital heart disease. Neurology 10: 452—456, 1960.

Cottrill, C. M., Kaplan, S.: Cerebral vascular accidents in cyanotic congenital heart disease. Amer. J. Dis. Child. 125: 484—494, 1973.

Courville, C. B.: Case studies in cerebral anoxia. VII. Focal cortical necrosis superimposed upon a malformed brain in a case of congenital heart disease. Bull. Los Angeles Neurol. Soc. 20: 69—73, 1955.

Dellille, A., Lhermitte, I., Lesobre, R.: Ramollissement hémorrhagique d'origine veineuse chez un enfant atteint de malformation cardiaque. Rev. Neurol. 66: 754—759, 1936.

Eppinger, A.: Stenosis aortae congenita seu isthmus persisteus. Vjschr. prakt. Heilk. 112: 31—67, 1871.

Erbslöh, F.: Das Zentralnervensystem bei Krankheiten des Herzens und der Lungen. In: Handb. Spec. Path. 13/2/B, Henke Lubarsch, Berlin-Göttingen-Heidelberg: Springer 1958.

Farre, J. R.: On Malformation of the Human Heart. London: Longmans 1814.

Gluck, R., Hall, J., Stevenson, H.: Brain abscess associated with congenital heart disease. Pediatrics 9: 192—203, 1952.

Graser, F., Burkhard, I.: Die marantische Sinusthrombose als Komplikation des Morbus caeruleus im Säuglingsalter. Medizinische (Stuttgart) 1953: 1195—1195.

Hanna, R.: Cerebral abscess and paradoxic embolism associated with congenital heart disease. Amer. J. Dis. Child. 62: 555—567, 1941.

Lhermitte, J., Lerebouillet, J., Kaplan, B.: Ramollissement hémorrhagique d'origine veineuse chez un enfant atteint de malformation cardiaque. Rev. Neurol. 65: 305—312, 1936.

Le Roux, B. T.: Pulmonary arteriovenous fistulae. Quart. J. Med. 28: 1—19, 1959.

Marone, R. F.: Brain abscess and congenital heart disease. Ann. Int. Med. 33: 602—606, 1950.

Matson, D., Salam, M.: Brain abscess in congenital heart disease. Pediatrics 27: 772—788, 1961.

Meessen, H., Storchdorph, O.: Gehirnbefunde bei Morbus caeruleus. Proc. I. Int. Congr. Neuropath. III, pp. 469—477. Torino: Rosenberg & Sellier 1952.

Mymin, D.: Carotid thrombosis in childhood, Arch. Dis. Child. 35: 515—518, 1960.

Newton, E. J.: Hematogenous brain abscess in cyanotic congenital heart disease. Quart. J. Med. (Oxf.) 25: 201—220, 1956.

Pollter, J.: Untersuchungen an Blutgefäßen der Leptomeninx bei kongenitalen Herzfehlern mit Mischungszyanose. Virchow Arch. Path. Anat. 329: 73—93, 1956.

Sancetta, S. M., Zimmerman, H. A.: Congenital heart disease with septal defects in which paradoxical brain abscess causes death. Circulation 1: 593—601, 1950.

Stevens, H.: Carotid artery occlusions in childhood. Pediatrics 23: 699—709, 1959.

Terplan, K. L.: Patterns of brain damage in infants and children with congenital heart disease. Association with catheterization and surgical procedures. Amer. J. Dis. Child. 125: 175—185, 1973.

Weber, G.: Hirnabszesse und cerebrale venöse Thrombosen bei kongenitalen Herzfehlern. Schweiz. med. Wschr. 87: 159—162, 1957.

Wolfman, H. W., Shelden, W. D.: Neurologic complications associated with congenital stenosis of the aorta. Arch. Neurol. Psychiat. 17: 303—316, 1927.

Yater, W. M., Finnegan, J., Giffin, H. M.: Pulmonary arteriovenous fistula (varix); review of literature and report of 2 cases. J.A.M.A. 141: 581—589, 1949.

15. Cranio-Cerebral Trauma in Infancy

Infants comprise only a small fraction of the total number of cases of cranio-cerebral trauma encountered in neuropathology. The lesions found in infants and children older than 1 or 2 years do not differ in principle from those seen in adults. Numerous excellent descriptions of the pathologic features of lacerations, contusions, and of the various types of traumatic hemorrhages—epidural, subdural, subarachnoid and intracerebral—are available in the medical literature, and describing them here would exceed the

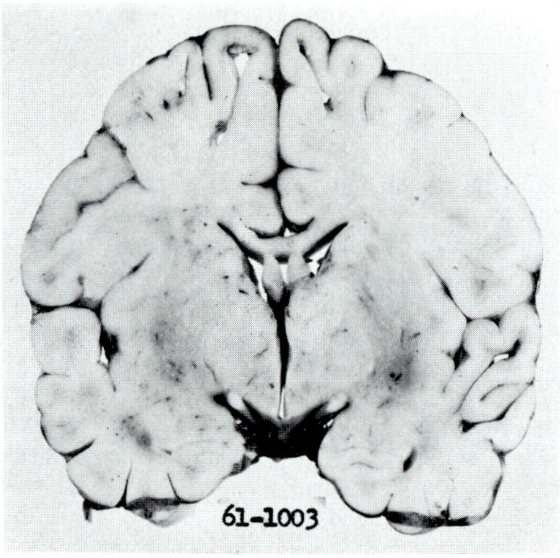

Fig. 54. Traumatic tears in the hemispheric white matter (courtesy of Dr. Lindenberg)

limitations of this text; reference is made only to lesions characteristic of infancy.

Cerebral Lesions from Blunt Trauma in Early Infancy. Contusions in the adult brain result from a mechanical interaction between the rigid cranium and the apposing cerebral tissue. The characteristics of the interaction are modified in early infancy by the open fontanels and the pliability of the bones which allow for much greater deformation of the cranium and brain than is possible later in life. These mechanical properties of the immature skull evidently account for the fact that typical cortical contusions are rarely seen in infants less than 1 year old.

Cerebral lesions characteristic of trauma in early infancy were described by Lindenberg and Freytag (1969) who found them in autopsies of 16 infants, all younger than 5 months, but could not find them in 52 older infants, 6 months to 2 years. The latter group showed contusions, hemorrhages and necrosis of the brain similar to those found in adults. The young infants had suffered closed head injuries from a blunt force, due either to falling or to being struck on the head. Their lesions consisted of tears of the white matter, which formed grossly visible slit-like or irregular cavities (Fig. 54), mostly in the orbital and temporal white matter and in the first or second frontal convolutions. Tears were commonly bilateral and extended occasionally from the white matter into the cortex or into the walls of the lateral ventricles, or into both. Bleeding into the torn tissue was usually slight, and hemorrhagic lesions outside of the tears were uncommon.

Recent tears in infants that had died upon the insult were difficult to distinguish from artefacts, except for the occurrence of local hemorrhages. Reactive changes consisting of astrocytic hypertrophy and microglial proliferation in the torn tissue had developed after 36 hours and became marked by the third day. Astrocytic fibrosis was marked after 1 month, but changes in myelin stains were slight at any phase of survival. Lindenberg and Freytag (1969) also mentioned a variant of this lesion, consisting of horizontal tears through the crests of gyri. Cerebral tears were attributed to shearing forces within the subcortical white matter produced by rapid and extreme deformation of the brain, made possible by the pliability of the infant's skull.

Growing Skull Fracture of Childhood. Persisting and enlarging skull fractures in infants have been described under the names of leptomeningeal cysts, growing skull fracture, cephalhydrocele, post-traumatic porencephaly, spurious meningocele and others. Most case reports are clinical observations in the neurosurgical literature, and there is a great deal of confusion of these lesions and arachnoid cysts (Chapter 20), meningoceles (Chapter 23) and porencephaly (Chapter 11). Growing skull fracture was first described by Howship (1816) for a child who fell down a flight of stairs at the age of 9 months. There was no wound in the scalp but the right parietal bone had an oblong impression 1 × 3 inches immediately after injury. The child was unconscious initially and was subsequently found to be paretic on the left side. Within 14 days a pulsation was noticed at the site of the impression. A smooth-edged defect was palpable at the age of 4 years and the pulsations of the brain were clearly felt through the scalp. Howship comments that the lesion is not very rare and that eventual regrowth of the bone may occur later in life. The first pathologic observations were reported by Rokitansky (1856) for an 8-month-old child having a cranial aperture, 6 × 4 cm, containing a fluid-filled membranous bag overlaying a dural opening; there was brain injury in the subjacent cortical tissue. There are numerous case reports on growing skull fractures in the literature, among them a series of 7 by Taveras and Ransohoff (1953). The comprehensive review by Lende and Erickson (1961) lists 61 quotations. It may be of interest that some of the defects found in prehistoric skulls have been attributed tentatively to growing fractures rather than to therapeutic or ritual trepanations.

The trauma producing growing skull fractures occurs within the first year of life for more than half of the cases, and under the age of 3 for 90 percent. The parietal bone or the parietal bone and one adjacent bone are most often affected. Occurrence in the occipital bone is rare. The initial traumatic event is a skull fracture without laceration of the scalp. Examination by X-ray as well as palpation evidence the formation of a defect and its subsequent enlargement during the ensuing weeks. The initial enlargement may proceed rapidly to near maximum size, followed by a slower continued widening. The resultant bone defect is irregular in shape, having scalloped margins, and there is some degree of sclerosis in the adjacent bone. The defect tends to be oblong, its axis corresponding to that of the fracture which may still be apparent at the poles of the defect. Both tables of the bone are involved, the inner often to a greater extent than the outer, but the reverse has been observed as well. The dura always shows a defect and may be deficient for an area larger than the bone defect; the opening may be filled by a fibrous neomembrane. The bone defect contains an arachnoid cyst of irregular configuration filled with a clear fluid which, on examination, has been found to be identical in composition to CSF. In some cases brain tissue herniates into the bone defect (Stein and Tenner, 1972). The leptomeninges show adhesions and collagen scarring, and brain damage is said to be consistently present. Compared with the numerous surgical reports, detailed neuropathologic studies of the coexistent brain damage are almost nil. Some of the cases reported as porencephaly in the older literature were evidently cerebral lesions associated with growing fractures: for example, large cystic defects of the cerebral hemispheres were found directly underneath an oblong parietal bone defect dating to early infancy (Meschede, 1866; von Kahlden, case 8, 1895). The case by the latter author is perhaps unique in that the skull fracture appeared to be the result of multiple attempts at instrumental delivery. A recent case reported by Döpper *et al.* (1972) showed, 99 days after the trauma, at the age of 10 months, a large hematoma in the left frontal lobe, and extensive bilateral cortical ischemic necrosis and hydrocephalus.

The development of growing skull fractures depends on the presence of an initial bone fracture with tearing of the dura, local hemorrhage and interposition of tissue between the fracture faces. It is not clear to what extent the associated cerebral injury contributes to the formation of the growing fracture; its significance may lie in local tissue damage, or in terms of a general increase in intracranial pressure facilitating herniation into the fracture. The factors responsible for formation of growing fractures were studied experimentally (Goldstein *et al.*, 1967). Simple craniotomy wounds in dogs and puppies healed without difficulty. The interposition of dura, pericranium or muscle into the craniotomy wound prevented healing in 96 percent without producing growing fractures. The latter developed in 53 percent of the experiments if a dural pouch was formed in the craniotomy and the arachnoid was opened. Additional damage to pia or brain did not increase the incidence of growing fractures. In another study (Rosenthal *et al.*, 1970) the authors demonstrated that the cyst in the craniotomy site was not in open communication with the cerebrospinal fluid spaces, and was not reached by india ink injected into the subarachnoid space.

References

Döpper, Th., Spaar, F. W., Orthner, H.: Zur Neuropathologie des posttraumatischen Hirndrucks im Kindesalter. Zugleich in „Beitrag zur Klinik und Pathogenese der wachsenden Schädelfraktur". Z. Neurol. 202: 37—51, 1972.

Goldstein, F. P., Sakoda, T., Kepes, J. J., *et al.*: Enlarging skull fractures: An experimental study. J. Neurosurg. 27: 541—550, 1967.

Howship, J.: Practical Observations in Surgery and Morbid Anatomy, pp. 33—35. London: Longman, Hurst, Rees, Orme, and Brown 1816.

Lende, R. A., Erickson, T. C.: Growing skull fractures in childhood. J. Neurosurg. 18: 479—489, 1961.
Lindenberg, R., Freytag, E.: Morphology of brain lesions from blunt trauma in early infancy. Arch. Path. 87: 298—305, 1969.
Meschede, F.: Über Classification der Geisteskrankheiten und über die essentielle Verschiedenheit paralytischer und gewisser epileptischer Blödsinnsformen, erläutert an einem Fall von Porencephalie. Virchow Arch. 34: 300—327, 1866.
Rokitansky, C.: Lehrbuch der pathologischen Anatomie, 3rd ed., p. 2. Wien: Braumüller 1856.
Rosenthal, W. A. E., Grieshop, J., Freeman, L. M., *et al.*: Experimental observations on enlarging skull fractures. J. Neurosurg. 32: 431—434, 1970.
Stein, B. M., Tenner, M. S.: Enlargement of skull fracture in childhood due to cerebral herniation. Arch. Neurol. (Chic.) 26: 137—143, 1972.
Taveras, J., Ransohoff, J.: Leptomeningeal cysts of the brain following trauma with erosion of the skull: A study of seven cases treated by surgery. J. Neurosurg. 10: 233—241, 1953.
Tenner, M. S., Stein, B. M.: Cerebral herniation in the growing fracture of the skull. Radiology 94: 351—355, 1970.
von Kahlden, C.: Porencephalie. Beitr. path. Anat. 18: 231—404, 1895.

16. Fetal Infections

A discussion of the pathology of fetal infections must be cognizant of the fact that infection of the fetus may cause two rather different types of lesions: First, there may be the inflammatory and destructive changes characteristic of infectious processes in general. Secondly, the tissue damage resulting from the infection may derange the subsequent development of the organ, leaving malformations in its wake. These two components may coexist or overlap. The first type of lesion is readily identified during the active phase of the disease when inflammatory changes are present, and when the causative organism may be seen in the tissue, or recovered from it. Diagnostic difficulties become greater once the active phase of the inflammation has subsided; the residual tissue damage may be morphologically similar to that caused by noninfectious processes damaging the brain at the same age. The periventricular tissue, for example, is rather prone to become involved from infections spreading through the cerebral ventricles, but it is also a site of predilection for various asphyctic lesions (Chapter 4; Differential Diagnosis); further, lesions of different etiologies may cause similar secondary tissue reactions, *e.g.*, mineralization. The etiologic classification of such residual tissue damage may be difficult, *e.g.*, for rubella infection of the fetus. There are, for example, reports on granulomatous encephalitis in infancy (Wyatt and Tribby, 1952; Sturgill and Brown, 1966) referring to lesions that had all the features of asphyctic periventricular infarcts.

It is even more difficult to define, for a given case, the relation between fetal infection and cerebral malformation. The association of certain malformations, such as polymicrogyria, with active or residual fetal infectious processes has been reported, and such observations are consistent with experimental data on the induction of malformations by fetal infections, as reviewed later in this chapter. Such data, however, do not permit generalization. Many malformations can be induced by a variety of infectious as well as noninfectious agents and the factual evidence linking malformation of the human brain with infection during pregnancy is meager. Baron *et al.* (1969) searched for serologic evidence of fetal infection by cytomegalovirus, herpes simplex, rubella and toxoplasma in a series of 62 microcephalic, 42 retarded normocephalic and 44 normal infants and found no significant difference in the frequencies of infections. The authors concluded that most cases of mental retardation are of other causes, although fetal infections may be responsible for a few. Sixteen viral antigens were determined in 54 cases with congenital central nervous system anomalies and 104 matched controls without showing correlation between serologic evidence of maternal viral infection during pregnancy and fetal nervous system anomalies (Elizan *et al.*, 1969). Evidence of viral infection during pregnancy was found in a considerable number of mothers that had normal babies. These selected references illustrate some of the difficulties involved in relating malformations of the nervous system to fetal infection.

Rubella Embryopathy. Gregg (1942) recognized the relation between an increased incidence of congenital cataracts and maternal infection with rubella during the Australian epidemic in 1940. His observations on the rubella syndrome of cataracts, deafness, congenital heart disease and dental anomalies were amply confirmed in the subsequent literature. The risk of fetal malformation from maternal rubella infection during the first trimester of pregnancy had been greatly exaggerated in early retrospective studies. Prospective studies indicated a risk of approximately 10 to 12 percent, but this is still about 6 times the risk of an uncomplicated pregnancy (Greenberg and Pelleteri, 1957; Ingalls and Purshottan, 1953; Blattner and Heys, 1961). Malformations occur most frequently for infection during the early phases of pregnancy. Dekaban *et al.* (1958) analyzed 108 patients and found highest incidence of malformations when the infection had occurred during the first 4 weeks of gestation; the incidence was much lower up to the 10th week of gestation; no instances were found after the 20th week. The spread of the infection to the fetus occurs during maternal viremia which may last up to 1 week during the initial stage of the maternal disease. Recovery of virus from the products of conception showed a much higher incidence of placental than of fetal infection (Alford *et al.*, 1964; Monif *et al.*, 1965), indicating the possibility that the fetus may be affected in different ways by either fetal infection or damage to the placenta (Ornoy *et al.*, 1973). Fetal infection apparently results in an extremely high incidence of clinical stigmata; the virus continues to replicate in the tissue once infection has taken hold. Histologic examination of 57 fetuses from therapeutic abortions for maternal rubella disclosed cell necrosis affecting the given organs only at certain stages of primordial differentiation and without apparent inflammatory response (Töndury and Smith, 1966). This investigation, however, disclosed a frequency of histologic changes far in excess of the established risk for fetal infection. The effect of the virus on cultures of human tissue consists of a tissue-selective inhibition of cell replication by the continued growth of the virus (Plotkin *et al.*, 1965); a higher incidence of chromosomal breaks was also observed, but its importance in human pathology is not established.

A series of 271 abnormal infants from the 1964 rubella epidemic in the United States (Cooper and Krugman, 1967) showed congenital heart disease at 52 percent, consisting mostly of patent ductus arteriosus, with or without stenosis of pulmonary artery or atrial and ventricular septal defects. Partial, unilateral or bilateral loss of hearing occurred at 52 percent, due to damage to the organ of Corti. Ocular changes, occurring at 40 percent, included cataracts and, less frequently, microphthalmus, buphthalmus or retinopathy. Psychomotor retardation was moderate to severe for 24 percent, slight for 16 percent, often associated with microcephaly. Other anomalies were talipes equinovarus, syndactyly, hypospadias, general muscular weakness, damage to olfactory bulb and dental anomalies.

In addition to these developmental defects, a high incidence of persistent chronic infection with rubella virus has been demonstrated by its recovery from the patients several months after birth (Monif and Sever, 1966), disappearing eventually during postnatal life. Manifestations of continued infection include neonatal thrombocytopenia, hepatosplenomegaly, meningoencephalitis, pneumonitis, myocarditis and hepatitis. An interference with cell replication by continued growth of the virus is probably responsible for retardation in the growth of various organs, with subnormal numbers of cells per organ (Naeye and Blanc, 1965).

Data on the neuropathologic aspects of the rubella syndrome are still limited; the most definite information refers to the changes resulting from persistent viral infection. The clinical picture of meningoencephalitis consists of lethargy, bulging fontanel, increased protein content of CSF with presence of virus therein, retardation of cranial growth and a wide range of neurologic abnormalities (Desmond *et al.*, 1967). The process may be quiescent for as long as 13 months after birth and activated by postnatal stress (Michaels, 1966). Surviving infants show microcephaly, intracranial calcifications, severe mental retardation, seizures, deafness and focal neurologic defects. The cerebral lesions consist of chronic meningitis with moderately dense infiltrates of mononuclear cells, lymphocytes and plasma cells in the leptomeninges and in perivascular spaces. Small foci of necrosis occur in the nervous parenchyma and were tentatively attributed to vasculitis (Yow, 1965; Singer *et al.*, 1967). The 6 infants described by Rorke and Spiro (1967) had inactive lesions consisting of vascular mineralization and intima proliferation, conceivably as part of a general rubellar vasculopathy (Chapter 12) and multiple foci of necrosis, thought to differ from periventricular infarcts in terms of their wide dissemination. However, 4 of the infants had multiloculated subependymal cysts in the matrix tissue similar to those resulting from subependymal hemorrhage (Chapter 2). Singer *et al.* (1967) also illustrate lesions indistinguishable from periventricular infarcts produced by perinatal asphyxia (Chapter 4). Pneumencephalographic evidence of aqueduct occlusion in a case was reported recently by Sarwar *et al.* (1974). Naeye and Blanc (1965) list unilateral atresia of the foramen of Luschka, a frontal cyst interpreted as periventricular infarct, vascular mineralization, hydrocephalus and subarachnoid hemorrhage; many of these lesions must be considered of questionable relation to the rubella syndrome. These reports attest to the difficulties of separating specific lesions attributable to the rubella syndrome from those of nonspecific perinatal damage.

The brain weight is affected by the general retardation of organ growth, probably caused by continued viral replication. The average brain weight of affected newborns was 72 percent of normal; that of infants 1 to 3 months, 79 percent of normal (Naeye and Blanc, 1965). Delayed myelination of fiber tracts described by Rorke and Spiro (1967) is probably component of this general growth retardation.

Evidence for the causation of specific cerebral malformations by fetal rubella infection is inconclusive. Kappers (1957) described cranioschisis and exencephaly for a 7 week fetus infected at the age of 33 days, but this case cannot be considered exemplary since anencephaly and meningomyelocele are conspicuously absent from the stigmata of rubella embryopathy. Swan (1949) lists a number of lesions in sporadic cases, the most definite of which is the infant with agenesis of corpus callosum described by Friedman and Cohen (1947); in this case attribution to rubella infection rests merely on the mother's report of a rash on her lower extremities during the second month of pregnancy. There is no evidence, therefore, for the relationship between the rubella syndrome and specific cerebral malformations, except micrencephaly.

Generalized Cytomegalic Inclusion Disease. Generalized infection with cytomegalovirus or generalized salivary virus disease is almost entirely confined to newborns; its occurrence in older children or adults is rare. The fetus seems to become infected during the initial viremia of a mostly asymptomatic maternal infection which occurs in about 6 percent of pregnancies; affectation of the fetus in subsequent pregnancies is virtually unknown. In several instances only one of twins was affected (Shearer *et al.* 1972). Routine autopsy studies disclose a fairly high incidence of 10 to 32 percent of nonsymptomatic infection of the salivary glands in children, but it is not clear whether this indicates that a fetal infection takes a localized, nonsymptomatic course for many or else a restriction and lesser severity of the process when the infection occurs during early infancy (Weller and Hanshaw, 1962). The presence of generalized disease in autopsy series is 1 or 2 percent, and about half of the affected infants are premature (Seifert and Oehme, 1957), compared to about one-fourth prematurity for toxoplasma (Feldman and Miller, 1956). Generalized cytomegalic inclusion disease simulates fetal erythroblastosis, including extreme hepatosplenomegaly, jaundice, erythroblastic anemia, thrombocytopenia, petechiae and diarrhea. Symptoms appear shortly after birth, and the disease usually runs a fatal course within days or weeks. An acute fatal course involves the central nervous system in approximately 10 percent of cases (Medearis, 1957), but the incidence of cerebral affection appears to be much higher in survivors. Neurologic abnormalities were found in more than half of the infants in the series of Weller and Hanshaw (1962) and McCracken *et al.* (1969), mostly microcephaly, mental retardation and cerebral calcification, or diplegia, seizures, deafness and chorioretinitis. The course of the disease is more variable in cases in whom the symptoms first appear during the postnatal period. Infection in older children or adults often occurs superimposed on other chronic disease processes. There is no evidence of sex preference.

The infection locates preferentially in the epithelia of ducts of excretory organs, particularly the convoluted tubules of the kidney, in the bronchial epithelia and alveolar linings of the lung, and in the pancreatic and salivary ducts, but it has also been found in endocrine glands and other organs. The predilection for ducts facilitates clinical diagnosis, as proposed by Wyatt *et al.* (1950), by locating the affected enlarged cells, often called "owl eye cells", in the urine. Confirmation is obtained by recovery and cultivation of the virus. The disease was reviewed by Smith and Vellios (1950), Seifert

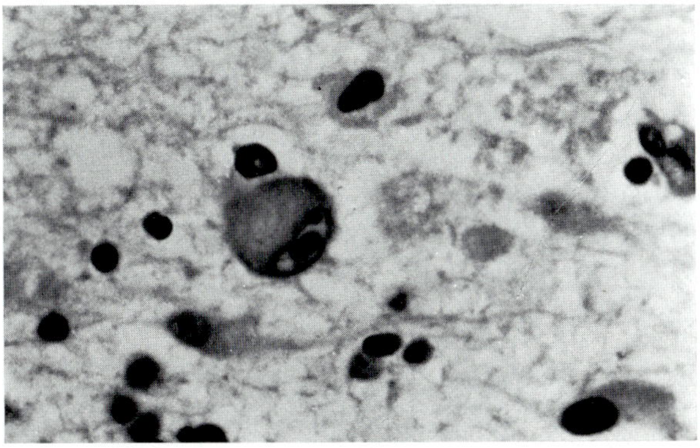

Fig. 55. Intranuclear inclusion in cytomegalic inclusion disease (courtesy of Dr. Schochet)

and Oehme (1957), Medearis (1957), Smith (1959), Wolf and Cowen (1959) and others.

A comprehensive description of the cerebral lesions was given by Haymaker *et al.* (1954) who emphasized the preferential distribution in the olfactory bulb and the walls of the lateral ventricles, far less frequently in the walls of the third and fourth ventricles. This peculiar pattern was explained by a predilection of the infection for the germinal matrix tissue. Periventricular lesions occur in more than half of the cases, but lesions are also common in the cerebral cortex and white matter, cerebellum, brain stem and cord. There is considerable variance in the intensity of tissue changes, ranging from sporadic enlarged cells with nuclear inclusions in the subependymal tissue to massive subependymal glial proliferation with extensive periventricular mineralization and relatively sparse inflammatory infiltrates lacking multinucleated giant cells. Destruction of ependyma results in a nodular glial proliferation which, however, does not reach the extent found in toxoplasmosis and, also, does not result in obliteration of the aqueduct. Also, toxoplasmosis characteristically shows widespread dissemination of the lesions throughout the central nervous system and more frequent retinal involvement.

Cytomegalic inclusions are found in various cells identified, at times tentatively, as astrocytes, microglia or ependyma, or in leptomeninges, vascular epithelia and, occasionally, in neurons. The inclusion-bearing cells have considerably enlarged nuclei and an increased mass of cytoplasm (Fig. 55). Intranuclear inclusions are extremely large, up to 15 μ, acidophilic, and round or oval, sometimes kidney-shaped or irregular; a granular substructure is found in some. Inclusions are separated by a clear halo from the nuclear membrane which shows small condensations of chromatin, called orbital or polar bodies, opposite to which the inclusions may appear indented. One inclusion per nucleus is the rule. The acidophilic nuclear inclusions are negative for PAS and stain positive with the Feulgen reaction. In addition there are numerous basophilic cytoplasmic inclusions usually localized in one portion of the cytoplasm. These are uniform in size (2 to 4 μ) and spherical in shape, staining bluish-purplish with H & E, positive with PAS and negative with the Feulgen reaction. Cytoplasmic inclusions never occur in the absence of nuclear inclusions, while the reverse may be true (Smith and Vellios, 1950; Diezel, 1954; Haymaker *et al.*, 1954). Electron microscopic demonstration of the virions in the brain tissue was reported by Anzil *et al.* (1970). They consisted of spherical, hexagonal or pentagonal cores, averaging 93 mμ in diameter, with a single membrane-like envelope separated from the core by a clear interspace.

A different pattern of cerebral lesions of cytomegalovirus infection was recognized more recently for 2 premature infants, 2 months old, which showed a widespread nodular encephalitis of brain stem, cerebellum, basal ganglia and cerebral hemispheres. The histologic changes consisted of microglial nodules without central mineralization containing, occasionally, typical cytomegalic cells (Vortel *et al.*, 1968). The authors considered these changes concomitant infections of cytomegalovirus and coxsackie virus. Similar lesions were found in immune-suppressed patients who had undergone human organ transplantation (Schneck, 1965). These modifications of the pathologic lesions may relate to the frequent association of cytomegalovirus infection with other infections, such as its frequent association with pneumocystis infection of the lung (Hamperl, 1956). Cytomegalic inclusion disease in a 9-day-old boy appeared to be grafted postnatally on a neonatal meningitis by E. coli in the case of Anzil *et al.* (1970).

The association of cytomegalic inclusion disease with cortical malformations was recognized by Diezel (1954) who observed widespread polymicrogyria of the neocortex, sparing the paleocortex, in a 24-day-old boy who also showed bilateral temporal defects, massive ventricular enlargement and acute inflammatory necrotizing changes with numerous inclusion bodies in the tissue. Large foci of mineralization, and aplasia of cortex, were found in the cerebellum. Diezel also reviewed another case with polymicrogyria, and several similar instances have been published since (Born, 1955; Verron, 1955; Wolf and Cowen, 1959; Crome and France, 1959; Navin and Angevine, 1968). All the cases had polymicrogyria, variably associated with porencephalic defects and with local inflammatory changes in the tissue. The case of Born resembles Diezel's case in showing cerebellar hypoplasia. Crome and France in their report of a 31-hour-old infant found cytomegalovirus inclusions in kidney and submaxillary glands but none in brain while Navin and Angevine and others observed granulomatous encephalitis and inclusion bodies in the tissue adjacent to the porencephalic defect. Crome and France caution against generalization of a cause-effect relation between the infection and the induction of malformation. Cerebral cavitation may reach the degree of hydranencephaly (Chapter 11).

Other Viral Infections. Blattner and Heys (1961) and Hardy (1965) reviewed the available evidence for the causation of fetal malformations by maternal viral infection. Smallpox, herpes zoster, influenza, measles, mumps, hepatitis virus, enteroviruses and adenoviruses were considered; at least some of these may result in an increased risk of fetal damage or death when occurring during the early stages of pregnancy. Sporadic cases of mental retardation, microcephaly, microphthalmia and hydrocephalus have been described following maternal virus infection, but these instances are too rare to permit definite conclusions. An instance suggestive of intrauterine infection with herpes virus during early gestation was reported for a newborn infant with clinical findings of microcephaly, intracranial calcifications, microphthalmus and retinal dysplasia (South *et al.*, 1969). The infant had vesicular lesions of the skin from which herpes virus, type II, was recovered. Type II virus commonly infects the genital tract, type I the oral mucosa. The mode of transmission was thought to be by way of maternal genital infection. The authors speculate that this may require the unusual circumstance in which the spread of type II virus infection is not confined to the genital tract by antibodies from a previous type I infection. Postnatal herpes encephalitis is dealt with in Chapter 18.

Two clinical observations of prenatal infection with lymphocytic choriomeningitis virus, transmitted by contact with golden hamsters during the second half of pregnancy were reported by Ackermann *et al.* (1974); both infants had congenital hydrocephalus and extensive chorioretinitic scarring.

Toxoplasmosis. Toxoplasma is a protozoan parasite recently classified as coccidian, having its sexual and asexual stages in cat intestinal mucosa (Hutchinson and Dunachie, 1971); the role of the cat in human infection remains unresolved. Toxoplasma was discovered first in a North African rodent, the gondi, and simultaneously in the rabbit in Brazil. The parasite has worldwide distribution and has been detected in a great number of mammalian, reptilian and avian species. Initially it had been named successively after each host from which it had been isolated, but it is now recognized that the species has very low host specificity. Infection of the human fetus appears to occur transplacentally, at or after the 3rd month of gestation, from a maternal infection, with minimal or without clinical signs. Transplacental infection is evident from the extent and chronicity of the lesions found at the time of birth. The organism has been identified occasionally in the placenta of mothers of infants with congenital toxoplasmosis. The disease may also become manifest during postnatal life; it is often not clear whether these cases are postnatal infections or activation of a latent fetal infection. The disease was first described by Janků (1923) who reported an infant with encephalitis and chorioretinitis and described the organism without being able to identify it. Toxoplasma was recognized as the causative organism by Wolf *et al.* (1939) who isolated the parasite from the patient and described the cerebral lesions in detail. Numerous cases have been published, but the disease is comparatively uncommon and is responsible for only a small percentage of infants with mental deficiency. Reviews were published by Callahan *et al.* (1946), Wolf and Cowen (1959) and, more recently, by Frenkel (1971).

Symptoms of connatal toxoplasmosis are usually present at birth or manifest within the first 6 weeks. There is a high incidence of hydrocephalus which is progressive and may, rarely, be already present at the time of birth. Microcephaly is less common. Ophthalmoscopic examination shows chorioretinal lesions; cerebral calcifications are evident on X-ray. Neurologic deficits are those of widespread involvement of the central nervous system with convulsions, opistotonus and paralysis, accompanied at times by a mild fever, a rash, jaundice, hepatosplenomegaly, vomiting or diarrhea. The spinal fluid is xanthochromic and turbid, with elevated protein content and pleocytosis. The disease is progressive to death within the first month of life in approximately one-fifth of the cases, the rest survives, mostly with serious defects. About one-fourth of the cases is premature, and these have a higher death rate, at 20 percent, than mature infants, at 7 percent (Feldman and Miller, 1956). Adult infection occurs most frequently in the form of toxoplasmic lymphadenitis, clinically resembling mononucleosis; chronic relapsing encephalitis occurs in immune-depressed patients.

Gross inspection of the brain shows numerous depressed, soft, yellowish lesions, a few mm to several cms in size, distributed at random over the hemispheric surface. They are well demarcated at the cut surface and have soft centers, some containing gritty material, others forming cysts. They occur in random disposition throughout cerebral cortex, basal ganglia and subjacent white matter and may occupy the entire width of the hemispheric wall. The ventricular system is enlarged from obstructive hydrocephalus as well as from loss of tissue from the numerous destructive lesions. Marked periventricular inflammation results in a lining of the ventricles with friable necrotic tissue, and with coarse granular ependymitis in less severely affected portions of the ventricular walls. Lesions of a similar type are found in the pons and medulla oblongata, but involvement of the cerebellum is less intense. The spinal cord is frequently involved and may be necrotic for much of its cross-section.

Microscopic examination discloses a chronic focal meningoencephalitis; large necrotic areas with macrophages are encompassed by a rich granulation tissue, with capillary proliferation and reactive astrocytosis and by infiltrates of leukocytes, lymphocytes, plasma cells, macrophages and a moderate number of eosinophils (Fig. 56). There is good preservation of the adjacent gray matter outside of the inflammatory foci, but perivascular cuffing may be seen at a distance. The leptomeninges overlying the lesions show similar inflammatory infiltrates. Mineralization is frequent and extensive, in the form of coarse masses or a fine dusting of the tissue; or, mineralization of cells may outline neuronal dendrites and axons. The necrotizing lesions cause large cystic spaces in the later stages of the disease. In addition, miliary granulomas are common in the less severly affected portions of the tissue, frequently in contact with small blood vessels. They contain epitheloid cells with abundant cytoplasm, scattered lymphocytes and microglia and are encompassed by reactive gliosis; granulomas show no tendency of central necrosis. Denudation of ependyma and massive productive inflammation are found in the periventricular tissue; severe nodular ependymitis results in obliteration of the aqueduct. Chorioretinitis consists of focal swelling, edema, necrosis and inflammatory infiltrates in all layers of the retina, being generally

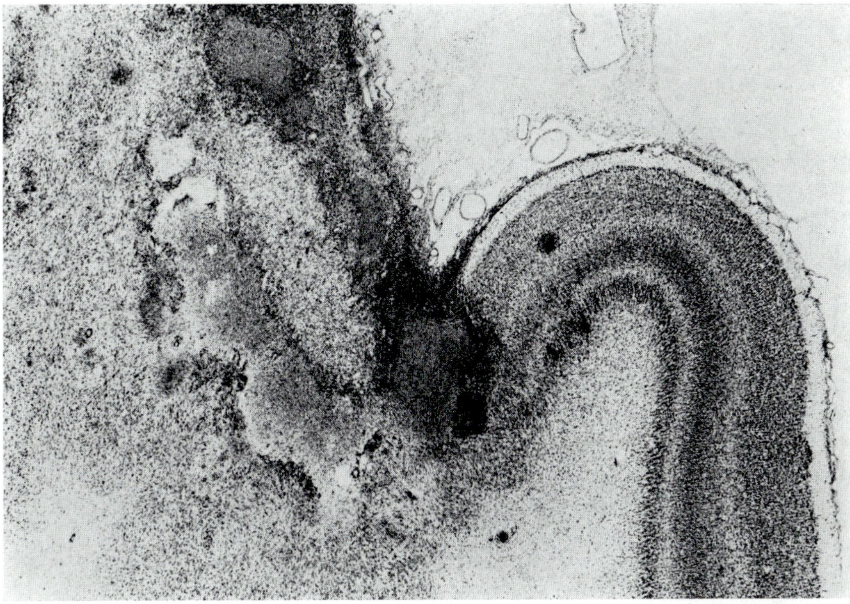

Fig. 56. Toxoplasmosis; necrosis and granuloma formation in cortex and white matter; cresyl violet ×7

most advanced in the inner layers. Evidence of infection is found in many other organs, most frequently in lung, heart and adrenals.

Organisms are found in association with the lesions, single or enclosed in cysts (Fig. 57). The cysts themselves elicit no inflammatory response, but their bursting releasing single organisms causes intense inflammatory changes. Single organisms appear in paraffin-embedded tissue as small, rounded or short, oval bodies, 2 to 3 μ long and 1.5 to 2 μ wide, having distinct margins and a small, usually eccentrically placed basophilic nucleus. Elongate or fusiform shapes are less frequent in tissue sections but predominate in smears where the organisms are larger and crescentic or curved. Single or small groups of organisms are found free in the tissue or enclosed in mononuclear or epitheloid cells, less frequently in polymorphonuclear leukocytes, rarely in endothelial cells. Cysts occur often in areas of comparatively mild inflammatory changes, forming rounded aggregates, 20 to 30 μ in diameter, of organisms slightly smaller than the free forms. Electron microscopic demonstration of the parasite in human brain tissue (Ghatak and Zimmerman, 1973) reveals a multiforme organism having a cone-shaped anterior end, a nucleus near a rounded posterior end, a double layered pellicle and occasional cytoplasmic organelles. The parasite is obligate intracytoplasmic, but cysts may be either intra- or extracellular. Various stages of replication are seen in host cells as well as in cysts.

Prior to Wolf *et al.* (1939) toxoplasmosis had been confused with encephalitozoon encephalitis. Encephalitozoon has never been documented as an infective agent in man but causes encephalitis in laboratory animals. The

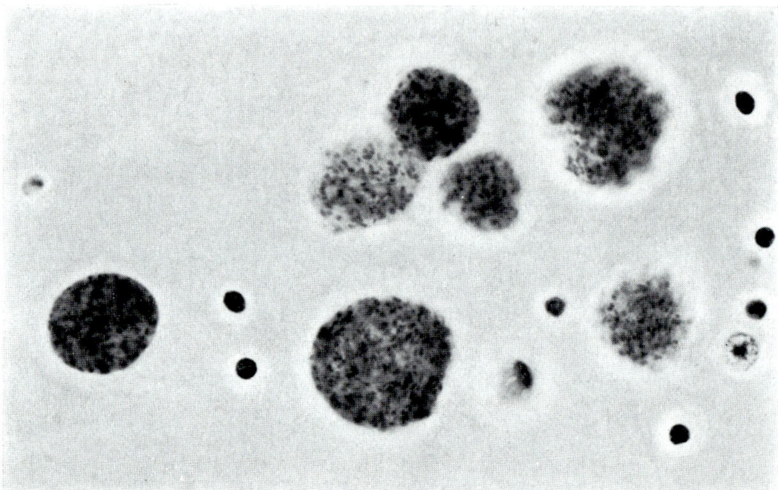

Fig. 57. Toxoplasmosis; multiple pseudocysts in nonreactive tissue; H & E ×600

criteria for the light microscopic distinction of the two organisms in tissue sections were worked out by Perrin (1943).

Toxoplasma encephalitis may be associated with developmental lesions similar to those for cytomegalic inclusion disease. Its coexistence with hydranencephaly has been described in several instances (Chapter 11), and there may be polymicrogyria in the residual cortical tissue. The case 1 of de Leon (1972) also showed cerebral and cerebellar polymicrogyria though without hemispheric defects; no reference was made to the retina and there was no proof of toxoplasma infection.

Connatal Syphilis. Syphilitic infection in infancy is nearly always the result of infection of the fetus *in utero* on the basis of placental infection and transplacental transmission of treponema pallidum. The fetus probably becomes infected between the fourth and seventh month of pregnancy. The incidence of connatal syphilis amounted to 2 to 4 percent in the pediatric cases before 1920. It had decreased to approximately one-tenth in the survey by Ullrich (1939), published 2 years before the first trial of penicillin was reported, and has been nearly eliminated by antibiotic therapy.

The pathologic lesions germaine to this chapter are those of the disseminated intrauterine fetal infection, which need to be distinguished from the manifestations of latent connatal syphilis in infancy. Active fetal infection is characterized by exanthema, chronic hemorrhagic rhinitis, hepatosplenomegaly, osteochondritis and other stigmata. It may result in premature abortion or stillbirth. The changes in the fetal nervous system were described on hand of 50 cases by Ranke (1907) and 21 cases by Wohlwill (1918), although the former report includes nonspecific lesions such as asphyctic leptomeningeal hemorrhages. Microscopic examination disclosed scattered infiltrates, mostly lymphocytes, plasma cells and mast cells in the leptomeninges and in the form of perivascular cuffing in brain tissue, associated with intima proliferation of blood vessels. Masses of spirochetes occurred in the leptomeninges and superficial portions of brain tissue. Parenchymal damage was slight, but focal cortical infiltrates were occasionally associated with focal necrosis. Inflammatory changes were most intense in the premature infants and diminished toward term.

The lesions of disseminated fetal infection differ pathologically from those of latent connatal syphilis in infants (lues tarda) characterized clinically by Hutchinson's triad of keratitis parenchymatosa, loss of hearing and peculiar deformation of upper incisors as well as radial scars of lips, saddle nose and deformity of the tibia. General paresis may develop toward the end of the first or during the second decade, and its lesions are more severe than those in adults, particularly in the cerebellum. Meningoencephalitic syphilis of infants results in basal meningitis which may cause obstructive hydrocephalus. Tabes is rare in infancy. Description of these lesions exceeds the scope of this text.

Malformations Produced by Experimental Fetal Infections. The ample literature on lesions produced by experimental viral infection of laboratory animals includes a number of particularly impressive reports on highly selective lesions in the central nervous system. Atresia of the aqueduct and hydrocephalus are caused by fetal infection with a non-neuropathic strain of mumps, parainfluenza-2 and influenza A viruses in suckling hamsters and with influenza A virus in suckling mice. The infection is selectively localized to the ependyma, resulting in its necrosis, followed by narrowing of the aqueduct and hydrocephalus in a high percentage of cases. The residual lesions resemble congenial atresia of the aqueduct in man (Chapter 22), showing no evidence of past inflammatory lesions. Ependymal denudation occurs with infection of older animals (Johnson and Johnson, 1969, 1972). Similar ependymal lesions resulting in obstruction of aqueduct and hydrocephalus were also produced by reo virus type I (Margolis and Kilham, 1969).

Fetal infections by various strains of rat virus (Kilham and Margolis, 1964) and by lymphocytic choriomeningitis virus (Monjan *et al.*, 1972) may localize selectively in the actively proliferating germinal layer of the cerebellum. The residual lesions in survivors consist of aplasia of the cerebellar granular layer (Chapter 31).

These reports document conclusively that fetal viral infection can cause lesions having all the histopathologic features of malformations. However, a review of these lesions in the respective chapters shows that each can unquestionably also result from a variety of other causes. Hence, the significance of fetal infection for causing malformations in the human brain remains to be decided on an individual basis, considering the merits of a given case.

References

Ackermann, R., Körver, G., Turss, R., *et al.*: Prenatale Infektion mit dem Virus der Lymphozytären Choroimeningitis. Dtsch. med. Wschr. 99: 629—631, 1974.

Alford, C. A., Neva, F. A., Weller, T. H.: Virologic and serologic studies on human products of conception after maternal rubella. New Engl. J. Med. 271: 1275—1281, 1964.

Anzil, A. P., Blinzinger, K., Dožić, S.: Cerebral form of generalized cytomegaly of early infancy. Light and electron microscopic findings. Virchow Arch. 351: 233—247, 1970.

Baron, J., Youngblood, L., Siewers, M. E., Medearis, D. N., Jr.: Incidence of cytomegalovirus, herpes simplex, rubella, and toxoplasma antibodies in microcephalic children. Pediatrics 44: 932—939, 1969.

Blattner, R. J., Heys, F. M.: Roles of viruses in the etiology of congenital malformations. Progr. med. Virol. 3: 311—362, 1961.

Born, E.: Über frühkindliche Hirnschädigung bei der Cytomegalie und ihre Abgrenzung gegenüber der Toxoplasmose. Arch. Psychiat. 193: 557—568, 1966.

Callahan, W. P., Russell, W., Smith, M. G.: Human toxoplasmosis. Medicine 25: 343—397, 1946.

Cooper, L. Z., Krugman, S.: Clinical manifestations of postnatal and congenital rubella. Arch. Ophthal. 77: 434—439, 1967.

Crome, L., France, N. E.: Microgyria and cytomegalic inclusion disease in infancy. J. clin. Path. 12: 427—434, 1959.

Dekaban, A., O'Rourke, J., Corman, T.: Abnormalities in offspring related to maternal rubella during pregnancy. Neurology 8: 387—392, 1958.

de Leon, G. A.: Observations on cerebral and cerebellar microgyria. Acta Neuropath. 20: 278—287, 1972.

Desmond, M., Wilson, G., Melnick, J., Singer, D., Zion, T., Rudolph, A., Pineda, R., Ziai, M., Blattner, R.: Congenital rubella encephalitis. J. Pediat. 71: 311—331, 1967.

Diezel, P. B.: Mikrogyrie infolge cerebraler Speicheldrüsenvirusinfektion im Rahmen einer generalisierten Cytomegalie bei einem Säugling. Virchow Arch. 325: 109—130, 1954.

Elizan, T. S., Ajero-Froehlich, L., Fabiyi, A., *et al.*: Viral infection in pregnancy and congenital CNS malformations in man. Arch. Neurol. 20: 115—119, 1969.

Feldman, H. A., Miller, L. T.: Congenital human toxoplasmosis. Ann. N.Y. Acad. Sci. 64: 180—184, 1956.

Frenkel, J. K.: Toxoplasmosis. Current Topics Path. 54: 28—75, 1971.

Friedman, M., Cohen, P.: Agenesis of corpus callosum as possible sequel to maternal rubella during pregnancy. Amer. J. Dis. Child. 73: 178—185, 1947.

Ghatak, N. R., Zimmerman, H. M.: Fine structure of toxoplasma in the human brain. Arch. Path. 95: 276—283, 1973.

Greenberg, M., Pelleteri, O.: Frequency of defects in infants whose mothers had rubella during pregnancy. J.A.M.A. 165: 675—678, 1957.

Gregg, N. M.: Congenital cataract following German measles in the mother. Trans. ophthal. Soc. Aust. 3: 35—46, 1942.

Hamperl, H.: Pneumocystis infection and cytomegaly of the lungs in the newborn and adult. Amer. J. Path. 32: 1—13, 1956.

Hardy, J. B.: Viral infection in pregnancy. A review. Amer. J. Obstet. Gynec. 93: 1052—1065, 1965.

Haymaker, W., Girdany, B. R., Stephens, J., *et al.*: Cerebral involvement with advanced periventricular calcification in generalized cytomegalic inclusion disease in the newborn. J. Neuropath. exp. Neurol. 13: 562—586, 1954.

Hutchinson, W. M., Dunachie, J. F.: The life cycle of the coccidian parasite toxoplasma gondii, in the domestic cat. Trans. roy. Soc. trop. Med. Hyg. 65: 380—399, 1971.

Ingalls, T. H., Purshottan, N.: Fetal risks from rubella during pregnancy. New Engl. J. Med. 249: 454—455, 1953.

Janků, J.: Pathogenesa a pathologická anatomie tak nazvaného v vozeného kolombu žluté sbvrany v oku normálně velikém a microphalmickém s nálezem parasitu v sítnici. Časop. lék. Česk. 62: 1021—1027, 1054—1059, 1081—1085, 1111—1115, 1138—1143, 1923.

Johnson, K. P., Johnson, R. T.: Granular ependymitis. Occurrence in myxovirus infected rodents and prevalence in man. Amer. J. Path. 67: 511—522, 1972.

Johnson, R. T., Johnson, K. P.: Hydrocephalus as a sequela of experimental myxovirus infections. Exp. Molec. Path. 10: 68—80, 1969.

Kappers, J. A.: Developmental disturbance of the brain by German measles in an embryo of the 7th week. Acta Anat. 31: 1—20, 1957.

Kilham, L., Margolis, G.: Cerebellar ataxia in hamsters inoculated with rat virus. Science 143: 1047—1047, 1964.

— — Hydrocephalus in hamsters, ferrets, rats and mice following inoculations with reovirus type I. I. Virologic studies. Lab. Invest. 21: 183—188, 189—198, 1969.

McCracken, G. H., Jr., Shinefield, H. R., Cobb, R., Rausen, A. R., Dische, M. R., Eichenwald, H. F.: Congenital cytomegalic inclusion disease. Amer. J. Dis. Child. 117: 522—539, 1969.

Margolis, G., Kilham, L.: Hydrocephalus in hamsters, ferrets, rats and mice following inoculations with reovirus type I. II. Pathologic studies. Lab. Invest. 21: 189—198, 1969.

— — Experimental virus-induced hydrocephalus. Relation to pathogenesis of the Arnold-Chiari malformation. J. Neurosurg. 31: 1—9, 1969.

Medearis, D. N., Jr.: Cytomegalic inclusion disease: analysis of clinical features based on literature and six additional cases. Pediatrics 19: 467—480, 1957.

Michaels, R.: Encephalitis and persistent infection in congenital rubella. J. Pediat. 68: 842—842, 1966.

Monif, G. R. G., Sever, J. L.: Chronic infection of the central nervous system with rubella virus. Neurology (Minneap.) 111—112, 1966.

— — Schiff, G. M., Traub, R. G.: Isolation of rubella virus from products of conception. Amer. J. Obstet. Gynec. 91: 1143—1146, 1965.

Monjan, A. A., Gilden, D. H., Cole, G. A., Nathanson, N.: Cerebellar hypoplasia in neonatal rats caused by lymphocytic choriomeningitis virus. Science 171: 194—196, 1972.

Naeye, R. L., Blanc, W.: Pathogenesis of congenital rubella. J.A.M.A. 194: 1277—1283, 1965.

Navin, J. J., Angevine, J. M.: Congenital cytomegalic inclusion disease with porencephaly. Neurology (Minneap.) 18: 470—472, 1968.

Oehme, J.: Cerebrale Verlaufsform der Cytomegalie. Mschr. Kinderheilk. 105: 366—367, 1957.

Ornoy, A., Segal, S., Nishmi, M., *et al.*: Fetal and placental pathology in gestational rubella. Amer. J. Obstet. Gynec. 116: 949—956, 1973.

Perrin, T. L.: Toxoplasma and encephalitozoon in spontaneous and experimental infections in animals. Arch. Path. 36: 568—578, 1943.

Plotkin, S. A., Boué, A., Boué, J. G.: The in vitro growth of rubella virus in human embryo cells. Amer. J. Epidem. 81: 71—85, 1965.

Ranke, O.: Über Gewebsveränderungen im Gehirn luetischer Neugeborener. Neurol. Zbl. 26: 112—123, 157—165, 1907.

Rorke, L., Spiro, A.: Cerebral lesions in congenital rubella syndrome. J. Pediat. 70: 243—255, 1967.

Sarwar, M., Azar-Kia, B., Mannie, F. F. R., *et al.*: Aqueductal occlusion in the congenital rubella syndrome. Neurology (Minneap.) 24: 198—201, 1974.

Schneck, S. A.: Neuropathological features of human organ transplantation. J. Neuropath. exp. Neurol. 24: 415—429, 1965.

Seifert, G., Oehme, J.: Pathologie und Klinik der Cytomegalie. Abhandl. Gebiet. prakt. Kinderheilk., Vol. 2. Leipzig: Thieme 1957.

Shearer, W. T., Schreiner, R. L., Marshall, R. E., Barton, L. L.: Cytomegalovirus infection in a newborn dizygous twin. J. Pediat. 81: 1161—1164, 1972.

Singer, D. B., Rudolph, A. J., Harvey, S., Rosenburg, H. S., Rawls, W., Boniuk, M.: Pathology of the congenital rubella syndrome. J. Pediat. 71: 665—675, 1967.
Smith, M. G.: Salivary gland viruses of man and animals (cytomegalic inclusion disease). Progr. med. Virol. 2: 171—202, 1959.
— Vellios, F.: Inclusion disease or generalized salivary gland virus infection. Arch. Path. 50: 862—884, 1950.
South, M. A., Tompkins, W. A. F., Morris, C. R., Rawls, W. E.: Congenital malformation of the central nervous system assosiated with genital type (type 2) herpesvirus. J. Pediat. 75: 13—18, 1969.
Sturgill, B., Brown, A.: Congenital cerebral granulomas. Pediatrics 37: 769—775, 1966.
Swan, C.: Rubella in pregnancy as an aethiological factor in congenital malformation, stillbirth, miscarriage and abortion. J. Obstet. Gynaec. Brit. Emp. 56: 341—363, 1949.
Töndury, G., Smith, D.: Fetal rubella pathology. J. Pediat. 68: 867—879, 1966.
Ullrich, O.: Lues congenita. Med. Welt 13: 4—7, 1939.
Verron, G.: Klinische Beiträge zur generalisierten Cytomegalie. Ann. Paediat. (Basel) 185: 293—302, 1955.
Vortel, V., Fingerland, A., Placky, V.: Glial-nodule encephalitis associated with generalized cytomegalic inclusion body disease. J. clin. Path. 49: 319—324, 1968.
Weller, T. H., Hanshaw, J. B.: Virologic and clinical observations on cytomegalic inclusion disease. New. Engl. J. Med. 266: 1233—1244, 1962.
Wohlwill, F.: Pathologisch anatomische Untersuchungen am Zentralnervensystem klinisch gesunder Syphilitiker (mit Einschluß der kongenitalen Syphilis). Arch. Psychiat. 59: 733—772, 1918.
Wolf, A., Cowen, D.: Perinatal infections of the central nervous system. J. Neuropath. exp. Neurol. 18: 191—243, 1959.
— — Paige, B. H.: Toxoplasmic encephalomyelitis. Amer. J. Path. 15: 657—694, 1939.
Wyatt, J. P., Saxton, J., Lee, R. S., Pinkerton, H.: Generalized cytomegalic inclusion disease. J. Pediat. 36: 271—294, 1950.
— Tribby, W. W.: Granulomatous encephalomyelitis in infancy. Arch. Path. (Chic.) 53: 103—120, 1952.
Yow, M.: Discussion at rubella symposium, 1964 rubella epidemic. J. Pediat. 67: 987—988, 1965.

17. Leptomeningitis in Newborns and Infants

Neonatal Leptomeningitis. Scherer (1895) described leptomeningitis in 3 newborns with bacteriologic identification of E. coli as the causative organism. Barron (1918) reviewed 42 cases from early reports on this common disease. The clinico-pathologic features of neonatal leptomeningitis were defined in more detail in the series published by Craig (1936), Watson (1957), Ziai and Haggerty (1958), Groover *et al.* (1961), Yu and Grauaug (1963), Overall (1970) and others.

Usage of the term neonatal meningitis is usually restricted to cases for which the onset of the disease occurs within the first 28 days of life; meningitis complicating meningoceles or encephaloceles has been excluded from many series although the clinico-pathologic features are the same. The overall incidence of the disease has been calculated as 0.42 to 0.46 per 1,000 live births. Premature infants are significantly more susceptible than full term babies: 1.36 to 0.37 per 1,000 (Overall, 1970) or 2.24 to 0.13 per 1,000 (Groover *et al.*, 1961) respectively. Other predisposing factors are maternal infection and complications during labor or delivery. Various studies indicate either no sex preference or a slight preference for males.

The onset of the disease is most frequent during the first 2 weeks of life.

The clinical picture is vague and nonspecific, with lethargy, fever or subnormal temperature, anorexia or vomiting, and irritability. Stiffness of the neck is an uncommon sign. Coma, convulsions, opisthotonus and a bulging fontanel herald the final phase of the disease. The prognosis is poor and has improved only little with antibiotic therapy. Overall mortality has been as high as 60 to 75 percent; the mortality for prematures is still higher, above 80 percent. Death usually occurs within 4 days of onset of symptoms; one- to two-thirds of the survivors have complications, such as neurologic

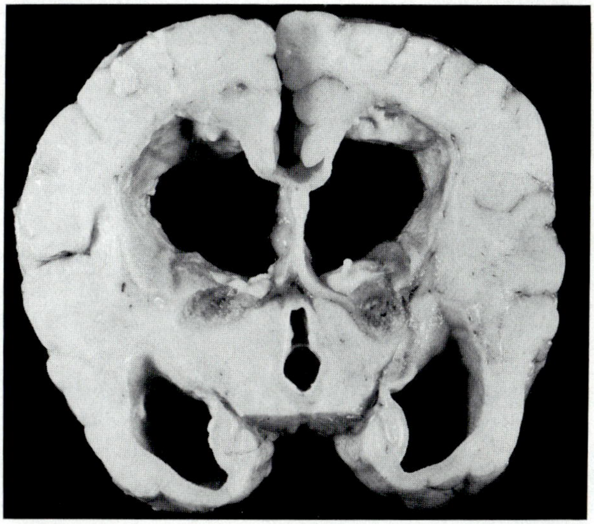

Fig. 58. Purulent neonatal leptomeningitis and ventriculitis, acute obstructive hydrocephalus

deficits or hydrocephalus. Fitzhardinge *et al.* (1974) report 40 percent mortality and an IQ below 90 percent for one-third of survivors.

Neonatal meningitis is often part of a general septicemic process, and the same organism may be cultured from the meninges and the blood for a majority of cases. Coexistent pneumonia, otitis, gastroenteritis, peritonitis, arthritis, urinary, umbilic or skin infections may form portals of entry or sites of septic dissemination. Practically any pyogenic organism may cause neonatal meningitis, but gram negative enteroorganisms are most common, mostly E. coli which may account for up to approximately one-third of all cases. Enteric organisms comprise approximately 60 percent of all cases and are still more frequent, above 80 percent, if the onset of the disease is within 14 days or for patients with abnormal perinatal history. Eradication of other bacterial populations by antibiotic treatment also increases the percentage of gram negative organisms. Infections by streptococcus and staphylococcus species are second in frequency and affect more often infants for which the onset of the disease occurs after the second week of life; however, there are marked fluctuations in the preponderance of certain types of organisms over an extended period of time. In instances of maternal infection the same organism is usually found as the cause of meningitis in the infant.

Neonatal meningitis is very rarely caused by those organisms which are observed most frequently in leptomeningitis in infants and children older than 2 months, namely hemophilus, pneumococcus and meningococcus. Only 1 of 276 infants with hemophilus meningitis was under 2 months of age (Fothergill and Wright, 1933). The clinical features of neonatal hemophilus meningitis were reviewed by De Berranger *et al.* (1973).

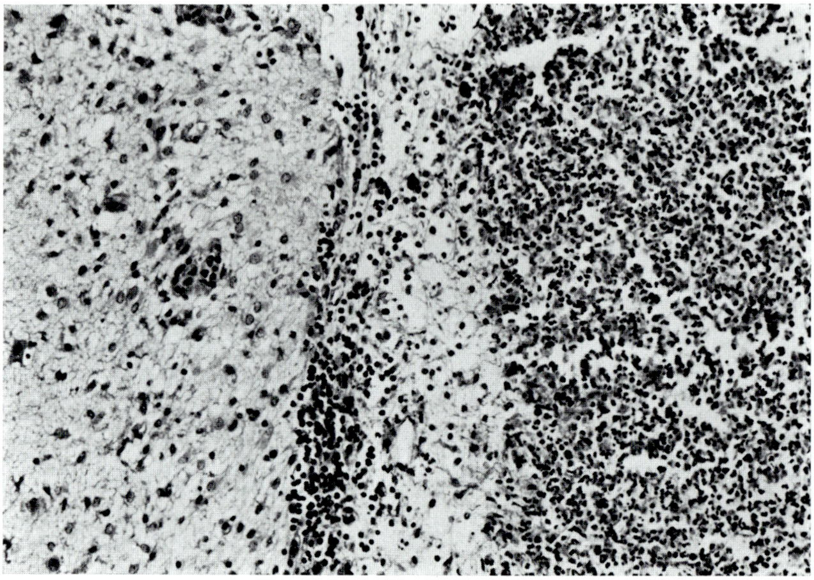

Fig. 59. Subacute leptomeningitis; bilaminar texture of the exudate due to its organization from the pial surface; H & E ×150

Gross and Microscopic Features. Pathologic findings in neonatal meningitis were described by Craig (1936) and Berman and Banker (1966). There is general congestion of blood vessels; a purulent exudate is usually most marked over the cerebral hemispheres, filling the depth of the sulci and lining leptomeningeal veins. The exudate tends to be less extensive in the spinal cord, unless the meningitis is ascending from a spina bifida. The ventricular walls and choroid plexus may be free of inflammatory changes during the first days but become involved later. The cerebral ventricles may be small, compressed by swelling of the brain; acute distension of the ventricles may develop upon plugging of the aqueduct, the cerebellar foramina or the basal cysterns by purulent exudate (Fig. 58). Meningitis caused by proteus or paracolon organisms often results in extensive softening and liquefaction of the fowl smelling tissue because of a high incidence of infarcts and, also, because of histolysis produced by extensive postmortem multiplication and swarming of the mobile proteus bacillus (Rance *et al.*, 1962; Shortland-Webb, 1968).

The exudate found during the first weeks of the disease consists predominantly of polymorphonuclear leukocytes and scattered histiocytes; the amount of fibrin varies, and aggregates of bacteria are found disseminated or within the leukocytes or macrophages. The number of mononuclear cells, mainly histiocytes and macrophages, increases during the second and third week of the disease. Organization of the exudate begins with proliferation of fibroblasts forming scattered strands of collagen. Organization seems to progress from the pial surface outwards, and the exudate becomes bilayered

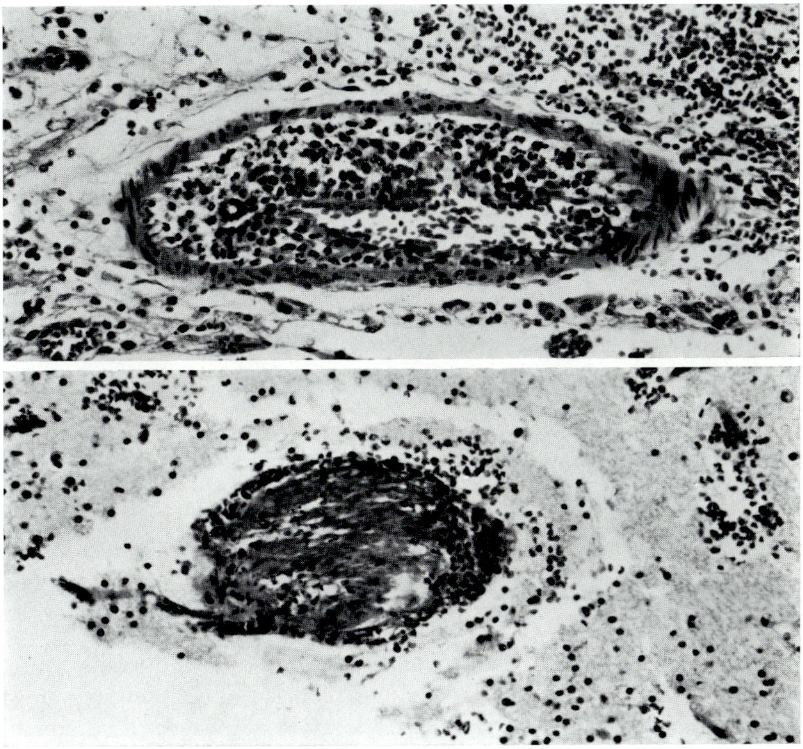

Fig. 60. Vascular affection in neonatal leptomeningitis. Top: Infiltrates in arterial intima, usually nonocclusive; H & E ×200. Bottom: fibrinous thrombus occluding cortical vein; H & E ×200

with more fibroblasts and macrophages in the inner portion (Fig. 59). There is proliferation of glia in the superficial subpial portions of cortical tissue. Exudate is found in choroid plexus and ventricular walls, and there is focal loss of ependyma and nodular or patchy proliferation of subependymal glia. Sleeves of exudate around the roots of cranial and spinal nerves may be accompanied with focal areas of degeneration. Chronic changes in patients surviving the initial onslaught of the disease consist of increasing numbers of lymphocytes and mononuclear cells. Residual strands or tubules of ependyma become buried under a thick layer of glial proliferation. Dense collagen fibrosis develops in the leptomeninges.

Cerebral infarcts often complicate neonatal leptomeningitis, at a frequency of approximately 30 percent (Friede, 1972). They are caused by fibrinous thrombi in distended veins and occur often at multiple sites in leptomeningeal, cortical or subependymal veins. Thrombosis of cortical veins is usually not secondary to thrombosis of an intracranial sinus, as is typical for phlebothrombosis complicating general disease processes (Chapter 13). It is customary to attribute the thrombi to thrombophlebitis, although there is often no correlation between their presence and the intensity of inflammatory changes about the veins. Thrombosis and infarction often develop during the first days of the disease; the inference from observations in adults that thrombosis is a late complication resulting from prolonged exposure of

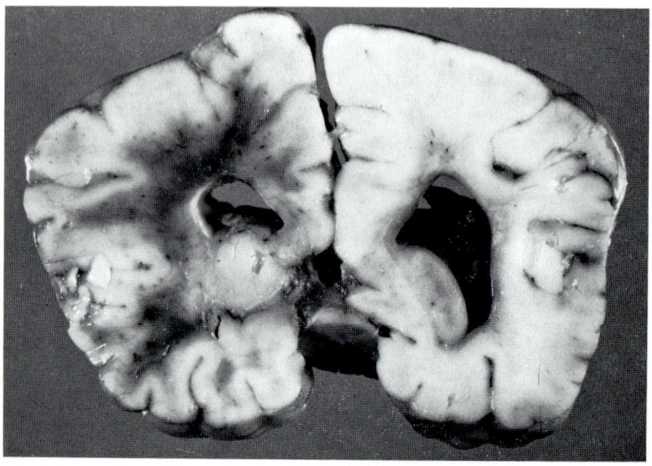

Fig. 61. White matter infarcts complicating neonatal leptomeningitis

arteries to the exudate (Cairns and Russell, 1946) is not applicable to neonatal meningitis. Inflammatory arterial changes consist of thickening and leukocytic infiltrates in the intima; the media is always spared. Endarteritis may result in narrowing of the arterial lumen but as a rule does not precipitate thrombotic occlusion. There are no comparable proliferative changes in the intima of thrombosed or nonthrombosed veins (Fig. 60).

The infarcts complicating leptomeningitis are often large and hemorrhagic and involve cortex and underlying white matter in random distribution over the convexity of the hemispheres. In addition, periventricular infarcts are common in the basal ganglia and the deep portions of the hemispheric white matter (Fig. 61), as described by Wertham (1931) who compared the distribution of infarcts in 14 children having leptomeningitis with that in 10 adults. Deep white matter infarcts result from thrombosis of subependymal veins (Berman and Banker, 1966). In other instances of periventricular infarction thrombosis may be found in the internal cerebral veins or their tributaries; these may be encompassed by a massive exudate in the cysterna ambiens while relatively little inflammatory change is seen in the ventricular walls. Superinfection of the infarcted tissue results in abscess formation (Munslow *et al.*, 1957). White matter infarcts complicating leptomeningitis are rare in adults

(Stammler, 1969; Buchan and Alvord, 1969; Minauf and Pateisky, 1971); they differ from the neonatal lesions in having irregular shape, perivascular distribution, and in lacking periventricular arrangement.

Residual Lesions. Eicke (1947) claimed that 76 percent of the lesions found in a series of 50 cases of infantile cerebral damage were postmeningitic, but he based this conclusion entirely on the frequency of nonspecific intima fibrosis of cerebral arteries. Residual lesions with verified history of neonatal meningitis (Bovet-Dubois, 1956; Friede, 1973; Schultz and Leeds, 1973) show a disposition of large cavities in cortex, subcortical white matter and peri-

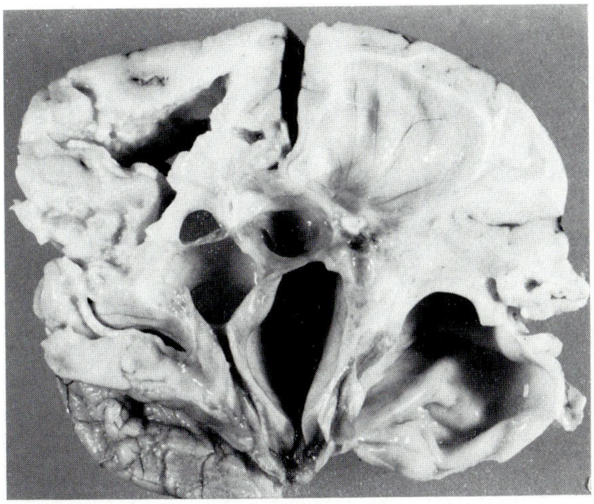

Fig. 62. Extensive cavitation and septations of ventricles and periventricular tissue, residual to neonatal leptomeningitis

ventricular tissue of the cerebral hemispheres. The cavities are at times separated from the ventricles by a layer of fibrillary glial scar tissue, or they may communicate, forming large diverticles of the ventricle. The entire central portion of the hemispheres may be transformed into a multiloculated cluster of noncommunicating cavities, formed from loculated segments of the ventricles, ventricular diverticles, and periventricular cysts (Fig. 62). The walls of these cavities and septa traversing the loculated ventricles are composed of intense fibrillary gliosis; mineralization is absent. Destruction of periventricular structures includes fornix and corpus callosum, and cavities in basal ganglia. Cavities derived from noninfected infarcts may coexist with chronic or healed abscesses. The ventricles, or their residual segments, are dilated, their walls showing extensive gliosis, and there is collagen fibrosis in the leptomeninges, especially in the basal cysterns.

Neonatal leptomeningitis has not been widely recognized as a cause of cavitated cerebral lesions; accordingly, its residual lesions may have been classified as having derived from other processes. Courville (1971) illustrated a brain (case 40) with cysts in the basal ganglia and obliteration of midline structures in an infant who ruptured a meningocele at the age of 1 month and died at 2 months. Similar changes were illustrated by Malamud (1957) for an infant with a history of acute illness at the age of 3 weeks, clinically diagnosed as meningitis. A cystic dilation of the cavum septi pellucidi in a hydrocephalic 6½-year-old child associated with ventricular diverticula and intense gliosis of the ventricular walls (Dooling *et al.*, 1972) also suggests postmeningitic lesions. Northfield and Russell (1939) and Russell (1949) described diverticula of the lateral ventricles as a complication of hydrocephalus, which they attributed to mechanical rupture of ventricular walls. These resemble the diverticula seen with postmeningitic lesions. It may be mentioned in this context that ventricular diverticula may also form from the needle tract of a ventriculography (Jenkins, 1967).

Obstructive hydrocephalus as a postmeningitic complication is generally recognized, and is dealt with in Chapter 22. Subdural accumulation of fluid is another complication of meningitis which has received considerable attention in the clinical literature. Nearly all of the reported cases were children older than 2 months. The complication seems rare for neonatal meningitis; it was not observed in the series of Berman and Banker (1966), which agrees with the present author's experience.

Pathogenetic Considerations. The organisms responsible for leptomeningitis in infants undergo a striking reversal in frequency at approximately the second month of life. Enteroorganisms and streptococci are the most common causes of leptomeningitis in neonates, while hemophilus, pneumococci and meningococci are the most common causes in infants older than 2 months. This reversal in susceptibility is explained best by differences in placental permeability for various antibodies and by changes in antibody formation in the newborn. Antibodies to hemophilus readily pass the placenta, resulting in passive immunity of the newborn, which subsides *pari passu* with the expected turnover and decay of antibodies. A lack of immunity between approximately the second month and the second year of life corresponds to the peak occurrence of hemophilus meningitis (Fothergill and Wright, 1933). Serum gamma globulin levels also decrease within the first few weeks after birth, dropping to one-third of normal and then rising between the first and third month, reaching adult levels by the second year (Orlandini *et al.*, 1955). The 19-S macroglobulin fraction of the serum which contains the aglutinine antibodies to coliform bacteria does not pass through the placenta (Gitlin *et al.*, 1963), thus resulting in a lack of passively acquired immunity to gram negative organisms at a time when they massively colonize the intestinal tract (Vahlquist, 1960). Prematures generally are less protected by immune mechanisms as their gamma globulin levels vary in direct proportion with birth weights (Saito *et al.*, 1956). The human infant is capable of responding to an antigenic impulse within the first weeks of life, but there is a delay in response when compared to the adult. Other factors have been invoked for the explanation of neonatal meningitis, such as less than normal phagocytic ability of neonatal leukocytes or mononuclear cells, immature immune responses, and higher permeability of leptomeninges. These factors may contribute to the course of the disease but they do not explain the striking variance in susceptibility to various organisms.

Neonatal Listeriosis. Listeria monocytogenes is a small, flagellated, gram positive or gram labile rod which elicits monocytosis when injected into rodents. Infection in man has marked predilection for the very young and the very old. Nicholls and Woolley (1962) in reviewing listeria meningitis found it most frequent in infants up to 1 month old, less frequent in adults above 60, and still less in infants up to 1 year. The most common manifestation of listeriosis in newborns is that of an acute, purulent leptomeningitis with clinical and pathologic features similar to those of neonatal leptomeningitis caused by other organisms. Listeriosis, however, may also affect the fetus or the pregnancy in several other ways. Listeria infection of either male or female genital tracts of man, as well as of wild and domesticated animals, has been recognized as a cause of habitual abortion (Rost *et al.*, 1958; Rappaport *et al.*, 1960). The fetus may also become infected transplacentally from maternal septicemia, with resulting fetal death and abortion (Barber and Okubajedo, 1965). Disseminated infection of the fetus occurs after the 5th month of gestation and results in "granulomatosis infantiseptica". It consists of numerous disseminated, pin-head sized, necrotizing granulomatous lesions affecting placenta, amnionic membrane and umbilical cord; the lesions also involve liver, lung, the posterior pharyngeal wall, tonsils, esophagus, adrenals and other parenchymal organs of the fetus. The central nervous system may become involved in the disseminated form of listeriosis. Miliary focal granulomatous lesions in the meninges and brain substance consist of foci of necrosis with leukocytic and lymphocytic infiltrates which may lead to formation of microabscesses. Organisms are demonstrated in the necrotic portions of the lesions with gram stain or Levaditti silver impregnations. Perivascular cuffing and leptomeningeal infiltrates with lymphocytes and monocytes are seen near the lesions (Reiss, 1953). In adults central nervous system involvement by listeriosis may produce a suppurative encephalitis (Eck, 1957) or a nonmeningitic, purulent, necrotizing encephalitis with predilection for pons and medulla oblongata (Duffy *et al.*, 1964); this localized form has not been observed in newborns or children. A comprehensive review of listeriosis was published by Seelinger (1961).

Residual cerebral lesions after infantile infection with listeria have been observed in rare instances. Hirasawa (1958) described an infant surviving meningitis for several months with marked hydrocephalus and extensive periventricular cavitating lesions. A most peculiar lesion was found in a 5-year-old boy in whom listeria was cultured on two occasions from the CSF during neonatal meningitis with onset on the 10th day (Lu *et al.*, 1962). Marked hydrocephalus was present at autopsy and the posterior portion of the aqueduct, the anterior medullary velum, and the lingula and central lobe of the superior vermis formed a huge cyst having a wall composed of glial tissue partly lined with ependyma. The cyst was in broad communication with the fourth ventricle.

Intrauterine Meningitis. Leptomeningitis in the newborn is commonly the result of intra- or postpartum infection and less frequently of ascending infection of the fetus *in utero;* transplacental infection of the fetus may occur in instances of overwhelming maternal septicemia. An alleged instance of intrauterine bacterial leptomeningitis reported by Crosby *et al.* (1958) has been widely quoted, but the interpretation of this case is in doubt. It pertains to an infant in whom intrauterine development of hydrocephalus was diagnosed radiologically at the 8th month of gestation and the infant was delivered 2 weeks premature by Cesarian section. The head circumference at birth was 44.5 cm; there was no fever or distress. A spinal tap on the third day showed xanthochromic fluid without white cells. Craniotomy on the 23rd day disclosed 55 cc of xanthochromic fluid overlying a greenish-yellowish tissue extending to a depth of 6.5 cm. Pure staphylococcus aureus hemolyticus was grown from the latter and microscopic examination showed granulation tissue consistent with neomembrane. The authors interpreted this case as intrauterine infection producing hydrocephalus. It is more likely, however, that this was an instance of secondary infection of a subdural hematoma complicating connatal hydrocephalus (Chapter 19).

Leptomeningitis in Infancy. The most frequent organisms causing leptomeningitis in young infants are hemophilus influenzae and meningococcus, having a maximum incidence at 1 to 2 years of age, and pneumococcus, with a less restricted age distribution (Smith, 1954). Adams *et al.* (1948) described pathologic findings in 14 cases of influenza meningitis. The exudate was uniformly distributed during the first 2 weeks of life and had thickened at the base of the brain with longer survival. Hydrocephalus had developed in all of 7 cases that had survived for more than 1 month. Thrombophlebitis had developed in 4 cases, but not before the second week of the disease. A high frequency of cortical lesions was reported, but these authors considered simple shrinkage of neurons diagnostic of cell death. Another series of 34 fatal cases of hemophilus meningitis (Smith and Landing, 1960) includes 6 instances of thrombophlebitis of cortical veins and 12 of phlebitis without thrombosis. Four of the cases had developed intracerebral abscesses or suppurative encephalitis and one a subdural abscess. Seven had cortical necrosis. One showed bilateral frontal remnants of neomembranes and atrophy with laminar cortical necrosis of the underlying frontal poles. Widespread neuronal loss having the features of anoxic encephalopathy was attributed to toxic factors or to compression of the tissue by the exudate, but the development of progressive sclerosing cortical atrophy due to febrile convulsions should also be considered (Chapter 12). Infarction of periventricular tissue of the type seen in neonatal leptomeningitis is also found as a complication of meningitis in older infants and children (Wertham, 1931), but its frequency appears to decrease with age.

Subdural effusions as a complication of bacterial meningitis in infancy attracted considerable attention. These lesions were described by McKay *et al.* (1950) who later (1953) reviewed their experience with 50 children. Subdural effusions were diagnosed by the aspiration of fluid of high protein content from subdural taps through the fontanel. Burr holes were made in 42 infants; 14 had bilateral and 10 had unilateral neomembranes; the majority was less than 1 year old. Positive taps for 20 of 43 infants with meningitis were also reported by Smith *et al.* (1951) who recommended that subdural tapping be done routinely on admission. Many other reports on these lesions have been published during the fifties. A high frequency of subdural effusion was not confirmed by Smith (1954) who observed effusions in 19 of 409 meningitic infants; craniotomy was performed on 4 and neomembranes were found in 3. Smith suggested that diagnostic or therapeutic techniques may induce the effusions, as taps in several infants were negative on the first attempt, and subsequent taps were positive. Escape of CSF into the subdural space may result from perforation of the arachnoid by tapping, but Williams and Stevens (1957) suggest that extreme spinal drainage of CSF may also produce effusions due to stretching of parasagittal tissue structures (compare Chapter 19); they observed a diminished frequency of effusions when spinal tapping was restricted to 3 cc. Mathies and Wehrle (1968) estimated the frequency of subdural effusions at 10 percent, but there are postmortem series in which subdural effusions complicating meningitis were never seen (Christensen and Husby, 1962).

It appears very likely, therefore, that the formation of subdural effusions is related to the management of cases of meningitis. Clinical descriptions are nearly always rudimentary, often referring only to a positive aspiration of fluid. The accumulation of fluid in the subdural space may occur without membrane formation or, less frequently, may be associated with neomembrane. For example, Epstein and Goldsier (1953) provide microscopic descriptions of typical neomembranes removed from an infant with leptomeningitis having been tapped subdurally four times during the 2 weeks preceding craniotomy.

Little information is available on residual cerebral lesions of infantile leptomeningitis in childhood except for the common complication of leptomeningeal fibrosis with hydrocephalus (Chapter 22). Extensive cerebral defects were described in a 13-year-old girl who had pneumococcus meningitis at the age of 1½ years (Smith *et al.*, 1957). Both frontal and parietal lobes were replaced by thin-walled cystic cavities; the temporal lobes were spared except for cortical scarring adjacent to the defects. There was extensive retrograde degeneration in the thalamus. Partly recanalized thrombi were found in the anterior and middle cerebral arteries. The cerebral lesions were associated with loss of pontine neurons, bilateral neocerebellar atrophy affecting the granular layer, and recent focal lesions in the cervical cord. The hemispheric defects in this child resemble "postnatal hydranencephaly" (Chapter 11). Lesions of this type appear to result from impairment of circulation in both carotid arteries, with ensuing infarction, a process which may be precipitated by febrile diseases. The case of Smith *et al.* (1957) is exceptional in showing recanalized vascular lesions and other coexistent lesions in the brain stem and cerebellum.

Abscesses and Empyemas. The pathologic features of intracerebral abscesses or subdural empyemas in infancy do not differ significantly from those in adults and are not described here in detail. Cerebral abscesses in newborns may complicate a variety of underlying diseases, some of which are discussed in the chapters on cerebral phlebothrombosis (13) and congenital cardiac disease (14).

Subdural empyemas may develop from the propagation of infections from the nasal sinus, the inner ear, osteomyelitis, or infections of pericranial soft tissues; occasionally there may be secondary infection of a subdural hematoma or hygroma with abscess formation. The lesions were common in adults before the antibiotic era but were rare in infants; only 2 of the 42 cases studied by Courville (1944) were less than 1 year old, the rest older than 8 years. Subdural empyema in infants may develop as a complication of purulent leptomeningitis (Farmer and Wise, 1973), which is uncommon at higher ages. The pathological features of subdural empyema in adults were described in detail by Kubik and Adams (1943) and Courville (1944).

Primary epidural spinal abscesses occur in infants of 1 month to 2 years of age (Baker, 1971), the youngest at 3 weeks (Palmer and Kelly, 1972); most are located at mid-thoracic or lower lumbar level and are caused by staphylococcus.

References

Adams, R. D., Kubik, C. S., Bonner, F. J.: The clinical and pathological aspects of influenza meningitis. Arch. Pediat. 65: 354—376, 408—441, 1948.

Baker, C. J.: Primary spinal epidural abscess. Amer. J. Dis. Child. 121: 337—339, 1971.

Barber, M., Okubajedo, O. A.: Maternal and neonatal listeriosis: Report of case and brief review of literature of listeriosis in man. Brit. med. J. 2: 735—738, 1965.

Barron, M.: Meningitis in the newborn and in early infancy. Amer. J. med. Sci. 156: 358—369, 1918.

Berman, P. H., Banker, B. Q.: Neonatal meningitis. A clinical and pathological study of 29 cases. Pediatrics 38: 6—24, 1966.

Bovet-Dubois, N.: Etude anatomoclinique des séquelles d'une méningoencéphalite à l'époque de la naissance. Ann. Pediat. 187: 161—167, 1956.

Buchan, G. C., Alvord, E. C.: Diffuse necrosis of subcortical white matter associated with bacterial meningitis. Neurology (Minneap.) 19: 1—9, 1969.

Cairns, H., Russell, D. S.: Cerebral arteritis and phlebitis in pneumococcal meningitis. J. Path. Bact. 58: 649—665, 1946.

Christensen, E., Husby, J.: Chronic subdural hematoma in infancy. Acta Neurol. Scand. 39: 324—342, 1962.

Courville, C. B.: Subdural empyema secondary to purulent frontal sinusitis. Arch. Otolaryngol. 32: 211—230, 1944.

— Birth and Brain Damage. Pasadena, Cal.: M. Farnsworth Courville 1971.

Craig, W. S.: Meningitis in the newborn. Arch. Dis. Child. 11: 171—186, 1936.

Crosby, R. M. N., Mosberg, W. H., Smith, G. W.: Intrauterine meningitis as a cause of hydrocephalus. J. Pediat. 52: 94—101, 1958.

Cussen, L., Ryan, B.: Hemorrhagic cerebral necrosis in neonatal infants with enterobacterial meningitis. J. Pediat. 71: 771—776, 1967.

De Berranger, P., Decobert, G., Sans, P., Gillot, F.: Hemophilus influenzae meningitis in the newborn. Semaine Hop. 49: 745—754, 1973.

Dooling, E. C., Barlow, J. F., Murphy, J. V., Richardson, E. P.: Cyst of the cavum septi pellucidi. Arch. Neurol. (Chic.) 27: 79—84, 1972.

Duffy, P. E., Sassin, J. F., Summers, D. S., Lowrie, H.: Rhombencephalitis due to listeria monocytogenes. Neurology (Minneap.) 14: 1067—1072, 1964.

Eck, H.: Encephalomyelitis listeriaca apostematosa. Schweiz. med. Wschr. 87: 210—214, 1957.

Eicke, W. J.: Gefäßveränderungen bei Meningitis und ihre Bedeutung für die Pathogenese frühkindlicher Hirnschäden. Virchow Arch. 314: 88—124, 1947.

Epstein, J. A., Goldsier, S. E., II: Bilateral encapsulated subdural effusion complicating bacterial meningitis in infancy. Arch. Neurol. Psychiat. 69: 242—249, 1953.

Farmer, T. W., Wise, G. R.: Subdural empyema in infants, children and adults. Neurology (Minneap.) 23: 254—261, 1973.

Fitzhardinge, P. M., Kazemi, M., Ramsay, M., Stern, L.: Long-term sequelae of neonatal meningitis. Develop. Med. Child. Neurol. 16: 3—10, 1974.

Fothergill, L. D., Wright, J.: Influenzal meningitis. J. Immunol. 24: 273—284, 1933.

Friede, R. L.: Cerebral infarcts complicating neonatal leptomeningitis. Acute and residual lesions. Acta Neuropath. 23: 245—253, 1973.

Gitlin, D., Rosen, F. S., Michael, J. G.: Transient 19-S gamma globulin deficiency in the newborn infant and its significance. Pediatrics 31: 197—208, 1963.

Groover, R. V., Sutherland, J. M., Landing, B. H.: Purulent meningitis of newborn infants. Eleven-year experience in the antibiotic era. New Engl. J. Med. 264: 1115—1121, 1961.

Herzberger, E., Rotem, U., Braham, J.: Remarks on thirty-three cases of subdural effusions in infancy. Arch. Dis. Child. 31: 44—50, 1956.

Hirasawa, H.: Morphologischer Beitrag zur Kenntnis der Listeria Meningoencephalitis beim Erwachsenen und Säuglingen. Arch. Psychiat. (Berl.) 197: 449—462, 1958.

Jenkins, R.: Paraventricular porencephalic diverticulum with latent hemiparesis as a complication of ventriculography. J. Neurol. Neurosurg. Psychiat. 30: 261—263, 1967.

Kubik, C. S., Adams, R. D.: Subdural empyema. Brain 66: 18—42, 1943.

Lu, A. T., Yuen, T. G. H., Bassler, T. J.: Mesencephalic cyst in the fourth ventricle causing obstructive hydrocephalus. Bull. Los Angeles Neurol. Soc. 27: 79—86, 1962.

McKay, R. J., Ingraham, F. D., Matson, D. D.: Subdural fluid complicating bacterial meningitis. J.A.M.A. 152: 387—391, 1953.

— Morisette, R. A., Ingraham, F. D., Matson, D. D.: Collections of subdural fluid complicating meningitis due to hemophilus influenzae (Type B). New Engl. J. Med. 242: 20—21, 1950.

Malamud, N.: Atlas of Neuropathology, p. 440. Berkley-Los Angeles: Univ. Calif. Press 1957.

Mathies, A. W., Jr., Wehrle, P. F.: Management of bacterial meningitis in children. Pediat. Clin. N. Amer. 15: 185—195, 1968.

Minauf, M., Pateisky, K.: Peculiar white matter lesions associated with purulent meningitis. Acta Neuropath. 18: 262—266, 1971.

Munslow, R. A., Stovall, V. S., Price, R. D., Kohler, C. M.: Brain abscess in infants. J. Pediat. 51: 74—79, 1957.

Nicholls, W., Woolley, F. J.: Listeria monocytogenes meningitis. J. Paediat. 61: 337—350, 1962.

Northfield, D. W. C., Russell, D. S.: False diverticulum of lateral ventricle, causing hemiplegia with chronic internal hydrocephalus. Brain 62: 311—320, 1939.

Orlandini, O., Sass-Kortsak, A., Ebbs, J. H.: Serum gamma globulin levels in normal infants. Pediatrics 16: 575—583, 1955.

Overall, J. C.: Neonatal bacterial meningitis. J. Pediat. 76: 499—511, 1970.

Palmer, J. J., Kelly, W. A.: Epidural abscess in a 3-week-old infant. Pediatrics 50: 817—820, 1972.

Rance, L., Roy, T., Donohue, W., Sepp, A., Elder, R., Finlayson, M.: An epidemic of septicemia with meningitis and hemorrhagic encephalitis in premature infants. J. Pediat. 61: 24—32, 1962.

Rappaport, F., Rabinovitz, M., Toaff, R., Krochik, N.: Genital listeriosis as a cause of repeated abortion. Lancet 1: 1273—1275, 1960.

Reiss, J. H.: Zur pathologischen Anatomie der frühkindlichen Listeriose. Kinderärztl. Prax. 21: 92—99, 1953.

Rost, H. F., Paul, H., Seelinger, H. P. R.: Habitueller Abort und Listeriose. Dtsch. med. Wschr. 83: 1893—1897, 1958.

Russell, D. S.: Observations on the Pathology of Hydrocephalus. London: HMSO 1949.

Saito, M., Gittleman, I. F., Pincus, J. B., Sobel, A. E.: Plasma protein patterns in premature infants of varying weights on the first day of life. Pediatrics 17: 657—662, 1956.

Scherer, F.: Ein Beitrag zur Ätiologie der Leptomeningitis purulenta bei Säuglingen. Jb. Kinderheilk. 39: 1—11, 1895.

Schultz, P., Leeds, N. E.: Intraventricular septations complicating neonatal meningitis. J. Neurosurg. 38: 620—626, 1973.

Seelinger, H. P. R.: Listeriosis. New York: S. Karger 1961.

Shortland-Webb, W. R.: Proteus and coliform meningocephalitis in neonates. J. clin. Path. 21: 422—431, 1968.
Smith, E. S.: Purulent meningitis in infants and children. A review of 409 cases. J. Pediat. 45: 425—436, 1954.
Smith, H. V., Norman, R. M., Urich, H.: The late sequelae of pneumococcal meningitis. J. Neurol. Neurosurg. Psychiat. 25: 250—259, 1957.
Smith, J. F., Landing, B. H.: Mechanisms of brain damage in H. influenzae meningitis. J. Neuropath. exp. Neurol. 19: 248—265, 1960.
Smith, M. H. D., Dormont, R. E., Prather, G. W.: Subdural effusions complicating bacterial meningitis. Pediatrics 7: 34—43, 1951.
Stammler, A.: Perivenöse Markdestruktion bei eitriger Meningitis. Dtsch. med. Wschr. 94: 1529—1532, 1969.
Vahlquist, B.: Neonatal immunity. Amer. J. Dis. Child. 99: 729—734, 1960.
Watson, D. G.: Purulent neonatal meningitis. A study of fourty-five cases. J. Pediat. 50: 352—360, 1957.
Wertham, H.: Cerebral lesions in purulent meningitis. Arch. Neurol. Psychiat. 26: 549—582, 1931.
Williams, J. M., Stevens, H.: Post-meningitic subdural effusions. J. Int. Coll. Surg. Bull. 27: 590—594, 1957.
Yu, J. S., Grauaug, A.: Purulent meningitis in the neonatal period. Arch. Dis. Child. 38: 391—396, 1963.
Ziai, M., Haggerty, R. J.: Neonatal meningitis. New Engl. J. Med. 259: 314—320, 1958.

18. Meningoencephalitic Processes in the Perinatal Period

This chapter concerns types of meningoencephalitis in the newborn that typically develop from intra- or early postpartum infection; a detailed review of these processes was given by Wolf and Cowen (1959). Purulent leptomeningitis of the neonate was covered in the preceding chapter (17) and infections that typically affect the fetus *in utero* in Chapter 16. The disease processes described in the present chapter occur in children and adults as well, but the text is restricted to their features in early infancy.

Candida Albicans. Candidiasis is the most frequent type of fungal infection in newborns. The fungus is a common saprophyte of skin, mucous membranes and intestinal tract of healthy subjects (Dobia, 1957). The infant may become infected postnatally, or during passage through an infected maternal genital tract, or *in utero* from an ascending chorionic infection (Benirschke and Raphael, 1958; Lopez and Aterman, 1968). Chronic neoplastic or non-neoplastic debilitating diseases predispose to candidiasis; other predisposing factors are antibiotic or steroid therapy (Winter and Foley, 1956), diabetes, nonmalignant diseases of intestinal tract (Salter and Zinneman, 1967), or indwelling polyethylene catheters (Toala *et al.*, 1970).

Candida meningitis was reviewed by De Vita *et al.* (1966). A frequent type of affection of the central nervous system in newborns is purulent leptomeningitis with ventriculitis; a polymorphonuclear and lymphocytic exudate contains the hyphae of the fungus. Hydrocephalus is a common complication (Smith and Sano, 1933; Burry, 1957; Eckerberg, 1961). Invasion of the nervous parenchyma results in widespread, necrotizing encephalitis (Fig. 63), with large areas of necrosis, massive polymorphonuclear exudates, reactive glial proliferation and a granulomatous tissue response. Fungus is found in areas of necrosis and adjacent tissue in the form of round or oval, single or budding organisms and pseudomycelial fragments (Fig. 64). Cultures are necessary for a definite diagnosis. Candida infection in children and adults may also present in the form of large abscesses or as an encephalitis with multiple microabscesses and granulomata having necrotic or purulent centers and multinuclear giant cells. These granulomas tend to be larger and more destructive than those of viral or bacterial encephalitis (Eschwege, 1958; Roessmann and Friede, 1967; Issel, 1971).

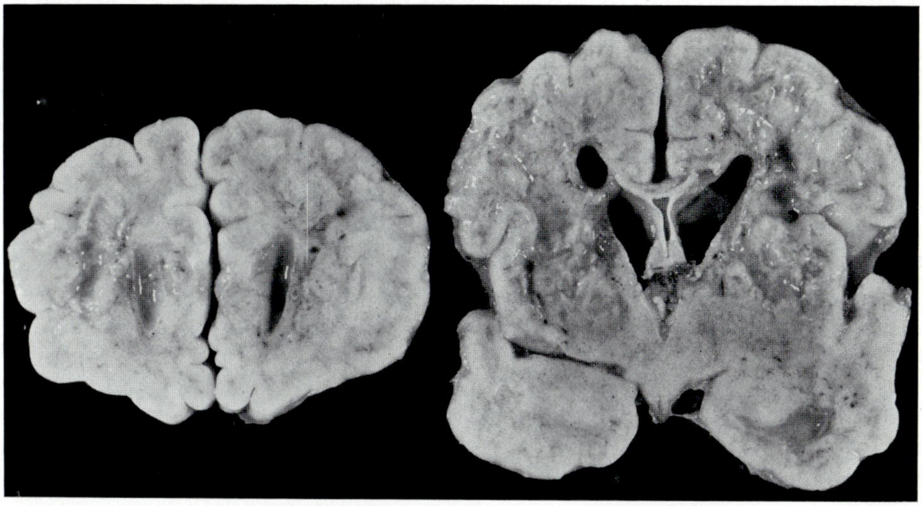

Fig. 63. Neonatal meningoencephalitis due to candida. Widespread necrosis with periventricular accentuation (superimposed asphyctic damage?)

Cryptococcus. Infection of the newborn with cryptococcus is extremely rare. The 3 premature boys described by Neuhauser and Tucker (1948) are controversial; toxoplasma has been identified in these slides (Wolf and Cowen, 1959), but cryptococcus neoformans had also been demonstrated in animal studies for 2 of them (Farber, 1950). The hydrocephalic brains showed an abundance of large mineralized plaques in the leptomeninges which were readily discernible on X-ray examination. There were also dense leptomeningeal infiltrates of mononuclear cells and eosinophils, amorphous mineral deposits, and a granulomatous encephalitis with focal infiltrates. Two of the three infants had chorioretinitis. The large hemispheric defects described for one are highly suggestive of a "basket brain" (Chapter 11). Meningoencephalitis due to torula histolytica in a 6-month-old boy was mentioned by Herzberger *et al.* (1956), but there are no neuropathologic reports of unequivocal instances of this infection in infancy.

Mucor Mycosis. Mucor mycosis in a 2½-month-old infant was reported by Martin *et al.* (1954); it presented with thrombosis of the internal carotid artery and infarction of the frontal pole. A review of the literature by Landau and Newcomer (1962) cites several instances of mucor mycosis in children. The microscopic features of the lesions consist of widespread necrosis from infarction as well as from direct fungal invasion of the parenchyma, edema and focal polymorphonuclear exudates. A granulomatous response, epitheloid cells, and caseation are less common. The fungus is dispersed through the necrotic tissue or is found in adjacent normal tissue, and has a tendency to invade the walls of blood vessels which are occluded by thrombi and masses of mycelia; the fungus also invades bone or nerves. Carotid occlusion occurs in one-third of cases. The hyphae are broad, nonseptate, frequently branching, and occur in single filaments or in interwoven masses; the average width ranges between 15 and 20 μ, but it may exceed that range considerably. Occasional small oval sporangiospores, 2–3 μ in diameter, are discharged from ruptured sporangia.

Aspergillus. A rare instance of perinatal infection by aspergillus was described in a 20-day-old boy by Akkoyunlu and Yucel (1957). The case of Iyer *et al.* (1952) survived to the age of 11 months, after the infection had apparently developed at the age of 4 months. Large bilateral areas of necrosis were found in cerebral cortex and white matter. A chronic meningeal exudate contained lymphocytes, monocytes and occasional plasma cells and multinucleated macrophages. Granulomatous foci contained multinucleated giant cells, and extensive mineralization had occurred in the tissue adjacent to the defects. Hyphae were identified as aspergillus on the basis of morphologic criteria. No evidence of infection was found in the rest of the body. Gaton and Gotlieb (1973) reported necrotizing, absceding, and granulomatous cerebral lesions caused by aspergillus in a 6-month-old child. The hyphae of aspergillus are branched, septate, 3–4 μ in width, and have small round spores, 2 to 3 μ in diameter, occasionally arranged in chains.

Herpes Simplex. Type II herpes virus commonly infects the genital tract, type I the oral mucosa. Infection with herpes simplex virus during infancy is commonly of type II (Pettay *et al.*, 1972); it may produce a severe generalized disease, or it may run a restricted encephalitic course.

Herpes simplex virus infection in newborns results in an acute, generalized, frequently fatal disease, with viremia and disseminated lesions in various organs. Transplacental infection *in utero* is evident in some instances by the presence of active lesions at the time of birth. Other infants may become infected during passage through an infected maternal genital tract; still others become infected postnatally. Prematurity disposes to infection. The disease manifests commonly by the 5th to 7th postnatal day with fever or hypothermia, respiratory difficulties, lethargy, jaundice, hepatosplenomegaly, vomiting, cyanosis and signs of rapidly developing circulatory collapse (Zuelzer and Stulberg, 1952). Cutaneous lesions or lesions of mucous membranes may be absent, negligible or widespread.

The most severe pathologic alterations occur in liver and adrenals, as first described by Hass (1935) who suggested herpes virus as the infective agent in a 7 months premature girl with necrosis of liver and adrenal cortex and numerous intranuclear inclusion bodies. Involvement of the central nervous system is common in general herpetic infection but the severity of the lesions varies. A disseminated focal meningoencephalitis affects pre-

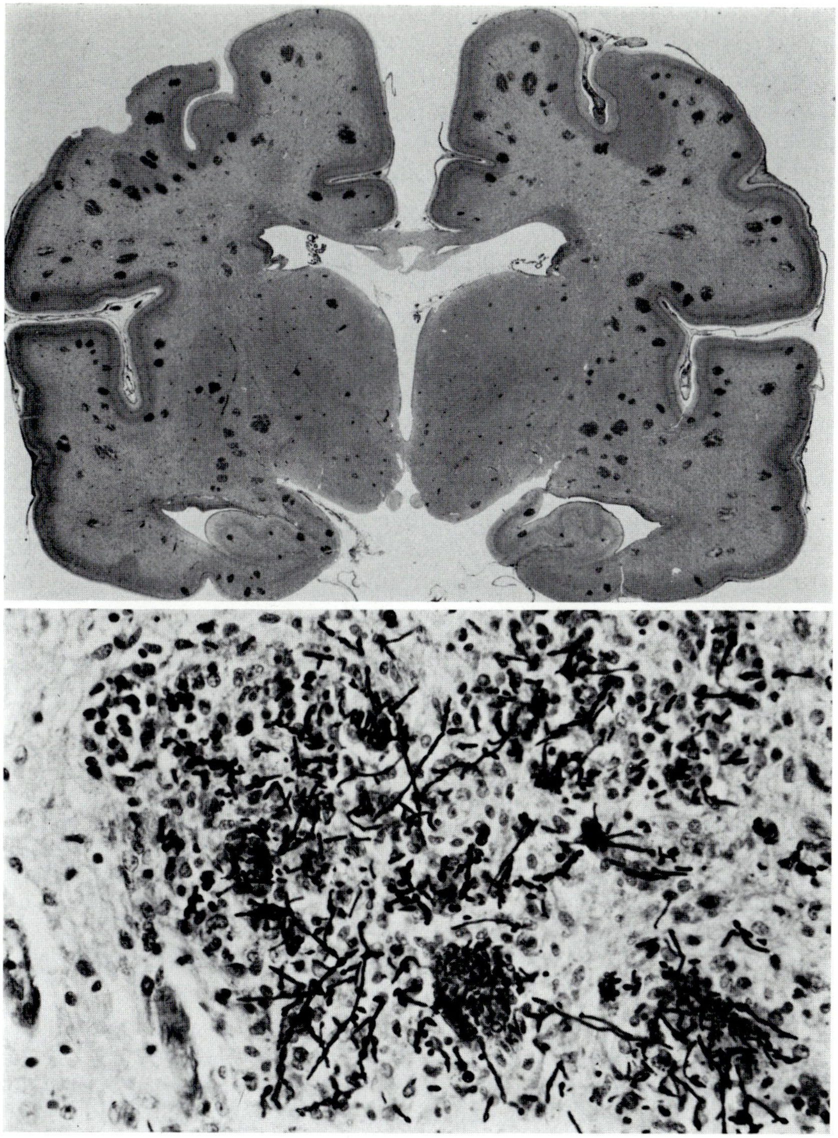

Fig. 64. Granulomatous lesions in candida encephalitis; H & E ×1.5; budding hyphae in a granuloma, partly included in multinucleated giant cells; PAS ×275

dominantly the brain stem and cerebellum (Zuelzer and Stulberg, 1952; Wolf and Cowen, 1959), showing fairly discrete nodular proliferations of microglia, mononuclear cells and a few lymphocytes. Endothelial swelling and early necrosis is seen in small vessels. Acidophil, homogeneous inclusions in neurons and glial cells in or near the inflammatory foci have sharply defined margins surrounded by a clear halo separating the inclusion for nearly all of its circumference from the thickened undulate nuclear membrane. Other inclusions stain slightly basophilic, having an indistinct granular texture that fills the entire nucleus. Focal lesions with small focal softenings are widely scattered throughout the gray and white matter and subependymal tissue (France and Wilmers, 1953). Leptomeningeal infiltrates of lymphocytes, mononuclear and polymorphonuclear leukocytes and hemorrhages tend to be more widely disseminated than the parenchymal lesions. Herpetic encephalitis may be survived without sequelae, but it often causes severe mental retardation, neurologic defects and chorioretinitis (Florman and Mindlin, 1952).

A purely encephalitic form of infantile herpetic infection was described and reviewed for 7 cases by Haymaker *et al.* (1958); 4 were 1 month or younger. Symptoms consisted of convulsions, fever, lymphocytosis and increased protein content of the CSF. Pathologic alterations were found mainly or exclusively in the central nervous system, consisting of widespread cerebral softening and massive microglial proliferation with macrophages; there was relatively little inflammatory response. A moderate number of lymphocytes, few plasma cells, macrophages and neutrophils were found in the leptomeninges and in perivascular spaces. An abundance of nuclear inclusions was seen in nerve cells and oligodendroglia. The encephalitic form of herpes infection in newborns is similar to herpes encephalitis in adults, but the lesions are more widespread, involving the basal ganglia, brain stem and cerebellum. In a case reported by Young *et al.* (1965), there was extensive cavitation of cortex and hemispheric white matter, as well as chorioretinitis. The infant had had an increasing titer of complement fixing antibodies to herpes simplex. The case is of interest in that it suggests an encephalitic etiology for lesions having the features of the so-called hydranencephaly of postnatal onset (Chapter 11). A necrotizing encephalitis with inclusion bodies affecting predominantly the temporal lobes, like the pattern found in adults, is seen in infants 2 years or older, but these also have focal lesions in pons and medulla oblongata (Bellanti *et al.*, 1968).

Coxsackie Virus. Coxsackie virus was named after its isolation from the feces of 2 children with paralytic poliomyelitis who lived in Coxsackie, New York. The virus is subclassified into groups A and B according to the histopathologic features induced by experimental inoculation in suckling mice (Gear, 1958; Kibrick, 1959). Infection with type B, groups 1 through 5 (Wright, 1963), produces a severe disseminated infection in human newborns. The disease is most common during the hot summer months and affects infants predominantly during the first week of life; nearly all cases occur during the first month of life. A sudden onset of fever, lethargy, cardiac signs and respiratory distress are characteristic. Affection of the central nervous system is indicated by meningismus, convulsions and pleocytosis of CSF. The disease often runs a fatal course.

Pathologic changes consist of a patchy necrotizing myocarditis, associated in more than half of the cases with meningoencephalitis, hepatic necrosis, pancreatitis and, less frequently, with adrenal necrosis (Kibrick and Benirschke, 1956, 1958). Gross changes of the central nervous system consist of edema and congestion. Microscopic examination discloses a meningoencephalitis with focal arachnoid infiltrates of polymorphonuclear leukocytes or lymphocytes and macrophages; there is perivascular cuffing in the nervous parenchyma, and a focal nodular encephalitis (Fig. 65) affects preferentially gray matter (Hosier and Newton, 1958; Fechner *et al.,* 1963). Moossy and Geer (1960) reviewed the distribution of encephalitic changes and emphasized their frequency in the inferior olivary nuclei and in the ventral horn of the spinal cord. A more widespread involvement of the brain stem, including pons and midbrain also occurs, and the encephalitic foci may be widely dispersed throughout the gray and white matter of the cerebral hemispheres,

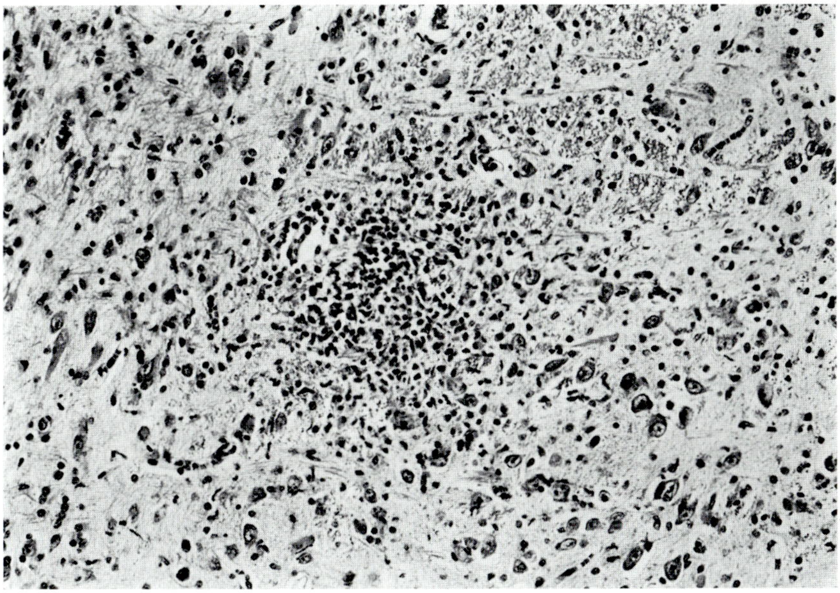

Fig. 65. Coxsackie encephalitis; glial nodule in the tegmentum; H & E ×275

ventricular walls, choroid plexus and cerebellum. The nodules consist of microglial proliferation and polymorphonuclear leukocytic infiltrates, with or without central necrosis, encompassed by reactive proliferation of astrocytes. Eosinophils, plasma cells or inclusion bodies are absent. Small vessels near the lesions show endothelial swelling and mixed perivascular infiltrates, but the encephalitic foci are often independent of blood vessels. The lesions in human brains are similar to those produced by experimental inoculation in suckling mice. Coxsackie encephalitis may resemble poliomyelitis, particularly if spinal cord involvement is severe. However, there is less tendency of neuronophagia, inclusion bodies are absent, and involvement of the brain stem prefers the inferior olivary nuclei whereas poliomyelitis prefers the tegmentum (Moossy and Geer, 1960).

Poliomyelitis. Many instances of poliomyelitis during the first 6 months of life were observed before the near eradication of the disease by vaccination. Bates (1955) reviewed 58 patients, most with an onset of symptoms between 4 and 21 days, which is consistent with peri- or postnatal infection considering a minimal incubation period of 5 or 6 days. Infection of the newborn may occur from active maternal disease, from infected siblings, or, often, from obscure sources (Mouton *et al.*, 1950). Infection of the fetus *in utero* is very rare but has been proven by virologic demonstration of placental and fetal infection with polio virus (Schaeffer *et al.*, 1954), by the recovery of virus from the meconium of stillborn infants of diseased mothers (Barsky and Beale, 1957) and for infants with manifest disease soon after birth (Bates, 1955). Elliott and McAllister (1956) described a flaccid newborn without spontaneous movement that had been born to a mother with acute poliomyelitis; it lived for only 32 minutes. The central nervous system revealed the typical microscopic changes of acute poliomyelitis in spinal cord and brain stem. The lesions in this and other cases were the same as those of poliomyelitis in adults (Baskin *et al.*, 1950; Pugh and Dudgeon, 1954), consisting of acute inflammatory infiltrates predominantly in the ventral horns of the cord, destruction of neurons and neuronophagia, occasional intranuclear inclusions, perivascular lymphocytic cuffings, intense reactive gliosis, and sparse meningeal infiltrates. The process extended into the medulla oblongata, pons, midbrain tegmentum, the roof nuclei of cerebellum, thalamus, hypothalamus and cerebral cortex with predilection for the motor region.

Aseptic Meningitis Due to Entero Viruses. Coxsackie and ECHO viruses (Enteric Cytopathogenic Human Orphan viruses) have been identified as responsible for outbreaks of aseptic meningitis (Kibrick, 1959). Meningitis in very young infants may be caused by Echo virus type 9 or Coxsackie virus B type 5 (Nogen and Lepow, 1967). An outbreak of aseptic meningitis in very young children was attributed to Echo virus type III (Peters *et al.*, 1972). No information is available on the pathology of these lesions which run a benign and self-limited course.

Arthropode-Borne Viruses. Viruses of the arthropode-borne group may occasionally cause encephalomyelitis in infancy (Wolf and Cowen, 1959). The virus of Western equine encephalomyelitis has a particular predilection for infants, affecting approximately one-half under the age of 10 (Bruyn and Lennette, 1953). Of the 17 infants described by Medovy (1943), 2 showed development of the illness during the 3rd or 4th day of life, probably due to transplacental infection from maternal disease. Both infants developed significant antibody titer against Western equine virus. Residual cerebral lesions causing spasticity, retardation, or slow development were found subsequently in these 2 infants as well as in the older ones, while the rest recovered completely. Other instances of early infection due to transplacental transmission of virus have been observed (Shinefield and Townsend, 1953), but the pathologic features of the acute lesions in infants are unknown. Residual lesions described by Noran and Baker (1943) consisted of multiple cystic cavities replacing much of the cortex and white matter of the right frontal lobe and less severe changes in the left cerebral hemisphere. The defects communicated with the frontal horn of the left lateral ventricle. The temporal and occipital lobes, brain stem and cerebellum were spared. The lesions in this case resemble those of multilocular cystic encephalopathy (Chapter 11) which is typically found as a perinatal lesion. A brief report by Bruyn and Lennette (1953) on residual lesions of infantile Western equine encephalitis describes pale sclerotic areas, 1 to 2 cm in diameter, in the basal ganglia and in the cerebral hemispheres and pronounced sclerosis of cerebellar white matter.

Tuberculosis. Numerous instances of connatal tuberculosis have been described, a few of which had involvement of the central nervous system in the form of leptomeningitis or leptomeningeal tubercles (Hughesdon, 1946). Tuberculous meningitis in young infants is often complicated by encephalomalacia due to arteritic involvement of leptomeningeal vessels (Wagner and Menon, 1954).

References

Akkoyunlu, A., Yucel, F. A.: Aspergillose broncho-pulmonarie et encéphalo-meningée chez un nouveau-né de 20 jours. Arch. franç. Pédiat. 14: 615—622, 1957.

Barsky, P., Beale, A. J.: The transplacental transmission of poliomyelitis. J. Pediat. 51: 207—211, 1957.

Baskin, J., Soule, E. H., Mills, S. D.: Poliomyelitis of the newborn. Amer. J. Dis. Child. 80: 10—21, 1950.

Bates, T.: Poliomyelitis in pregnancy, fetus and newborn. Amer. J. Dis. Child. 90: 189—195, 1955.

Bellanti, J. A., Guin, G. H., Grassi, R. M., Olson, L. C.: Herpes simplex encephalitis: Brain biopsy and treatment with 5-iodo-2'deoxyuridine. J. Pediat. 72: 266—275, 1968.

Benirschke, K., Raphael, S. L.: Candida albicans infection in the amniotic sac. Amer. J. Obstet. Gynec. 75: 200—202, 1958.

Blattner, R.: Congenital damage to the CNS as a result of intrauterine infection. Comments on current literature. J. Pediat. 52: 620—626, 1958.

Bruyn, H. B., Lennette, E. H.: Western equine encephalitis in infants, a report on 3 cases with sequelae. Calif. Med. 79: 362—366, 1953.

Burry, A. F.: Hydrocephalus after intrauterine fungal infection. Arch. Dis. Child. 32: 161—163, 1957.

De Vita, V. T., Utz, J. P., Williams, T., Carbone, P. P.: Candida meningitis. Arch. intern. Med. (Chic.) 117: 527—535, 1966.

Dobia, B.: Moniliasis in pediatrics. J. Dis. Child. 94, 234—251, 1957.

Eckerberg, B.: A case of prenatal mycosis. Acta Paediat. 50: 317—317, 1961.

Elliott, G. B., McAllister, J. E.: Fetal poliomyelitis. Amer. J. Obstet. Gynec. 72: 896—902, 1956.

Eschwege, J.: Generalized moniliasis with coagulations of the brain. Arch. Neurol. Psychiat. 79: 250—263, 1958.

Farber, S.: Discussion. Amer. J. Dis. Child. 79: 367—368, 1950.

Fechner, R. E., Smith, M. G., Middelkamp, J. N.: Coxsackie B virus infection of the newborn. Amer. J. Path. 42: 493—504, 1963.

Florman, A. L., Mindlin, R. L.: Generalized herpes simplex in an eleven-day-old premature infant. Amer. J. Dis. Child. 83: 481—486, 1952.

France, N. E., Wilmers, M. J.: Herpes-simplex hepatitis and encephalitis in newborn twins. Lancet 1: 1181—1183, 1953.

Gaton, E., Gotlieb, A.: A case of aspergillotic meningo-encephalitis in an infant. Beitr. Path. 150: 197—204, 1973.

Gear, J. H.: Coxsackie virus infections of the newborn. Prog. Med. Virol. 1: 106—121, 1958.

Hass, G.: Hepato-adrenal necrosis with intranuclear inclusion bodies. Amer. J. Path. 11: 127—142, 1935.

Haymaker, W., Smith, M. G., van Bogaert, L., de Chenar, C.: Pathology of viral disease in man characterized by intranuclear inclusions. In: Viral Encephalitis (Fields, W. S., Blattner, R. J., eds.), pp. 95—204. Springfield: Thomas 1958.

Herzberger, E., Rotem, Y., Braham, J.: Remarks on thirty-three cases of subdural effusions in infancy. Arch. Dis. Child. 31: 44—50, 1956.

Hosier, D. M., Newton, W. A.: Serious coxsackie infection in infants and children. J. Dis. Child. 96: 251—267, 1958.

Hughesdon, M. R.: Congenital tuberculosis. Arch. Dis. Child. 21: 121—138, 1946.

Issel, W.: Über den Befall des Zentralnervensystems mit Candida albicans. Ärztl. Forsch. 25: 34—43, 1971.

Iyer, S., Dodge, P. R., Adams, R. D.: Two cases of aspergillus infection of the central nervous system. J. Neurol. Neurosurg. Psychiat. 15: 152—163, 1952.

Kibrick, S.: The role of coxsackie and ECHO viruses in human disease. Med. Clin. N. Amer. 43: 1291—1308, 1959.

— Benirschke, K.: Acute aseptic myocarditis and meningoencephalitis in newborn child infected with coxsackie virus Group B, Type 3. New Engl. J. Med. 255: 883—889, 1956.

— — Severe generalized disease (encephalohepatomyocarditis) occurring in newborn period and due to infection to coxsackie virus, Group B. Pediatrics 22: 857—874, 1958.

Klein, J. D., Yamauchi, T., Horlick, S. P.: Neonatal candidiasis, meningitis, and arthritis: Observations and a review of the literature. J. Pediat. 81: 31—34, 1972.

Landau, J. W., Newcomer, V. D.: Acute cerebral phycomycosis (mucormycosis). Pediatrics 61: 363—385, 1962.

Lopez, E., Aterman, K.: Intrauterine infection by candida. Amer. J. Dis. Child. 115: 663—670, 1968.

Martin, F. P., Lukeman, J. M., Ranson, R. F., Geppert, L. J.: Mucormycosis of the central nervous system associated with thrombosis of the internal carotid artery. J. Pediat. 44: 437—442, 1954.

Medovy, H.: Western equine encephalomyelitis in infants. J. Pediat. 22: 308—318, 1943.

Moossy, J., Geer, J. C.: Encephalomyelitis, myocarditis, and adrenal cortical necrosis in coxsackie B 3 virus infection: Distribution of the central nervous lesions. Arch. Path. 70: 614—622, 1960.

Mouton, C. M., Smillie, J. G., Bower, A. G.: Report of ten cases of poliomyelitis in infants under six months of age. J. Pediat. 36: 482—492, 1950.

Neuhauser, E. B. D., Tucker, A.: The Roentgen changes produced by diffuse torulosis in the newborn. Amer. J. Roentgenol. 59: 805—815, 1948.

Nogen, A. G., Lepow, M. L.: Enteroviral meningitis in very young infants. Pediatrics 40: 617—626, 1967.

Noran, H. H., Baker, A. B.: Sequels of equine encephalomyelitis. Arch. Neurol. Psychiat. 49: 398—413, 1943.

Peters, A. H., O'Grady, E., Milanovich, R. A.: Aseptic meningitis associated with echovirus type 3 in very young children. Amer. J. Dis. Child. 123: 452—456, 1962.

Pettay, O., Leinikki, P., Donner, M., Lapinleimu, K.: Herpes simplex virus infection in the newborn. Arch. Dis. Child. 47: 97—103, 1972.

Pugh, R. L., Dudgeon, J.: Fatal neonatal poliomyelitis. Arch. Dis. Child. 29: 381—384, 1954.

Roessmann, U., Friede, R. L.: Candidal infection of the brain. Arch. Path. 84: 495—498, 1967.

Salter, W., Zinneman, H. H.: Bacteremia and Candida septicemia. Review of 185 cases during a four year period. Minn. Med. 50: 1489—1499, 1967.

Schaeffer, M., Fox, M. J., Li, C. P.: Intrauterine poliomyelitis infection: report of a case. J.A.M.A. 155: 248—250, 1954.

Shinefield, H. R., Townsend, T. E.: Transplacental transmission of Western equine encephalomyelitis. J. Pediat. 43: 21—25, 1953.

Smith, L. W., Sano, M. E.: Moniliasis with meningeal involvement. J. infect. Dis. 53: 187—196, 1933.

Toala, P., Schroeder, S. A., Daly, A. K., Finland, M.: Candida at Boston City Hospital. Arch. intern. Med. (Chic.) 126: 983—989, 1970.

Wagner, J. A., Menon, P. G.: Encephalomalacia in children resulting from tuberculous meningitis and arteritis. The Antiseptic (Madras), p. 323, 1954.

Winter, W. D., Foley, G. E.: Candida infections in children with neoplastic disease. Influence of therapy with antibiotics and steroid hormones. Pediatrics 18: 595—603, 1956.

Wolf, A., Cowen, D.: Perinatal infections of the central nervous system. J. Neuropath. exp. Neurol. 18: 191—242, 1959.

Wright, H. T., Okuyama, K., McAllister, R. M.: An infant fatality associated with coxsackie B[1] virus. J. Pediat. 63: 428—431, 1963.

Young, G. F., Knox, D. L., Dodge, G. R.: Necrotizing encephalitis and chorioretinitis in a young infant. Arch. Neurol. (Chic.) 13: 15—24, 1965.

Zuelzer, W. W., Stulberg, C. G.: Herpes simplex virus as a cause of fulminating visceral disease and hepatitis in infancy. Amer. J. Dis. Child. 83: 421—439, 1952.

19. Subdural Hematomas, Hygromas and Effusions

Chronic subdural hematomas have been recognized since the middle of the nineteenth century, when these lesions were commonly referred to as "pachymeningitis hemorrhagica interna". However, the peculiarities of subdural hematomas in infancy received relatively little attention compared to the numerous publications on their occurrence in adults. The early literature on subdural hematomas in infants was reviewed by Rosenberg (1921). There are wide fluctuations in the indicated frequency of subdural hematomas in infants. Kowitz (1914) reports an 8 percent incidence of pathologic changes in the dura of 3,875 autopsies of infants between 8 days and 2 years; 4.9 percent had rust brown discoloration and 3.9 percent "pachymeningitis". Courville (1971), on the other hand, observed only 4 cases of chronic subdural hematoma for 50,000 consecutive autopsies of infants, and the lesions were also considered rare by Christensen and Husby (1962). Such variations in frequency may involve subjective factors in identifying and assessing the lesions, but there may also be true changes based on socio-economic factors and advances in obstetric management.

Chronic subdural hematoma has a distinct bimodal age distribution, being common in adults of middle and advanced age and in young infants; the disease is rarer in children and juveniles. Two-thirds of the infants with subdural hematomas treated by Ingraham and Matson (1944) were less than 6 months old. Pia (1966) reviewed 149 subdural lesions in infants requiring neurosurgical intervention during an 8 year period; 120 of these had occurred in babies, the rest in children up to 15 years. The lesions were classified as 54 acute, 16 subacute and 56 chronic subdural hematomas, and 23 acute hygromas.

Subdural hematoma of infancy occurs under a number of circumstances rarely encountered in adulthood. Classification of these in terms of etiologic factors is difficult because much of the information on pathogenetic mechanisms is based on conjecture; moreover, even the interrelations between hematoma, hygroma and effusion are not generally agreed upon. Hence, the general histopathologic features of the lesions are described first, followed by a provisional clinico-pathologic classification of the circumstances under which the disease occurs.

General Gross and Microscopic Features. The general pathology of chronic subdural hematomas in infancy (Ingraham and Matson, 1944;

Christensen and Husby, 1962; and others) is essentially the same as in adults (Fig. 66). The most characteristic histopathologic feature of chronic subdural hematoma is the neomembrane. Neomembranes consist of thin layers of vascular connective tissue at the inner surface of the dura; they occur in the form of a solid sheet of tissue or as double membranes enclosing a hematoma. In the former case, a dull, often richly vascularized tissue adheres to the inner surface of the dura mater containing small contorted blood vessels forming spiders or irregular patches; the course of the vessels does not follow that of the collagen bundles in the dura mater as normal intradural vessels do. Recent neomembranes easily scrape off the dura, exposing a smooth and apparently normal inner surface. Neomembranes frequently contain multiple, multicentric recent hemorrhages as well as evidence of old hemorrhage in form of rust-colored pigmentation. Neomembranes also form the envelope of large subdural hematomas, whereby one membrane is in contact with the dura, the other apposed to but not fused with the arachnoid. The two neomembranes merge at the edge of the hematoma. The hematoma itself may be dark red and of fairly recent date, or liquefied, forming a brownish fluid. Neomembranes encompassing still older hematomas are firm and fibrotic, enclosing cavities filled with a thin brownish or xanthochromic fluid. Extensive chronic subdural hematomas may show loculation with multiple layers of neomembranes.

Microscopic examination of recent neomembranes discloses a thin layer of loose connective tissue with a mesh of actively proliferating fibroblasts, few collagen fibers and many distended, thin-walled sinusoid capillary vessels. This tissue is often described as granulation tissue, but neomembranes differ from granulation tissue elsewhere in the body in the prevalence of distended sinusoid capillaries, and they may have a somewhat looser tissue structure. Neomembranes may contain variable amounts of scattered acute and chronic inflammatory infiltrates and multicentric recent and old hemorrhages with nests of hemosiderin-laden macrophages. It is often misleading to attempt dating neomembranes in terms of their thickness and their relation to the enclosed hematoma, since they commonly show evidence of repetitive bleeding, so that the age of the hematomas is not necessarily the same as that of the neomembrane. Neomembranes that had persisted for several months are characterized by increasing numbers and density of coarse collagen fibers. Such membranes may either be solid, replacing the hematoma completely, or they may form the rigid walls of liquid-filled cavities. Ultimately, they are transformed into layers of dense collagen tissue similar to dura mater. At this terminal stage, the microscopic structure of the membrane differs from normal dura mainly in the irregular intertwining of the collagen fibers, which contrasts with their regular layering in the normal dura. The sinusoid capillaries and the fibroblasts seen in the early stages of neomembrane formation are absent, but groups of hemosiderin-laden macrophages may persist. Mineralization frequently develops and may progress to the stage of ossification. These lesions are appropriately called post-hemorrhagic fibrosis of dura mater, reserving the term neomembrane for the earlier stages with active fibroblastic proliferation.

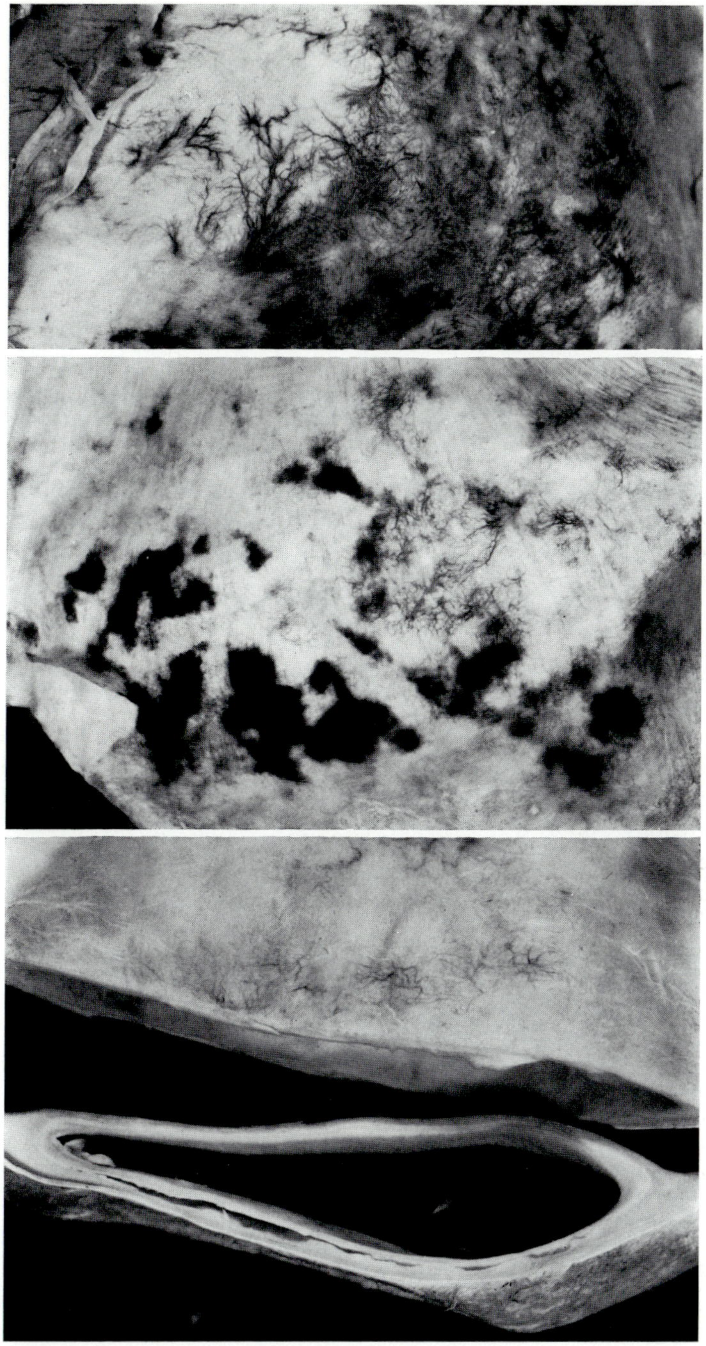

Fig. 66. Chronic subdural hematoma. Top: vascularized neomembrane. Middle: vascularized neomembrane with multifocal hemorrhages. Bottom: fibrosis of dura and encapsulated hygroma

Inflammatory changes in chronic subdural hematomas are usually restricted to small foci of lymphocytes and a few plasma cells; they are more common in older hematomas. However, a chronic subdural hematoma may become super-infected, resulting in a dense polymorphonuclear leukocytic infiltrate within the hematoma, with formation of an encapsulated subdural abscess or empyema, respectively.

The term subdural hygroma designates encapsulated subdural lesions filled with clear or xanthochromic fluid. Various pathogenetic mechanisms have been proposed for the formation of hygromas, also called hydroma by some authors. The most widely held assumption is that the hygroma is a residual cavity of a large, incompletely organized chronic subdural hematoma. Liquefaction of the hematoma transforms it into a fluid of low viscosity which, with the passage of time, turns from turbid dark brown to xanthochromic and finally to clear. The dense capsule of collagen tissue prevents the collapse of the cavity. This interpretation of hygromas is supported by the observation of hematomas in various stages of organization and transition to hygromas, and by microscopic evidence of old hemorrhage in the walls of hygromas. It has also been proposed, on the other hand, that the formation of hygromas differs in principle from that of hematomas, the hygroma resulting primarily from an exudate of clear fluid in the subdural space. This fluid may derive from the escape of CSF through a discontinuity of the arachnoid membrane due to craniocerebral trauma or hydrocephalus, or from a clear transudate caused by increased vascular or membrane permeability, *e.g.*, in the presence of inflammation (Dandy, 1955). It is impossible to distinguish these two modes of formation of subdural hygromas on the basis of the morphologic features of the residual lesions. However, chronic hygromas usually occur under conditions under which hematomas are found during the acute phase of the disease. This suggests that hemorrhage generally is a more important factor in hygroma formation than the escape of CSF or a clear transudate. The postulated primary mechanism of hygroma formation is not necessarily pertinent to the process involved in maintaining the fluid balance in an established hygroma, as discussed later in this text.

Acute and Chronic Subdural Hematomas in Babies and Young Infants. In considering these lesions it is convenient to distinguish between supra- and infratentorial hematomas. The symptoms of acute supratentorial subdural hemorrhage at birth include a bulging fontanel, shock with pallor, twitching or seizures, vomiting, irritability and restlessness and stupor (Ingraham and Matson, 1944; Schipke *et al.*, 1954). Most of these infants are born at term, commonly with a history of traumatic or instrumental delivery. Twenty of the 98 infants treated for subdural hematoma by Ingraham and Matson (1944) were known to have experienced severe trauma at birth, and another third had alleged postnatal trauma. A 75 percent incidence of abnormal or difficult labor was indicated in the series of Guthkelch (1953). Subdural hematomas of postnatal onset commonly develop upon craniocerebral trauma, often associated with linear skull fractures (Hendrick *et al.*, 1964). The development of a chronic subdural hematoma manifests during postnatal development by lack of normal weight gain, irritability, poor feeding and, sometimes, an accelerated increase in head size. Cranial enlargement may be asymmetrical, and transillumination may occur if there is a hygroma filled with clear fluid. Subdural hematomas were responsible for 9 percent of 310 babies with an enlarged head (Ingraham and Matson, 1944).

Subdural hematomas of early infancy are frequently bilateral, for example in 77 percent of 98 cases by Ingraham and Matson (1944), in 60 percent of 24 cases by Christensen and Husby (1962) and in 80 percent of 149 cases by Pia (1966). The most common distribution is biparietal, but the hematoma may extend over the entire hemisphere and into the interhemispheric fissure. The most probable mode of formation of supratentorial hematomas is the stretching and tearing of the bridging veins at their entrance in the superior sagittal sinus due to deformation of the head by traumatic birth or by postnatal craniocerebral trauma.

Infratentorial subdural hematomas cause changes in respiration in terms of rate, depth or rhythm, changes in cry, vomiting, poor suck and general hypotonia (Gilles and Shillito, 1970). Subdural hematomas at this site are most likely caused by laceration of the tentorium, as indicated by the attachment of organized hematomas to the falx or by the formation of neomembranes in association with an organized hematoma between the leaflets of the falx (Kowitz, 1914; Gilles and Shillito, 1970). Clinically identified subdural hematomas in the posterior fossa of newborns are rare (Coblentz, 1940); these lesions are much less common than supratentorial hematomas and fewer than ten cases are recorded in the literature (Pitlyk *et al.*, 1967; Gilles and Shillito, 1970). The lesions may be on the decline due to the improvement of obstetrical management, but the frequency of subdural hemorrhage was probably also greatly overrated in the older literature in which asphyctic subarachnoid or cerebellar hemorrhages were commonly mistaken for lesions of birth trauma. The report of subdural hematomas in the posterior fossa of 3 infants by Gilles and Shillito (1970) is of interest in showing that upward herniation of the cerebellum through the tentorial hiatus may cause compression and local sclerosis of the cerebellar cortex at the edge of the tentorium; these changes were associated with tonsillar sclerosis due to herniation into the foramen magnum.

Chronic Subdural Hematoma and Hydrocephalus. Infratentorial subdural hematomas may cause hydrocephalus by obstructing CSF flow. Hydrocephalus in infants also often coexists with large supratentorial chronic subdural hematomas or hygromas (Dandy, 1955). This combination may be interpreted as posthemorrhagic hydrocephalus due to traumatic birth. However, there is very little evidence to show that supratentorial subdural hemorrhage or encapsulated subdural hematomas cause hydrocephalus. The cause-effect relationship may actually be reverse, as demonstrated by Anderson (1952) who observed the formation of unilateral or bilateral subdural hemorrhages in 3 hydrocephalic infants following a sudden collapse of the brain from the draining of intraventricular fluid by shunting or by intraventricular surgery. The subdural bleeding was evidently caused by the stretching and tearing of the bridging veins near the sinus due to the retraction of the collapsing cerebral hemispheres. Another example of this mechanism was described by

Williams (1957) for an infant that had undergone sacral meningocele repair in a prone position with the head to the left side. On opening the meningocele sac a considerable quantity of CSF escaped. After the repair the head started to increase in circumference but with irregular configuration; craniotomy disclosed a subdural accumulation of 35 cc fluid enclosed by neomembranes on the left side, that is the side that was up during the meningocele repair. Emery (1965) described chronic subdural hematomas in shunted hydrocephalic infants and demonstrated the dimpling of the cortical surface by the stretching of blood vessels in brains that were fixed *in situ.* Becker and Nulsen (1968) observed subdural hemorrhages as a complication of shunting in 5 percent of 140 hydrocephalic patients. The mechanism responsible for the formation of subdural hemorrhages is potentially repetitive, and one may observe bilateral chronic subdural hematomas with many layers of neomembranes, or recent hemorrhages into definitely older fibrotic hygromas.

Subdural Hemorrhage upon Dehydration. The mechanism causing subdural hemorrhage in hydrocephalic infants may potentially be activated by retraction of the cerebral hemispheres from other causes, particularly if one considers that an open fontanel permits much greater deformation and stretching of parasagittal structures than is possible in adults. Subdural effusions or neomembranes were observed in dehydrated infants with severe diarrhea or general disease (Williams and Stevens, 1954; Freundlich and Beller *et al.,* 1956); Herzberger *et al.* (1956) reported subdural effusions in 12 infants with gastroenteritis and malnutrition, 7 of which had neomembranes, and 2 complicated by cerebral phlebothrombosis. Girard (1956) produced hemorrhages at the inner surface of the dura of cats and dogs by severe dehydration from injection of a 20 percent solution of sodium chloride in the blood stream. This mechanism, nonetheless, is a matter of conjecture, as several other factors such as general disease and repeated tappings need to be considered. Also, the available pathologic documentation of subdural hemorrhage upon dehydration is still fragmentary.

Chronic Subdural Hematomas Coexisting with Atrophic Hemispheric Lesions. Chronic subdural hematomas may be found in infants having a variety of atrophic or destructive cortical lesions, and the problem of the causal relationship between the two lesions recurs. Instances of unilateral subdural hematomas associated with unilateral ulegyria, or with unilateral progressive sclerosing cortical atrophy (hemiatrophy), are quoted in the respective chapters. Bilateral subdural hematomas associated with progressive sclerosing cortical atrophy were reported by Christensen and Højgaard (1964); Griepentrog (1952) reported chronic subdural hematomas with hydranencephaly.

The shrinkage of atrophic cerebral hemispheres may result in the stretching of cortical bridging veins which traverse the greatly enlarged subdural space, as shown instructively by Herzberger *et al.* (1956). Hughes and Oppenheimer (1969, case 9) reported a bilateral subdural hematoma in a 7-month-old boy whose illness started with febrile disease and general convulsions at the age of 6 weeks. Surgical exposure revealed shrunken cerebral hemispheres that had retracted from the falx, the bridging veins being absent. This finding was later confirmed at autopsy; there was also widespread cavitation of white matter and cortex in the cerebral hemispheres. The assumption that chronic subdural hematomas may be secondary to hemispheric atrophy may also pertain to the observation that subdural hematomas form as a complication of shunting procedures for the so-called "normal pressure hydrocephalus" in adults (Samuelson *et al.*, 1972).

Other authors, however, assumed a reverse cause-effect relationship, assuming that cerebral damage results from compression of the cerebral tissue by the hematoma; this interpretation was presupposed in the reports of Noetzel (1961) and Entzian and Gullotta (1972). Their cases, however, did not show the clear-cut topographic relationship between the hematoma and cerebral damage reported by Phillips (1955): A 4-month-old infant had died after a stormy course with repeated convulsions. Autopsy disclosed bilateral frontal chronic subdural hematomas which corresponded in regional distribution to lesions in the cerebral cortex which ranged from necrosis of the upper layers to total cortical necrosis.

Subdural Effusions in Leptomeningitis. Subdural effusions of clear fluid complicating purulent leptomeningitis in infants are discussed in Chapter 17. These lesions may result from therapeutic measures such as repeated subdural taps or excessive draining of cerebrospinal fluid or from abnormal transudates. Neomembranes have been found frequently in association with these subdural effusions, but there is little evidence to suggest that they progress to form encapsulated hygromas. Subdural effusions of clear fluid may also result from the presence of an infective process in the epidural space, such as in otitis media.

Traumatic Subdural Effusions. Formation of subdural hygromas has been attributed to rupture of the arachnoid membrane in craniocerebral trauma, whereby a ball valve action results in hygroma formation (Dandy, 1955). It is unlikely that such lesions occur in the absence of subarachnoid or subdural hemorrhage, which renders the distinction between the respective roles of hemorrhage and escaping CSF difficult. Some instances of fluid accumulation attributed to this mechanism may represent misinterpretations of arachnoid cysts (Chapter 20).

Subdural Hemorrhages in General Disease Processes. Subdural hematomas in the course of general disease processes typically affect older infants and children, corresponding to the age distribution of the underlying diseases. Subdural hematomas or neomembranes are caused by blood dyscrasia including hemophilia, anticoagulant therapy and others (Chapter 46). The extent of these lesions varies, ranging from asymptomatic thin neomembranes with small subdural petechiae to larger symptomatic hematomas; these apparently form from the confluence of multiple petechiae from small intradural vessels, rather than from the rupture of bridging veins. Gilman and Tanzer (1932) reported a subdural hematoma in an infant with scurvy and found 7 other instances in the literature, 5 of which were also infants. This cause of subdural bleeding needs to be kept in mind in reviewing data from the older literature. Neomembrane formation and subdural hemorrhage may also ensue from various kinds of neoplastic processes lodging in the dura mater; the most frequent cause in infants are microscopic leukemic infiltrates in the dura mater, the presence of which is often heralded by thin neomembranes.

Pathogenetic Considerations. The pathogenesis of chronic subdural hematoma in adults has been embroiled in controversy since the nineteenth century. The points of view are: 1. that formation of a neomembrane is always secondary to traumatic subdural hemorrhage or 2. that the neomembrane may itself be the cause of repetitive bleeding and hematoma formation upon minimal trauma (Friede, 1971, refs.). On reviewing chronic subdural hematoma of infancy, there appears to be little question that these lesions nearly always result from subdural hemorrhage. The role of subdural transudates from increased vascular permeability in meningitis or the traumatic escape of CSF into the subdural space remain matters of conjecture, but these mechanisms are, at best, responsible for only a small minority of the encapsulated subdural hematomas or hygromas found in infants or children.

Why a subdural hematoma becomes chronic rather than undergo quick organization and removal has attracted considerable speculation. The osmotic uptake of fluid into the cavity due to the molecular breakdown of the hematoma components has been proposed as a pathogenic mechanism, but is not supported by determinations of the osmolality of hematoma fluid (Weir, 1971). Also, the breakdown of the hematoma is not truly pertinent to the maintenance of fluid balance in a hygroma cavity: Gitlin (1955) showed that the albumin-gamma globulin, and the albumin-total protein ratios of the subdural fluids of 18 patients were considerably higher than the ratios in corresponding serum samples, suggesting that the fluids were effusates through capillary walls. This point was supported in studies with I^{131} labelled serum albumin (Rabe *et al.*, 1962), demonstrating an equilibrium of the protein content of subdural hematoma fluid with that of serum. Probably the most important primary factor inducing chronicity is the delayed reabsorption of macromolecular material from the subdural space which commonly requires organization; macromolecular material is readily removed from the subarachnoid space by the so-called "bulk flow" of CSF. The structural integrity of the arachnoid membrane separating these two compartments would seem to be an important factor in the development of chronicity.

References

Anderson, F. M.: Subdural hematoma. A complication of operation for hydrocephalus. Pediatrics 10: 11—17, 1952.

Becker, D. P., Nulsen, F. E.: Control of hydrocephalus by valve-regulated venous shunt: avoidance of complications in prolonged shunt maintenance. J. Neurosurg. 28: 215—277, 1968.

Christensen, E., Højgaard, K.: Poliodystrofia cerebri progressiva infantis. Acta Neurol. Scand. 40: 21—40, 1964.

— Husby, J.: Chronic subdural hematoma in infancy. Acta Neurol. Scand. 39: 324—342, 1962.

Coblentz, R. G.: Cerebellar subdural hematoma in infant 2 weeks old with secondary hydrocephalus operation with recovery. Surgery 8: 771—776, 1940.

Courville, C. B.: Birth and Brain Damage. Pasadena, Cal.: M. F. Courville, Pub. 1971.

Dandy, W. E.: Chronic subdural hydroma. In: Practice of Surgery (Lewis, D., ed.), Chapter 12, p. 291. Hagerstown, Md.: W. F. Prior Co. 1955.

Emery, J. E.: Intracranial effect of long standing decompression of the brain in children with hydrocephalus and meningocele. Develop. Med. Child. Neurol. 7: 302—309, 1965.

Entzian, W., Gullotta, F.: Hydrocephalus, subdural effusion and sclerotic brain atrophy in infancy. Neuropädiatrie 3: 313—318, 1972.

Freundlich, E., Beller, A. J., Berman, S.: Subdural hematoma in infancy. Amer. J. Dis. Child. 91: 608—613, 1956.

Friede, R. L.: Incidence and distribution of neomembranes of dura mater. J. Neurol. Neurosurg. Psychiat. 34: 439—446, 1971.

Gilles, F., Shillito, J.: Infantile hydrocephalus. Retrocerebellar subdural hematoma. J. Pediat. 76: 529—537, 1970.

Gilman, B. B., Tanzer, R. C.: Subdural hematoma in infantile scurvy. J.A.M.A. 99: 989—991, 1932.

Girard, F.: Les hématomes sous duraux. Acta Paediat. 45: 618—632, 1956.

Gitlin, D.: Pathogenesis of subdural collections of fluid. Pediatrics 16: 345—352, 1955.

Griepentrog, F.: Die Bedeutung subduraler Ergüsse für die Pathologie der Pachymeningitis haemorrhagica interna (an Hand eines Falles von frühkindlicher Hirnschrumpfung). Arch. Psychiat. Nervenkr. 189: 373—379, 1952.

Guthkelch, A. N.: Subdural effusions in infancy: Twenty-four cases. Brit med. J. 1: 233—239, 1953.

Hendrick, E. B., Harwood-Hash, D. C. F., Hudson, A. R.: Head injuries in children: a survey of 4465 consecutive cases at the Hospital for Sick Children. Clin. Neurosurg. 11: 46—65, 1964.

Herzberger, E., Rotem, Y., Braham, J.: Remarks on thirty-three cases of subdural effusions in infancy. Arch. Dis. Child. 31: 44—50, 1956.

Hughes, T., Oppenheimer, D. R.: Superficial siderosis of the central nervous system. Acta neuropath. 13: 56—74, 1969.

Ingraham, F. D., Matson, D. D.: Subdural hematoma in infancy. J. Pediat. 24: 1—37, 1944.

Kowitz, H. L.: Intracranielle Blutungen und Pachymeningitis haemorrhagica chronica interna bei Neugeborenen und Säuglingen. Virchows Arch. 215: 233—246, 1914.

Noetzel, H.: Gehirnveränderungen bei raumfordernden Durahaematomen bzw. Hydromen im Kindesalter. Acta Neurochir. (Wien) Suppl. 7: 501—509, 1961.

Phillips, J. Y.: Cerebral cortical damage incident to chronic subdural hematoma in infancy. Bull. Los Angeles neurol. Soc. 20: 30—36, 1955.

Pia, H. W.: Hirnverletzungen bei Kindern und ihre akuten Komplikationen. Münch. med. Wschr. 108: 760—768, 1966.

Pitlyk, P. J., Miller, R. H., Stayura, L'. Á.: Subdural hematoma of the posterior fossa: Report of a case. Pediatrics 40: 436—439, 1967.

Rabe, E. F., Flynn, R. E., Dodge, P. R.: A study of subdural effusions in an infant: With particular reference to the mechanisms of their persistence. Neurology (Minneap.) 12: 79—93, 1962.

Rosenberg, O.: Pachymeningitis haemorrhagica interna im Kindesalter. Erg. inn. Med. Kinderheilk. 20: 549—638, 1921.

Samuelson, S., Long, D. M., Chou, S. N.: Subdural hematoma as a complication of shunting procedures for normal pressure hydrocephalus. J. Neurosurg. 37: 548—551, 1972.

Schipke, R., Riege, D., Scouville, W. B.: Acute subdural hemorrhage at birth. Pediatrics 14: 468—474, 1954.

Weir, B.: The osmolality of subdural hematoma fluid. J. Neurosurg. 34: 528—533, 1971.

Williams, J. M., Stevens, H.: The surgical management of subdural effusions and their accompanying neomembranes in infancy. Ann. Surg. 139: 287—292, 1954.

— — Post-meningitic subdural effusions. J. int. Coll. Surg. (Bull.) 27: 590—594, 1957.

20. Meningeal Cysts

Arachnoid and Glio-Ependymal Cysts, General Features and Classification. Cystic lesions filled with clear fluid and located within the arachnoid membrane may be classified in terms of their localization along the neuraxis, or in terms of the structure of the cyst wall which may consist of either arachnoid connective tissue or of glio-ependymal tissue. There is overlap for these classifications, as arachnoid and glio-ependymal cysts may occur in the same locations, though not with the same frequency at any given location. Further, some cysts may combine features of arachnoid and glio-ependymal cysts, or light microscopic identification of the elements forming the cyst wall may be doubtful. Some cysts, for example, are lined with flattened or cuboidal, nonciliated cells whose derivation from ependyma or from metaplastic arachnoid tissue is a matter of conjecture. Some of the cysts described in the present chapter also resemble other types of cysts, such as neurenteric cysts (Chapter 26), or colloid cysts. The following text refers to the general histologic features of arachnoid and glio-ependymal cysts first, followed by a review of their occurrence at typical sites along the neuraxis.

Arachnoid cysts consist of local, circumscribed, bulging loculations of CSF within the arachnoid membrane; microscopic examination shows that the walls of the cysts are formed from a splitting of the arachnoid membrane into an inner and an outer layer bounding the cyst cavity. The layers consist of fibro-connective tissue which may be slightly denser than normal arachnoid and may show hyaline changes. There is no indication of past inflammation or hemorrhage, and few, if any, blood vessels are found in the cyst wall. There is no epithelial lining in typical arachnoid cysts. The outer surface of the cyst may be loosely adherent to the dura. The gross and microscopic features of these lesions are known best for supratentorial arachnoid cysts, as described by Scherer (1935) and Starkman *et al.* (1958) who proposed that these cysts form on the basis of a congenital malformation of the arachnoid membrane.

Glio-ependymal cysts are grossly similar to arachnoid cysts, but on microscopic examination they show walls composed of glial tissue with or without ependymal lining. The presence of glial tissue in the cyst wall may be considered evidence that the cyst derives from dysgenetic processes involving neuroectodermal tissue, contrary to the entirely mesodermal derivation of arachnoid cysts. Other cysts have a wall of connective tissue lined with columnar ciliated epithelium, and these are more difficult to classify. They are often considered of ependymal origin, but light microscopic examination alone may not suffice to distinguish between a ciliated ependyma and a respiratory epithelium or a ciliated epithelium of fetal esophagus. The difficulties are still greater for cysts lined with a flattened or low cuboidal epithelium having no ciliae. A low cuboidal lining may be derived from proliferation of arachnoid cap cells, or it may be simulated by metaplasia, or by compression and flattening of the innermost tissue of the cyst wall. This type of cyst has been described as epithelial cyst without further qualifications.

Glio-ependymal cysts have been linked tentatively to several other types of midline epithelial cysts, such as those originating from Rathke's pouch, or to the intraventricular colloid cysts of the third and fourth ventricles (Shuangshoti *et al.*, 1965). In the spine they need to be distinguished from the enteric or neurenteric cysts (Chapter 26), or from cystic teratomas (Ingraham and Bailey, 1946).

The frequency of arachnoid and of glio-ependymal cysts differs in different portions of the neuraxis. Cysts on the convexity of the cerebral hemispheres and in the spinal canal are nearly always arachnoid; whereas, either arachnoid or glio-ependymal cysts are found in supracollicular and retrocerebellar localization.

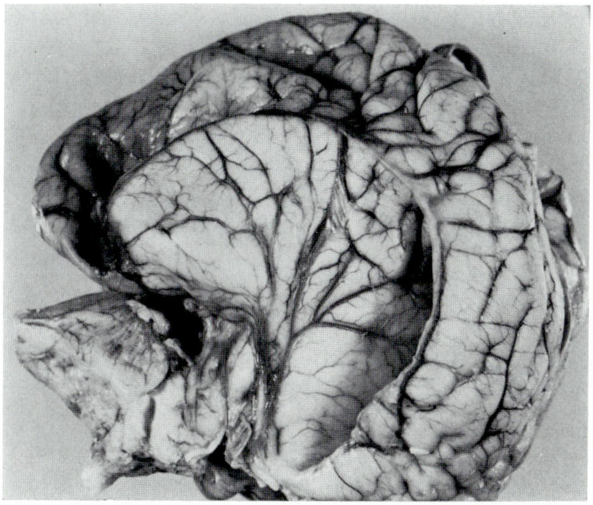

Fig. 67. Arachnoid cyst distending the Sylvian fissure

Cysts of the Cerebral Hemispheres. Arachnoid cysts of the cerebral hemispheres are often found incidentally at autopsy in adults. Some may cause local symptoms or increased intracranial pressure necessitating surgical intervention. The clinico-pathologic features of supratentorial arachnoid cysts in infancy were described by Anderson and Landing (1966) who reported 9 cases, 8 of whom were between 6 weeks and $3^1/_2$ years. There were no histories or gross findings suggestive of a preceding craniocerebral trauma. The infants had a tense fontanel and widened cranial sutures. The head was enlarged, either diffusely or in the form of a local protrusion showing transillumination and thinning of the bone on X-ray examination; other symptoms varied.

Common localization of arachnoid cysts are the Sylvian fissure (Fig. 67), parasagittal in the interhemispheric fissure or other portions of the hemispheric convexity. Most cysts are unilateral and they adhere loosely to dura or falx. The cyst tends to be rounded where it abuts and compresses nerve tissue; it indents deeply into the hemisphere or invaginates into its major fissures, displacing and flattening the underlying cortex. However, there are no local lesions or defects in the hemispheric wall, nor is there atrophy or scarring of the compressed cortex *. Most cysts are filled with a clear, colorless fluid of low protein content comparable to normal CSF, but some may show elevated protein content. The cavity of the cyst may be single or loculated by septations, and its wall is usually smooth. Microscopic examination shows an avascular connective tissue consistent with arachnoid, lacking hemosiderin, capillary proliferation or epithelial lining.

Glio-ependymal cysts of the cerebral hemispheres are much rarer than arachnoid cysts. Their gross features resemble arachnoid cysts in that they do not communicate with the lateral ventricle and compress adjoining normal cortex. Loeser and Alvord (1968) described a cluster of interhemispheric cysts attached to the falx in a newborn girl of a diabetic mother; the cysts were lined with ependyma and contained choroid plexus. Other instances were intracerebral, lined with ciliated ependyma (Bouch *et al.*, 1973). The frontal and parietal cysts described by Jakubiak *et al.* (1968) were lined with glial tissue and ciliated ependyma and with local papillary tufts consistent with choroid plexus; one contained 280 mg per 100 ml of protein. Two very similar lesions reported by Tandon *et al.* (1972) also showed ciliated ependyma and a high protein content. Further examples were described by Šimek and Gutman (1949) and by Patrick (1971). An ependyma-lined cyst of the olfactory bulb was reported by Baillie and Littler (1973). Electron microscopic examination of an intracerebral cyst disclosed a lining similar to ependyma, though situated on a basement membrane (Ghatak *et al.*, 1974).

Several lesions need to be considered in the differential diagnosis of hemispheric arachnoid cysts. The deep invagination of an arachnoid cyst into the cerebral hemisphere may simulate porencephaly, to the extent that Davison and Friedman (1946) spoke of "pseudoporencephaly". However, the bottom of an arachnoid cyst displaces intact cerebral cortex; whereas, porencephaly (Chapter 11) consists of a hemispheric defect involving cortex and white matter, fringed by abnormal cortex. Chronic subdural hygromas (Chapter 19) are located in the subdural rather than in the subarachnoid space, are commonly bilateral, and have a flat or lentiform profile. Hygromas tend to compress the hemispheric surface without invaginating into it. The hygroma fluid may be xanthochromic, and the cyst wall is formed by vascularized neomembranes or dense fibrotic tissue. The difference between a subdural hygroma and an arachnoid cyst is usually obvious on postmortem examination, but it may be less evident on surgical exposure, which may account for a tendency in the neurosurgical literature to compound the two types of cysts. Growing skull fractures (Chapter 15) have often been quoted as examples of traumatic arachnoid cysts in children; these lesions differ from arachnoid cysts in that a prolapse of arachnoid tissue occurs into a bone defect secondary to skull fracture, commonly in association with severe cerebral lesions.

Basal Cysts. Arachnoid cysts are uncommon at the base of the brain.

* Only rarely is there cortical compression of a degree causing necrosis.

They were documented in the chiasmatic or the interpeduncular cisterns of infants; the walls of the cysts were lined with glial or ependymal tissue (Harrison, 1971).

Supracollicular Cysts (Cysts of Cisterna Ambiens). Supracollicular cysts often lead to early clinical manifestations because they compress the quadrigeminal plate and aqueduct, causing severe, obstructive hydrocephalus. Approximately two-thirds of the recorded cases were infants less than 1 year old, although instances in children (Hamby and Gardner, 1935) and in adults (Noetzel, 1940; Katagiri, 1960) were also observed. The cysts are located

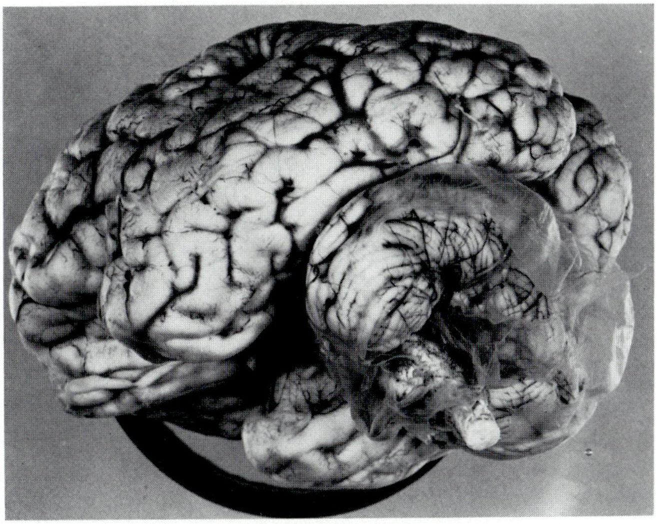

Fig. 68. Retrocerebellar arachnoid cyst

at the tentorial hiatus and do not communicate with the ventricular system. There is no attachment to the falx or tentorium. The majority of these cysts have a glial wall (Alvord and Marcuse, 1962), or a glial wall with ependymal lining (Hamby and Gardner, 1935; Kruyff, 1955). The 7-month-old boy described by Lewis (1962) had a cyst wall of connective tissue which contained in one place papillary tufts lined by cuboidal cells closely resembling choroid plexus. True arachnoid cysts also occur in supracollicular localization (Alexander, 1953; Kruyff, 1955; Harrison, 1971).

Retrocerebellar and Basal Infratentorial Cysts. These cysts are found often in the midline, compressing the vermis and dislocating the cerebellar hemispheres laterally (Fig. 68). Little *et al.* (1973) classify 20 infratentorial cysts as follows: Cerebellopontine: 6; inferior midline: 6; superior midline: 1; hemispheric: 4; clivus: 1; tentorial notch: 2. Large cysts may extend through the tentorial hiatus into the middle cerebral fossa or through the foramen magnum into the spinal canal. Retrocerebellar arachnoid cysts are described more frequently in the surgical than in the pathologic literature. These lesions are easily overlooked on postmortem examination as they are nearly always disrupted on removal of the brain; their presence is evident from the characteristic indentation of the cerebellar surface and fragments of the disrupted cyst wall. Small retrocerebellar arachnoid cysts may be asymptomatic, found as incidental observations at autopsy. Larger cysts obstruct the flow of CSF, and hydrocephalus may develop soon after birth or later in life. Eleven infants and children, 2 weeks to 9 years old, with retrocerebellar arachnoid cysts, were described by Gilles and Rockett (1971). The majority of these cysts are true arachnoid cysts, but some contain tufts of choroid plexus in their wall (Cloward and Bucy, 1937). Others have walls lined with glia and ependyma and were interpreted as evidencing derivation of the cysts from an outpouching of the embryonal roof of the fourth ventricle (Gilles and Rockett, 1971). Retrocerebellar arachnoid cysts need to be distinguished from atresia of the cerebellar foramina and from the Dandy-Walker malformation; see Chapter 30 for differential diagnosis.

Spinal Arachnoid Cysts. The vast majority of leptomeningeal cysts in the spinal column are true arachnoid cysts. Arachnoid cysts, or arachnoid diverticula, respectively, may be located in the subdural space or in the epidural space.

Subdural arachnoid cysts are uncommon and most were reported for juveniles and young adults (Perret *et al.*, 1962). The cysts are typically located at the dorsal surface of the cord, forming single, elongated, smooth-walled bags of fluid which, upon reaching a certain size, are capable of producing cord compression. Arachnoid diverticules are single or multiple pendant outpouchings of the arachnoid at the dorsal surface of the cord. The diverticules communicate with the subarachnoid space and are filled with CSF; all reported instances have been identified by means of radiologic contrast studies (Teng and Papatheodorou, 1966; Stewart and Red, 1971). Large arachnoid diverticules may cause cord compression, while smaller ones may be asymptomatic. Microscopic examination of the membranes enclosing these cysts or diverticules discloses membranous fibroconnective tissue consistent with arachnoid. Arachnoid cysts also occur as a component of myelodysplasia in spinal dysraphic lesions.

Epidural arachnoid cysts often occur in kyphoscoliotic juveniles (Cloward and Bucy, 1937). The average age of 34 cases reviewed by Wise and Foster (1955) was 22.6 years; there was a more than 2 to 1 preference for males and 19 had kyphoscoliosis. An occurrence in twins was recorded by Zander *et al.* (1967). Epidural arachnoid cysts typically occur at mid-thoracic levels, less frequently at lumbo-sacral or sacral levels (Bodosi, 1970). They consist of elongated membranous sacs of clear CSF in the epidural space dorsal to the cord. The spinal canal is widened and there may be erosion of the pedicles. Some cysts have no connection to the dura, while others communicate with the subarachnoid space by means of a thin stalk penetrating through the dura.

The differential diagnosis of intradural arachnoid cysts includes multiple cystic loculations of CSF in adhesive arachnitis. The latter are usually multiple and their origin from arachnitis is evident from the dense fibrosis, proliferation and residual inflammatory changes in the adjacent arachnoid. Epidural arachnoid cysts need to be distinguished from acquired cysts caused by trauma or surgery. The basic structure of the lesion also resembles meningoceles; the latter, however, are most common in the lumbosacral region; they are associated typically with spina bifida; they involve dura as well as arachnoid, often including nerve roots (Chapter 24). Cysts of the dorsal root ganglia are observed in 8 to 24 percent of autopsies, though not in children (Dickenman and Chason, 1964). Extradural ganglion cysts are filled with a gelatinous material which presumably arises from the bursae of the vertebral joints; these lesions occur at an advanced age (Chung *et al.*, 1968).

The occurrence of glio-ependymal cysts in the spinal canal is not firmly established. A 6-year-old boy reported by Moore and Book (1966) had a cyst, lined with what they considered ependyma without ciliae, on a connective tissue wall; there was a coexistent defect of the vertebral arches. Hyman *et al.* (1938) described a similar cyst in a 7-year-old boy. A ventral cyst at the level of C_{2-4} in a 6-year-old boy was said to be lined by meningothelial tissue (Hoffman, 1960). Wisoff and Ghatak (1971) reported a low sacral cyst lined with ciliated ependyma; however, later electron microscopic examination of the specimen disclosed features consistent with respiratory epithelium (Hirano *et al.*, 1971). The data available on the small number of epithelium-lined cysts in the spinal canal cast some doubt as to their classification as either enteric cysts (Chapter 26) or cysts of neuroectodermal derivation.

Choroid Plexus Cysts. Cystic or hydropic degeneration of the stroma of the choroid plexus, particularly at its glomus, is common in adults and is observed in more than half of the necropsies in which these changes are searched for. These cysts rarely exceed a few mm to 1 cm in size and are always without clinical importance in adults. Symptom causing choroid plexus cysts in children are very rare. Neblett and Robertson (1971) reported one in a 9-year-old girl and reviewed two previous reports on a 4- and a 10-year-old child. The cysts were located in the lateral ventricle, originating from the glomus of the choroid plexus. The cyst cavity was filled with clear CSF and was bounded by a thin membrane of connective tissue without choroid plexus epithelium.

Dural Cysts. Only a few instances of cysts within the dura mater are recorded in the literature. Haymaker and Foster (1944) described a case in whom a duplication of the dura formed a symmetric midline cavity in the posterior fossa. The bone covering the cavity was eroded and the cavity communicated with the posterior fossa through an opening on the left side. The cerebellar surface, covered with normal arachnoid, protruded only slightly through the opening into the cavity. The walls of the cavity were lined with granulation tissue, presumably because the patient had died from meningitis. The authors attribute the lesion to a failure of union of the two layers of the dura during fetal life. Robertson (1949) described a similar dural pocket which protruded between the occipital lobes and communicated with the posterior fossa. Its cavity contained a diverticule of arachnoid membrane. The present author observed a posterior fossa intradural cyst in a 6-year-old girl with multiple congenital anomalies including an atrioventricular defect and a double ureter. The cyst was formed from a duplication of the dura, was filled with clear CSF, and communicated with the posterior fossa through a broad opening. The overlying bone was eroded. The cerebellar cortex did not protrude into the cyst, and the leptomeninges were attached to the cerebellar cortex rather than to the wall of the cyst. The few available observations on intradural cysts suggest that they are developmental anomalies of little or no clinical significance.

The interesting lesion reported by Dunkser and McCreary (1971) resembles an intradural cyst only superficially. A cystic cavity was found within the occipital squame of an 18-year-old man. The cavity had eroded the diploe, and its walls were formed by the inner and outer tables of the bone. The patient had suffered an occipital fracture 16 years earlier, which suggests strongly that the lesion was more akin to growing skull fractures than to intradural cysts.

References

Alexander, E.: Benign subtentorial supracollicular cyst as a cause of obstructive hydrocephalus. J. Neurosurg. 10: 317—323, 1953.

Alvord, E. C., Jr., Marcuse, P. M.: Intracranial cerebellar meningo-encephalocele (posterior fossa cyst) causing hydrocephalus by compression at the incisura tentorii. J. Neuropath. exp. Neurol. 21: 50—69, 1962.

Anderson, F. M., Landing, B. H.: Cerebral arachnoid cysts in infants. J. Pediat. 69: 88—96, 1966.

Baillie, E. E., Littler, E. R.: Olfactory bulb cyst. Univ. Mich. Med. Center J. 39: 172—173, 1973.

Bodosi, M.: Die angeborene spinale extradurale Zyste. Acta Neurochir. (Wien) 23: 275—283, 1970.

Bouch, D. C., Mitchell, I., Maloney, A. F. J.: Ependymal lined paraventricular cerebral cysts; a report of three cases. J. Neurol. Neurosurg. Psychiat. 36: 611—617, 1973.

Chung, C. K., Uihlein, A., Bickel, W., Soule, E.: Lumbar intraspinal extradural ganglion cysts. J. Neurosurg. 29: 168—172, 1968.

Cloward, R. B., Bucy, P. C.: Spinal extradural cyst and kyphosis juvenilis. Amer. J. Roentgenol. 38: 681—706, 1937.

Davison, C., Friedman, A. P.: A cortical anomaly with some porencephalic features. J. Neuropath. exp. Neurol. 5: 225—232, 1946.

Dickenman, R. C., Chason, J. L.: Cysts of the dorsal root ganglia. Arch. Path. (Chic.) 77: 366—370, 1964.

Dunkser, S. B., McCreary, H. S.: Leptomeningeal cyst of the posterior fossa. J. Neurosurg. 34: 687—692, 1971.

Ghatak, N. R., Hirano, A., Kasoff, S. S., Zimmerman, H. M.: Fine structure of an intracerebral epithelial cyst. J. Neurosurg. 41: 75—82, 1974.

Gilles, F., Rockett, F.: Infantile hydrocephalus: Retrocerebellar arachnoidal cyst. J. Pediat. 79: 436—443, 1971.

Hamby, W. B., Gardner, W. J.: An ependymal cyst in the quadrigeminal region; report of a case. Arch. Neurol. Psychiat. (Chic.) 33: 391—398, 1935.

Handa, H., Bucy, P. C.: Benign cysts of the brain simulating brain tumor. J. Neurosurg. 13: 489—499, 1956.

Harrison, M. J.: Cerebral arachnoid cysts in children. J. Neurol. Neurosurg. Psychiat. 34: 316—323, 1971.

Haymaker, W., Foster, M. E.: Intracranial dural cyst. J. Neurosurg. 1: 211—218, 1944.

Hirano, A., Ghatak, N., Wisoff, H. S., Zimmerman, H. M.: An epithelial cyst of the spinal cord. An electron microscopic study. Acta Neuropath. (Berl.) 19: 214—223, 1971.

Hoffman, G. T.: Cervical arachnoidal cyst. J. Neurosurg. 17: 327—330, 1960.

Hyman, I., Hamby, W. B., Sanes, S.: Ependymal cysts of the cervicodorsal region of the spinal cord. Arch. Neurol. Psychiat. 40: 1005—1012, 1938.

Ingraham, F. D., Bailey, O. T.: Cystic teratomas and teratoid tumors of the central nervous system in infancy and childhood. J. Neurosurg. 3: 511—532, 1946.

Jakubiak, P., Dunsmore, R. H., Beckett, R. S.: Supratentorial brain cysts. J. Neurosurg. 28: 129—136, 1968.

Katagiri, A.: Arachnoidal cysts of the cysterna ambiens. Neurology (Minneap.) 10: 783—786, 1960.

Kruyff, E.: Paracollicular plate cysts. Amer. J. Roentgenol. 95: 899—916, 1955.

Lewis, A. J.: Infantile hydrocephalus caused by arachnoid cyst. J. Neurosurg. 19: 431—434, 1962.

Little, J. R., Gomez, M. R., MacCarty, C. S.: Infratentorial arachnoid cysts. J. Neurosurg. 39: 380—386, 1973.

Loeser, J. D., Alvord, E. C.: Clinicopathological correlations in agenesis of the corpus callosum. Neurology (Minneap.) 18: 745—756, 1968.

Lourie, H., Berne, A. S.: Radiological and clinical features of arachnoid cyst of quadrigeminal cystern. J. Neurol. Neurosurg. Psychiat. 24: 374—378, 1961.

Moore, M. T., Book, M. H.: Congenital cervical ependymal cyst. J. Neurosurg. 24: 558—561, 1966.

Neblett, C. R., Robertson, J. W.: Symptomatic cysts of the telencephalic choroid plexus. J. Neurol. Neurosurg. Psychiat. 34: 324—328, 1971.

Noetzel, H.: Arachnoidalcysten in der Cisterna ambiens. Zbl. Neurochir. 5: 281—294, 1940.

Patrick, B. S.: Ependymal cyst of the Sylvian fissure. J. Neurosurg. 35: 751—754, 1971.

Perret, G., Green, D., Keller, J.: Diagnosis and treatment of intradural arachnoid cysts of the thoracic spine. Radiology 79: 425—429, 1962.

Robertson, E. G.: Developmental defects of the cisterna magna and dura mater. J. Neurol. Neurosurg. Psychiat. 12: 39—51, 1949.

Scherer, E.: Über Zystenbildungen der weichen Häute im Liquorraum der Sylvischen Furche mit hochgradiger Deformation des Gehirns. Z. ges. Neurol. Psychiat. 152: 787—799, 1935.

Shuangshoti, S., Roberts, P., Netsky, M. G.: Neuroepithelial (colloid) cysts. Arch. Path. (Chic.) 80: 214—224, 1965.

Šimek, J., Gutman, E.: Kongenitální cysta mozková. Časopis lékařů českých Prague 88: 926—933, 1949.

Starkman, S. P., Brown, T. C., Linell, A. E.: Cerebral arachnoid cysts. J. Neuropath. exp. Neurol. 17: 484—500, 1958.

Stewart, D. H., Jr., Red, D. E.: Spinal arachnoid diverticula. J. Neurosurg. 35: 65—79, 1971.

Tandon, P. N., Roy, S., Elvidge, A.: Subarachnoidal ependymal cyst. Report of two cases. J. Neurosurg. 37: 741—745, 1972.

Teng, P., Papatheodorou, C.: Spinal arachnoid diverticula. Brit. J. Radiol. 39: 249—254, 1966.

Wise, B. L., Foster, J. J.: Congenital spinal extradural cyst. J. Neurosurg. 12: 421—427, 1955.

Wisoff, H. S., Ghatak, N. R.: Ependymal cyst of the spinal cord: Case report. J. Neurol. Neurosurg. Psychiat. 34: 546—550, 1971.

Zander, E., Jéquier, M., Perrig, A.: Contribution à l'étude des kystes méningés extra-duraux de la region dorso-lombaire. Neurochirurgie 13: 585—594, 1967.

21. Hydrocephalus—Basic Concepts and General Pathology

The term hydrocephalus, in its broadest sense, means an increased amount of fluid in the CSF spaces, particularly in the cerebral ventricles, as opposed to local accumulations of fluid in subdural hygromas, arachnoid cysts, or cavities within the cerebral parenchyma. Enlargement of the cerebral ventricles may result from their distension by increased intraventricular pressure, or from the loss of tissue caused by disease processes destroying nervous parenchyma; it is customary to distinguish "increased pressure hydrocephalus" from "hydrocephalus e vacuo". It needs to be emphasized from the start that these two mechanisms of ventricular dilation are not mutually exclusive and that they often combine and interact. For example, long-standing distension of the cerebral hemispheres because of increased intraventricular pressure eventually induces tissue damage and superimposed hemispheric atrophy. Conversely, massive destruction of the hemispheres, such as in hydranencephaly (Chapter 11), may result in secondary impairment of CSF circulation, whereby pressure hydrocephalus becomes grafted upon encephaloclastic lesions. In adult brains there may be difficulties in deciding whether a mild ventricular enlargement results from increased pressure or from hemispheric atrophy, particularly if there are no additional clues as to the causative mechanism. This problem usually does not arise for the hydrocephalus in infants and children. An increase in intracranial pressure produces enlargement of the growing skull having unfused cranial sutures, while destructive cerebral lesions are more likely to cause microcephaly if there is no additional impairment of CSF circulation. The usage of the term "hydrocephalus" in this text, therefore, is essentially synonymous with "increased pressure hydrocephalus". The term "e vacuo hydrocephalus" is useful in general pathogenetic discussions, but it has no place in the diagnostic vocabulary of the pathologist. It is more appropriate to describe and classify these lesions in terms of the disease process that caused hemispheric atrophy, rather than in terms of the resultant ventricular enlargement.

Selected aspects of CSF circulation are briefly reviewed in this chapter as a base line for the understanding of the disturbances in the production, circulation or resorption of CSF causing increased pressure hydrocephalus, and to elucidate the compensatory mechanisms available for the reduction of a pathologically increased pressure. Davson's (1967) comprehensive text provides an indispensable foundation for all deeper considerations of the subject. The present chapter also concerns the general, nonspecific alterations in the brain tissue caused by hydrocephalic distension of the ventricular system.

Circulation of CSF in Small, Primitive Brains. The circulation of CSF in small, thin-walled, primitive brains, such as in fishes and amphibia, differs from that in the brains of higher species. The general architecture of the brain of lower species reflects its derivation from the neural tube, in that the various subdivisions of the brain form local thickenings of the wall of an essentially tubular structure, being only 1 to 2 mm thick for most portions. The supporting tissue consists, in large part, of primitive ependymo-glial cells combining the morphologic features of ependyma and astrocytes. The perikarya are indistinguishable from ependymal cells of higher species, but the basal process traverses the entire width of nervous tissue and terminates in a typical astrocytic footplate at the pial surface. Ependymo-glia cells persist in the mammalian brain in certain thin portions of the ventricular walls, such as in the tuber cinereum; elsewhere they are replaced by astrocytes. The most primitive stage of vascular supply of nervous tissue consists of a superficial meningeal plexus of thin-walled sinusoid capillaries which do not enter the parenchyma. This type of vascularization is a normal feature of the spinal cord of cyclostoma, but a meningeal plexus of sinusoid capillaries remains in many lower species after capillaries have penetrated into the brain tissue. Persistence of a primitive meningeal plexus is a common trait in malformed nervous tissue (Chapter 34).

The ventricles of small primitive brains do not communicate with the meningeal fluid spaces. The fourth ventricle is closed off by a membrane which forms, centrally, a primitive choroid plexus having papillary fronds at its inner surface, while the outer surface is flat, highly vascularized and continuous with the leptomeninges. The flow of the intraventricular CSF is controlled by the beating of ependymal ciliae: In frog larvae the CSF is propelled in a cranial direction in the dorso-lateral portions of the ventricle and it flows caudally in the ventro-median portions (Adam, 1953). No directional flow of fluid occurs in the meningeal compartment, which contains fluid enmeshed in a loose mesenchymal tissue. The meningeal fluid may be considered either lymphatic or CSF, but the distinction is irrelevant as its composition is the same as that of the ventricular CSF.

The only available pathways for communication between ventricular and meningeal fluid compartments are the narrow extracellular spaces in the brain tissue and in the choroid plexus. The narrowest passages are at the cell junctions (Brightman and Reese, 1969) which abound especially between the ependymal cells where they are situated at the intercellular clefts near the ventricular surface. These cell junctions do not block the exchange of fluids between the ventricles and the extracellular tissue compartment, and they were shown to permit the passage of markers of fairly large molecular size, such as ferritin or peroxidase, from one compartment into the other (Brightman, 1967). It was also shown (Friede and Hu, 1971) that the concentration of various electrolytes in the CSF equilibrates within 5 minutes with that in the extracellular compartment of fish brain incubated *in vitro* and that equilibration of markers of large molecular size, such as sorbitol, requires up to 45 minutes. The size of the extracellular compartment was calculated from these studies, and a value of 23 percent was obtained for several markers.

The rate of production of CSF by the choroid plexus of primitive brains having a closed ventricular system is unknown. Hence, it is difficult to estimate the extent of normal flow of CSF from the ventricle through the brain tissue into the outer meningeal fluid spaces. However, diffusion of electrolytes clearly occurs between the ventricular and meningeal compartments, and it was shown that dyes injected into the ventricles of carps (Van Rijssel, 1946) or teleosts or lizards (Bakay, 1947) find their way into the meningeal fluid and *vice versa*.

In conclusion, the fluid movement in small, thin-walled brains is characterized by noncommunication between ventricular and meningeal fluid spaces, directional streaming of the ventricular fluid propelled by ciliary activity, and a diffusion equilibrium between the ventricular and the meningeal fluid which communicate through the extracellular compartment of the cerebral tissue. It can be assumed that the fluid dynamics of the early fetal mammalian brain is essentially the same.

Circulation of CSF in Large Brains. The circulation of CSF is significantly modified during growth and development of the brain, although some of the features characteristic of small brains remain in rudimentary form. Most important is the establishment of direct communication between the ventricular and the meningeal fluid spaces through the foramina of Luschka and Magendie at the caudal end of the fourth ventricle. This communication, probably augmented by an increase in the rate of CSF production, causes spreading of CSF throughout the leptomeninges. The studies of Weed (1917) have shown that this occurs in pig embryos at a length of 14 mm and concurrent with a transformation of the small-meshed meningeal mesenchyme into larger spaces which provide ample room for the flow of CSF. The residual mesenchymal tissue forms the trabecules of the arachnoid. The canalization of pig leptomeninges is completed at a fetal length of 26 mm, and the flow of CSF characteristic of mature mammalian brain is presumably established by that time. Ciliary motion persists in fetal ependyma (Friede, 1955; Hild, 1957) and even in adult man (Worthington and Cathcart, 1963). The direction of ciliary beating is toward the ventricular orifices (Cathcart and Worthington, 1964), but it is of secondary significance as a force for the propulsion of CSF, which results mainly from the vis a tergo from its continuous secretion at the choroid plexus, possibly aided by pulsations transmitted from the blood stream. These forces propel the fluid through the ventricles and the cerebral subarachnoid space toward its reabsorption, chiefly at the arachnoid granulations (Davson, 1967). The CSF of the spinal column does not partake in this directional flow, forming a backwater that mixes with the rest of the CSF by diffusion and pulsatile movements (Grundy, 1962).

The CSF bathing the surfaces of nervous tissue is in a diffusion equilibrium with the fluid in the extracellular tissue compartment, similar to that in small, primitive brains. However, a direct diffusion equilibrium between the ventricular and the meningeal fluid can no longer be established because of the thickness of the brain tissue separating them. Ventriculo-cisternal perfusion of dogs with inulin showed a marker concentration of 7.6 percent in the innermost 2 mm of ventricular wall, decreasing with the distance from the ventricular wall to 3.7, 1.5, and 0.5 percent (Rall *et al.*, 1962). The diffusion equilibrium between CSF and extracellular fluid is further modified by the presence in the brain tissue of numerous capillaries, each capillary having its own diffusion equilibrium with the surrounding extracellular fluid. The constant exchange between the extracellular compartment and the CSF flowing past the cerebral surfaces is known as the "sink action" of CSF which is an important factor in modifying the concentration of a given marker in brain tissue.

The size of the extracellular compartment in large brains is difficult to determine. Various sources of error enter the available techniques; these include changes in cell volume and redistribution of electrolytes between cells and extracellular fluid in determinations *in vitro,* types of equilibria in marker concentration between blood and CSF *in vivo,* or dilution of the marker in the extracellular space of the brain by the "sink action" of CSF. For a comprehensive review of the subject the reader is referred to Van Harreveld (1966) who estimated the size of the mammalian cerebral extracellular compartment to be in the order of 18 percent.

Pathophysiology of Disturbed CSF Circulation. A disturbance in the circulation of CSF is often loosely attributed either to its increased production or to its reduced reabsorption. However, any change in production will not cause disturbances if it is offset by a corresponding change in reabsorption and *vice versa.* A disturbance in circulation of CSF, therefore, results from a disproportion or a disequilibrium between the rates of production and absorption. In normal subjects, reabsorption of CSF increases linear with its pressure (Mortensen and Weed, 1934).

The classic investigations of Dandy and Blackfan (1914), and of many others, showed that hydrocephalus is commonly caused by impaired circulation or impaired reabsorption of CSF. Lorenzo *et al.* (1970) found two types of disturbances on perfusion of the CSF spaces of hydrocephalic infants. In one type no reabsorption of CSF took place until its pressure rose to considerably above normal, but reabsorption occurred at an approximately normal rate thereafter. In the other, reabsorption began at approximately normal pressure, but occurred at a subnormal rate at any pressure. Studies of the flow of fluids through formalin-fixed aqueducts showed a greatly reduced rate of flow through stenotic aqueducts, increasing only moderately as perfusion pressure was increased (Alvord, 1961). An increase in CSF pressure, therefore, is to some extent compensatory in speeding up the movement of fluid through constricted passages such as stenotic luminae or a fibrosed subarachnoid space.

The diffusion of CSF from the ventricle into the extracellular compartment of the brain tissue also is accelerated by increased intraventricular pressure. Acute experimental hydrocephalus increases the water content of periventricular tissue (Lux *et al.,* 1970). The penetration of dyes is also increased (Hochwald *et al.,* 1970), as is the diffusion of markers up to 2.5 to 3 mm depth before they are absorbed and removed by the capillary blood stream (Sahar *et al.,* 1969). The increased penetration of CSF into the extracellular compartment of the brain tissue provides a compensatory mechanism for increased reabsorption of CSF within the ventricular walls. Consequently, the intraventricular pressure may return to normal although the ventricles remain enlarged (Edvinsson and West, 1971; Hochwald *et al.,* 1972). Cutler *et al.* (1973) reported an infant in whom overproduction of CSF was compensated by increased transventricular absorption in the enlarged ventricles.

The following morphologic alterations in the ventricular walls may facilitate an adaptive increase in CSF reabsorption: Distension of the ventricle increases the tissue surface available for reabsorption. Flattening and stretching of the ependymal cells and the enlargement of the extracellular compartment facilitate the entrance of CSF into the tissue (Weller and Wisniewski, 1969; Weller *et al.,* 1971; Ogata *et al.,* 1972). Denudation of ependymal cells has the same effect as it reduces the number of tight junctions; relatively few junctions exist between the subependymal astrocytes. Increased reabsorption of CSF in the distended ventricular walls may explain the phenomenon of "normal pressure hydrocephalus" (Adams *et al.*, 1965), although in a different way than that proposed by the authors.

Another, less well documented, compensatory mechanism consists of a reduced production of CSF in chronic hydrocephalus. Lorenzo *et al.* (1970) found a slight decrease of 14 percent in the mean rate of CSF production in hydrocephalic patients; a 30 percent decrease was found in hydrocephalic cats and dogs (Hochwald *et al.*, 1969); no changes in production were observed by Bering and Sato (1963). Reversible alterations in the fine structure of choroid plexus epithelium were found in hydrocephalic dogs (Dohrmann, 1971). Generally, however, there is no gross or microscopic evidence of atrophy of choroid plexus in hydrocephalic brains. The secretion of CSF may conceivably be impaired if the choroid plexus becomes encased in a dense connective tissue in the course of chronic ventriculitis.

Changes in the composition of the CSF may also affect its circulation or reabsorption. Increased protein content normally has little or no effect on CSF pressure as it is removed by the bulk flow of CSF (Cutler *et al.*, 1967). However, when the reabsorption of CSF is strained to capacity, an increase in its protein content may conceivably decompensate adaptive mechanisms. For example increased viscosity of CSF may reduce its flow rate through restricted channels, or it may interfere with the penetration of CSF into the extracellular compartment of the periventricular tissue. The latter is evident when considering that the rate of diffusion of inulin molecules from the CSF into the extracellular spaces is approximately 10 times slower than that of electrolytes (Friede and Hu, 1971). The relation between the protein content of CSF and hydrocephalus is discussed further in Chapter 22.

The preceding considerations of abnormal CSF flow concern only steady elevations in CSF pressure; in addition to these, the effects of fluctuation in CSF pressure need to be considered. Continuous recording of intraventricular pressure in hydrocephalic infants demonstrates variations with time, as large as 100 mm of water, having no relation to physical activity or posture (Hayden *et al.*, 1970). Rapid changes in CSF pressure have a different effect on the ventricular walls than steady elevations in pressure. The ventricular walls behave like a solid membrane on impact of a pressure wave although they are actually quite permeable to fluids. The arterial pulse is the main source of rapid fluctuations in CSF pressure (Adolph *et al.*, 1967). Such fluctuations cause to and fro movement of contrast material in the CSF spaces in man (du Boulay, 1966). The choroid plexus is the most important site for the transfer of arterial pulsation onto the CSF (Bering, 1955). If the choroid plexus is removed from one lateral ventricle, the foramen of Monro left open, and experimental hydrocephalus induced, there is unilateral distension of the ventricle which contains choroid plexus, while the contralateral ventricle without plexus does not enlarge (Bering, 1962). These interesting experiments suggest that pressure pulses have a role in ventricular enlargement.

General Morbid Anatomy of Hydrocephalus. Hydrocephalus in infancy is characterized by progressive enlargement and ballooning of the head, with separation and delayed closure of the cranial sutures, and by tense, enlarged fontanels sometimes having intercalate bones. The distended skull shows sparse hair growth and congestion of subcutaneous veins. The eyeballs are dislocated downward and outward by the depressed orbital roof. Neurologic signs include spasticity of legs and, to a lesser extent, of arms, ataxia, tremor, imbalance and clumsiness of fine finger movements. Intellectual impairment is closely related to the degree of physical disability (Laurence, 1969).

On postmortem examination the cranial bones are thin and eroded. The cerebral hemispheres are greatly distended and fluctuant and collapse upon

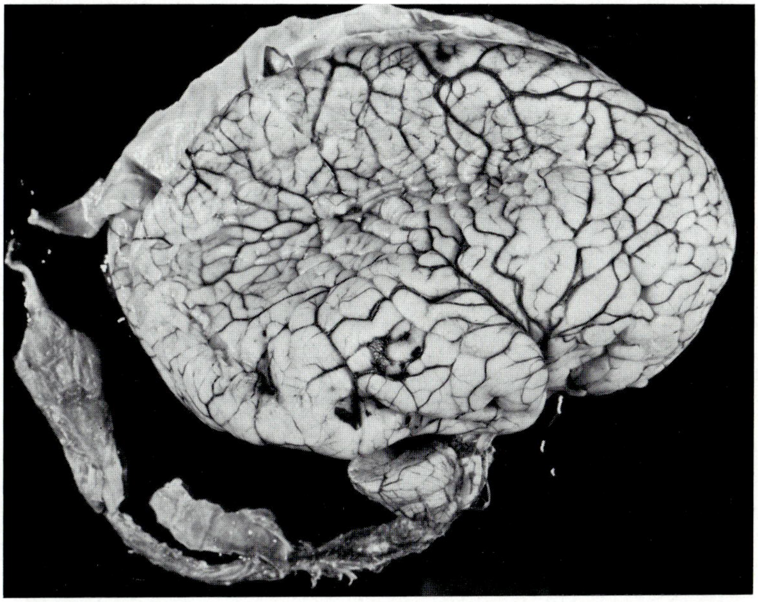

Fig. 69. Redundant gyration of the collapsed hydrocephalic hemispheres of an infant with Arnold-Chiari malformation

draining the CSF. The ventricles are enlarged, and the septum pellucidum is stretched and thin and often fenestrated by atrophy. All the thin portions of the ventricular wall bulge outwards, *e.g.*, the anterior wall of the third ventricle which may become perforated in long-standing, severe hydrocephalus. The ventricular surfaces are irregular and often exhibit a pattern of transverse, rib-like arches running perpendicular to the sagittal sinus. Dyke and Davidoff (1939) found a blood vessel at the top of each arch and concluded that the vessel offers greater resistance to ventricular distension than the white matter.

The hemispheres of brains distended by hydrocephalus in early infancy often show numerous small, irregularly arranged convolutions (Fig. 69) which have been described as polymicrogyria although they have no relationship to the cortical malformation bearing this name (Chapter 29). The microscopic architecture of gyri is normal, except for stretching or atrophy in severe, long-standing hydrocephalus. The redundant gyration of hydrocephalic brains is understood best by referring to the postnatal growth rate of cortical surface and of cerebral hemispheric surface (Scammon and Hesdorfer, 1935). The cortical surface of the normal newborn approximates 700 cm^2, which is about 43 percent of the adult value; the latter is reached by the second year of life. The postnatal growth in cortical surface normally occurs in proportion to the growth in hemispheric surface, so that approximately 66 percent of the newborn cortex and 65 to 67 percent of the adult cortex are intrasulcal. The abnormal distension of the hemispheres in hydrocephalus causes an abnormal rate of increase in hemispheric surface, while the growth in cortical surface may be normal. Consequently, a much greater portion of the intrasulcal cortex is exposed, resulting in redundant gyration, particularly during the first two years of life when the growing cortex can still adapt to the abnormal distension in hemispheric surface.

The walls of the distended hydrocephalic hemispheres are thinner than normal and may become reduced to a few mm thickness. Such thinning may result from a simple rearrangement of the hemispheric tissue around the enlarged ventricles without actual loss of tissue or reduction in brain weight. It may also result from tissue damage and atrophy with ensuing reduction in brain weight. Differentiating hemispheric distension without atrophy from hemispheric atrophy is important in assessing the capacity for restitution following treatment by surgical shunting. Encephalographic studies indicate that a hemispheric thickness of 2 cm will permit average intellectual development if CSF pressure is corrected by shunting (Scarff, 1952).

If the hydrocephalus remains untreated, the chronic distension of the cerebral hemispheres inevitably induces tissue damage and hemispheric atrophy. The brunt of the atrophy is borne by the white matter. Microscopic examination shows scattered degenerative changes in myelinated fibers, reactive axonal swellings, neutral fat, macrophages and reactive gliosis (Penfield and Elridge, 1932). The changes are usually slight because they develop in succession over a prolonged period of time. Loss of fibers may account, at least in part, for a decrease in the lipid content of hydrocephalic hemispheric white matter (Bachs and Walker, 1953; Fishman and Greer, 1963). Chemical changes may be found in the white matter in the absence of evidence of loss of nerve cells in gray matter (Rubin *et al.*, 1972).

Several mechanisms may be involved in producing the degenerative changes in the white matter: 1. Stretching and tearing of nerve fibers affect particularly those of long tracts. Preferential displacement and stretching of the upper portion of the internal capsule by the bulging ventricles explains the paraplegia and spasticity of hydrocephalic patients (Yakovlev, 1947). 2. An increased diffusion of CSF into the periventricular white matter causes chronic edema and local damage to nerve fibers (Weller and Wisniewski, 1969). 3. Edema of the periventricular white matter may be locally superimposed by the mechanical stress of rounding, stretching and flattening of the ventricular corners. If the deformation of ventricular corners occurs with sufficient speed, there may be tearing and laceration of the ventricular walls, such as in intraventricular hemorrhages in adults (Harris *et al.*, 1968) and in newborns (Chapter 2). 4. Diffuse atrophy of white matter has also been attributed to chronic compression, or to ischemia from compression, but this factor is probably overrated. A quantitative study of 22 hydrocephalic brains, from newborn to 17 years, showed a normal start and progression of myelin formation in the white matter even though the thickness of the hemispheric walls was reduced from 25 to 3 mm (Friede, 1962).

The cerebral cortex of greatly distended hydrocephalic brains is stretched and narrowed, but a thin ribbon of cortical tissue covering a thin layer of white matter is found even if the hemispheric wall measures only a few mm. The stretching of cortex is particularly manifest in the Ammon's horn, in which the pyramidal layer is unrolled and extended, distorting the normal architecture of this region. The myelinated hemispheric white matter is usually sharply delineated from a thickened layer of fibrous subependymal glia covered, at the ventricular walls, with islands of flattened, atrophic ependyma. Ependymal cells generally do not proliferate upon ventricular distension, so that large portions of the ventricular walls are denuded, with moderate reactive proliferation of subependymal glia. These nonspecific changes caused by ventricular distension may be superseded by massive gliosis if the hydrocephalus is post-inflammatory.

Atrophy of the hemispheric wall generally does not progress to the state of its complete obliteration. However, scrutiny of greatly distended hydrocephalic brains discloses, most often in the occipital, parietal and temporal lobes, circumscribed defects in which the hemispheric wall is reduced to a thin translucent membrance. Russell (1949) considered such defects local herniations of the ventricular wall through the cortex, but microscopic examination often discloses evidence for their derivation from cortical infarcts. The membranous portion is formed by leptomeninges and by a persistent molecular layer which blends with the intact cortex at the edge of the defect; some defects may still show organization of necrotic tissue or residual macrophages. Cortical infarcts may result from excessive stretching or compression of superficial arteries. Brains having relatively large defects may give the misleading impression that hydranencephaly forms on the basis of extreme hydrocephalic atrophy of the hemispheres; the relationship between hydranencephaly and hydrocephalus is more fully discussed in Chapter 11.

The ventricular dilation of hydrocephalic brains can regress completely upon correction of excess CSF pressure by early shunting, as shown by encephalographic studies of human patients (Shenkin and Perry, 1946; Nulsen and Spitz, 1952) as well as in animal experiments (Granholm, 1966). Postmortem examinations of children with long-standing decompression by shunting show the hemispheres restituted to near normal with some evidence of residual damage: The corpus callosum may be thin, and there may be cortical atrophy and widening of sulci. The leptomeninges may be thickened and gelatinous, apparently serving as a space-filling tissue. Evidence of chronic subdural hematoma is common (Emery, 1965). Early shunting is of the utmost importance for the prevention of secondary tissue damage. Patients treated early may show, after long-standing decompression, completely normal hemispheres and the ventricles may be normal, or even slightly below normal size (Kaufman *et al.*, 1973), although markedly distended ventricles had been demonstrated encephalographically at the time of shunting. Radiologic studies also show that the erosion and atrophy of squamous bones and of the basis of the skull and the enlargement of the sella turcica are capable of restitution after surgical shunting, and the size of the sella may even become reduced (Kaufman *et al.*, 1970).

References

Adam, H.: Kugelförmige Pigmentzellen als Anzeiger der Liquorströmung in den Gehirnventrikeln von Krallenfroschlarven. Z. Naturforsch. (B) 8: 250—258, 1953.

Adams, R. D., Fisher, C. M., Ojemann, R. G., Sweet, W. H.: Normal-pressure hydrocephalus. New Engl. J. Med. 273: 117—126, 1965.

Adolph, R. J., Fukusumi, H., Fowler, N. O.: Origin of cerebrospinal fluid pulsations. Amer. J. Physiol. 212: 840—846, 1967.

Alvord, E. C., Jr.: The pathology of hydrocephalus. In: Disorders of the Developing Nervous System (Fields, W. S., Desmond, M. M., eds.), chapter 14. 1961.

Bachs, A., Walker, A. E.: Experimental hydrocephalus. J. Neuropath. exp. Neurol. 7: 283—292, 1953.

Bakay, L.: Phylogenesis of the perivascular spaces of the brain. Nature (Lond.) 160: 789—790, 1947.

Bering, E. A., Jr.: Choroid plexus and arterial pulsation of cerebrospinal fluid. Arch. Neurol. Psychiat. 73: 165—172, 1955.

— Circulation of the cerebrospinal fluid. J. Neurosurg. 19: 405—413, 1962.

— Sato, O.: Hydrocephalus: Changes in formation and absorption of cerebral spinal fluid within the cerebral ventricles. J. Neurosurg. 20: 1050—1063, 1963.

Brightman, M. W.: Movement within the brain of ferritin injected into the cerebral spinal fluid compartments. In: Brain Edema (Klatzo, I., Seitelberger, F., eds.), pp. 271—284. Wien-New York: Springer 1967.

— The intracerebral movement of proteins injected into blood and cerebrospinal fluid of mice. In: Brain Barriers Systems (Lajtha, A., Ford, D. H., eds.). Progr. Brain Res. 29: 19—37, 1967.

— Reese, T. S.: Junctions between intimately apposed cell membranes in the vertebrate brain. J. Cell Biol. 40: 648—677, 1969.

Cathcart, R. S., Worthington, W. C., Jr.: Ciliary movement in the rat cerebral ventricles: Clearing action and directions of currents. J. Neuropath. exp. Neurol. 28: 69—618, 1964.

Cutler, R. W., Deuel, R. K., Barlow, C. F.: Albumin exchange between plasma and cerebrospinal fluid. Arch. Neurol. (Chic.) 17: 261—270, 1967.

— Murray, J. E., Moody, R. A.: Overproduction of cerebrospinal fluid in communicating hydrocephalus. Neurology (Minneap.) 23: 1—6, 1973.

Dandy, W. E., Blackfan, K. D.: Internal hydrocephalus. Amer. J. Dis. Child. 8: 406—482, 1914.

Davson, H.: Physiology of the Cerebrospinal Fluid. London: Churchill 1967.

Dohrmann, J. G.: The choroid plexus in experimental hydrocephalus. A light and electron microscopic study in normal, hydrocephalic, and shunted dogs. J. Neurosurg. 34: 56—69, 1971.

du Boulay, G. H.: Pulsatile movements in the CSF pathways. Brit. J. Radiol. 39: 255—262, 1966.

Dyke, G. G., Davidoff, L. M.: An explanation for the ribbing seen in the walls of dilated cerebral ventricles. Yale J. Biol. Med. 11: 485—487, 1939.

Edvinsson, L., West, K.: Relation between intracranial pressure and ventricular size at various stages of experimental hydrocephalus. Acta Neurol. Scand. 47: 451—457, 1971.

Emery, J. E.: Intracranial effects of long standing decompression of the brain in children with hydrocephalus and myelomeningocele. Develop. Med. Child. Neurol. 7: 302—309, 1965.

Fishman, R. A., Greer, M.: Experimental obstructive hydrocephalus: changes in the cerebrum. Arch. Neurol. (Chic.) 8: 156—161, 1963.

Friede, R. L.: Untersuchungen an flimmerndem Ependym in Kultur. Arch. Psychiat. (Berl.) 193: 205—392, 1955.

— A quantitative study of myelination in hydrocephalus. J. Neuropath. exp. Neurol. 21: 645—648, 1962.

— Hu, K. H.: A new approach for determining the volume of cerebral extracellular fluid and demonstration of its communication with CSF. J. Physiol. (Lond.) 218: 477—493, 1971.

Granholm, L.: Induced reversibility of ventricular dilation in experimental hydrocephalus. Acta Neurol. Scand. 42: 581—588, 1966.

Grundy, H. F.: Circulation of cerebrospinal fluid in the spinal region of the cat. J. Physiol. (Lond.) 163: 457—465, 1962.

Harris, L. S., Roessmann, U., Friede, R. L.: Bursting of cerebral ventricular walls. J. Path. Bact. 96: 33—38, 1968,

Hayden, P., Shurtleff, D. B., Foltz, E. L.: Ventricular fluid pressure recordings in hydrocephalic patients. Arch. Neurol. (Chic.) 23: 147—154, 1970.

Hild, W.: Ependymal cells in tissue culture. Z. Zellforsch. 46: 259—271, 1957.

Hochwald, G. M., Lux, W. E., Jr., Sahar, A., Ransohoff, J.: Experimental hydrocephalus. Arch. Neurol. (Chic.) 26: 120—129, 1972.

— Sahar, A., Sadik, A. R., Ransohoff, J.: Cerebrospinal fluid production and histological observations in animals with experimental obstructive hydrocephalus. Exp. Neurol. 25: 190—199, 1969.

Kaufman, B., Sandstrom, P. H., Young, H. F.: Alteration in size and configuration of the sella turcica as the result of prolonged cerebrospinal fluid shunting. Radiology 97: 537—542, 1970.

— Weiss, M. H., Young, H. F., Nulsen, F. E.: Effects of prolonged cerebrospinal fluid shunting on the skull and brain. J. Neurosurg. 38: 288—297, 1973.

Laurence, K. M.: Neurological and intellectual sequelae of hydrocephalus. Arch. Neurol. (Chic.) 20: 73—81, 1969.

Lorenzo, A. V., Page, L. K., Watters, G. V.: Relationship between cerebrospinal fluid formation, absorption and pressure in human hydrocephalus. Brain 93: 679—692, 1970.

Lux, W. E., Jr., Hochwald, G. M., Sahar, A., Ransohoff, J.: Periventricular water content. Arch. Neurol. (Chic.) 23: 475—479, 1970.

Milhorat, T. H., Clark, R. G., Hammock, M. K., McGrath, P. P.: Structural, ultrastructural, and permeability changes in the ependyma and surrounding brain favoring equilibration in progressive hydrocephalus. Arch. Neurol. (Chic.) 22: 397—407, 1970.

Mortensen, O. A., Weed, L. H.: Absorption of isotonic fluids from subarachnoid space. Amer. J. Physiol. 108: 458—468, 1934.

Nulsen, F. E., Spitz, E. B.: Treatment of hydrocephalus by direct shunt from ventricle to jugular vein. Surg. Forum 2: 399—403, 1952.

Ogata, J., Hochwald, G. M., Cravioto, H., Ransohoff, J.: Distribution of intraventricular horseradish peroxidase in normal and hydrocephalic cat brains. J. Neuropath. exp. Neurol. 31: 454—463, 1972.

Penfield, W. L., Elridge, A. R.: Hydrocephalus and the atrophy of cerebral compression. In: Cytology and Cellular Pathology of the Nervous System (Penfield, W., ed.), chapter 28. New York: Hoeber 1932.

Rall, D. P., Oppelt, W. W., Patlak, C. S.: Extracellular space of brain as determined by diffusion of inulin from the ventricular system. Life Sci. 2: 43—48, 1962.

Rubin, R. C., Hochwald, G. M., Liwnicz, B., Tiell, M., Mizutani, H., Shulman, K.: The effect of severe hydrocephalus on size and number of brain cells. Develop. Med. Child. Neurol. 14, Suppl. 27: 117—120, 1972.

Russell, D. S.: Observations on the Pathology of Hydrocephalus. Med. Res. Council Special Rep. Series No. 265. London: HMSO 1949

Sahar, A., Hochwald, G. M., Ransohoff, J.: Alternate pathway for cerebrospinal fluid absorption in animals with experimental obstructive hydrocephalus. Exp. Neurol. 25: 200—206, 1969.

Scammon, R., Hesdorfer, H.: Growth of the human nervous system. Proc. Soc. exp. Biol. 33: 415—421, 1935.

Scarff, J. E.: Nonobstructive hydrocephalus; treatment by endoscopic cauterization of choroid plexus. Long term results. J. Neurosurg. 9: 164—176, 1952.

Shenkin, H. A., Perry, C. R.: Reversibility of cerebral ventricular dilatation. J. Neurosurg. 3: 234—238, 1946.

Van Harreveld, A.: Brain Tissue Electrolytes. Washington, D.C.: Butterworth 1966.

Van Rijssel, J. G.: Circulation of cerebrospinal fluid in carassius gibelio. Arch. Neurol. Psychiat. (Chic.) 56: 522—543, 1946.

Weed, L. H.: Developments of the cerebrospinal spaces in pig and man. Contrib. Embryol. Publ. Carnegie Inst. Washington 5, No. 14, 1917.

Weller, R. O., Wisniewski, H.: Histological and ultrastructural changes with experimental hydrocephalus in adult rabbits. Brain 92: 819—828, 1969.

— — Shulman, K., Terry, R. D.: Experimental hydrocephalus in young dogs: Histological and ultrastructural study of the brain tissue damage. J. Neuropath. exp. Neurol. 30: 613—626, 1971.

Worthington, W. C., Jr., Cathcart, R. S.: Ependymal cilia: Distribution and activity in the adult human brain. Science 139: 221—222, 1963.

Yakovlev, P. I.: Paraplegias in hydrocephalics. Amer. J. ment. Defic. 51: 561—576, 1947.

22. Hydrocephalus—Special Pathology

The recognition of hydrocephalus dates back to ancient times (Dandy, 1920, review), but no insights were obtained into the pathogenesis of the disease until the physiology of flow of CSF, reviewed in Chapter 21, was understood. Disturbances in the flow of CSF may result from its altered secretion, circulation or reabsorption. A comprehensive review of the morbid anatomy of hydrocephalus by Russell (1949) led her to conclude that at least 99 percent of her cases had resulted from impaired circulation of CSF caused by mechanical obstructions of the CSF spaces. Neoplasia is a common cause of obstruction, but description of these lesions is beyond the scope of the present text and they are mentioned only occasionally for reference. The most common nonneoplastic types of obstructions are shown in Table 3 from the statistics of Ford (1926) and Gilles and Shillito (1970). The description of lesions causing hydrocephalus in this chapter is arranged as to follow the normal flow of CSF: The problem of overproduction of CSF by the choroid plexus is considered first; next, the various obstructive lesions within and outside of the ventricles; and, last, impaired mechanisms of CSF reabsorption.

Hypersecretory Hydrocephalus. The concept of hypersecretory hydrocephalus is based on observations of intracranial hypertension and progressive hydrocephalus in infants with choroid plexus papillomas. Nearly half of these tumors occur during the first decade of life, occasionally connatal, with preference for males. In infants papillomas occur most frequently in the lateral ventricles, occasionally in the third, rarely in the fourth ventricle; the pattern is reversed at higher ages (Matson and Crofton, 1960). Hydrocephalus complicating choroid plexus papillomas may occur without evident obstruction of CSF pathways; there is diffuse symmetrical dilation of the entire ventricular system as well as of the basal cisterns. These changes were attributed to overproduction of CSF: Ray and Peck (1956) observed enormous abdominal distension immediately following intra-abdominal shunting in an infant with choroid plexus papilloma, and daily flow rates of 800 or 300 to

Table 3. *Common Causes of Hydrocephalus*

	Ford, 1926: 100 cases of infantile hydrocephalus	Gilles and Shillito, 1970: 97 cases of hydrocephalus among 1,050 consecutive autopsies
Meningitis and arachnoid fibrosis	53	25
Syphilitic meningitis	3	—
Arnold-Chiari malformation	16	22
Aqueduct stenosis alone	14	6
Subdural hematoma	2	3 [1]
Arachnoid cyst, posterior fossa	—	2
Major malformations	3	3
Fresh ventricular hemorrhage	2	—
Associated with porencephaly	3	—
Cryptogenic	4	9
Neoplasia	—	27

[1] Posterior fossa.

400 cc of CSF have been reported (Vigouroux, 1908; Laurence, 1958). The intracranial pressure returns to normal upon removal of the tumor (Kahn and Luros, 1952; Matson and Crofton, 1960). In some instances, however, the hydrocephalus fails to regress (McDonald, 1969), and arachnoid fibrosis may be found in the basal cisterns at autopsy (Harris, 1962; Jellinger *et al.*, 1970). Fibrosis of the arachnoid may be induced by a sterile inflammatory reaction to necrotic material discharged from the neoplasm or to the absorption of proteinaceous transudates.

Obstruction of the Foramen of Monro. Selective distension of one or both lateral ventricles may result from obstruction of CSF flow through the foramina of Monro. The most common cause of obstruction is neoplasia, such as colloid cysts or craniopharyngiomas. Long-standing ventriculitis, particularly neonatal meningitis (Chapter 17), or the organization of massive intraventricular hematomas may also obstruct the foramina of Monro; in these instances pathologic changes are usually evident throughout the ventricular walls and may reach the extent of loculation or septation of the lateral ventricles. Several instances reported as "atresia of the lateral ventricles" (Cloward, 1969; Russell, 1949, case 29) were posthemorrhagic ventricular loculations. Aplasia of the foramen Monro has been diagnosed on surgical exploration (Anderson *et al.*, 1974), but the lesion is not well documented pathologically. Hydrocephalic distension of the ventricles may coexist with a very large cavum septi pellucidi or cavum Vergae respectively (Chapter 28), but there is no evidence to substantiate that a large cavum may induce hydrocephalus by obstructing the foramina of Monro. A hydrocephalic infant reported by Dooling *et al.* (1972) had a cystic cavum septi pellucidi, but there was also granular ependymitis probably residual to a neonatal meningitis ascending from a meningocele.

Obstruction of the Third Ventricle. Hydrocephalus from obstruction of the third ventricle in infants is usually caused by neoplasms compressing or invading the ventricle, such as craniopharyngiomas, gliomas, or implanted tumors; intraventricular neuroepithelial or choroid plexus cysts obstructing the third ventricle are extremely uncommon in infants (Henschen, 1955). Fusion of the walls of the third ventricle was observed in a 6-month-old hydrocephalic boy (Kepes *et al.*, 1969), but the aqueduct was obliterated as well, and the authors interpreted the case as an extreme degree of spreading of the process of aqueductal obliteration. Fusion of the basal ganglia often occurs in holoprosencephaly without causing hydrocephalus. An exceptionally large massa intermedia with broad fusion of the thalami has been considered a developmental stigma because many animal species have a very large massa intermedia; no obstruction of CSF flow results from this variant.

Obstruction of the Cerebral Aqueduct; General Pathology. The cerebral aqueduct is the most common site of intraventricular obstruction of CSF flow, evidently because it is the longest and narrowest passage and, perhaps, also because there is no choroid plexus in it. A brief introduction on the normal anatomy and development of the human aqueduct may help in the interpretation of pathologic changes.

The fetal aqueduct develops from a ventricle-like distension of the lumen of the neural tube underneath the tectal plate; the distented portion is separated from the third and fourth ventricles by narrow passages and there are deep dorsal recesses in the tectal plate. The caudal portion of the embryonal aqueduct, in particular, forms a large pouch which overrides the anterior medullary velum. The adult configuration of the aqueduct results from its gradual narrowing during fetal development (Turkewitsch, 1935). Microscopic examination of the walls of the fetal aqueduct reveals interesting areas of tissue differentiation (Keene and Hewer, 1935): The subcommissural organ covers the ventricular surface of the posterior commissure; it consists of a layer of high cylindrical epithelium with secretory features. The organ undergoes involution near term in man, but persists throughout adult life in all other vertebrate species. Residual islands of high columnar epithelial cells are still discernible in the ependymal lining of the posterior commissure of newborns. Reisner's fiber, a most curious structure, originates at the surface of the subcommissural organ and extends through the fourth ventricle into the spinal canal. A narrow ependyma-lined recess, the recessus mesocoelicus, extends deeply into the tectal plate immediately caudal to the posterior commissure. This recess can still be found in newborns; it normally obliterates during postnatal life, but persists occasionally as a thin tube of ependymal cells in adults. Very little is known on the functional significance of these structures although the pertinent literature is quite voluminous.

The configuration of the aqueduct of newborns approximates that of adults. It is triangular at the cranial orifice underneath the posterior commissure, is rounded or oval under the superior colliculi, and assumes the shape of an inverted "U" at the posterior colliculi. The caudal third of the aqueduct usually shows a deep median slit in its floor, extending midline into the raphe. The walls of this ventral slit may be fused in its dorsal portion, forming a narrow ependyma-lined channel that projects in a cranial direction, in the midline, under the main lumen of the aqueduct (Fig. 70). This channel is a common feature in serial sections of normal human aqueducts (Friede, 1961) but is seen only on occasion in random sections; it has been misinterpreted as pathologic forking of the aqueduct when found in instances of aqueduct stenosis. The narrowest portion of the normal adult aqueduct measures 0.8 cm^2 with a range of 0.4 to 1.5 cm^2 (Woollam and Millen, 1953). The mean cross sectional area of the narrowest portion of the formalin-fixed

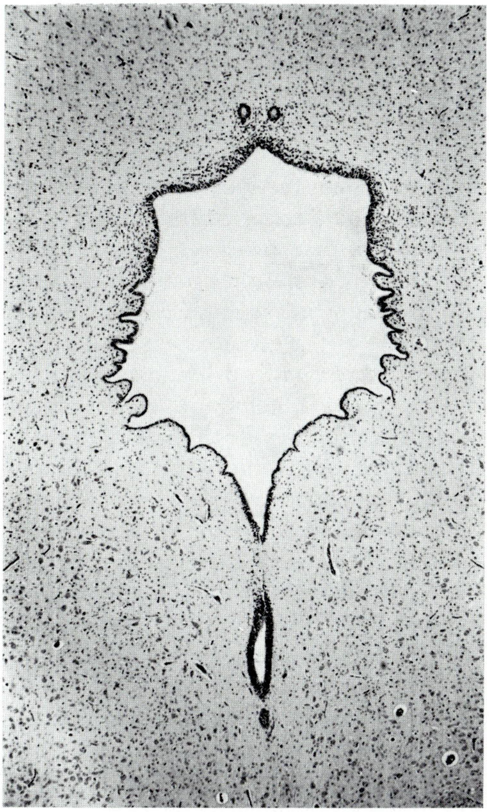

Fig. 70. Channel ventral to the aqueduct (forking) in a normal newborn; H & E ×32

aqueduct of 83 children was 0.5 cm^2; a lumen below 0.15 cm^2 can be considered abnormal, although a minimal lumen of 0.1 cm^2 is still consistent with a normal size of the ventricle (Emery and Staschak, 1972).

Complete obstruction of the aqueduct is referred to as *atresia*, incomplete obstruction as *stenosis*. The type of obstruction is also commonly classified as congenital or acquired according to the microscopic features of the lesions. In congenital obstruction the lumen of the aqueduct is either absent or greatly malformed and replaced by multiple tenuous channels in irregular disposition. In acquired obstruction the outlines of a normal lumen are discernible by residual nests of ependyma, and the lumen is filled up with reactive gliosis

(Fig. 71). The histopathologic classification of these two types of lesion is controversial, however. Drachman and Richardson (1969) in reviewing the literature found wide disagreement as to the histopathologic criteria used for classification; they also presented a case which showed different types of lesions at different levels of the aqueduct. The difficulties in distinguishing acquired from connatal obstruction of the aqueduct are further increased by the rather common notion that congenital atresia, in the meaning of nonpassage from birth on, is synonymous with aplasia, meaning nonformation. Dandy (1920) pointed out the fallacy of this concept: The neural tube has a lumen from its very origin on, and all strictures of this lumen must be secondary and acquired; the term "aplasia" is a misnomer when applied to obstructions of the aqueduct. Experimental evidence, quoted later in this text, has shown that lesions of the type of congenital atresia can be induced during fetal development with a variety of infectious or noninfectious agents. The difference between "congenital" and "acquired" obstruction, therefore, is probably more in the timing of the disease processes than in any other factor. With these limitations in mind, the distinction of congenital from acquired aqueduct stenosis retains a certain diagnostic usefulness, and most lesions can easily be classified as belonging to one or the other category.

Stenosis of the aqueduct results in dilation of lateral and third ventricles, while the fourth ventricle and cerebellum are of normal size or are compressed by the expansion of the hemispheres in the supratentorial compartment. The onset of hydrocephalus depends on the nature of the disease process and on the degree to which the aqueduct is obstructed. Congenital atresia induces progressive hydrocephalus *in utero* or shortly after birth and runs a fatal course, usually within one year, unless corrected by surgical shunting.

Congenital Sex-Linked Stenosis of the Aqueduct. Stenosis of the aqueduct occurs as a familiar, sex-linked trait, affecting males only, but being transmitted by unaffected females (Bickers and Adams, 1949). The severity of hydrocephalus varies considerably. This disease accounts for only a small fraction of all cases of aqueductal obstruction, but its recognition is important in genetic counselling. Several families having this trait have been reported (Warren *et al.,* 1963; Needleman and Root, 1963). In the one described by Edwards *et al.* (1961) there was coexistent deformity of the thumbs, spasticity and contractions, but hydrocephalus was not a dominating lesion in this family. The association of thumb deformity with hydrocephalus was also noted by Jezequel *et al.* (1973).

Only a fraction of the cases of sex-linked stenosis were studied neuropathologically, and these had a stenotic aqueduct with a very narrow lumen in the form of a thin slit with its long axis in the sagittal plane. The lumen was lined with ependyma throughout, often with marked local folding; the scattered nests and aberrant channels of ependyma seen in nonhereditary congenital stenosis were not observed (Holmes *et al.,* 1953).

Congenital Obstruction of the Aqueduct. Congenital atresia, or stenosis, of the aqueduct may occur as the only cerebral lesion, or it may coexist with other deformities, most often with the Arnold-Chiari malformation or with hydranencephaly. Obstruction of the aqueduct with the Arnold-Chiari mal-

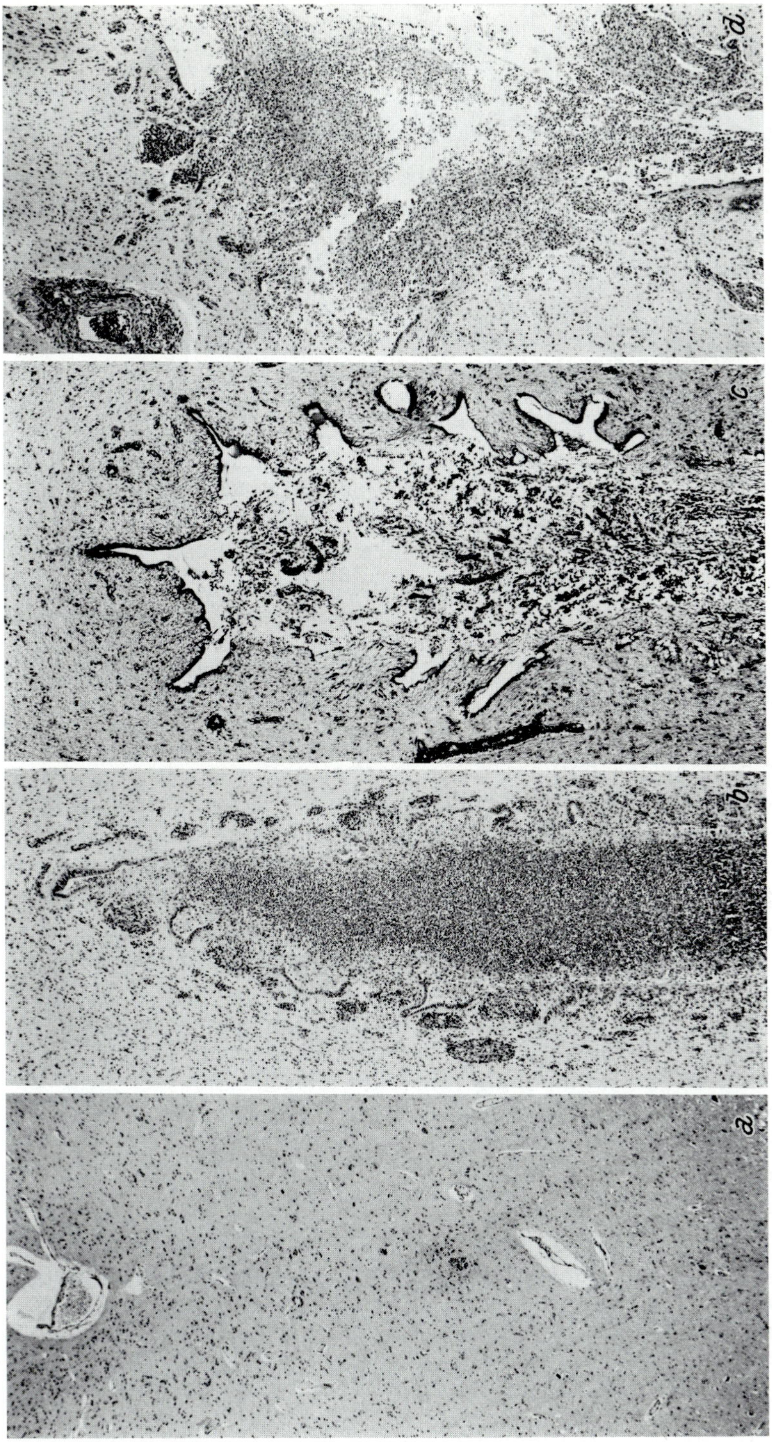

Fig. 71. Types of aqueductal obstruction. a: congenital atresia: site of lumen is marked by minute ependymal nests. b: plugging of aqueduct by acute fibrinopurulent exudate. c: fibrovascular organization of exudate. d: subependymal gliosis invading the lumen of the aqueduct. H & E ×36

formation (Chapter 25) is usually of the congenital type, but it may also be an acquired gliotic obstruction from an ascending leptomeningitis. Obstruction of the aqueduct in hydranencephaly may be either of the congenital or of the acquired type (Chapter 11).

In congenital atresia the aqueduct may not be discernable on gross inspection of the cut surface of the midbrain. Microscopic examination discloses clusters of ependymal nests or ependymal channels embedded in a loose glial tissue. The arrangement of these structures does not conform in any way to the normal outlines of the aqueduct. The aqueduct may be atretic for the entire length, or for a short segment, its cranial orifice forming a dilated diverticle. There is no evidence of active or past inflammatory changes. The surrounding midbrain structures are usually normal, but there may be slight deviations in the arrangement of nuclear groupings. Congenital atresia of the aqueduct is often referred to as "forking", suggesting a deviation and nonjunction of CSF channels. This concept is embryologically incorrect; it is often based on a misinterpretation of the normal anatomy of the aqueduct, as described above. MacFarlane and Maloney (1957) proposed to call the ventral cul de sac of the normal aqueduct "simple forking" to distinguish it from the intertwining channels in congenital atresia which they called "complex forking". In view of this overlapping usage, the term forking is of debatable value.

Acquired Gliotic Obstruction of Aqueduct. Acquired stenosis, or atresia, of the aqueduct is commonly part of a widespread ependymitis throughout the ventricular walls. On microscopic examination one finds residual nests of ependyma along the outlines of the normal profile of the aqueduct, but its lumen is partly or completely obliterated by proliferated glial tissue which has invaded the aqueduct through breeches in the ependyma. Strands of glial tissue may subdivide the lumen. Neonatal or infantile meningitis is the most common cause of this type of obstruction; the lumen of the aqueduct may have been plugged during the acute or subacute phase of the disease by a semi-solid fibrinopurulent exudate being successively organized from the surrounding subependymal tissue; in other instances stenosis had developed gradually from the progressive proliferation and fusion of glial nodules in diffuse nodular ependymitis. Less common causes of acquired obstruction of the aqueduct are organization of an intraventricular hemorrhage, or the spilling into the ventricles of large amounts of necrotic debris from extensive hemispheric lesions. The latter mechanism appears to be operative in at least some of the cases of hydranencephaly.

Obstruction of the aqueduct by nonneoplastic reactive gliosis needs to be differentiated from the small, subependymal astrocytomas, usually of piloid type, which cause progressive aqueduct stenosis in children and young adults in the absence of pathologic changes elsewhere at the ventricular surfaces.

Septum of Aqueduct. Hydrocephalus due to a thin septum across the aqueduct is rare. Turnbull and Drake (1966) reviewed 16 cases including 4 of their own. Enlargement of the head was found for most, and all except one were older than 2 years, the oldest 46 years. The prognosis of a septum of the aqueduct, therefore, is much better than that of congenital stenosis or of atresia of the aqueduct, presumably because CSF flow is less severely impaired by the thin septum. The septum was found at the caudal end of the aqueduct in all cases and some showed small openings or ependymal canaliculi in the septum. The septum is usually formed by a loose glial tissue having sparse ependymal cells (Russell, 1949). Turnbull and Drake (1966) consider a septum a minimal form of aqueduct stenosis rather than a specific disease entity.

Experimentally Induced Obstruction of the Aqueduct. A large number of teratogenic agents are known to induce hydrocephalus in experimental animals, but a precise mode of action has been defined for only a few. Congenital stenosis of the aqueduct was induced in rats born to mothers fed with a diet deficient in vitamin B 12 or folic acid. The aqueduct became completely closed during gestation and reopened by the 16th day; there was also aplasia of the subcommissural organ (Overholser *et al.*, 1954; Woodard and Newberne, 1967). Stenosis of the aqueduct is also induced in rats by subcutaneous injection of trypan blue into the mothers during early gestation (Stempak, 1964). Fetal infection with myxovirus localizes selectively to the ependyma, inducing necrosis of ependymal cells and subsequent congenital stenosis of the aqueduct in the absence of residual inflammatory changes (Johnson and Johnson, 1969; Chapter 16). Congenital stenosis of the aqueduct has also been observed as a hereditary trait in mice (Clark, 1934). These data show that a variety of nutritional, infectious or hereditary factors can induce aqueductal stenosis during fetal life, but they do not allow for definite conclusions as to the etiologic factors operative in man.

Obstruction of the Aqueduct by Vascular Malformations. Obstruction of the aqueduct by vascular malformations is rare at any age (Courville, 1961). A 7-month-old boy, hydrocephalic since the first month, had the aqueduct occluded by a cluster of thin-walled vascular channels with interspaced scattered nervous tissue elements (Bailey and Woodward, 1959). An 11-year-old girl described by Rowbotham (1938) had a septum across the aqueduct just caudal to an aneurysm.

Compression of the Aqueduct. Compression of the aqueduct causing hydrocephalus in infancy may be the result of neoplasia such as tumors of pineal gland or tumors infiltrating the midbrain. It is also a typical manifestation of arteriovenous aneurysm of the vein of Galen (Chapter 34) and of arachnoid or glioependymal cysts in the cisterna ambiens (Chapter 20). Very large aneurysms of the basilar artery may also compress the aqueduct (Ekbom *et al.*, 1968), but this cause has been observed in adults only.

Obstruction at the Cerebellar Foramina. A variety of posterior fossa lesions other than neoplasia may interfere with the normal communication of the cerebral ventricles with the subarachnoid space. Some of these lesions are described in the chapter on atresia of the cerebellar foramina and the Dandy-Walker malformation (Chapter 30), on retrocerebellar arachnoid cysts (Chapter 20) and on infratentorial subdural hematomas (Chapter 19). These lesions interfere with the normal draining of the ventricular system either by obstructing or by deforming the cerebellar foramina without dislocating them in a caudal direction.

Another type of obstruction results from dislocation of the cerebellar foramina into the foramen magnum in acute or in chronic cerebellar herniations. Impaction of the cerebellum into the foramen magnum with acute cerebellar tonsillar herniation probably closes the median aperture (foramen of Magendie) first, or it may permit its communication with the spinal canal without allowing for backflow into the cranial vault. The lateral apertures are sealed later and less completely by compression of the flocculus and of the cerebellum caudal to the flocculus as these structures become pressed against the adjoining bone. A fluctuating ventricular distension may result varying with the degree of compression (Howell, 1959).

Cerebellar tonsillar herniation may cause increased intraventricular pressure by directly impairing the drainage of the ventricles, but it may also eliminate the dampening effect of the spinal dural sac on the fluctuations of the CSF pressure. It has been shown that the spinal dural sac acts as an elastic reservoir for CSF, which flows back and forth through the foramen magnum, allowing for rapid adaptations to changes in intracranial blood volume and to changes in CSF volume (Martins *et al.*, 1972).

A more severe type of obstruction of CSF spaces at the foramen magnum occurs in the Arnold-Chiari malformation (Russell and Donald, 1935; Russell, 1949), in which the caudal portion of the fourth ventricle and the cerebellum as well as all the cerebellar foramina are displaced into the cervical spinal canal. The herniated fourth ventricle communicates directly with the spinal subarachnoid space, but the latter does not communicate with the cranial subarachnoid space. The two subarachnoid compartments are separated by the impaction of the cerebellar tissue at the foramen magnum and by the dense leptomeningeal fibrosis that typically develops at that site. This type of noncommunication is dramatized when an ascending leptomeningitis involves the spinal leptomeninges and the cerebral ventricles without spreading into the cranial leptomeninges. The same type of obstruction was demonstrated in hydrocephalus induced in rabbits with hypovitaminosis A, by showing the passage of colloidal carbon from the ventricles into the spinal subarachnoid space, but no passage into the cerebral subarachnoid space (Millen and Woollam, 1958).

Noncanalization of the Subarachnoid Space. It may be stated from the start that noncanalization of subarachnoid space has never been documented as a cause of hydrocephalus in man; nonetheless, the potential existence of this process has been discussed in the literature. Canalization of the leptomeninges develops in the fetus subsequent to the opening of the cerebellar foramina and the ensuing flow of CSF from the ventricles into the subarachnoid space (Chapter 21). Milhorat *et al.* (1971) studied the leptomeninges of 52 hydrocephalic patients and observed a subarachnoid space in all. However, the emphasis in this study was misplaced, in that the authors searched for congenital absence of the leptomeninges, which is unlikely, rather than for absence of canalization of the subarachnoid space, which is merely a change in the mesh-size of the meningeal mesenchyme which is very difficult to assess or document on microscopic examination of fixed tissue specimens. One may speculate that there is insufficient canalization of the subarachnoid space in some instances of the Arnold-Chiari malformation or other malformations—such as the meningeal tissue of the area cerebrovasculosa. Green (1970) interpreted increased density of leptomeninges in congenital hydrocephalus of type (ch) in mice as noncanalization of the subarachnoid space; this strain of mice also shows other anomalies such as impairment of basicranial cartilage (Grüneberg, 1953). The question of noncanalization of subarachnoid space, thus, remains an intriguing concept whose documentation would seem to require other methods than inspection of sections of tissue fixed after much of the CSF had been drained from the meninges.

Fibrotic Obstruction of Subarachnoid Space. Fibrotic obstruction of the subarachnoid space is the most common cause of hydrocephalus in infancy (Table 3). Fibrosis develops most often from the organization of a fibrinopurulent exudate in the subarachnoid space (Chapter 17), but it may also result from the organization of subarachnoid hemorrhages, such as the intraventricular and subarachnoid hemorrhages complicating asphyxia in prematures (Chapter 2) or hemorrhages from disturbances in blood clotting mechanisms, as described in Chapter 46. Fibrosis may also be induced by the organization of massive proteinaceous exudates or necrotic debris spilling into the subarachnoid space. The hydrocephalus found in mucopolysaccharidoses (Chapter 35) appears to be the result of impaired CSF circulation in the subarachnoid space, but the precise pathogenetic roles of meningeal fibrosis or of meningeal polysaccharide deposition are not established.

Early stages of arachnoid fibrosis in purulent leptomeningitis are characterized by the aggregation of macrophages and proliferating fibroblasts in the deep epipial portions of the subarachnoid space; the exudate may become bilayered, being organized in its deeper portion, while strictly purulent, often with necrosis, in its outer portion. Upon longer survival the organization of the exudate proceeds across its entire width, with an increased density of collagen fibers and scattered residual focal lymphocytic infiltrates. The changes tend to be most severe in the basal cisterns.

Posthemorrhagic fibrosis of the leptomeninges may be accompanied with very little gross pigmentation of the leptomeninges. Microscopic examination of the meninges of infants surviving perinatal asphyxia for weeks or months may disclose fibroblastic proliferation in the leptomeninges of the basal cisterns and cerebellum, identified as posthemorrhagic from scattered hemosiderin-laden macrophages. There are usually no lesions or pigmentation in the adjacent nervous parenchyma, in distinction to its characteristic affection in posthemorrhagic superficial siderosis (Chapter 9).

Fibrosis of the subarachnoid space with subsequent obstruction of CSF circulation is readily induced by the injection of irritant foreign materials, being the most convenient and reliable method for inducing hydrocephalus in experimental animals. The effective agents were reviewed by Pudenz *et al.* (1960) and include bacteria, toxins, india ink, kaoline, paraffin, powdered wood, gelatin and others; Wisniewski *et al.* (1969) added silicone oil to this list.

Diseases Affecting Arachnoid Granulations. Weed's (1914) concept that the CSF is reabsorbed at the arachnoid granulations is now widely accepted, although some uncertainty remains as to the relative importance of ancillary sites of reabsorption. The history of the discovery of arachnoid granulations was reviewed by Turner (1961). It is customary to distinguish the arachnoid granulations visible to the naked eye from the arachnoid villi which are discernible only with the microscope. Both structures are basically the same; arachnoid granulations are considered hypertrophic arachnoid villi. Arachnoid villi appear in man at approximately the 12th week of gestation (Turner, 1961). No granulations are discernible in the newborn; they become evident by the 18th month and are numerous and widely disseminated by the 3rd and 4th year of life (Clark, 1920). Granulations are most common along the superior sagittal sinus, but they occur at any other intracranial sinus as well. Arachnoid villi were also found at the spinal root sleeves of monkeys (Welch and Pollay, 1963).

It has been suggested that the arachnoid granulations serve as one-way valves permitting direct flow of CSF into the blood stream, but none in the reverse direction (Welch and Friedman, 1960). The valves were considered large enough to permit passage of particulate material (Welch and Pollay, 1961) or even intact erythrocytes (Simmonds, 1953). Shabo and Maxwell (1968) and Alksne and Lovings (1972) challenged the existence of such large pores on the basis of electron microscopic data showing no direct passage of markers through the limiting endothelium; passage did occur by active transport through the cells. More recently, the distension of the villi and the size of the intercellular gaps were found to depend directly on fixation pressure (Gomez *et al.*, 1973). Reexamination of the characteristics of flow of CSF tended to confirm an unrestricted passage of proteins through pores of meningeal draining channels (Hollingsworth *et al.*, 1970).

Congenital aplasia of arachnoid granulations has been reported as a cause of communicating hydrocephalus for 2 infants (Gilles and Davidson, 1971). One, a boy over 3 years old, had only a few rudimentary granulations near the sagittal sinus. The other, 31 months old, had no granulations at all, and a few villi, considered abnormal in structure, were found on serial sectioning of the superior sagittal sinus. The number of granulations in these infants was considered significantly less than normal and was thought to be the cause of hydrocephalus. We have recently observed complete agenesis of granulations and of villi in a 5-year-old hydrocephalic child having no other cerebral lesions, and subtotal agenesis in a nonhydrocephalic 7-year-old (Gutierrez *et al.*), indicating the difficulties involved in assessing the importance of a well developed Pacchionian system.

Acute blockage of the arachnoid granulations by hemorrhage has also been proposed as a mechanism impairing CSF reabsorbtion (Ellington and Margolis, 1969). The arachnoid villi of patients with subarachnoid hemorrhage were packed with red cells. Electron microscopic examination of villi in experimental animals demonstrated entrapment and *in situ* degeneration of erythrocytes within the villi (Alksne and Lovings, 1972). These interesting data still need to be reconciled with the usually rapid and eventless resorbtion of hemorrhages from the subarachnoid space which, at least for the vast majority, occurs without blockage or demonstrable residual fibrosis of the granulations, or impairment of CSF circulation.

Functional Impairment of the Reabsorption of CSF. Functional disturbances of the reabsorption of CSF do not appear to be a significant factor in the production of hydrocephalus in man. The reabsorption of CSF may be impaired by changes in its composition or by changes in venous pressure. An increase in the protein content of CSF may impair its reabsorption by decreasing the osmotic gradient between CSF and plasma. However, experimental studies show that the outflow of an artificial CSF from the cranial vault is independent of the colloid osmotic pressure of the fluid (Hollingsworth *et al.*, 1970). Increased CSF protein was thought to be responsible for the concurrence of nonobstructive hydrocephalus or increased intracranial pressure with small tumors located anywhere along the cerebrospinal fluid axis (Gardner *et al.*, 1954) or with Guillain-Barré syndrome (Morley and Reynolds, 1966). Yet, the significance of the elevated protein content in these instances may not be in terms of a reduction in the rate of reabsorption of CSF; high protein content may induce meningeal fibrosis (Harris, 1962) or it may compromise compensatory mechanisms of CSF reabsorbtion, such as its drainage into the ventricular walls (Chapter 21).

A second mode of impairment of CSF reabsorbtion consists of an increase in venous pressure. Ventriculo-lumbar perfusion of children has shown that reabsorbtion of CSF ceases if its pressure falls below 68 mm, that is if the CSF pressure becomes lower than the pressure of blood in the superior sagittal sinus (Cutler *et al.*, 1968). Elevation in venous pressure, therefore, would raise the threshold for CSF absorbtion. However, there are few observations indicating a causal relationship between hydrocephalus and systemic or local increases in venous pressure in man. Thrombotic occlusion of intracranial sinus may cause a transient increase in intracranial pressure, a symptom that has been referred to as "otitic hydrocephalus" (Symonds, 1931; Chapter 13). Ventricular enlargement coexistent with thrombotic occlusion of the superior sagittal sinus (Emery and Zachary, 1956) or thrombosis of superficial cortical veins (Russell, 1949) has been considered indicative of hydrocephalus caused by venous occlusion. However, ventricular enlargement was asymmetric, and the hemispheres were not searched in detail for lesions accounting for atrophy.

Attempts to induce hydrocephalus by clamping the great vein of Galen succeded in one of 10 dogs, and the one successful experiment resulted from placing the clamp proximal to the principal tributaries of the vein (Dandy and Blackfan, 1914). Guleke (1930) reported positive results in 1 of 8 dogs in similar experiments. Hydrocephalus was produced in 13 of 21 dogs by occlusion of all venous drainage channels in the neck, including the anastomoses with the spinal canal. Even with such excessive impairment of venous drainage, the resultant hydrocephalus was not steadily progressive, reaching a maximum in 2 to 3 weeks (Berling and Salibi, 1959). It is unlikely that such extreme degrees of obstruction of venous outflow are duplicated by human disease processes.

Another mode of production of hydrocephalus by increased venous pressure was recently proposed by Cronqvist *et al.* (1972). They had observed regression of hydrocephalus in 2 infants after removal of large arterio-venous malformations which had resulted in enormous shunting of blood into the superior sagittal sinus and ensuing cardiac failure. Hydrocephalus complicating arteriovenous aneurysm of the vein of Galen may also involve this mechanism, although it usually results from compression of the quadrigeminal plate and aqueduct by the aneurysm.

Hydrocephalus Concurrent with Dysplasia of Cranial Bones. Hydrocephalus is known to complicate various dysplasias of the cranial bones, but the pathogenetic mechanism and pathologic features are insufficiently documented. Hydrocephalus in achondroplasia (Dandy, 1921) is probably related to basilar impression, and to impairment of CSF flow at the foramen magnum (Wise *et al.*, 1971). Hydrocephalus may occur with craniosynostosis (Fishman *et al.*, 1971) or with craniosynostosis as a component of the syndrome of acrocephalosyndactyly (Alperts' syndrome); stenosis of the aqueduct was recorded in one instance of Alperts' syndrome (Hogan and Bauman, 1971).

Disturbances in Intracranial Pressure Induced by an Abnormal Supply of Vitamin A. Chronic hypervitaminosis A may cause increased intracranial pressure in infants (Marie and See, 1953) with papilledema and neurological symptoms consistent with "pseudo tumor" (Morrice *et al.*, 1960) and widening of cranial sutures (Siegel and Spackman, 1972). Neither the morbid anatomy nor the mechanism leading to this disturbance is well understood. Hypervitaminosis A is also known to be a potent teratogenic agent in rats, inducing exencephaly, eye malformations, cleft palate, spina bifida, myelocele and hydrocephalus when given during the 7th to 10th day of gestation (Cohlan, 1954).

Hypovitaminosis A may also lead to increased intracranial pressure (Millen and Woollam, 1958). Carton and Pascal (1961) reviewed the extensive literature on this subject and classified the experimental lesions into four groups: Neurologic lesions; neurologic lesions secondary to bone overgrowth and neural compression; neurologic lesions secondary to cessation of bone growth and disproportionate brain growth; increase in cerebrospinal pressure and/or hydrocephalus. Their review provides numerous references on the effects of hypo- and hypervitaminosis A in man.

References

Alksne, J. F., Lovings, E. T.: The role of the arachnoid villus in the removal of red blood cells from the subarachnoid space. An electron microscope study in the dog. J. Neurosurg. 36: 192—200, 1972.

— — Functional ultrastructure of the arachnoid villus. Arch. Neurol. (Chic.) 27: 371—377, 1972.

Anderson, H., Carlsson, C.-A., Gomes, S. P.: Unilateral hydrocephalus. Neurochirurgie 17: 63—65, 1974.

Bailey, O. J., Woodward, J. S.: Small vascular malformations of the brain: Their relationship to unexpected death, hydrocephalus and mental deficiency. J. Neuropath. exp. Neurol. 18: 98—108, 1959.

Berling, E. A., Jr., Salibi, B.: Production of hydrocephalus by increased cephalic-venous pressure. Arch. Neurol. (Chic.) 81: 693—698, 1959.

Bickers, D. S., Adams, R. D.: Hereditary stenosis of the aqueduct of Sylvius as a cause of congenital hydrocephalus. Brain 72: 246—262, 1949.

Borit, A., Sidman, R. L.: New mutant mouse with communicating hydrocephalus and secondary aqueductal stenosis. Acta Neuropath. 21: 316—331, 1972.

Carton, C. A., Pascal, R. R.: Hydrocephalus and vitamin-A-deficiency in the rabbit: General considerations. In: Disorders of the Developing Nervous System (Fields, W. S., Desmond, M. M., eds.), chapter XI, pp. 214—266. Springfield, Ill.: Ch. C Thomas 1961.
Clark, F. H.: Anatomical basis of hereditary hydrocephalus in the house mouse. Anat. Rec. 58: 225—233, 1934.
Clark, W. E. L.: On the Pacchionian bodies. J. Anat. 55: 40—48, 1920.
Cloward, R. B.: Atresia of the lateral ventricle. J. Neurol. Neurosurg. Psychiat. 32: 624—629, 1969.
Cohlan, S. Q.: Congenital anomalies in the rat produced by excessive intake of vitamin A during pregnancy. Pediatrics 13: 556—567, 1954.
Courville, C. B.: Obstructive internal hydrocephalus incident to small vascular anomaly of midbrain. Bull. Los Angeles neurol. Soc. 26: 41—45, 1961.
Cronqvist, S., Granholm, L., Lundström, N.-R.: Hydrocephalus and congestive heart failure caused by intracranial arteriovenous malformations in infants. J. Neurosurg. 36: 249—254, 1972.
Cutler, R. W. P., Page, L., Galicich, J., Watters, G. V.: Formation and absorption of cerebrospinal fluid in man. Brain 91: 707—720, 1968.
Dandy, W. E.: Diagnosis and treatment of hydrocephalus resulting from stricture of the aqueduct of Sylvius. Surg. Gynec. Obstet. 31: 340—358, 1920.
— Hydrocephalus in chondrodystrophy. Bull. Johns Hopk. Hosp. 32: 5—10, 1921.
— Blackfan, K. D.: Internal hydrocephalus. Amer. J. Dis. Child. 8: 406—482, 1914.
Dooling, E. C., Barlow, J. F., Murphy, J. V., Richardson, E. P., Jr.: Cyst of the cavum septi pellucidi. Arch. Neurol. (Chic.) 27: 79—84, 1972.
Drachman, D. A., Richardson, E. P.: Aqueductal narrowing, congenital and acquired. A critical review of the histologic criteria. Arch. Neurol. (Chic.) 5: 552—559, 1961.
Edwards, J. H., Norman, R. M., Roberts, J. M.: Sex-linked hydrocephalus: report of a family with 15 affected members. Arch. Dis. Child. 36: 481—485, 1961.
Ekbom, K., Greitz, T., Kugelberg, E.: Hydrocephalus due to ectasia of the basilar artery. J. Neurol. Sci. 8: 465—477, 1968.
Ellington, E., Margolis, G.: Block of arachnoid villus by subarachnoid hemorrhage. J. Neurosurg. 30: 651—657, 1969.
Emery, J. L.: Intracranial effects of long-standing decompression of the brain in children with hydrocephalus and meningomyelocele. Develop. Med. Child. Neurol. 7: 302—309, 1965.
— Staschak, M. C.: The size and form of the cerebral aqueduct in children. Brain 95: 591—598, 1972.
— Zachary, R. B.: Hydrocephalus associated to obliteration of the longitudinal sinus. Arch. Dis. Child. 31: 288—292, 1956.
Fishman, M. A., Hogan, G. R., Dodge, P. R.: The concurrence of hydrocephalus and craniosynostosis. J. Neurosurg. 34: 621—629, 1971.
Ford, F. R.: Cerebral birth injuries and their results. Medicine 5: 121—194, 1926.
Friede, R. L.: Surface structures of the aqueduct and the ventricular walls: a morphologic, comparative and histochemical study. J. comp. Neurol. 116: 229—247, 1961.
Gardner, W. J., Spitler, D. K., Whitten, C.: Increased intracranial pressure caused by increased protein content in the cerebrospinal fluid. New Engl. J. Med. 250: 932—936, 1954.
Gilles, F. H., Davidson, R. I.: Communicating hydrocephalus associated with deficient dysplastic parasagittal arachnoidal granulations. J. Neurosurg. 35: 421—426, 1971.
— Shillito, J.: Infantile hydrocephalus: retrocerebellar subdural hematoma. J. Pediat. 76: 529—537, 1970.
Gomez, D. G., Potts, G., Deonarine, V., Reilly, K.: Effect of pressure gradient changes on the morphology of arachnoid villi and granulations in the monkey. Lab. Invest. 28: 648—657, 1973.
Green, M.: The developmental effects of congenital hydrocephalus (ch) in the mouse. Develop. Biol. 23: 585—608, 1970.
Grüneberg, H.: Genetic studies on the skeleton of the mouse. VII. Congenital hydrocephalus. J. Genet. 51: 327—358, 1953.

Guleke, N.: Über die Entstehung des Hydrocephalus internus. Arch. klin. Chirurgie 162: 533—550, 1930.

Gutierrez, Y., Friede, R. L., Kaliney, W. J.: Agenesis of arachnoid granulations and its relationship to communicating hydrocephalus. J. Neurosurg., in press.

Harris, P.: Chronic progressive communicating hydrocephalus due to protein transudates from brain and spinal tumors. Develop. Med. Child. Neurol. 4: 270—278, 1962.

Henschen, F.: Tumoren des Zentralnervensystems und seiner Hüllen. In: Handbuch der speziellen pathologischen Anatomie und Histologie (Lubarsch, Henke, and Rössle, eds.), 13/3, pp. 413—1083. Berlin-Göttingen-Heidelberg: Springer 1955.

Hogan, G. R., Bauman, M. L.: Hydrocephalus in Alperts' syndrome. J. Pediat. 79: 782—787, 1971.

Hollingsworth, G., Davson, H., Segal, M. B.: The mechanism of drainage of the cerebrospinal fluid. Brain 93: 665—678, 1970.

Holmes, L. B., Nash, A., Zu Rhein, G. M., Levin, M., Opitz, J. M.: X-linked aqueductal stenosis: clinical and neuropathological findings in two families. Pediatrics 51: 697—704, 1973.

Howell, D. A.: Upper brain-stem compression and foraminal impaction with intracranial space-occupying lesions and brain swelling. Brain 82: 525—550, 1959.

Jellinger, K., Grunert, V., Sunder-Plassman, M.: Choroid-plexus papilloma associated with hydrocephalus in infancy. Report of two cases. Neuropädiatrie 1: 344—348, 1970.

Jezequel, Ch., Belloir, D., Jehan, P., *et al.*: Congenital hydrocephalus. Bilateral abnormality of the thumbs and eye changes. Semaines Hopitaux 49: 927—934, 1973.

Johnson, R. T., Johnson, K. P.: Hydrocephalus as a sequela of experimental myxovirus infections. Exp. Molec. Path. 10: 68—80, 1969.

Kahn, E. A., Luros, J. T.: Hydrocephalus from overproduction of cerebrospinal fluid. J. Neurosurg. 9: 59—67, 1952.

Keene, M. F. L., Hewer, E. E.: The sub-commissural organ and mesocoelic recess in the human brain, together with a note on Reissner's fibers. J. Anat. 69: 501—507, 1935.

Kepes, J. J., Clough, C., Villanueva, A.: Congenital fusion of the thalami (atresia of the third ventricle) and associated anomalies in a 6 months old infant. Acta Neuropath. 13: 97—104, 1969.

Laurence, V. M.: Discussion. In: Ciba Foundation Symposium on Cerebrospinal Fluid (Wolstenholm, G. E., O'Conner, C. M., eds.), pp. 310—326. Boston, Mass.: Little, Brown and Co. 1958.

McDonald, J. V.: Persistent hydrocephalus following the removal of papillomas of the choroid plexus of the lateral ventricles. Report of two cases. J. Neurosurg. 30: 736—740, 1969.

MacFarlane, A., Maloney, A. F. J.: The appearance of the aqueduct and its relationship to hydrocephalus in the Arnold-Chiari malformation. Brain 80: 479—491, 1957.

Marie, J., See, G.: Hydrocéphalie aigue bénigne du nourrisson après ingestion d'une dose massive unique de vitamine A. Ann. Pediat. (Paris) 180: 308—314, 1953.

Martins, A. N., Wiley, J. K., Myers, P. W.: Dynamics of the cerebrospinal fluid and the spinal dura mater. J. Neurol. Neurosurg. Psychiat. 35: 468—473, 1972.

Matson, D. D., Crofton, F. D. L.: Papilloma of the choroid-plexus in childhood. J. Neurosurg. 17: 1002—1027, 1960.

Milhorat, T. H., Hammock, M. K., Chandra, R. S.: The subarachnoid space in congenital obstructive hydrocephalus. Part 2. Microscopic findings. J. Neurosurg. 35: 7—15, 1971.

Millen, J. W., Woollam, D. H. M.: Vitamins and the cerebrospinal fluid. In: Ciba Foundation Symposium on the Cerebrospinal Fluid, pp. 168—188. Boston, Mass.: Little, Brown and Co. 1958.

Morley, J. B., Reynolds, E. H.: Papilloedema and the Landry-Guillain-Barré syndrome. Brain 89: 205—222, 1966.

Morrice, G., Havenes, W. H., Kapelansky, F.: Vitamin A intoxication as a cause of pseudotumor cerebri. J.A.M.A. 173: 1802—1805, 1960.

Needleman, H. L., Root, A. W.: Sex-linked hydrocephalus. Pediatrics 31: 396—399, 1963.

Overholser, M. D., Whitley, J. R., O'Dell, B. L., Hogan, A. G.: The ventricular system in hydrocephalic rat brains produced by a deficiency of vitamin B_{12} or of folic acid in the maternal diet. Anat. Rec. 120: 917—933, 1954.

Pudenz, R. H., Russell, F. E., Agnew, W. F.: Experimental hydrocephalus: a historical summary. Bull. Los Angeles neurol. Soc. 25: 118—129, 1960.

Ray, B. S., Peck, F. C.: Papilloma of the choroid plexus in the lateral ventricles causing hydrocephalus in an infant. J. Neurosurg. 13: 405—410, 1956.

Rowbotham, G. F.: Small aneurysm completely obstructing lower end of aqueduct of Sylvius. Arch. Neurol. Psychiat. (Chic.) 40: 1241—1243, 1938.

Russell, D. S.: Observations on the Pathology of Hydrocephalus. Medical Res. Council, Special Report Series No. 265. London: HMSO 1949.

— Donald, C.: Mechanism of internal hydrocephalus in spina bifida. Brain 58: 203—215, 1935.

Shabo, A. L., Maxwell, D. S.: Electron microscopic observations on the fate of particulate matter in the cerebrospinal fluid. J. Neurosurg. 29: 464—474, 1968.

Siegel, N. J., Spackman, T. J.: Chronic hypervitaminosis A with intracranial hypertension and low cerebrospinal fluid concentration of protein. Two illustrative cases. Clin. Pediat. (Phila.) 11: 580—584, 1972.

Simmonds, J. W.: The subarachnoid space: some experimental approaches to its pathology. Med. J. Aust. 19: 452—456, 1953.

Stempak, J. G.: Etiology of trypan blue induced antenatal hydrocephalus in the albino rat. Anat. Rec. 148: 561—571, 1964.

Symonds, C. P.: Otitic hydrocephalus. Brain 54: 55—71, 1931.

Turkewitsch, N.: Die Entwicklung des Aquaeductus cerebri des Menschen. Jb. f. Morphologie u. mikroskop. Anat. 76: 421—447, 1935.

Turnbull, I. M., Drake, C. G.: Membranous occlusion of the aqueduct of Sylvius. J. Neurosurg. 24: 24—36, 1966.

Turner, L.: The structure of arachnoid granulations with observations on their physiological and pathological significance. Ann. roy. Coll. Surg. Eng. 29: 237—264, 1961.

Vigouroux, A.: Ecoulement de liquide céphalo-rachidien. Hydrocéphalie papillome de plexus choroids du IVe ventricle. Rev. Neurol. 16: 281—285, 1908.

Warren, M. C., Lu, A. T., Ziering, W. H.: Sex-linked hydrocephalus with aqueductal stenosis. J. Pediat. 63: 1104—1110, 1963.

Weed, L. H.: Studies on the cerebrospinal fluid III. The pathways of escape from the subarachnoid spaces with particular reference to the arachnoid villi. J. Med. Res. 31: 51—91, 1914.

— Development of the cerebrospinal spaces in man. In: Contributions to Embryology, Vol. V, No. 14. Carnegie Institute of Washington, Pub. 1917.

— An anatomical consideration of the cerebrospinal fluid. Anat. Rec. 12: 461—496, 1917.

Welch, K., Friedman, V.: The cerebrospinal fluid valves. Brain 83: 454—469, 1960.

— Pollay, M.: Perfusion of particles through arachnoid villi of the monkey. Amer. J. Physiol. 201: 651—654, 1961.

— — The spinal arachnoid villi of the monkeys *Cercopithecus aethiops sabaeus* and *Macaca irus.* Anat. Rec. 145: 43—48, 1963.

Wise, B. L., Sondheimer, F., Kaufman, S.: Achondroplasia and hydrocephalus. Neuropädiatrie 3: 106—113, 1971.

Wisniewski, H., Weller, R. O., Terry, R. D.: Experimental hydrocephalus produced by the subarachnoid infusion of silicone oil. J. Neurosurg. 31: 10—14, 1969.

Woodard, J. C., Newberne, P. M.: The pathogenesis of hydrocephalus in newborn rats deficient in vitamin B_{12}. J. Embryol. exp. Morph. 17: 117—187, 1967.

Woollam, D. H. M., Millen, J. W.: Anatomical considerations in the pathology of stenosis of the cerebral aqueduct. Brain 76: 104—112, 1953.

Part 2. Malformations

23. Anencephaly, Rachischisis, and Encephaloceles

Anencephaly. The rather grotesque malformation of anencephaly has been recognized since medieval times; many references to published cases are found in the report of Warren (1951), and the comprehensive review of the literature by Nakano (1973) provides a wealth of specific epidemiological and other information. The frequency of the disease varies between approximately 0.5 and 2.0 per thousand births in the United States and most of Europe; it is locally higher in Britain and lower in Africa, Asia, and South America. Anencephaly may comprise 29.5 percent of all major abnormal births (Coffey and Jessop, 1957). Epidemiologic studies have shown that the variation relates to geography, race, social standing, seasons and many other factors; many of the reported variations in the frequency of anencephaly are concordant with similar variations for spina bifida. Epidemic waves of both lesions have been recorded (Janerich, 1973).

Most anencephalics are born during the last 3 months of pregnancy. The history of pregnancy is inconclusive, with no illness indicated for about 80 percent; if illness had occurred, a statistically significant predilection for the first 3 months of gestation was noted (Coffey and Jessop, 1957). Anencephaly is frequently associated with polyhydramnion, found in up to 50 percent of the cases in some series (Böök and Rayner, 1950). There is a striking preference for the female sex, ranging 3 to 1 or more than 4 to 1, particularly for fetuses of early gestation; the proportion of males was found to increase with increasing length of gestation. The malformation is incompatible with life and anencephalics are either stillborn or die within a few days after birth.

Extensive epidemiological studies have so far failed in identifying an etiologic agent (Nakano, 1973). Studies in twins show a very low rate of concordance of anencephaly. Vogel (1958) reported a cojoined double twin having two heads attached to a single torso with anencephaly in one head and a normal cranium and brain in the other. Iniencephaly was observed in 1 of biamnionic monochorionic twins (Lewis, 1897). There is no consistent anomaly of chromosome patterns, although anencephaly has been observed coexistent with chromosomal anomalies on occasion (Nakano, 1973).

Embryological considerations date the origin of anencephaly to the early part of pregnancy, near the period of closure of the neural tube which is thought to occur during the 4th week. The fact that the eyes had developed normally in most instances appears to set a lower limit for the date of origin, at approximately the 18th day, when the optic vesicles form. The early onset of anencephaly is verified from its observed occurrence in very young aborted human embryos. There are numerous reports of anencephaly in embryos 14 to 18 mm crown-rump length (Dodds and De Angelis, 1937; Stroer and van der Zwan, 1939; Warren, reporting 9 cases, 1951; Erskine, 1955) as well as in embryos 20 mm or longer (Böhmig, 1927; de Vries, 1927). Anencephaly was described in a human embryo of 9 mm crown-rump length (Lebedeff, 1881), and anencephaly with complete rachischisis has been dated still earlier

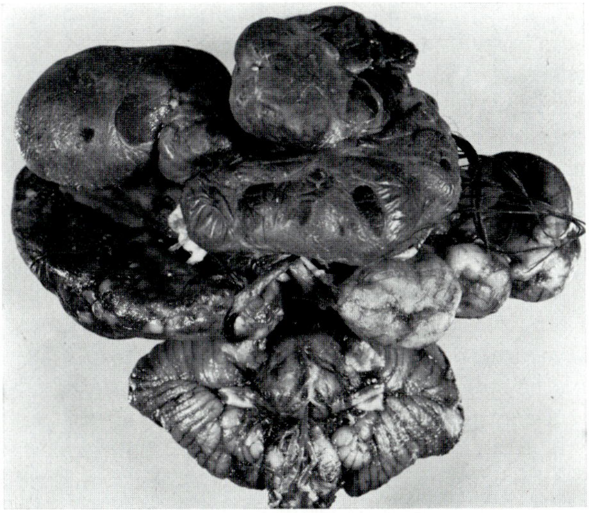

Fig. 72. Anencephaly: cerebral remnants, area cerebrovasculosa and attached segments of scalp

(Chapter 24). These studies provide insight into the pathogenesis of anencephaly and, in addition, confirm its onset during or before the 2nd month of gestation. Anencephaly is not restricted to the human species and was found in calves, mice and dogs (Innes and Saunders, 1962) and in *Macaca fascicularis* (Price and Gilles, 1971).

Gross Features. Anencephaly is characterized by an absence of most or all of the brain tissue associated with deficiency or underdevelopment of the squamous bones forming the cranial vault (acrania). The skin of the bulging eyelids and the enlarged nose extends directly backwards over the base of the skull, which, along with shallow orbits, results in typical protruding exophthalmic eyes. These features have been referred to as "toad's head". The skin of the temples and occiput likewise turns over the basis of the skull, encircling a mass of amorphous, reddish, highly vascularized neural and mesenchymal tissue, commonly referred to as area or substantia cerebrovasculosa (Fig. 72). This basic organization of the lesion, that is a bone defect, malformed neural tissue, and a skin defect, is quite similar to that of myelomeningoceles. The volume of residual cerebral tissue varies greatly; an uncommon variant consists of a pedunculated mass of brain tissue attached to the base of the skull. The bases of the skull is abnormal, being convex in its anterior portion and lacking demarcation of the middle cerebral fossa, while the posterior fossa may be funnel-shaped. The tentorium and the cerebellar hemispheres are absent. The lamina cribrosa is usually nonperforate but a small sella turcica is found between the petrous bones. Eyes and orbital muscles are well developed, but the optic nerves terminate blindly in the orbit. Cranial nerves are usually identifiable from the trigeminal downward.

Involvement of the spine is a consistent feature of anencephaly, but its degree varies. In the cases without skin defect at the back there is nearly always nonfusion of the arches (spina bifida) of the uppermost cervical vertebra (Barson, 1970). In the others an open defect of the spine extends from the cranium downward along the cervical, thoracic or lumbar spine (craniorachischisis). It is customary to use the term "rachischisis" for severe, extensive lesions in which an open defect at the back extends over many spinal segments; the term "spina bifida" is used for less severe and more localized lesions forming a cyst, or for bone defects concealed by a skin covering. This nomenclature is merely a matter of convention as "rachis" stands for spinal column. Rachischisis, therefore, is strictly speaking synonymous with spina bifida. Cases of anencephaly with rachischisis exhibit a characteristic retroflexion of the head, the face being tilted upward and the base of the cranium set tightly against the shoulders; the vertebral column shows an anterior curvature, probably in consequence of lack of growth of the dorsal aspects of the spine. More severe defects of nervous tissue are common in these cases, and complete absence of brain tissue may coexist with dysplasia or absence of the spinal cord. The spinal canal forms an open gutter at the back or at the neck, and the severely deformed spinal cord may present as a splayed-out layer of nervous tissue which may lack a central canal. If the spinal cord is absent (amyelia), the defect exposes dura mater with or without residual vascular arachnoid tissue; arachnoid may persist at the origin of the nerve roots in the form of small floccules. The ligamenta denticulata may persist as longitudinal fibrous strands. Spinal nerves are always demonstrable outside of the dura and, at times, as stumps within the defect.

Anencephaly with rachischisis is about as frequent as it is without rachischisis; in both instances it is associated with other disproportions in body growth, including overgrowth of the tongue and hypoplasia of the bones related to the cranial vault, while the bones related to the face remain relatively normal. The neck is extremely short, and the upper extremities are abnormally large and long when compared with the lower extremities (Nañagas, 1925). Abnormalities of vertebral segmentation are common.

A less common group of malformations are referred to as iniencephaly (inion for nape of the neck). In these the cranial vault is intact except for a bone defect at the occiput, the predominant lesion being spina bifida or rachischisis of the cervical spine. The extent of the cervical lesion varies from spina bifida with intact, nonprotruding skin to a meningomyeloencephalocele or to open rachischisis. The classification of iniencephaly as a separate type of lesion or as a variant of anencephaly with spinal retroflexion has been disputed (Lemire *et al.*, 1972). It is evidently inappropriate to classify these lesions as anencephaly since the brain is present, but there is no valid reason to believe that both lesions are fundamentally different; their biologic statistics are similar. Published cases of iniencephaly were reviewed by Lewis (1897), Brodsky (1939), and Paterson (1944). We were unable to find detailed studies of the brains of iniencephalics in the literature.

Microscopic Features. The area cerebrovasculosa of anencephalics consists microscopically of irregular nests or masses of malformed brain tissue containing predominantly glial as well as scattered neuronal elements in a dis-

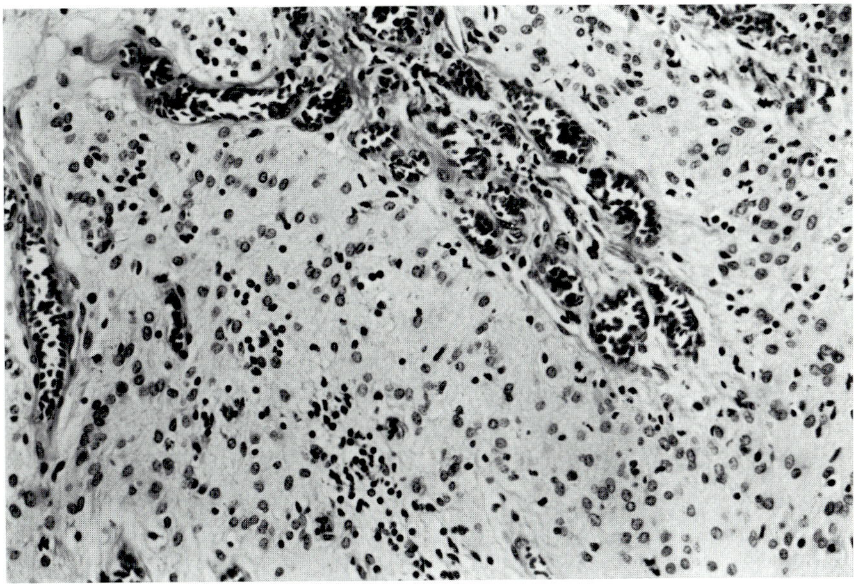

Fig. 73. Area cerebrovasculosa; intermingling of malformed glia tissue, immature cells, and vascular meninges; H & E ×200

ordered arrangement. This tissue includes nests or layers of ependyma and, frequently, portions of choroid plexus. The masses of malformed nervous tissue are sharply delineated from a surrounding loose but densely vascularized connective tissue representing leptomeninges (Fig. 73). The cornified squamous epithelium of the rudimentary scalp adjoins the malformed nervous tissue at the lateral aspects of the area cerebrovasculosa. Disorganized remnants of cerebellar cortex may be found in the caudal portions of the area cerebrovasculosa. The most cranial portions of the neuraxis having a reasonably well preserved structure are midbrain, pons or medulla oblongata, but their gross configuration and nuclear grouping may be distorted. Cranial nerves and intraosseous ganglia are normal. The medulla oblongata as well as the cervical cord may be absent if anencephaly is combined with rachischisis. The spinal cord of anencephalics is thinner than normal; examination discloses aplasia of ventral and lateral fiber tracts and relative overgrowth of the dorsal columns (Fig. 74), resulting in a characteristic outward rotation of the dorsal horns (Környey, 1928; Warren, 1951). The significance of these deformities for the potential dating of the cerebral lesions is discussed in Chapter 11 on hydranencephaly. Heterotopic islands of glia tissue may be found in the spinal leptomeninges.

The dense vascularity that gave the area cerebrovasculosa its name has been considered evidence of concurrence of a neuroectodermal and of a vascular malformation (Vogel, 1958). However, this type of increased vascu-

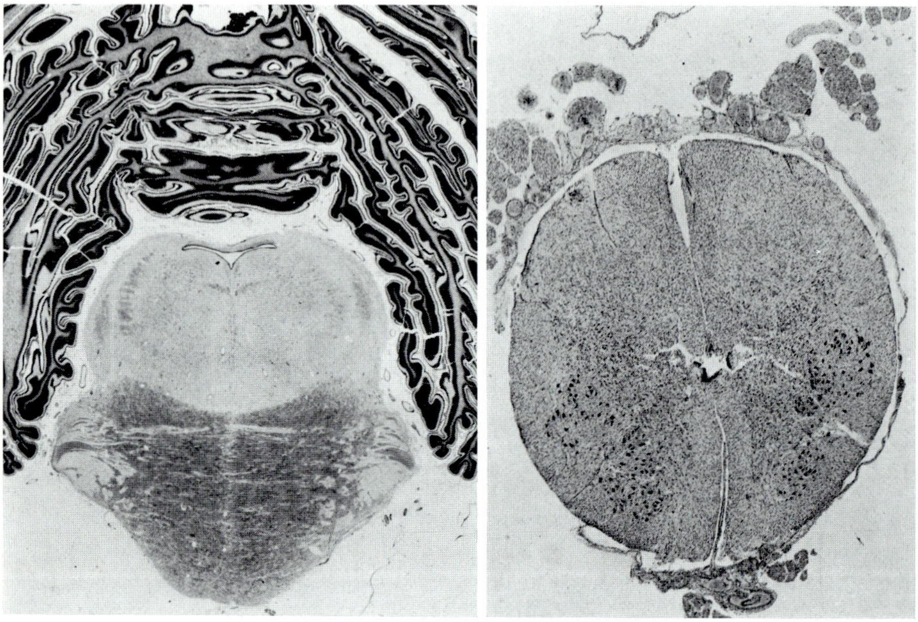

Fig. 74. Aplasia of descending fiber system in the pons and the spinal cord in anencephaly; in the cord there is lateral rotation of dorsal horns and hypoplasia of ventral and lateral spinal tracts

larity is a nonspecific trait often seen in malformations such as encephaloceles and myelomeningoceles. It represents persistence of embryonal meningeal vascularization, characterized by a dense plexus of sinusoid capillaries at the pial surface. In anencephalics it is often found, other then within the area cerebrovasculosa, in the leptomeninges covering the medulla oblongata and spinal cord (Környey, 1928; Warren, 1951; and Vogel, 1958).

Minor anomalies occur in the origin of craniobrachial vessels at the aortic arc (Epstein and Kolker, 1965), but the carotid and vertebral arteries are commonly present and normal. Much variance is encountered in the course of these arteries after they enter the cranial vault; there are irregularities in their union and absence of major ramifications (Vogel and McClenahan, 1952). This disorganization may be secondary to the severe malformation of neural tissue.

The anterior lobe of the pituitary gland can always be found in the deformed base of the skull, but the posterior lobe is often absent, depending on the degree of cerebral defects (Angevine, 1938). Electron microscopic studies of the pituitary gland of anencephalics demonstrate differentiation into thyrotrophs, gonadotrophs, somatotrophs and lactotrophs, apparently in absence of secretory activity (Salazar *et al.*, 1969). Hypoplasia of the adrenals had been described in the 19th century (Nakano, 1973, references; Angevine, 1938). It is caused by premature involution of the fetal zone of the adrenal cortex, after the 24th week of gestation, probably because of failure of the fetus to take over after the production of placental chorionic gonadotropin declines (Bernirschke, 1956). The significance of adrenal hypoplasia lies in its clinical manifestation in terms of a reduced urinary excretion of estrogen in the mother.

A variety of other malformations may be associated with anencephaly and iniencephaly (Brodsky, 1939; Warren, 1951; Coffey and Jessop, 1957); iniencephaly has been found associated with cyclopia (Oakley and Grimshaw, 1961). Of particular interest is the occurrence of heterotopic nervous tissue in the lungs of anencephalics (Potter and Young, 1942), probably due to bloodborne dislocation of neuroectodermal tissue from the lesions.

Pathogenetic Considerations. Anencephaly clearly belongs in the group of lesions that constitute the dysraphic complex, being linked to spina bifida by its occurrence in various combinations with other cranial and spinal lesions. There are also many common traits in the biological statistics of anencephaly and other dysraphic lesions (Chapter 24). Theories proposed for the formal pathogenesis of anencephaly include failure of formation of the forebrain anlage; failure of closure of the anterior neuropore; or opening of the neural tube after its closure, in analogy with the mechanisms postulated for spina bifida. Anencephaly has been induced experimentally during early gestation with a variety of techniques, for example X-irradiation of fetal rats between fertilization and the 9th day of gestation (Rugh and Grupp, 1959).

A primary failure or derangement of the development of the brain in anencephaly does not preclude the possibility that the malformed tissue becomes later on mechanically damaged *in utero* as there is no protective cranial vault. Mechanical trauma may aggravate the lesions and may cause the profound disorganization of neural tissue found in the area cerebrovasculosa. Repetitive trauma may also account for apparent discrepancies between the early onset of the deformity and observations indicating that some portions of the brain had differentiated to a certain degree before they became affected. The pulmonary heterotopias in anencephalics may also result from tissue trauma, as pulmonary emboli of brain tissue are known to occur during traumatic birth even if the skull is intact (Chapter 3).

The causes of hydramnion associated with anencephaly are a matter of dispute. Disturbances in the production or in the emptying of fetal urine (Bernirschke and McKay, 1958) and insufficient swallowing of amnionic fluid by the fetus which impedes transfer of fluids to the maternal circulation have been considered. The theory of Angevine (1938) is of neuropathologic interest in postulating that the hydramnion results from the secretory activity of the choroid plexus in the area cerebrovasculosa. Comparison of amnionic fluid volumes in a variety of experimentally induced malformations demonstrated a relation of hydramnion to anencephaly or to exencephaly rather than to agenesis of the kidney (Ferm and Saxon, 1971).

Encephaloceles and Cranial Meningoceles. These lesions are considerably less frequent than anencephaly or spina bifida cystica, occurring in 1 to 3 cases per 10,000 live births, but there is a similar preference for the female sex. Lesions are referred to as encephaloceles if they contain herniated or displaced cerebral tissue; cerebral tissue is absent in the much less common

Table 4. *Site of Herniated Sac in 1076 Cases of Encephalocele, Cranial Meningocele and Spina Bifida Cystica*

Site	Fisher *et al.*, 1952	Ingraham and Swan, 1943
Nasal cavity	8	5
Frontal	8	6
Temporal	1	—
Parietal	6	9
Occipital	34	63
Occipitocervical	11	—
Nasopharyngeal	—	1
Cervical	34	23
Cervico-thoracic	4	—
Thoracic	29	39
Thoraco-lumbar	14	43
Lumbar	233	205
Lumbosacral	94	87
Sacral	56	46
Pelvis	4	1
Thoracolumbosacral	—	10
Undesignated	—	8
Total	536 [1]	546

[1] Two sacs were present in each of 6 cases.

cranial meningoceles. Most encephaloceles occur as the only deformity, but occipital encephaloceles may also occur as components of Meckel syndrome associated with microcephaly, microphthalmia, cleft lip and palate, polydactily, polycystic kidneys, small genitalia and other deformities (Hsia *et al.*, 1971).

Typical Sites of Encephaloceles. The most common occurrence of encephaloceles is occipital (Table 4), either in the occipital squame, leaving the posterior fossa intact, or in the basal occiput, resulting in an enlarged foramen magnum and, at times, agenesis of the first vertebral arch. Frontal encephaloceles are less common and appear to be relatively more frequent in Southeast Asia than in Western Europe and North America; a series of 12 cases, 7 of which were females, was reported by Suwanwela and Suwanwela (1972) along with a classification of sites of encephaloceles. Anterior (or frontal) encephaloceles are most commonly found at the fronto-ethmoidal junction and protrude at the nose, into the ethmoid or orbit, less frequently between the frontal bones. Frontal encephaloceles almost invariably include olfactory tissue along with variable amounts of the frontal lobes. Encephaloceles are less common at other midline sites, such as at the anterior or posterior fontanel or interparietal. The rarest type occurs at the base of the skull and manifests as a pharyngeal mass, the bone defect being transethmoidal, sphenoethmoidal or transphenoidal (Wiese *et al.*, 1972). Encephaloceles occasionally occur off the midline, such as in the parietal region. In a series of 13 parietal lesions 4 were encephaloceles and 9 meningoceles, 2 of the latter containing heterotopic glial tissue (McLaurin, 1964). This proportion between encephaloceles and meningoceles is inverse to that observed for midline lesions.

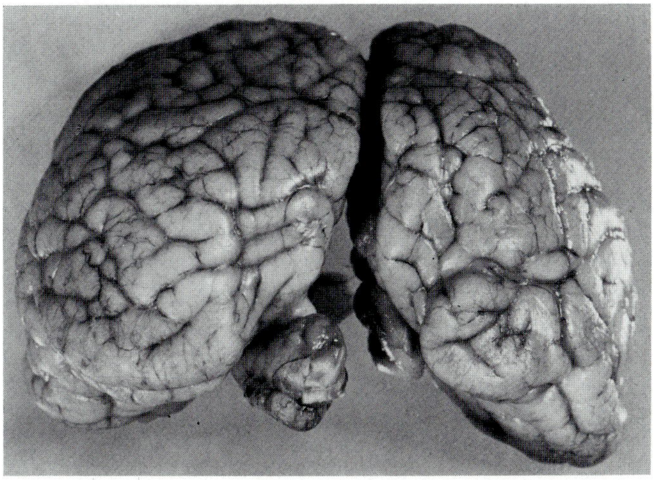

Fig. 75. Herniation of the occipital lobe in occipital encephalocele

Morbid Anatomy of Encephaloceles. Encephaloceles are typically associated with deformities of cranial bones beyond the existence of a local defect. The cranial fossae are smaller than normal; there is hypoplasia of the squamous bones of the cranial vault, while the facial bones tend to be less severely affected, similar to the findings in anencephalics. Falx and tentorium are absent or hypoplastic.

Encephaloceles form broad-based or pedunculated masses of cerebral tissue covered with dura and skin which may be haired depending on the site of the encephalocele. There is usually no evidence of a primary skin defect, although the skin may become ulcerated. In this regard the encephaloceles are homologous to spinal meningoceles; whereas, the spinal myelomeningocele resembles anencephaly in having a central area of exposed meningeal and neural tissue. The nervous tissue in the encephalocele usually connects to the underlying hemisphere through a narrow neck of cerebral tissue or a strand of glial tissue. Large encephaloceles may present as herniated portions of the corresponding cerebral lobes, including white matter and cortex with a normal gyral pattern. The lateral ventricle of the hemisphere may extend into the encephalocele and may contain choroid plexus; loculation of this portion of the ventricular system may result in its hydrocephalic distension.

Other encephaloceles show greater disorganization of the cerebral tissue, and there may be fragments of cerebral cortex or islands of glioneuronal tissue variably including ependyma or choroid plexus. Disorganized cerebellar cortical tissue is found in occipital encephaloceles. Islands of malformed neuroectodermal tissue are encompassed by leptomeninges with abundant sinusoid capillaries, consistent with persistent fetal leptomeningeal vascularization.

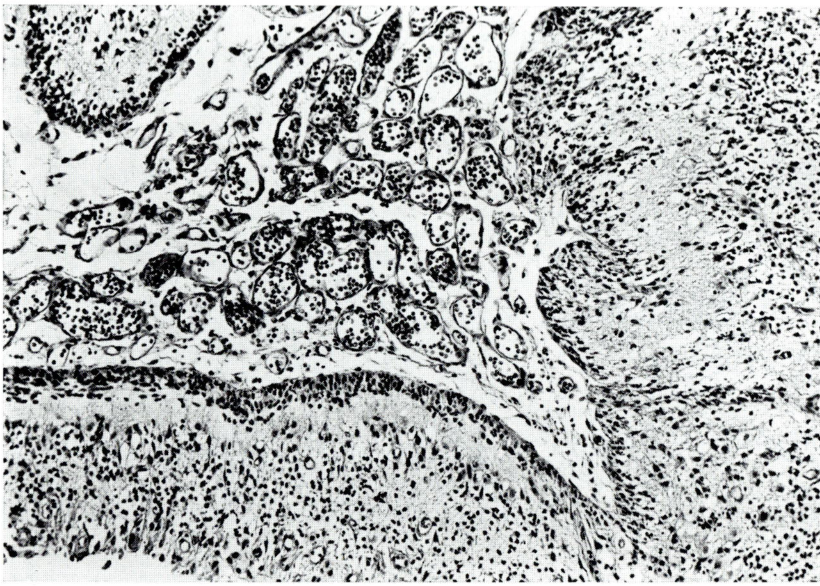

Fig. 76. Malformed cerebellar cortex and excessively vascularized meninges in an occipital encephalocele; H & E ×85

Encephaloceles are commonly associated with marked deformities of the cerebral hemispheres (Karch and Urich, 1972). Most encephaloceles connect to only one of the hemispheres, and the affected one is usually smaller than the other. The hemispheres are dislocated from their respective intracranial compartments (Fig. 75), the contralateral hemispheres often extending beyond the midline; the contralateral frontal lobe, for example, may occupy both anterior fossae. These dislocations cause stretching, kinking or retroversion of cranial nerves, most notably of the optic nerve which may be atrophic. Distortion of the hypothalamus and stretching or angulation of cerebral arteries are also common. The gross and microscopic architecture of the cerebral cortex is usually not disturbed, except for convergence of gyri toward the bone defect from which the encephalocele protrudes; polymicrogyria is not a characteristic feature. The lateral ventricles are deformed, either by communication with the encephalocele or by compression, distortion of fusion of the ventricular walls, or by hydrocephalic dilation of all or part of the ventricular system. Agenesis of the corpus callosum (Chapter 28) may coexist. Occipital encephaloceles cause severe deformities or agenesis of the cerebellum, and there is distortion or disorganization of the brain stem as well as aplasia of certain nuclear groups. Anomalies in the crossing of corticospinal tracts (Chapter 32) appear to be fairly common. Hydromyelia or other malformations may be found in the spinal cord. Persistent fetal vascularization may be found not only in the malformed tissue within the encephalocele (Fig. 76) but also in anatomically normal portions of brain stem and cord, similar to anencephaly.

Encephaloceles form portals of entry for infection, causing purulent leptomeningitis and abscess formation in the encephalocele as well as in the brain tissue. The nervous tissue in encephaloceles also often exhibits evidence of circulatory disturbances in the form of acute or organizing infarcts or secondary cystic lesions.

Cranial meningoceles may present as relatively small nodular subcutaneous masses overlying a smooth-walled bone defect; there are usually no other bone deformities. Microscopic examination of these lesions discloses a mass of loose mesenchymal tissue consistent with leptomeninges, being delineated sharply from the encompassing dermis. Nests of heterotopic glial tissue may be found in the meninges which usually lack the luxuriant vascularization observed in encephaloceles. The series of McLaurin (1946) indicates a considerably better prognosis for cranial meningoceles than for encephaloceles.

References

Angevine, P. M.: Pathologic anatomy of the hypophysis and adrenals in anencephaly. Arch. Path. 26: 507—518, 1938.

Barson, A. J.: Spina bifida: The significance of the level and extent of the defect to the morphogenesis. Develop. Med. Child. Neurol. 12: 129—144, 1970.

Bernirschke, K.: Adrenals in anencephaly and hydrocephaly. Obstet. Gynec. 8: 412—425, 1956.

— McKay, D. G.: The antidiuretic hormone in fetus and infant. Obstet. Gynec. 1: 638—649, 1958.

Böhmig, R.: Über das Primordialcranium eines menschlichen Embryos aus dem zweiten Monat mit Cranio-Rhachischisis. Z. Anat. Entwickl.-Gesch. 65: 570—590, 1927.

Böök, J. A., Rayner, S.: A clinical and genetical study of anencephaly. Amer. J. hum. Genet. 2: 61—84, 1950.

Brodsky, I.: Four examples of iniencephalus, with a statistical review of the literature. Med. J. Aust. 2: 795—800, 1939.

Coffey, V. P., Jessop, W. J. E.: Study of 137 cases of anencephaly. Brit. J. prev. soc. Med. 11: 174—189, 1957.

de Vries, E.: Description of a young human anencephalic and amyelic embryo. Anat. Rec. 36: 293—317, 1927.

Dodds, G. S., De Angelis, E.: An anencephalic human embryo 16.5 mm long. Anat. Rec. 67: 499—505, 1937.

Epstein, B. S., Kolker, P.: Congenital variations in cephalobrachial vessels in anencephaly. Amer. J. Roentgenol. 93: 339—341, 1965.

Erskine, C. A.: Human anencephaly in early developmental stages. Acta anat. 23: 251—258, 1955.

Ferm, V. H., Saxon, A.: Amniotic fluid volume in experimentally induced renal agenesis and anencephaly. Experientia 27: 1066—1067, 1971.

Hsia, Y. E., Bratu, M., Herbordt, A.: Genetics of the Meckel syndrome (dysencephalia splanchnocystica). Pediatrics 48: 237—247, 1971.

Innes, J. R. M., Saunders, L. Z.: Comparative Neuropathology. Academic Press 1962.

Janerich, D. T.: Epidemic waves in the prevalence of anencephaly and spina bifida in New York State. Teratology 8: 253—256, 1974.

Karch, S. B., Urich, H.: Occipital encephalocele: a morphological study. J. Neurol. Sci. 15: 89—112, 1972.

Környey, S.: Physiologisch-anatomische Beobachtungen bei merencephalen Mißbildungen. Arch. Psychiat. 85: 304—328, 1928.

Lebedeff, A.: Entstehung der Anencephalie bei Vögeln und Menschen. Virchow Arch. 86: 263—298, 1881.

Lemire, R. J., Beckwith, J. B., Shepard, T. H.: Iniencephaly and anencephaly with spinal retroflexion. A comparative study of eight human specimens. Teratology 6: 27—36, 1972.

Lewis, H. L.: Iniencephalus. Amer. J. Obstet. 35: 11—53, 1897.

McLaurin, R. L.: Parietal cephaloceles. Neurology (Minneap.) 14: 764—772, 1964.

Nakano, K. K.: Anencephaly: A review. Develop. Med. Child. Neurol. 15: 383—402, 1973.

Nañagas, J. C.: A comparison of the growth of the body dimensions of anencephalic human fetuses with normal fetal growth as determined by graphic analysis and empirical formulae. Amer. J. Anat. 35: 455—494, 1925.

Oakley, N. W., Grimshaw, J. S.: A case of iniencephaly associated with cyclopia. Brit. J. clin. Pract. 15: 845—849, 1961.

Paterson, S. J.: Iniencephalus. J. Obstet. Gynaec. Brit. Emp. 51: 330—333, 1944.

Potter, E. L., Young, R. L.: Heterotopic brain tissue in the lungs of two anencephalic monsters. Arch. Path. 34: 1009—1015, 1942.

Price, R. A., Gilles, F. H.: Telencephalic remnants in simian an human anencephaly. Arch. Path. 91: 529—536, 1971.

Rugh, R., Grupp, E.: Exencephalia following X-irradiation of the pre-implantation mammalian embryo. J. Neuropath. exp. Neurol. 18: 468—481, 1959.

Salazar, H., MacAulay, M. A., Charles, D., Pardo, M.: The human hypophysis in anencephaly. Arch. Path. 87: 201—211, 1969.

Stroer, W. F. H., van der Zwan, A.: Anencephaly and rhachischisis posterior, with description of a human hemicephalus of 18 mm. J. Anat. 73: 441—450, 1939.

Suwanwela, C., Suwanwela, N.: A morphological classification of sincipital encephalomeningoceles. J. Neurosurg. 36: 201—211, 1972.

Vogel, F. S.: The association of vascular anomalies with anencephaly. Amer. J. Path. 34: 169—175, 1958.

— McClenahan, J. L.: Anomalies of major cerebral arteries associated with congenital malformations of the brain. Amer. J. Path. 28: 701—711, 1952.

Warren, H. S.: Acrania induced by anencephaly. Anat. Rec. 111: 653—667, 1951.

Wiese, G. M., Kempe, L. G., Hammon, W. M.: Transsphenoidal meningohydroencephalocele. J. Neurosurg. 37: 457—478, 1972.

24. Spina Bifida and Related Spinal Lesions

Spina Bifida; Classification and Biologic Statistics. Spina bifida has been described in the medieval literature and was recognized before that time. Indeed, the association of foot deformities with sacral hypertrichosis may represent the source of the mythological figure of satyr (von Recklinghausen, 1866). The common occurrence and social importance of the disease is reflected in an extremely voluminous literature; a bibliography of 2,000 references was compiled by Ingraham *et al.* (1943). Brocklehurst (1971) gave a lucid review of early descriptions of the disease, and other comprehensive studies include those of Leveuf (1937), Doran and Guthkelch (1961), Smith (1965), and others.

The lesions of spina bifida consist of a combination of malformations of the vertebral column and the neuraxis. The mesodermal and the neuroectodermal malformations are usually of comparable magnitude but the relation is not precise, and either of the lesions may predominate or present as the sole feature. The disease may be classified in terms of either the spinal or the cord deformity. It is most widely accepted, and clinically most useful, to use the degree of the spinal defect for classification: 1. Spina bifida occulta consists of nonclosure of the vertebral arches without an externally visible cystic lesion in the back. These lesions differ from spina bifida cystica, in which a vertebral defect combines with a cystic lesion on the back. Spina bifida cystica is commonly subdivided into 2. meningoceles that do not involve the cord tissue and 3. myelomeningoceles in which the spinal cord is component of the cyst wall. 4. Rachischisis is the most severe defect, in which there is widely patent dorsal opening of the spine with or without residual cord tissue. As rachischisis is usually associated with anencephaly it is described in Chapter 23 and is mentioned here only for classification and comparison.

The deformities of the neuraxis that combine with the mesodermal lesions may be classified as amyelia, nonfusion of the dorsal half of the cord, diastematomyelia, hydromyelia, overgrowth of cord or nonspecific dysplasia. These categories are less useful in clinical classification. Either type of classification may lead to misconceptions if either the mesodermal or the neuroectodermal lesions are emphasized to the degree that sight is lost of its association with the other.

It may be briefly interjected at this point that some reviews on spina bifida include data on lateral intrathoracic meningoceles in patients with neurofibromatosis or kyphoscoliosis. These lesions consist of saccular meningeal herniae through the intervertebral foramen extending anteriorly between the ribs into the thoracic cavity. The lesions are uncommon and most occurred at the thoracic level, with rare exceptions in the lumbar region; the 64 cases reviewed by Ya Deau *et al.* (1965) were nearly all adults. These lateral intrathoracic meningoceles are more closely related to the spinal arachnoid cysts (Chapter 20), and their similarity to the dysraphic lesions is only superficial.

Statistics on the frequency of spina bifida occulta vary as much as from 2 to 24 percent of patients. The extent of this variation is, at least in part, age related: Spina bifida occulta of the first sacral vertebra was found in 51.6 percent of the 7 to 8 year group and 26.4 percent of adults; that of the fifth lumbar vertebra occurred in 16.1 percent of the 7 to 8 year group and only 2.2 percent of adults (Sutow and Pryde, 1956). Routine radiologic examination of 1,172 consecutive autopsies, most adults, showed a 5 percent incidence of spina bifida occulta (James and Lassman, 1972).

The frequency of spina bifida cystica was reviewed by Alter (1962), showing an average between 1 and 2.5 per 1,000 live births; there are, however, racial and/or geographic variations as it is approximately 2.5 times more frequent in Caucasians than in Negroes and is particularly high (above 4.0) in Belfast, Liverpool and Dublin and uncommon (0.2) in Japan. There are also reports of local epidemic rises of 2 to 6 times normal (Boris *et al.*, 1963; Lucey *et al.*, 1964).

Spina bifida occulta in adults shows nearly equal distribution between sexes (Sutow and Pryde, 1956). Spina bifida cystica shows a slight but definite female preference. Timson (1969) collected 3,521 cases from 9 studies and found an average female predilection of 65.5 percent, being statistically significant when compared with the general population or with their sibs. The predilection for females appears to be the greater the more severe the lesion. A larger female excess was found for stillbirths than for live births (Record and McKeown, 1949); female excess occurred entirely among myelomeningoceles but was absent for meningoceles (Doran and Guthkelch, 1961).

Clinical Features. The symptoms of the disease depend to a large extent on the degree of deformity of the neuraxis. Spina bifida occulta is often an asymptomatic lesion, though it may be associated with foot deformities, peculiar gait, shortening of one leg, incontinence, reflex anomalies or pain (James and Lassman, 1972). Meningoceles tend to have little or no neurologic deficits and offer good chances for cure and normal survival; hydrocephalus or infection are unlikely to develop (Laurence and Tew, 1971). Myelomeningoceles are invariably associated with neurologic defects, particularly when occurring in the lumbosacral region. Manifestations include weakness or flaccid paralysis of the lower extremities, particularly below the knee, and foot deformities. There is lack of response to painful or thermal stimuli, though sensory qualities may be less affected than motility. Loss of sphincter control results in vesicle and rectal incontinence. Total rachischisis is not compatible with postnatal life.

The majority of instances of spina bifida cystica are sporadic, although occurrence in families or in twins has been observed. The risk for the sibling after a case of anencephaly or spina bifida is 4.6 percent, which is significantly higher than the risk of occurrence in general (Yen and MacMahon, 1968). Lorber (1965) determined the risk at 8 percent, increasing to 24.1 percent in sibships of 5 or more.

The most common complications of myelomeningoceles are meningitis, hydrocephalus or pneumonia. Life expectancy to the eleventh birthday is 12.8 percent in the absence of modern surgical treatment (Laurence and Tew, 1971). Meningitis ascends from the myelomeningocele and is particularly frequent if the latter is localized within the area covered by the diaper; less frequently it develops from diagnostic or therapeutic measures for hydrocephalus. The causative organisms and the clinicopathologic features are the same as for neonatal leptomeningitis in anatomically normal infants (Lorber and Segall, 1962). The development of hydrocephalus is referred to in the chapter on the Arnold-Chiari malformation (25). The increasing efficacy of surgical treatment has brought the renal complications of spina bifida to greater attention. Among 50 infants with myelomeningocele, 6 had renal dysplasia with primitive ducts or metaplastic cartilage, often associated with hydronephrosis presumably on the basis of lower urinary tract obstruction during the fetal period; pyelonephritis was present in 6 (Forbes, 1972).

Bone Lesions of Spina Bifida. Vertebral changes of spina bifida consist of a lack of fusion or absence of the vertebral arches, resulting in bilateral broadening of the vertebrae and lateral displacement of pedicles and a widened spinal canal. Typical patterns in the distribution of the bone defects

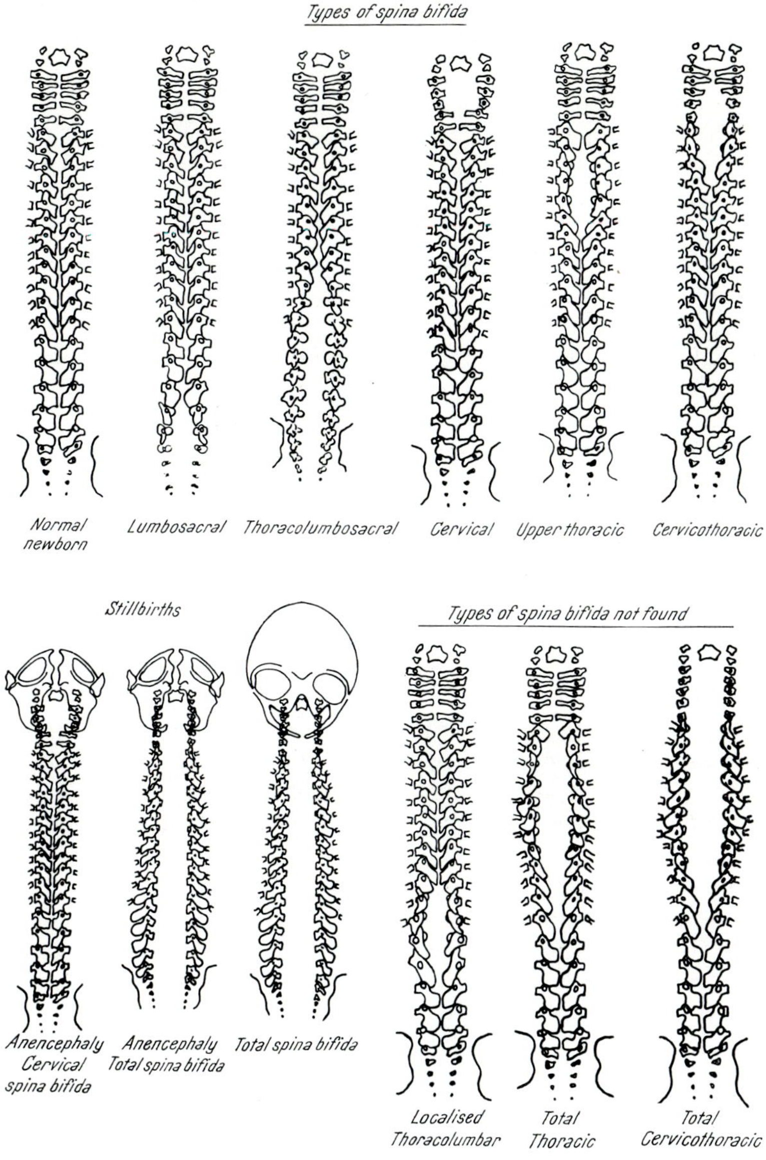

Fig. 77. Types of defects of the spinal column in spina bifida. (Courtesy Dr. Barson. Develop. Med. Child Neurol. 12: 129, 1970)

were reported by Barson (1970), who also emphasized the occurrence of kyphosis with thoracolumbar or lumbar spina bifida, but not with other localizations (Fig. 77). Many other vertebral anomalies may be associated with the vertebral defects, including sagittal splitting of vertebral bodies, hemivertebrae, fused vertebrae, or a median spur protruding into the spinal canal which suggests the presence of diastematomyelia. Other bone anomalies observed occasionally in patients with spina bifida include Klippel-Feil syndrome, Sprengel deformity, deformities of ribs, absence of radius, deformities of forearm, fragilitas osseum, cervical ribs or absence of sacrum (Ingraham and Swan, 1943; Fisher *et al.*, 1952).

Neoplasms of maldevelopmental origin may be found in association with the spinal lesions. Lipomas occur as subcutaneous or deep nodular masses with spina bifida occulta; they also present as diffuse fibrolipomatous tissue adherent to the cord and its roots. Fibrolipomatous tissue was found in 8 percent of the cases of spina bifida cystica by Ingraham and Swan (1943), who referred to these lesions as lipomyelomeningocele. Sacral teratomas may occur in association with spina bifida or meningocele; in rare instances they may occur within the meningocele sac (Mitgang, 1972).

Spina Bifida Occulta. Spina bifida occulta is often marked by cutaneous stigmata including hypertrichosis, a skin dimple or sinus, lipoma or a capillary nevus; these lesions may occur single or in various combinations (James and Lassman, 1972). A median sagittal cord of fibrous tissue may extend from the skin toward the spinal canal. The frequency of spinal cord lesions in spina bifida occulta is difficult to assess. James and Lassman (1972) reviewed surgical findings in spina bifida occulta for 100 cases with clinical symptoms. Seventy-one showed traction lesions in the form of small or atretic sclerosed meningoceles; there was fibrous attachment of the spinal cord or of spinal roots near or within the sac of the meningocele, preventing the normal ascent of the caudal end of the cord which was affixed below the level of L_2. Diastematomyelia was present in 42, which is comparable to its occurrence in 40 of the 85 children reviewed by Till (1968). Less common lesions were dermoid cysts, hydromyelia, coccygeal cysts, dermal sinus, and myelodysplasia presenting as a bulbous enlargement of the cord.

Spina Bifida Cystica. Von Recklinghausen (1886) described the morbid anatomy of spina bifida cystica and its variants in considerable detail on hand of 32 cases, and his observations form the basis of our knowledge on the morbid anatomy of the disease; there are numerous subsequent brief descriptions in the literature, and another comprehensive series was published by Keiller (1922). Spina bifida cystica occurs most frequently, in 80 to 90 percent of cases, in the lumbo-sacral region, and occasionally at other levels of the spinal column (Table 4, p. 236). The common lumbosacral localization of the cystic skin lesion is not representative of that of the bone defect which always extends to the extremity of the vertebral column and is most frequent in the sacrum (Barson, 1970). Multiple lesions are rare and were found in only 6 of 536 cases in the series of Fisher *et al.* (1952); a combination of a cervical with a sacral spina bifida cystica was reported by Bailey (1971).

Approximately 10 to 20 percent of cases of spina bifida cystica are meningoceles, the rest myelomeningoceles. The meningoceles are most commonly low lumbar or sacral and may be broad based or pedunculated; they are usually covered with normal skin, although there may be ulceration. The channel connecting the cyst with the vertebral canal is much narrower than the cyst itself, and the lumen of the latter is usually single but may be multilocular. The cyst wall is composed of skin, dura and arachnoid, the meningeal layers either being fused or separated. The spinal cord does not extend into the cyst, but it may be hydromyelic, diastematomyelic or otherwise deformed. Nerve roots may loop through the cyst or be attached to its walls.

The myelomeningoceles are nearly always broad based; the cyst wall shows a characteristic central area without epithelialization, where a highly vascular tissue is exposed from which CSF or tissue transudate may ooze.

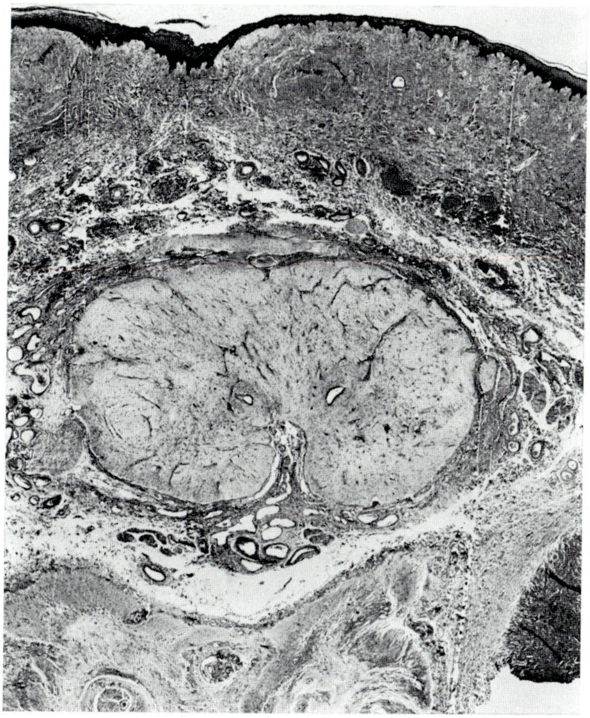

Fig. 78. Duplication of the central canal in a subcutaneous cord; surgical specimen from a myelomeningocele; ×9.5

This exposed tissue consists of highly vascularized meninges and neuroectodermal tissue; it resembles closely the area cerebrovasculosa of anencephaly and has been called area medullovasculosa (von Recklinghausen, 1886); it should not be mistaken for ulceration. The area medullovasculosa may become epithelialized *in utero,* but epithelialization occurs more commonly postnatally in infants surviving for more than 2 weeks, with resulting scarring in the central portion of the cyst wall (Cameron, 1956). On opening the cyst the spinal cord is found to be fused with the area medullovasculosa, being usually flattened and dorsally opened. The cyst cavity, hence, typically lies ventral to the cord and within the arachnoid and may be sealed off from the rest of the CSF spaces by arachnoid. Spinal roots originating from the malformed cord either traverse the cyst cavity on their course to the intervertebral foramina or run along the cyst wall. Their course after entering the spinal canal is modified by the tethering of the spinal cord; roots originating in the cranial pole of the meningomyelocele may ascend, while the caudal ones descend. The peripheral nerves can always be identified in the lower extremities. The motor disabilities of the infants are commonly attributed to ventral horn damage, but Stark and Drummond (1971) showed that electric stimulation of the cyst wall elicits movement in most muscle groups of the lower extremities and concluded that upper motor neuron damage at the level immediately cranial to the cyst was the most important cause of disabilities.

Microscopic examination of the area medullovasculosa discloses a highly vascularized, loose connective tissue, with sinusoid leptomeningeal capillaries forming a vascular plexus at the surface of the dysplastic cord tissue. The degree of cord deformity varies; there may be flattening or lack of fusion in the dorsal portion, duplication of the central canal, or complete disorganization with irregularly disposed nests of glioneuronal tissue in which motor neurons or ependyma are discernible. The nervous tissue may exhibit secondary changes including softening and cyst formation. In extreme lesions neuroectodermal tissue may be absent, the apex of the cyst being formed by a layer of arachnoid only, while dura and dermis terminate in the lateral portions of the cyst wall. Emery and Lendon (1973) classified the spinal cord lesions in 100 meningomyeloceles. Hydromyelia was found proximal to the main lesion in 29 percent and syringomyelia (an extension of the central canal into the cord parenchyma) in 14 percent. Within the myelomeningocele there was total or partial diastematomyelia in 36 percent and 35 percent showed an open neural plate; some cords were compressed to wing-shape by arachnoid cysts. Double or multiple central canals (Fig. 78) were present caudal to the myelomeningocele in 42 percent and diplomyelia in 25 percent. Cameron (1957) had earlier reported diastematomyelia in as much as 45 percent of cases. Jakobs *et al.* (1961) found amniotic fluid squames, lanugo hairs and mucus in the spinal subarachnoid space, in the central canal or in the cord of such infants, which demonstrates continuity between CSF spaces and amniotic fluid *in utero.* This phenomenon may be of diagnostic significance as it permits the escape of CSF-specific proteins into the amnionic fluid, where they may be detected by immune electrophoresis (Macri *et al.*, 1973).

A variant consists of a hydromyelic dilation of the central canal, the cyst cavity being within the cord and the spinal roots originating at the ventral and dorsal outer surfaces of the cyst wall. This lesion, called myelocystocele, occurs often in association with defects of vertebral bodies or intestinal fistula; also, lesions in the cervical and upper thoracic cord are often of this type, with distention of the central canal occurring locally at the level of the bone defect (Doran and Guthkelch, 1961; Barson, 1970).

Pathogenetic Considerations. The central nervous system originates from the medullary plate, a thickening of surface ectoderm along the dorsal midline of the embryo. The neural tube begins to form by the rising of the edges of this plate forming the neural groove, first discernible at 17 to 18 days. The neural tube forms from fusion of the upper edges of the neural groove, which begins in the cervical region and spreads in a cranial and caudal direction. Closure is completed slightly earlier at the cranial end (twenty-third day) than at the caudal end (twenty-fifth day). Tiny openings, the neuropores, persist for some time before the ends become completely sealed off. The neural tube ultimately sinks below the surface of the embryo, as the mesodermal elements ventral and lateral to it begin to proliferate and interpose themselves between the tube and the ectoderm. The vertebrae develop from this tissue, and vertebral arches are normally closed from the first cervical to the third or fourth sacral segment in the 50 mm (eleven weeks) embryo.

The normal course of these embryonal events appears to be rather susceptible to disturbances, as dysraphic lesions are the most common malformations in man and other species. The early developmental origin of the lesions agrees with numerous observations on dysraphic lesions in young fetuses, including spina bifida, rachischisis, anencephaly, encephalocele, or doubling of the neural tube (Wrete, 1959). Very early stages for which these lesions were described are 7 to 8 mm fetal length (Ingalls, 1933; Patten, 1953) and 5.5 mm length (Lemire *et al.*, 1965). The latter describe lesions, at the calculated gestational age of 28 days, characterized by eversion of the neural plate, loss of polarity of its nuclei and increase in the volume of neural tissue. Complete rachischisis at a still earlier stage—a 2.75 mm embryo—was reported by Dekaban and Bartelmez (1964).

Spina bifida may be induced in laboratory animals, particularly in chicks and rats. The critical period for the induction in rat is between the seventh and tenth day after conception, using trypan blue (Gunberg, 1956; Warkany *et al.*, 1958), excessive doses of vitamin A (Cohlan, 1954; Kalter and Warkany, 1961) or salicylate poisoning (Warkany and Takacs, 1959). There is also evidence for a hereditary occurrence of spina bifida, which is observed as part of a complex of malformations in certain strains of rats (Dun and Gluecksohn-Schonheimer, 1944) or in rabbits (Crary *et al.*, 1966), or as a relatively pure inherited anomaly in the manx cat (Kitchen *et al.*, 1972).

The most widely accepted theory on the pathogenesis of spina bifida attributes the lesions to failure of closure of the neural tube. Several subtheories have been invoked to explain the mechanism of this failure: Nonclosure of the neural tube was attributed to a primary developmental failure (von Recklinghausen, 1886) or to adhesions between the amnion and the edges of the neural groove (Padget, 1970). Patten (1952) attributed failure of closure to an overgrowth of neuroectodermal tissue near the defect; this author's measurements (1953) in an 8 mm human embryo with rachischisis showed that there was enough abnormal cord tissue to comprise two normal cords. The cause-effect relationship between neural overgrowth and nonclosure is not clear, however; Fowler (1953) observed overgrowth of spinal tissue secondary to experimental slitting of the neural tube. Another line of thinking assumes that closure of the neural tube proceeds normally, but that the closed tube is disrupted later by the propagation along the central canal of increased CSF pressure from hydrocephalus (Gardner, 1961). This concept has failed to gain wide acceptance as it is inconsistent with experimental data and observations in early human fetuses (Lemire *et al.*, 1956; Dekaban and Bartelmez, 1964) which demonstrate nonclosure of the neural tube at a time when the embryo has neither a choroid plexus nor a hydrocephalus (Warkany *et al.*, 1958). The same type of criticism has been leveled at theories explaining anencephaly on the basis of nonjunction of cerebral vessels with the general circulation (Dekaban and Bartelmez, 1964).

Most theories on the pathogenesis of spina bifida neglect the disturbances of mesodermal tissue, considering them secondary to lesions of the neural tube. This assumption is consistent with the normal order of development in which the closure of the neural tube is earlier than the dorsal proliferation of mesodermal tissue; yet it does not explain why mesodermal tissue does not eventually cover the defect, nor is it applicable to spina bifida occulta. Gallera (1951) concluded from experiments in chick embryos grown at elevated concentrations of CO_2 that a retardation of the normal elongation of the caudal mesodermal tissue precedes the formation of the meningocele. Considering the features common to the various lesions of the dysraphic complex, the most universal trait appears to be a lack of coordination between mesodermal and neuroectodermal growth, involving an abnormal growth of either or both of these tissues. There is indication that retardation of mesodermal growth may associate with either retardation or acceleration of neuroectodermal growth. To what degree one disturbance depends on the other, or is induced by the other, cannot be decided on the basis of available evidence (Barson, 1970).

Diastematomyelia. Diastematomyelia (diplomyelia) commonly associates with rachischisis, myelomeningocele, meningocele or spina bifida occulta as referred to in the preceding text. Of twenty-four patients in whom diastematomyelia was the predominant lesion, 18 had spina bifida and 6 had other types of bone anomalies (Moes and Hendrick, 1963; Dale, 1969). If the cases of these authors are added to those reviewed by Herren and Edwards (1940), there is a female preference of 28 among the 38 cases for which sex was indicated.

Herren and Edwards (1940) reviewed the morbid anatomy of diastematomyelia for 43 cases. It occurs in the caudal portion of the cord, usually affecting no more than 10 segments; in no instance did duplication occur at the level higher than mid-thoracic. The cord is separated into two segments by a bone spur or by a ligament of fibrous tissue protruding from the dorsal surface of the vertebral body into the spinal canal. The two halves of the cord are nearly always positioned lateral to each other; positioning above each other is exceedingly rare in man (Santha, 1930) but appears to be common in experimental animals. The two portions of the cord are rotated by 90°, facing each other with their ventral surfaces. Each portion shows a ventral fissure and an anterior spinal artery, a separate meningeal investment, and a full complement of ventral and dorsal horns and roots. The two halves of each cord may be symmetric and equal, or the median half of each cord may be hypoplastic including their dorsal and ventral horns and rootlets. Hydromyelic dilation of the central canal usually occurs at the level of the bifurcation of the cord.

Diastematomyelia is an extreme degree of cord dysraphia; lesser degrees consist of duplication of the central canal, dorsal extension of the central canal, duplication of the dorsal halves of the cord having a common set of ventral horns or divergence of the dorsal halves of the cord.

Hydromyelia. Hydromyelia consists of a dilation of the central canal of the spinal cord, usually in the lumbosacral region. It is often an incidental finding at autopsy, but is also common as a component of dysraphic lesions. The dilated central canal is completely lined by ependyma, but the latter may become dehiscent upon extreme dilation. The central canal varies from oval to irregular or slit-shaped, extending either in a bilateral or in a dorsal direction. These configurations may be considered persistence of fetal traits as the profile of the central canal of embryos is typically wide and angulated (Kolmer and Marburg, 1929). Myelocystocele, described earlier, represents an excessive degree of dilation of the central canal.

Dermoid Sinus. A dermoid sinus forms a small opening in the skin leading into a narrow duct, often marked by protruding hairs. It may be associated with hypertrichosis or a vascular nevus. Most dermoid sinuses occur in the midline, and their distribution along the neuraxis corresponds closely to the regional distribution of meningoceles and encephaloceles; in other words, dermal sinus is most frequent in the lumbo-sacral region, much less common in midline localization at the cranium, and occurs sporadically in other portions of the neuraxis.

A lumbo-sacral dermoid sinus may terminate in the subcutaneous tissue, or in the epidural or intradural space, or it may terminate intramedullary being attached to the dorsal surface of the cord by a thin strand of fibrous tissue. Bone anomalies may be absent, but spina bifida occulta is common if the sinus extends into the spinal canal. The dermatome containing the skin orifice of the sinus tract, the involved vertebral body and the level of contact with the spinal cord always belong to the same segment; the sinus tract, thus, runs in a caudo-cranial direction, passing several vertebral bodies on its course. The tract may terminate in a strand of fibrous tissue, or it may be attached to a lipoma or a dermoid cyst; approximately 20 percent of all dermoid cysts show an attached sinus tract. Occipital sinus tracts may connect to dermoid cysts in extradural localization, or to intracerebellar dermoid cysts situated within the fourth ventricle (Matson and Ingraham, 1951). Logue and Till (1952) reviewed 32 cases of posterior fossa dermoid cysts including 7 of their own: Three were extradural with a complete sinus tract; of the 29 intradural cysts 7 had a complete sinus tract, 4 an incomplete tract and 18 none. Congenital dermoid fistulas of the nose relate to a considerable variety of cystic lesions localized in the nose, palate or the nasal sinuses (Szalay and Bledsoe, 1972). Dermoid sinuses are rarely found away form the midline, but association of a sinus with an intradiploid dermoid cyst has been recorded in the temporal region (Neblett *et al.*, 1970).

Extension of the dermoid sinus tracts beyond the dura facilitates the spread of infection to the leptomeninges, and recurrent leptomeningitis of occult origin should induce careful search of the skin in the entire midline region for a small sinus tract (Matson and Jerva, 1966). Spread of infection from the tract into a dermoid cyst may induce acute spinal cord compression by rapid enlargement of the cyst. Dermoid cysts may also induce chemical leptomeningitis from the rupture of their wall, with release of the cyst contents into the cerebrospinal fluid, and keratin squames may be found in the CSF with polarized light (Cantu and Wright, 1968).

Microscopic examination of dermoid sinus tracts shows single or multiple channels lined with cornifying squamous epithelium (Fig. 79). The lumen of

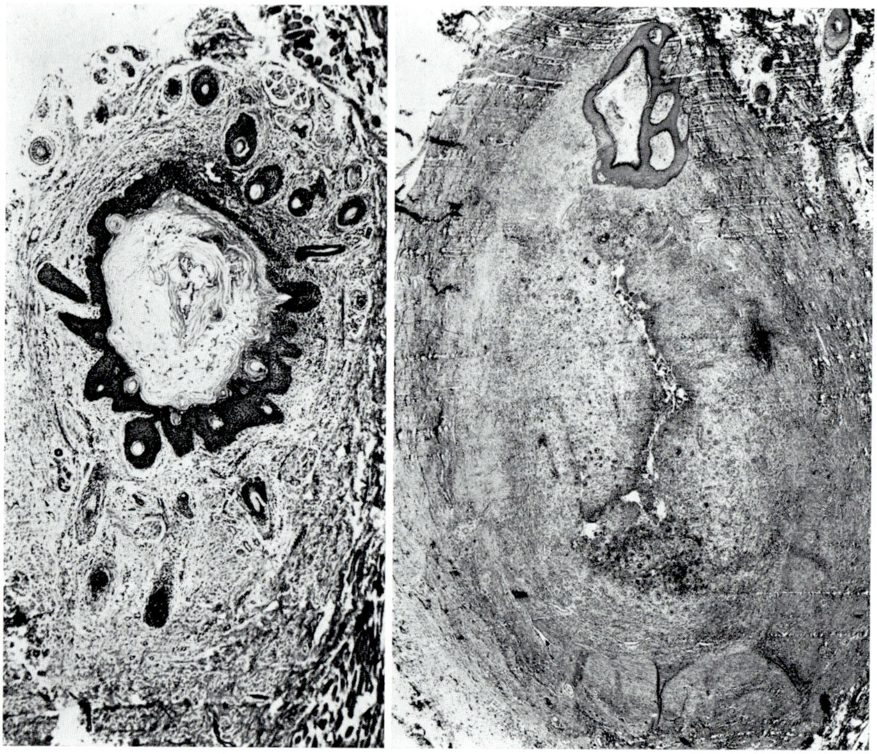

Fig. 79. Lumbosacral sinus tract. Left: lumen filled with cornified squames; H & E ×32. Right: lumen partially replaced by granulation tissue; H & E ×11.5

the tract contains desquamated keratin and hair; the surrounding collagen tissue may contain follicles and skin appendages, and there are usually scattered acute or chronic inflammatory infiltrates. Massive infection of a sinus tract may result in its complete necrosis and subsequent abscess formation.

References

Alter, M.: Anencephalus, hydrocephalus and spina bifida. Arch. Neurol. 7: 411—422, 1962.

Bailey, I. C.: Double meningocele. Arch. Dis. Child. 46: 549—550, 1971.

Barson, A. J.: Spina bifida: The significance of the level and extent of the defect to the morphogenesis. Develop. Med. Child. Neurol. 12: 129—144, 1970.

Boris, M., Blumberg, R., Feldman, D. B., Sellers, T. F.: Increased incidence of meningomyeloceles. J.A.M.A. 184: 768—768, 1963.

Brocklehurst, G.: The pathogenesis of spina bifida. Develop. Med. Child. Neurol. 13: 147—163, 1971.

Cameron, A. H.: The spinal cord lesion in spina bifida cystica. Lancet 2: 171—174, 1956.

— Malformations of the neurospinal axis, urogenital tract and foregut in spina bifida attributable to disturbance of the balstomere. J. Path. Bact. 73: 213—221, 1957.

Cantu, R., Wright, R.: Aseptic meningitic syndrome with cauda equina epidermoid tumor. J. Pediat. 73: 114—116, 1968.

Cohlan, S. Q.: Congenital anomalies in the rat produced by excessive intake of vitamin A during pregnancy. Pediatrics 13: 556—567, 1954.

Crary, D. D., Fox, R. R., Sawin, P. B.: Spina bifida in the rabbit. J. Hered. 57: 236—243, 1966.

Dale, A. J. D.: Diastematomyelia. Arch. Neurol. 20: 309—317, 1969.

Dekaban, A. S., Bartelmez, G. W.: Complete dysraphism in 14 somite human embryos. Amer. J. Anat. 115: 27—38, 1964.

Doran, P. A., Guthkelch, A. N.: Studies in spina bifida cystica. J. Neurol. Neurosurg. Psychiat. 24: 331—345, 1961.

Dun, L. C., Gluecksohn-Schonheimer, S.: A specific abnormality associated with a variety of genotypes. Proc. nat. Acad. Sci. 30: 173, 1944.

Emery, J. L., Lendon, R. G.: The local cord lesion in neurospinal dysraphism (meningomyelocele). J. Path. 110: 83—96, 1973.

Fisher, R. G., Uihlein, A., Keith, H. M.: Spina bifida and cranium bifidum: study of 530 cases. Proc. Mayo Clinic 27: 33—38, 1952.

Forbes, M.: Renal dysplasia in infants with neurospinal dysraphism. J. Path. 107: 13—20, 1972.

Fowler, I.: Responses of the chick neural tube in mechanically produced spina bifida. J. exp. Zool. 123: 115—151, 1953.

Gallera, J.: Influence de l'atmosphère artificiellement modifiée sur le dévelopment embryonaire du poulet. Acta anat. 11: 549—585, 1951.

Gardner, J. W.: Rupture of the neural tube. Arch. Neurol. 4: 1—7, 1961.

Gruenwald, P.: Tissue anomalies of probable neural crest origin in a twenty millimeter embryo with myeloschisis. Arch. Path. 31: 489—500, 1941.

Gunberg, D. L.: Spina bifida and the Arnold-Chiari malformation in the progeny of trypan blue injected rats. Anat. Rec. 126: 343—367, 1956.

Herren, R. Y., Edwards, J. E.: Diplomyelia. Arch. Path. 30: 1203—1214, 1940.

Hsu, C. Y., Van Dyke, J. H.: An analysis of growth rates in neural epithelium of normal and spina bifidous (myeloschisis) mouse embryos. Anat. Rec. 100: 745—745, 1948.

Ingalls, N. W.: Studies in pathology of development. II. Some aspects of defective development in the dorsal midline. Amer. J. Path. 8: 525—555, 1932.

Ingraham, F. D., Swan, H.: Spina bifida and cranium bifidum (encephalocele); a survey of 546 cases. New Engl. J. Med. 228: 559—563, 1943.

— — Hamlin, H., Lowrey, J. J., Matson, D. D., Scott, H. W.: Spina bifida and crania bifida. Cambridge: Harvard University Press 1943.

Jakobs, E. B., Landing, B. H., Thomas, W.: Vernicomyelia: Its bearing on theories of genesis of Arnold-Chiari complex. Amer. J. Path. 39: 345—351, 1961.

James, C. C. M., Lassman, L. P.: Spinal dysraphism: Spina bifida occulta. London: Butterworth 1972.

Kak, V. K., Chugh, K. S., Sodhi, J. S.: Occult intrasacral meningocele. Neurochirurgia 15: 148—152, 1972.

Kalter, H., Warkany, J.: Experimental production of congenital malformations in strains of inbred mice by maternal treatment with hypervitaminosis A. Amer. J. Path. 38: 1—21, 1961.

Keiller, V. H.: A contribution to the anatomy of spina bifida. Brain 45: 31—103, 1922.

Kitchen, H., Murray, R. E., Cockrell, B. Y.: Animal model for human disease: Spinal bifida, sacral dysgenesis and myelocele. Amer. J. Path. 68: 203—206, 1972.

Kolmer, W., Marburg, O.: Studien über die erste Entwicklung des Zentralkanals des Menschen. Z. Anat. Entwickl.-Gesch. 89: 54—70, 1929.

Laurence, K. M., Tew, B. J.: Natural history of spina bifida cystica and cranium bifidum cysticum. Major central nervous system malformations in South Wales, Part IV. Arch. Dis. Child. 46: 127—138, 1971.

Lemire, R. J., Shepard, T. H., Alvord, E. C.: Caudal myeloschisis (lumbosacral spina bifida cystica) in five millimeter human embryo. Anat. Rec. 152: 9—16, 1965.

Leveuf, J.: Etudes sur le spina bifida. Paris: Masson et Cie 1937.

Logue, V., Till, K.: Posterior fossa dermoid cysts with special reference to intracranial infection. J. Neurol. Neurosurg. Psychiat. 15: 1—12, 1952.

Lorber, J.: The family history of spina bifida cystica. Pediatrics 35: 589—595, 1965.

— Segall, M.: Bacterial meningitis in spina bifida. A review of 37 cases. Arch. Dis. Child. 37: 300—308, 1962.

Lucey, J. F., Mann, R. W., Simmons, G. M., Friedman, E.: An increased incidence of spina bifida in Vermont in 1962. Pediatrics 33: 981—984, 1964.

Mackenzie, N. G., Emery, J. L.: Deformities of the cervical cord in children with neurospinal dysraphism. Develop. Med. Child. Neurol. 13, Suppl. 25: 58—67, 1971.

Macri, J. N., Joshi, M. S., Evans, M. I.: An antenatal diagnosis of spina bifida in the Lewis rat. Nature New Biol. 246. 89—90, 1973.

Matson, D. D., Ingraham, F. D.: Intracranial complications of congenital dermal sinuses. Pediatrics 8: 463—474, 1951.

— Jerva, J. J.: Recurrent meningitis associated with congenital lumbo-sacral sinus tract. J. Neurosurg. 25: 288—297, 1966.

Mitgang, R. N.: Teratoma occurring within a myelomeningocele. Case report. J. Neurosurg. 37: 448—451, 1972.

Moes, C. A. F., Hendrick, E. B.: Diastematomyelia. Pediatrics 63: 238—248, 1963.

Neblett, C. R., Caram, P. C., Morris, R.: Lateral congenital dermal sinus tract associated with an intradiploic dermoid tumor. Case report. J. Neurosurg. 33: 103—105, 1970.

Padget, D. H.: Neuroschisis and human embryonic maldevelopment. J. Neuropath. exp. Neurol. 29: 192—216, 1970.

Passarge, E., Lenz, W.: Syndrome of caudal regression in infants of diabetic mothers. Pediatrics 37: 672—674, 1966.

Patten, B. M.: Overgrowth of the neural tube in young human embryos. Anat. Rec. 113: 381—393, 1952.

— Embryological stages in the establishing of myeloschisis with spina bifida. Amer. J. Anat. 93: 365—395, 1953.

Record, R. G., McKeown, T.: Congenital malformations of the central nervous system. I. A survey of 930 cases. Brit. J. soc. Med. 4: 183—219, 1949.

Santha, K. V.: Über das Verhalten des Kleinhirns in einem Fall von endogen familiärer Idiotie. Z. Neurol. Psychiat. 123: 717—793, 1930.

Smith, E. D.: Spina bifida and the total care of spinal myelomeningocele. Springfield: Ch. C Thomas 1965.

Stark, G. D., Drummond, M.: The spinal cord lesion in myelomeningocele (Casey Holter Memorial Lecture). Develop. Med. Child. Neurol., Suppl. 25: 1—14, 1971.

Sutow, W. W., Pryde, A. W.: Incidence of spina bifida occulta. Amer. J. Dis. Child. 91: 211—217, 1956.

Szalay, G. C., Bledsoe, R. C.: Congenital dermoid cyst and fistula of the nose. Amer. J. Dis. Child. 124: 392—400, 1972.

Till, K.: Spinal dysraphism: a study of congenital malformations of the back. Develop. Med. Child. Neurol. 10: 470—477, 1968.

Timson, J.: The sex ratio in spina bifida. Genetica 40: 427—433, 1969.

von Recklinghausen, F.: Untersuchungen über die Spina bifida. Virchows Arch. 105: 243—330, 373—455, 1886.

Warkany, J., Takacs, E.: Experimental production of congenital malformations in cats by salicylate poisoning. Amer. J. Path. 35: 315—331, 1959.

— Wilson, J. G., Geiger, J. F.: Myeloschisis and myelomeningocele produced experimentally in the rat. J. comp. Neurol. 109: 35—64, 1958.

Wrete, M.: Über die Kenntnis des abnormen Offenstehens des Neuralrohres bei menschlichen Embryonen und jungen Feten. Beitr. path. Anat. 121: 329—346, 1959.

Ya Deau, R. C., Clagett, O. T., Divertie, M. D.: Intrathoracic meningocele. J. Thorac. Cardiovasc. Surg. 49: 202—209, 1965.

Yen, S., MacMahon, B.: Genetics of anencephaly and spina bifida. Lancet 2: 623—626, 1968.

25. The Arnold-Chiari Malformation (Cleland-Chiari Malformation)

The deformities of brain stem and cerebellum generally known as Arnold-Chiari malformation were first described by Cleland (1883) for one infant of a series of 9 presenting with various combinations of spina bifida cystica, encephalocele and anencephaly. Cleland reports and illustrates the herniation of the vermis and the deformities of the medulla oblongata and tectal plate. Chiari (1891, 1896) described these lesions in considerable detail, including the ascending direction of nerve roots, and made reference to Cleland's article; excerpts of Chiari's (1891) original description were recently translated and republished (Wilkins and Brody, 1971). Chiari was concerned mainly with the types of cerebellar deformities, of which he distinguished three types: The first, consisting of herniation of the cerebellar tonsils is considered more closely under "Chronic Tonsillar Herniation" later in this chapter; type II is now widely recognized as the Arnold-Chiari malformation; type III was an instance of cervical spina bifida with cerebellar encephalocele. Twenty-four cases form the basis of the second report (1896), in which a fourth type, cerebellar hypoplasia, was added. Arnold's (1894) contribution consists of a report on an infant with myelomeningocele and absence of sacrum, sacral teratoma, and deformities of the lower extremities. A "ribbon-like" cerebellar herniation extending to the mid-cervical region was described, but the origin from vermis or tonsils was not specified and there is no record of a brain stem deformity. Arnold's coworkers, Schwalbe and Gredig (1907), proposed the name "Arnold-Chiari" malformation and specified further to use the name "Arnold's" malformation for the cerebellar hernia and "Chiari's" malformation for the brain stem deformity. Schwalbe and Gredig's paper had considerable impact on subsequent publications although the terminology proposed by these authors is clearly incorrect and contrary to the facts available to them. There may be little point in attempting to change a nomenclature that has lasted for the better part of a century; however, if an eponym is to be used, the term Cleland-Chiari malformation would be much more appropriate than that of Arnold-Chiari malformation. In any event, the distinction of "Arnold's" from "Chiari's" malformation should be discouraged.

The early reports on the morbid anatomy of the lesions were followed by sporadic case reports (Sandbank, 1955, references). The realization that the Arnold-Chiari malformation is an exceedingly common, if not consistent, feature in infants with lumbo-sacral spina bifida and myelomeningocele came through the reports on series of cases by Russell and Donald (1935) and Ingraham and Scott (1943), and with it came the widespread clinical recognition of the entity.

Clinical Features and Occurrence. Adams *et al.* (1941) distinguished five types of clinical symptoms: 1. Symptoms of increased intracranial pressure, 2. cranial nerve palsies, 3. symptoms due to compression of the brain stem against adjacent bone structures, 4. symptoms secondary to compression of the cervical cord, and 5. those of cerebellar involvement. Increased intracranial pressure with hydrocephalus is the most consistent aspect of the disease. The clinical statistics on hydrocephalus in children with spina bifida, however, are not representative of the frequency of the Arnold-Chiari malformation since the latter may occur without hydrocephalus, and since hydrocephalus may be of different causes, for example from stenosis of the aqueduct. Laurence (1960) observed hydrocephalus in 80 percent of his cases of lumbar spina bifida cystica; the frequency was 70 percent for thoraco-lumbar, 50 percent for sacral and 40 percent for thoracic localization of the spina bifida cystica. Lorber (1961) and Smith (1965) also observed hydrocephalus in 80 percent of cases of spina bifida; in Lorber's series the incidence of hydrocephalus was 89 percent for thoraco-lumbar and lumbo-sacral spina bifida cystica and 96 percent if the patients had paraplegia as well. Considerable interest has focussed on the development of hydrocephalus subsequent to surgical repair of myelomeningocele, and a cause-effect relationship has been implicated. Hydrocephalus, however, commonly develops in infants with myelomeningocele upon or shortly after birth; in the series of Doran and Guthkelch (1961) it was present in 46 percent at the time of admission; their statistics on untreated cases does not support the assumption that the development of hydrocephalus is triggered by surgical repair of the meningocele. It has been thought that the vascularized tissue of the myelomeningocele sac aids in the resorption of the CSF, but this is inconsistent with nearly equal rates of dye resorption from the CSF before and after surgical removal of the meningocele sac (Laurence, 1959).

Certain difficulties are encountered in defining exactly what constitutes the Arnold-Chiari malformation as the components of this syndrome of lesions may be found in various combinations. These include 1. a herniation of the cerebellar vermis or one of the tonsils, 2. various degrees in brain stem deformity combining with cerebellar herniation, and 3. the combination of cerebellar and of brain stem anomalies with various types of spina bifida. Although many combinations of these lesions are conceivable, the observed patterns of association are rather consistent, especially when considered in relation to the patient's age. The characteristic combination found in newborns and infants consists of lumbo-sacral myelomeningocele with herniation of the vermis and deformity of the brain stem. There may be herniation of tonsils rather than of vermis, prevalence of either the cerebellar or the brain stem deformity, or absence of the spina bifida, but these variants are uncommon or extremely rare. Generally, the severity of the deformity of the posterior fossa structures corresponds to the severity of lumbo-sacral spina bifida. A similar relationship is evident from the experimental data of Gunberg (1956) who observed lesions comparable to the Arnold-Chiari malformation in litters of trypan blue injected rats. There were no brain stem deformities with the least severe spinal lesion (spina bifida occulta). Brain stem deformities were found with spina bifida aperta, increasing in frequency to 100 percent with the severity of the latter.

When the Arnold-Chiari malformation afflicts adults, a different combination of lesions is typical: The deformity of the brain stem is more commonly associated with tonsillar herniation than with herniation of the vermis, and spina bifida cystica is absent. These types of lesions are considered under "Chronic Tonsillar Herniation" at the end of this chapter.

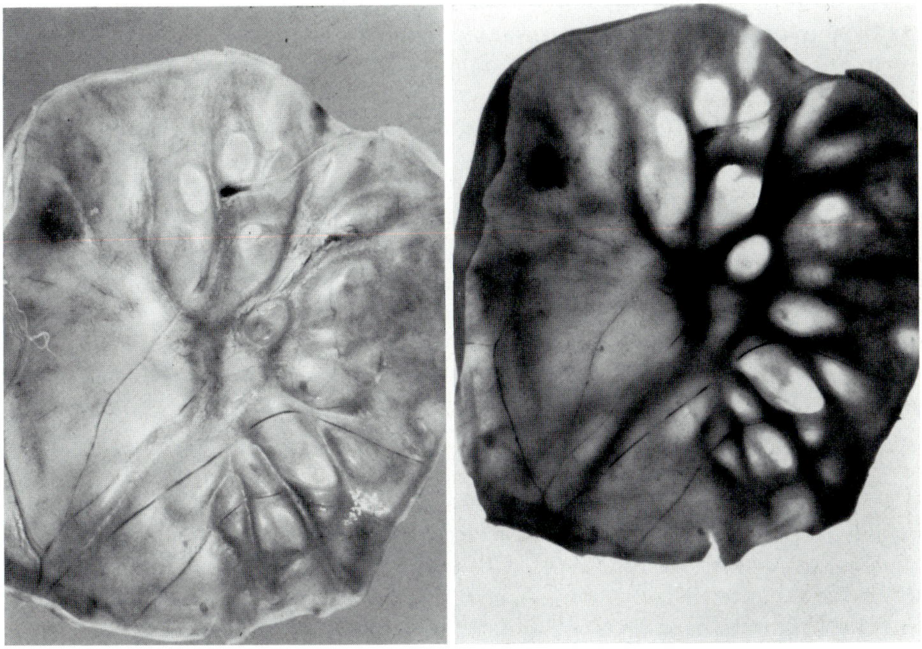

Fig. 80. Craniolacunia; bone defects are evident on transillumination

Morbid Anatomy. Most pathologic reports on the Arnold-Chiari malformation make only rudimentary reference to the anomalies of the cranial bones, although the latter are a characteristic component of the disease; indeed, most osseous changes were described by radiologists. The squamous bones of the cranial vault exhibit a characteristic variation in thickness known as craniolacunia, or Lückenschädel (Fig. 80). Radiologic evidence of craniolacunia was found in 43 percent of 120 patients with spina bifida, but was observed only twice among 5,000 patients without spina bifida cystica; it affected 53 percent of patients with myelomeningoceles, but only 12 percent of meningoceles (Vogt and Wyatt, 1941). Craniolacunia may occur in any of the squamous bones; it consists of an arborizing pattern of ridges which delineate irregularly shaped identations in the inner table. The latter may be eroded, or there may be a complete defect of bone, bridged by a tense membrane of fibrous tissue. The shape of the lacunae does not correspond precisely to that of the cortical gyri. Craniolacunia does not necessarily result from increased intracranial pressure or hydrocephalus as it has been observed with approximately equal frequency in patients with either fused or separated cranial sutures. Its occurrence had been considered an unfavorable prognostic sign (Vogt and Wyatt, 1941). Follow-up examinations of patients treated with surgical ventricular shunts show that the bone changes disappear beyond the age of 2 years. The falx is often short and may be fenestrated; shortness of the falx with fusion of the interhemispheric leptomeninges has been considered typical of the Arnold-Chiari malformation (Cameron, 1957), but this feature is quite common in otherwise normal brains.

In the posterior fossa an enlarged foramen magnum is observed as a constant feature by some and in a fraction of cases by others; the radiologic studies of Kruyff and Jeffs (1966) demonstrate enlargement of the foramen in 71 percent of cases. Radiologic examination also shows a shallow posterior fossa with low position of the torcular. The clivus is concave, with thinning of the bone particularly in its basal portion (Yu and Deck, 1971). Postmortem examination rather consistently reveals a small and shallow posterior fossa. The insertion of the tentorium is low, at times near the edge of the foramen magnum, and the tentorial hiatus is correspondingly wide; some cases have only a rudimentary tentorium. There is a low position of venous sinus, at times with an abnormal course near the foramen magnum. These changes are opposite in type to those in the Dandy-Walker malformation (Chapter 30) where the posterior fossa is large and the torcular elevated. Anomalies of the spinal column frequently include a defect in the posterior arch of the atlas bridged by a firm fibrous band; this defect was observed by Blaauw (1971) in 21 of 30 autopsies of infants with myelomeningocele, but occurred in only 3 percent of the 1,136 nonselected autopsies by Geipel (1930). The bone changes of spina bifida cystica in the lower parts of the spine are described in Chapter 24.

The brain stem and cerebellum exhibit tight crowding of all structures, being generally dislocated in a caudal direction and impacted firmly into the funnel-shaped foramen magnum and upper cervical canal. The fissures between the various anatomic subdivisions of the hindbrain, particularly the cisterna magna, are obliterated by the crowding of tissue. The caudal displacement of the brain stem causes a cranial course and elongation of the cranial nerves, particularly of those originating in the caudal portion of the medulla oblongata. Herniated cerebellar tissue extends into the spinal canal where it overlies the dorsal surface of the cord in the form of a peg or ribbon. It originates from the caudal portion of the vermis and involves uvula, nodulus and pyramis in that order (Daniel and Strich, 1958). The herniated tissue is firm, whitish and sclerotic and adheres to the opaque or gelatinous leptomeninges. A deformation of the brain stem (Fig. 81) is apparent on lateral view or on elevating the herniated cerebellar tissue; it consists of a caudal shifting of the entire dorsal aspects of the medulla oblongata, fourth ventricle and choroid plexus; the nuclear groups in the floor of the fourth ventricle are situated much farther caudal than would correspond to the landmarks at the ventral surface of the medulla. The caudal end of the fourth ventricle and its choroid plexus are dislocated into the spinal canal and the ventricle may show cystic dilation, the herniated cerebellar tissue being actually intraventricular in localization. The tissue caudal to the ventricle, containing the gracile and cuneate nuclei, forms a hump or a pedunculated mass which overrides and compresses the cervical cord, giving a characteristic Z-shaped configuration in median sagittal sections.

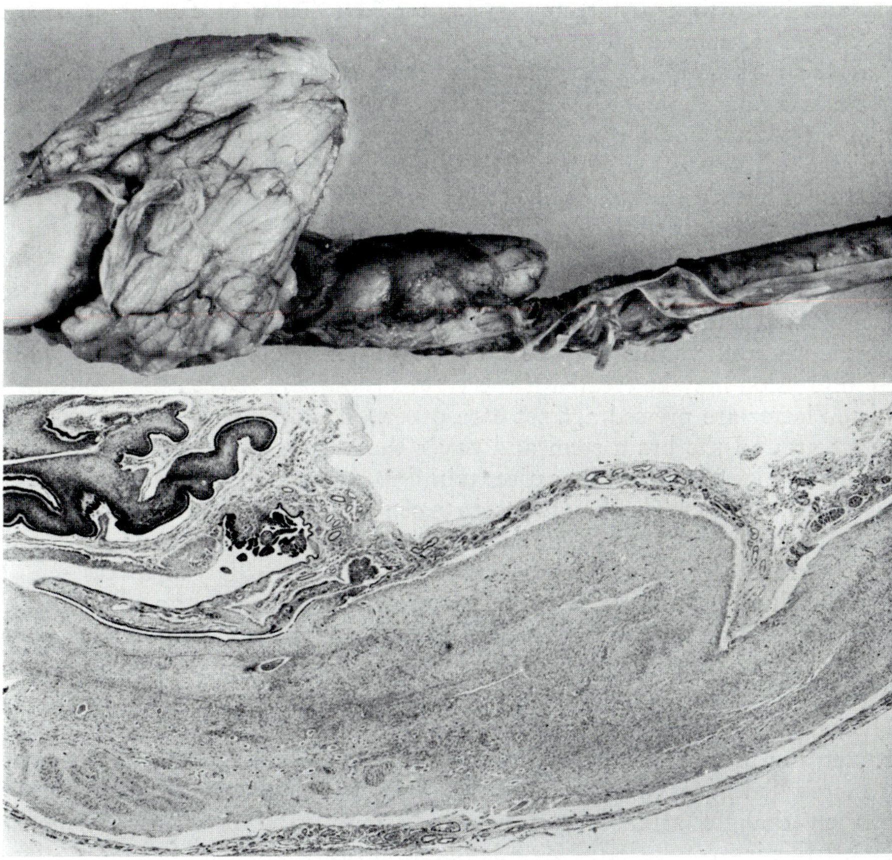

Fig. 81. Arnold-Chiari malformation; herniation of dorsal medullary tissue forms a peg overriding the cervical segments. The cerebellum is small and compressed. Longitudinal microscopic section shows the dorsal portions of medullary tissue displaced caudally in relation to the olivary nucleus (lower left). Choroid plexus, the caudal roof of the fourth ventricle and the cerebellum participate only slightly in the herniation in this case

The deformities of vermis and medulla typically occur in combination, although either may prevail—that is, either the cerebellar tissue or the deformed brain stem may extend farther caudal. In some instances the herniation is formed entirely by medullary tissue without herniation of cerebellum. In other instances the tonsils may herniate with the vermis, or the herniated cerebellum may form a broad mass of tissue with indistinct separation of vermis and tonsils. Herniation of the tonsils only is uncommon in infants but is the rule in adults; in these instances the tonsils project as two long pegs separated from each other.

Microscopic examination of the herniated cerebellar tissue shows loss of Purkinje and granular cells, with irregular sclerosis of folia and a residual layer of Bergmann-glia. The white matter is devoid of myelinated fibers. In addition to the changes of atrophy and sclerosis there may be focal dysplasia in cortical architecture (Chapter 31). Tufts of choroid plexus, at times fused in the midline, are often present and may exhibit various degrees of fibrosis and atrophy. Neuronal heterotopias are found on occasion in the cerebellar hemispheres. The brain stem shows extreme distortions of nuclei and fiber tracts, but the extensive scarring and gliosis that is found in the herniated cerebellar tissue is usually absent. Atrophy of brain stem nuclei has been described (Sieben *et al.*, 1971) but is difficult to substantiate because of the extent of distortion of cytoarchitecture.

Aside from the herniation into the spinal canal, there are numerous other deformities of posterior fossa structures. The cerebellar hemispheres are often asymmetrical and flattened at their dorsal surfaces. The separation between hemispheres and vermis may be incomplete (Russell and Donald, 1935), or this impression may be created if the vermis is buried between the hemispheres and the latter are pressed against each other. The cerebellar hemispheres also project around the brain stem and cover the ventral surface of the medulla oblongata (Fig. 82), in extreme cases touching each other in the midline (Daniel and Strich, 1958). The boundary between pons and medulla oblongata is flattened and indistinct. There is variation in the relationship between the upper surface of the cerebellar hemispheres and the enlarged hiatus tentorii. The cerebellum may be depressed below the hiatus, its dorsal surface flattened, and the occipital lobes may herniate into the posterior fossa with grooving at the edge of the tentorium (Daniel and Strich, 1958). In other instances herniation of the cerebellum into the supratentorial compartment is observed (Alvord, 1961). Such variations probably represent different balances in force between the pressure in the hydrocephalic hemispheres and that in the structures crowded into the infratentorial compartment. Emery's (1965) observations on changes after long-standing decompression by surgical shunting support this interpretation: He observed an upward growth of the cerebellum, which protruded like a tumor through the tentorial hiatus, along with an upward movement of the brain stem, lifting the hypothalamus and stretching the pituitary stalk. The deformities of the cerebellum at the tentorial hiatus commonly coexist with a characteristic beak-shaped deformity of the quadrigeminal plate, which Cleland (1883) described as "the testes being projected above the nates, and the nates being flattened". This configuration is rather similar to the shape of the tectum during early fetal development.

The cervical spinal roots are angulated at their origin and ascend cranially to their intervertebral foramina, rather than taking their normal lateral or descending course. This phenomenon has been interpreted as evidence of the causation of the brain stem deformity by caudal traction of the spinal cord. However, the displacement of roots dissipates within the upper four to six segments, the thoracic segments being in normal place and their roots descending in normal fashion (Barry *et al.*, 1957). One may interject at this point that angulated or ascending roots are a common feature at the low cervical and thoracic level of children and adults, where they are found in 71 to 76 percent of autopsies (Reid, 1960; Nathan and Feuerstein, 1970). The roots originating at the level of the myelomeningocele ascend from its dorsal pole and descend from its caudal pole. A variety of anomalies may

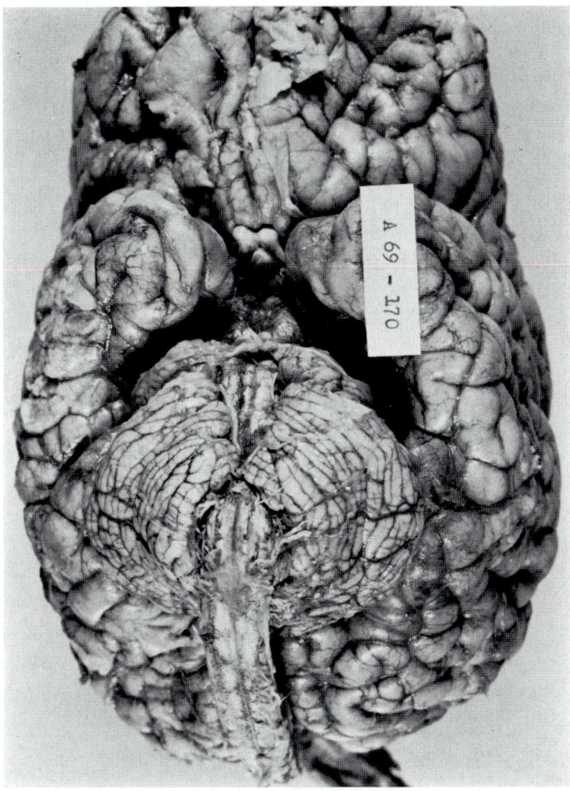

Fig. 82. Arnold-Chiari malformation; cerebellar hemispheres extend ventrally around the medulla to the point of touching each other in the midline

be found in the spinal cord. MacKenzie and Emery (1971) observed hydromyelia at approximately C_8 in 40 percent of 100 cords, as already recognized by Cleland (1883) and Chiari (1891). Hydromyelia presents as a dorsal slit-like extension or as a diffuse enlargement of the central canal. Syringomyelia was found in 20 percent of the cases; the cavities had usually formed just caudal to the herniations at the cervico-medullary junction and were considered secondary to the latter. Diastematomyelia was found in 6 cases, divergence of the dorsal halves of the cord in two, and multiple central canals in 9.

Various types of spina bifida cystica are associated with the Arnold-Chiari malformation; myelomeningocele is most common at a lumbo-sacral level, but any other portions of the spinal axis may be involved. Pure meningoceles, demonstrated by Russell (1968), are much less common than myelomeningoceles. Absence of spina bifida is exceedingly rare in infants (Peach, 1964) but is the rule for adults.

The most common change in the cerebral hemispheres consists of hydrocephalus, caused either by cervical herniation or by stenosis of the aqueduct, disregarding instances of secondary meningeal fibrosis from infection. Cervical herniation obstructs the communication of external CSF spaces between the spinal canal and the cranial vault by the impaction of brain stem and cerebellum into the foramen magnum and the associated leptomeningeal adhesions. The communication between the ventricles and the spinal CSF space may not be blocked as the cerebellar foramina are displaced into the spinal canal. This type of communication may be dramatized by the ascent of a spinal meningitis into the ventricles, sparing the cerebral subarachnoid spaces. The resultant hydrocephalus may be communicating or noncommunicating (Russell and Donald, 1935). Stenosis of the aqueduct was observed in one half of 20 cases of the Arnold-Chiari malformation by MacFarlane and Maloney (1957). It may be of the type of congenital atresia or of secondary gliosis (Chapter 22), implicating developmental disturbances as well as secondary changes from postnatal ascending meningitis. However, none of Emery's (1974) 100 cases had complete obstruction of the aqueduct, although the latter was nearly always shortened and probably acted as a valve due to its angulation from the tectal deformity.

The surface of the hydrocephalic cerebral hemispheres exhibits a pattern of redundant cortical gyration that has been described as microgyria (Ingraham and Scott, 1943) or as polymicrogyria (Alvord, 1961). Microscopic examination reveals normal laminar architecture without disorganization. The features characteristic of micropolygyria (Chapter 29) are consistently absent; claims to the contrary have not been documented convincingly. This abnormal gyral pattern has been considered evidence of a concurrent cortical malformation, an interpretation supported by rare cases having abundant small gyri in the absence of hydrocephalus. Alternatively one may assume that the hydrocephalic distention of the growing cortex produces abnormal proportions between the growth rate in cortical surface and in hemispheric surface (Chapter 21). Various malformations, such as heterotopias, may be found in the cerebral hemispheres, but none is observed with sufficient frequency to be considered typical.

Pathogenetic Considerations. There are numerous theories on the pathogenesis of the Arnold-Chiari malformation, as discussed in the reviews by Alvord (1961), Peach (1965), and Brocklehurst (1971). The traction theory has received wide attention, claiming that the brain stem deformity is produced by caudal traction of the cord due to its fixation in the myelomeningocele. This theory is inconsistent with the dissipation of root deviation within the upper cervical segments (Barry *et al.*, 1957) and with the characteristic deformation of the fourth ventricle. Sacral fixation of the spinal cord may occur without hindbrain deformity (Russell, 1964), and experimental fixation of the cord has failed to induce the latter (Goldstein and Kepes, 1965).

Another line of thinking considers the brain stem deformity secondary to hydrocephalus, that is as a result of the impaction of the posterior fossa structures into the foramen magnum (Gardner and Goodall, 1950). This theory is inconsistent with the presence of a brain stem deformity in the absence of hydrocephalus and with embryologic observations on the early phases of myelomeningocele formation (Chapter 24). However, it received new support from observations on the induction of the Arnold-Chiari malformation in experimental virus-induced hydrocephalus (Margolis and Kilham, 1969).

The theories cited above assume that the hindbrain deformity is secondary to primary maldevelopments of either spine or cerebral hemispheres. There seems to be greater merit in those theories which assume a primary developmental disturbance of the structures of the posterior fossa, either as component of a complex of malformations or in terms of a specific local type of derangement. Daniel and Strich (1958) assumed a failure of formation of the pontine flexure; however, the normal straightening of the pontine flexure involves rearrangement of pontine and olivary nuclei which are widely separated at early fetal stages (Essick, 1912). No corresponding disorganization of these nuclear groups is seen in the Arnold-Chiari malformation. Barry *et al.* (1957) introduced the concept of "overgrowth" of the cerebellum, akin to the overgrowth of spinal cord tissue near a myelomeningocele (Chapter 24). However, in Alvord's (1961) measurements the weights of brain stem and cerebellum and the volume of the posterior fossa were both below normal. Variend and Emery (1973) found uniformly reduced cerebellar weights for 100 infants with myelomeningocele. Measurements in a serially cut 95 mm fetus with spina bifida revealed a posterior fossa of less than one-third normal size containing just under half the normal volume of neural tissue; there was some indication of overgrowth of the spinal cord, but the mass of all neural tissue was about half normal (Brocklehurst, 1969). Doran and Guthkelch (1961) suggested that the term Arnold-Chiari malformation be replaced with "craniocerebral disproportion" and assumed that the disease was due to an increased volume of the cerebral hemispheres. The increase in hemispheric size, however, is due to hydrocephalic distension rather than to true megalencephaly; Jacobs *et al.* (1961) report increased brain weights but they do not comment on the need for draining all CSF before weighing. In Emery's (1964) measurements nearly all hemispheric weights of nonshunted infants were below normal, except for the first 2 weeks of life when above normal weights were noted. For shunted infants there was restoration to normal weight but no overgrowth. The term craniocerebral disproportion can also be understood as having a relative meaning; that is, a disproportion between the rate of expansion of the neural tissues in the posterior fossa and that of the mesodermal compartments enclosing them (Brocklehurst, 1969). Emery's (1965) observations on changes following long-standing surgical shunting are particularly revealing in this regard. They show that the direction of the growth of cerebellum and brain stem is reversed into the supratentorial compartment if the pressure in the latter is reduced by shunting and, at the same time, the cystic spinal defect closed. All the manifestations of the Arnold-Chiari malformation are readily explained by a disproportion between the posterior fossa and its contents; the posterior fossa is too small and expands too slowly to accomodate the rapid growth of the cerebellum.

There is no doubt that the hindbrain deformities originate during intrauterine life, as evident from their presence at birth, and from their occurrence in prematures, *e.g.*, a 22-week-old infant (Daniel and Strich, 1958). The earliest observed occurrences were at an estimated fetal age of 17 and 18 weeks; the malformation was found in an incipient stage at the age of 10 weeks (Barry *et al.*, 1957), that is considerably later than the earliest observations of spina bifida (Chapter 24). Early onset, nonetheless, does not preclude continued aggravation of the malformation. The growth of the cerebellum is late when compared to that of other portions of the brain (Chapter 1), and its disproportional growth continues well into the postnatal period; accordingly, a progression of the deformities may be anticipated as long as growth of neural tissue continues.

Chronic Tonsillar Herniation. The term "chronic tonsillar herniation" is introduced here to designate a group of lesions whose distinction from the Arnold-Chiari malformation has met with difficulty and confusion. Because of the uncertain state of classification, there has been a rather loose usage of the term Arnold-Chiari malformation particularly in regard to lesions found in adults. Some authors have applied it to any kind of chronic tonsillar herniation in the absence of space-occupying lesions, and still others even used it to describe pressure cones caused by tumors in the posterior fossa. The problem of distinguishing chronic herniations of the cerebellar tonsils from the Arnold-Chiari malformation traces back to Chiari's (1891, 1896) reports on the lesions which he called changes of type I, distinguishing them from herniation of vermis with brain stem deformity which he called type II. Chiari's description needs to be considered in a historical perspective. Tonsillar cerebellar herniation as consequence of increased intracranial pressure was first described by Cushing (1902) and Collier (1904), but it was not widely recognized until after Meyer's report (1920), who documented subfalcial and uncal herniation along with herniation of the cerebellar tonsils. The relationship between hydrocephalus and obstruction of flow of CSF was also not well understood at the time of Chiari's report. His description in 1896 refers to cerebellar tonsillar herniation in 14 cases, all having hydrocephalus; microscopic examination of the herniated tonsils showed definite sclerotic changes in 6. The retrospective interpretation of this group of cases is difficult; some of the cases may have been acute herniation due to increased intracranial pressure, but it is inappropriate to disregard the description of type I as being merely an early account of acute tonsillar herniation. Sclerosis of the tonsils was documented for many cases, and space-occupying lesions other than hydrocephalus were absent. The cause-effect relationship between the chronic herniations and hydrocephalus in these cases remains a matter of conjecture. Chiari thought that hydrocephalus must be present early in development to force the growth of the cerebellum into the spinal canal. The term malformation (or, rather, deformity) of Chiari's type I is, in principle, correct when applied to instances of chronic herniation affecting the cerebellar tonsils rather than the vermis. Its usage is undesireable, however, in that it opens the door to much ambiguity in suggesting that there is a specific disease entity by this name. The present text replaces it with "chronic tonsillar herniation"; the latter is used to designate all instances of chronic herniation of the cerebellar tonsils in the absence of space-occupying intracranial lesions, the tonsils showing atrophy, sclerosis and meningeal fibrosis.

A review of the literature on chronic states of herniation of the cerebellar tonsils allows for the distinction of two groups, that is the Arnold-Chiari

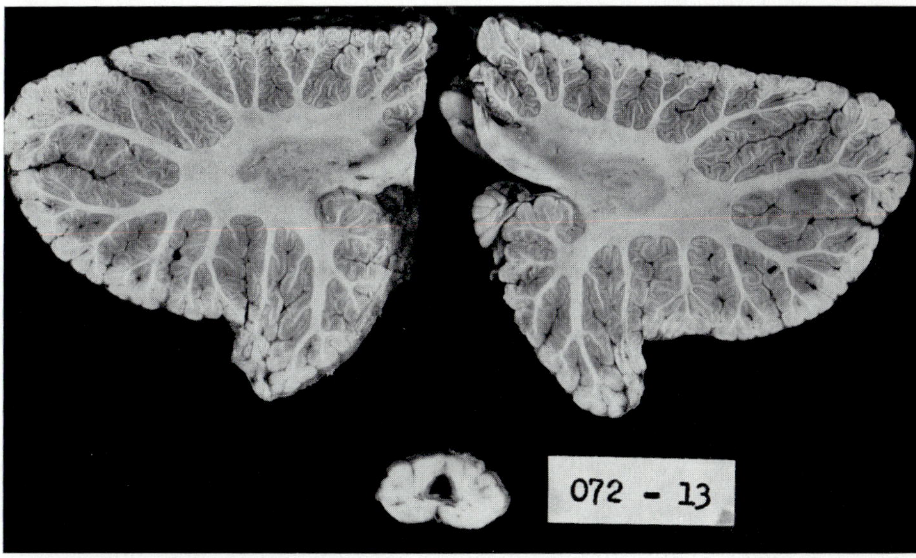

Fig. 83. Chronic herniation of cerebellar tonsils; sclerosis of the folia where they abutt the edge of the foramen magnum. A syringomyelia is present in the cervical cord

malformation in adults and the cases referred here as chronic tonsillar herniation. The Arnold-Chiari malformation in adults differs from the infantile form in that there is herniation of the cerebellar tonsils rather than the vermis, the latter being involved only as an exception. In the authors' opinion only those cases should be accepted as adult Arnold-Chiari malformation in whom at least one other component of the Arnold-Chiari complex is present, most often a medullar deformity in the form of a dorsal hump, or upward projecting cervical roots. The medullar deformity is usually less severe than for the infantile form. Spina bifida cystica or occulta is generally absent in the adult Arnold-Chiari malformation. These cases frequently manifest with symptoms of high cervical or posterior fossa compression during adult life. Pertinent observations were reported by McConnell and Parker (1938), Ogryzlo (1942) and, with increasing frequency, in the more recent literature.

If these cases of adult Arnold-Chiari malformation are excluded there remains another group in which chronic herniation of the cerebellar tonsils is the only identifyable cerebral lesion. Although some of these may conceivably represent minimal degrees or formes frustes of the adult Arnold-

Chiari malformation, there is no way of verification in the absence of other typical lesions. Some of these cases come to clinical attention during adult life because of symptoms of high cervical or posterior fossa compression, others go unnoticed and are found incidentally at autopsy. The present author collected, in addition, a group of 7 infants and children in whom chronic tonsillar herniation was found upon death following relatively minor cervical trauma, or unexpected death following normally non-fatal diseases or surgery.

Chronic tonsillar herniation may be mistaken for an acute pressure cone due to a "terminal brain edema" or for a variant in the configuration of the inferior cerebellar surface. However, the chronicity of herniation is evident upon careful gross inspection from the atrophy of foliae (Fig. 83). Microscopic examination discloses atrophy and sclerosis of foliae and fibrosis of meninges throughout the tonsil, at its tip, or at the indentation caused by the edge of the foramen magnum. No evidence of present or past cerebral lesions responsible for the chronic state of herniation is obtained.

There is overlap between the adult Arnold-Chiari malformation and chronic tonsillar herniation in regard to some of the associated findings. Hydrocephalus, usually of mild degree, may occur for both, though not consistently. Bone deformities of the basal cranium or of cervical vertebrae may be found for both. Some instances of chronic tonsillar herniations were associated with (and probably secondary to) platybasia (Gustafson and Oldenber, 1940; Ray, 1942; Spillane *et al.*, 1957), but a clearly defined basi-occipital anomaly is absent for most. Anomalies of the basiocciput or cervical vertebrae (List, 1941) also occur with the adult Arnold-Chiari malformation. Their actual frequency is difficult to assess as the classification of cases remains problematic. Sandbank (1955) found basilar impression for 23 of 101 cases of Arnold-Chiari malformation in adults, but his statistic does not separate cases of chronic tonsillar herniation. Another overlap of the two categories pertains to the occurrence of high cervical syringomyelia for both (Banerji and Millar, 1974).

References

Adams, R. D., Schatzki, R., Scoville, W. B.: Arnold-Chiari malformation: diagnosis, demonstration by intraspinal lipiodol and successful surgical treatment. New Engl. J. Med. 225: 125—131, 1941.

Alvord, E. C., Jr.: The pathology of hydrocephalus. In: Disorders of the Developing Nervous System, Chapter 14, pp. 343—412. Springfield, Ill.: Ch. C Thomas 1961.

Arnold, J.: Myelocyste, Transposition von Gewebskeimen und Sympodie. Beitr. path. Anat. 16: 1—28, 1894.

Banerji, N. K., Millar, J. H. D.: Chiari malformation presenting in adult life—Its relationship to syringomyelia. Brain 97: 157—168, 1974.

Barry, A., Patten, B. M., Stewart, B. H.: Possible factors in the development of the Arnold-Chiari malformation. J. Neurosurg. 14: 285—301, 1957.

Blaauw, G.: Defect in posterior arch of atlas in myelomeningocele. Develop. Med. Child. Neurol., Suppl. 25: 113—115, 1971.

Brocklehurst, G.: A quantitative study of a spina bifida foetus. J. Path. 99: 205—211, 1969.

— The pathogenesis of spina bifida: A study of the relationship between observation, hypothesis and surgical incentive. Develop. Med. Child. Neurol. 13: 147—163, 1971.

Cameron, A. H.: Arnold-Chiari malformation and other neuroanatomical malformations associated with spina bifida. J. Path. Bact. 73: 195—210, 1957.

Chiari, H.: Über Veränderungen des Kleinhirns, der Pons und der Medulla oblongata in Folge von congenitaler Hydrocephalie des Großhirns. Dtsch. med. Wschr. 27: 1172—1175, 1891.

— Über Veränderungen des Kleinhirns, Pons und der Medulla oblongata in Folge von congenitaler Hydrocephalie des Großhirns. Denkschr. Kaiserl. Akad. Wiss. Math. Naturw. Classe 63: 71—115, 1896.

Cleland: Contributions of the study of spina bifida, encephalocele and anencephalus. J. Anat. Physiol. 17: 257—292, 1883.

Collier, J.: The false localizing signs of intracranial tumor. Brain 27: 490—508, 1904.

Cushing, H.: Some experimental and clinical observations concerning states of increased intracranial tension. Amer. J. med. Sci. 124: 375—400, 1902.

Daniel, P. M., Strich, S. J.: Some observations on the congenital deformity of the central nervous system known as the Arnold-Chiari malformation. J. Neuropath. exp. Neurol. 17: 255—266, 1958.

Doran, P. A., Guthkelch, A. N.: Studies in spina bifida cystica. I. General survey and reassessment of the problem. J. Neurol. Neurosurg. Psychiat. 24: 331—345, 1961.

Emery, J. L.: Effects of continual decompression using Holter valve on weights of cerebral hemispheres in children with hydrocephalus and spina bifida cystica. Arch. Dis. Child. 39: 379—383, 1964.

— Intracranial effects of long-standing decompression of the brain in children with hydrocephalus and meningomyelocele. Develop. Med. Child. Neurol. 7: 302—309, 1965.

— Deformity of the aqueduct of Sylvius in children with hydrocephalus and myelomeningocele. Develop. Med. Child Neurol. Suppl. 32: 40—48, 1974.

Essick, C. R.: The development of the nuclei pontis and the nucleus arcuatus in man. Amer. J. Anat. 13: 25—54, 1912.

Gardner, J. W., Goodall, R. J.: The surgical treatment of Arnold-Chiari malformation in adults. J. Neurosurg. 7: 199—206, 1950.

Geipel, P.: Zur Kenntnis der Spina bifida des Atlas. Fortschr. Röntgenstr. 42: 583—589, 1930.

Goldstein, F., Kepes, J. J.: The relationship of the Arnold-Chiari malformation to lumbar meningomyeloceles. An experimental study. Vth Internat. Congr. Neuropath., Excerpta Medica Foundation, Amsterdam, 1965, pp. 734—737.

Gunberg, D. L.: Spina bifida and the Arnold-Chiari malformation in the progeny of trypan blue injected rats. Anat. Rec. 126: 343—367, 1956.

Gustafson, W. A., Oldenberg, E.: Neurological significance of platybasia. Arch. Neurol. Psychiat. 44: 1184—1198, 1940.

Ingraham, F. D., Scott, H. W.: Spina bifida and cranium bifidum; Arnold-Chiari malformation; a study of 20 cases. New Engl. J. Med. 229: 108—114, 1943.

Jacobs, E. B., Landing, B. H., Thomas, W., Jr.: Vernicomyelia. Its bearing on theories of genesis of the Arnold Chiari complex. Am. J. Path. 39: 345—353, 1961.

Kruyff, E., Jeffs, R.: Skull abnormalities associated with Arnold-Chiari malformation. Acta radiol. (Diagn.) (Stockh.) 5: 9—24, 1966.

Laurence, K. M.: Some applications of the urinary phenolsulphonphthalein excretion test in hydrocephalus and related conditions. Brain 82: 551—565, 1959.

— The natural history of spina bifida cystica. Proc. roy. Soc. Med. 53: 1055—1056, 1960.

List, C. F.: Neurologic syndromes accompanying developmental anomalies of occipital bone, atlas and axis. Arch. Neurol. Psychiat. 45: 577—616, 1941.

Lorber, J.: Systematic ventriculographic studies in infants born with meningomyelocele and encephalocele (The incidence and development of hydrocephalus). Arch. Dis. Child. 36: 381—389, 1961.

MacFarlane, A., Maloney, A. F. J.: The appearance of the aqueduct and its relationship to hydrocephalus in the Arnold-Chiari malformation. Brain 80: 479—491, 1957.

MacKenzie, N. G., Emery, J. L.: Deformities of the cervical cord in children with neurospinal dysraphism. Develop. Med. Child. Neurol. 13, Suppl. 25: 58—67, 1971.

McConnell, A. A., Parker, H. L.: Deformity of hind-brain associated with internal hydrocephalus; its relation to Arnold-Chiari malformation. Brain 61: 415—429, 1938.

Margolis, G., Kilham, L. K.: Experimental virus-induced hydrocephalus. J. Neurosurg. 31: 1—9, 1969.
Meyer, A.: Herniation of the brain. Arch. Neurol. Psychiat. 4: 387—400, 1920.
Nathan, H., Feuerstein, M.: Angulated course of spinal nerve roots. J. Neurosurg. 32: 349—352, 1970.
Ogryzlo, M. A.: Arnold-Chiari malformation. Arch. Neurol. Psychiat. 48: 30—46, 1942.
Peach, B.: Arnold-Chiari malformation with normal spine. Arch. Neurol. 10: 497—501, 1964.
— Arnold-Chiari malformation. Arch. Neurol. 12: 527—535, 1965.
Ray, B. S.: Platybasia with involvement of the central nervous system. Ann. Surg. 116: 231—250, 1942.
Reid, J. D.: Ascending nerve roots. J. Neurol. Neurosurg. Psychiat. 23: 148—155, 1960.
Russell, D. S.: Observations on the pathology of hydrocephalus. London: Her Majesty's Stationery Office 1968.
— Donald, C.: The mechanism of internal hydrocephalus in spina bifida. Brain 58: 203—215, 1935.
Sandbank, U.: Le syndrome d'Arnold-Chiari. Rev. Neurol. 93: 529—563, 1955.
Schwalbe, E., Gredig, M.: Über Entwicklungsstörungen des Kleinhirns, Hirnstamms und Halsmarks bei Spina bifida. Beitr. path. Anat. Ziegler 40: 132—194, 1907.
Sieben, R. L., Hamida, M. B., Shulman, K.: Multiple cranial nerve deficits associated with the Arnold-Chiari malformation. Neurology 21: 673—681, 1971.
Smith, E. D.: Spina Bifida and the Total Care of Spinal Myelomeningocele. Springfield, Ill.: Ch. C Thomas 1965.
Spillane, J. D., Pallis, C., Jones, A. M.: Developmental abnormalities in the region of the foramen magnum. Brain 80: 11—48, 1957.
Variend, S., Emery, J. L.: The weight of the cerebellum in children with myelomeningocele. Develop. Med. Child. Neurol. 15, Suppl. 29: 77—83, 1973.
Vogt, E. C., Wyatt, G. M.: Craniolacunia (Lückenschädel). A report of 54 cases. Radiology 36: 147—153, 1941.
Wilkins, R. H., Brody, I. A.: The Arnold-Chiari malformation. Arch. Neurol. 25: 376—379, 1971.
Yu, H. C., Deck, M. D. F.: The clivus deformity of the Arnold-Chiari malformation. Radiology 101: 613—616, 1971.

26. Ventral Dysraphic and Various Sacral Lesions

Neurenteric (Enterogenic) Cysts. Neurenteric cysts are malformations of early developmental origin, presenting as intraspinal cysts lined with mucosa of the alimentary tract. They vary considerably in size and in the type of mucosal lining. Their distinction from other cystic intraspinal lesions has caused diagnostic problems. Cystic teratomas, briefly described in a separate section of this chapter, have been confused with neurenteric cysts particularly in the older literature; spinal ependymal cysts, described in Chapter 20, also need to be considered.

Neurenteric cysts may be found as incidental lesions in newborns dying from other conditions, or they become symptomatic postnatally or during later life. Approximately three-fourths of the published cases were observed during the first six months of life, the rest in juveniles or young adults; the 20-year-old man reported by Scoville *et al.* (1963) appears to be the oldest case described in sufficient detail. Males outnumber females by 3 to 1. Clinical symptoms are caused by progressive compression of the spinal cord, occasionally with intermittent course. Meningitis may develop as a complication (Harriman, 1958; Rhaney and Barclay, 1959; Brun and Saldeen,

1968), and an intramedullary abscess had formed in the case of Millis and Holmes (1973). Infection may propagate from the intestinal tract; spontaneous rupture of the cyst with dissemination of its contents into the CSF may cause meningeal irritation.

Neurenteric cysts are most commonly located in the low cervical and upper thoracic segments of the spine, at the ventral surface of the cord. A case described by Puusepp (1934) is frequently quoted as a dorsally located enteric cyst, but the histologic features of the lesion more likely corroborate the author's designation of the case as a cystic teratoma. Enteric cysts may be attached to the vertebral body or to the dura respectively, or they may be located within the leptomeninges attached to the ventral surface of a grossly normal cord. Some are more intimately related to the cord, intramedullary or lodged between its separated halves which may be considerably displaced and flattened (Nemeth, 1965).

In instances where the cysts become symptomatic later in life, there may be no deformities of the spinal column or only slight alterations. Malformations of the spinal column are often extreme when the cysts are found in infants. There may be shortening of the neck, the chin abutting the chest, or complete splitting of spine with remnants of notocord in both halves of the divided vertebra (Feller and Sternberg, 1929). A less severe deformity consists of unfused or irregularly fused hemivertebrae, the defect being filled with cartilage and connective tissue. A tunnel or a thin strand of connective tissue may traverse the vertebral body; clinical detection of lesser deformities may require tomography. The vertebral defects allow for various types of communication between the intraspinal cysts and similar lesions occurring in the mediastinum or retroperitoneum. For example, an intraspinal cyst lined with esophageal epithelium was positioned opposite to a much larger mediastinal cyst with similar lining, both cysts extending with funnel-shaped diverticles into the fifth thoracic vertebra (Guillery, 1937). There may also be open communication between the prevertebral and intraspinal cysts through a tunnel passing the vertebral body (Rhaney and Barclay, 1959; Dorsey and Tabrisky, 1966). Mediastinal or retroperitoneal cysts with massive defects of the vertebral body may also occur in the absence of intraspinal cystic lesions (Veeneklaas, 1952).

Some cysts are thin walled, translucent and filled with a clear or milky viscous fluid. Microscopic examination of the cyst wall discloses loose fibrous connective tissue lined by a single layer of nonciliated columnar epithelium; the latter is attached in a regular row to a basement membrane, a feature not characteristic of ependyma. The epithelium contains an abundance of mucin-producing goblet cells, with their nuclei in the basal portion of the cell; the cytoplasm is distended and filled with clear material giving a positive reaction with PAS or with muci-carmine and other mucin stains (Harriman, 1958; Scoville *et al.*, 1963; Klump, 1971). The intraspinal portion of a given cyst may be lined with mucosa only, while the prevertebral portion may show, in addition, other layers of the intestinal wall. The walls of some of the intraspinal cysts contain all layers of the intestinal wall, including mucosa, submucosa and muscularis, the cyst forming a segment of gut attached to or impressed into the spinal cord. In the case reported by Korff (1937) a whole loop of intestine was wound through the split spinal cord. The epithelium lining the cyst wall may correspond to specific portions of the alimentary tract, such as esophagus (Guillery, 1937), stomach (Rhaney and Barclay, 1959), or small intestine (Korff, 1937; Nemeth, 1965). One type of epithelium may show transgression into another, such as gastric mucosa into esophageal squamous epithelium (Knight *et al.*, 1955; Brun and Saldeen, 1968). Pancreatic tissue may be present as well (Bale, 1973). The cyst wall may also be lined with ciliated epithelium undergoing squamous metaplasia (Knight *et al.*, 1955; Dorsey and Tabrisky, 1966); this is probably indicative of the normal transformation of the ciliated epithelium of fetal esophagus to the squamous epithelium of adult esophagus. This feature needs to be considered in the differential diagnosis of spinal ependymal cysts; the presence of ciliae in the latter has often been assumed to constitute proof of ependymal origin (Chapter 20). Yamashita *et al.* (1973) presented a case in whom the lining of a cervical intradural cyst was considered bronchiogenic.

Neurenteric cysts may coexist with a considerable variety of other CNS or systemic malformations including holoprosencephaly, anencephaly, heterotopias of gray matter, hydrocephalus or Klippel-Feil malformation; congenital cardiac anomalies have been found in several instances. Prevertebral or intraspinal enteric cysts were found coexistent with the Arnold-Chiari malformation (Cameron, 1957; Rhaney and Barclay, 1959).

Enteric cysts may also combine with anterior (or ventral) spina bifida and with posterior (or dorsal) spina bifida (or rachischisis) in many ways. Feller and Sternberg (1929) on reviewing 28 cases from the older literature distinguished four ways in which vertebral defects (anterior spina bifida) associate with other lesions: 1. Dorsal rachischisis with a direct opening of the intestine through the medullary plate in the defect at the back. 2. A dorsal opening of the intestine without exposure of the neuraxis which is split and is penetrated by the intestine. 3. Dorsal spina bifida without external opening of the intestine, but with an intestinal diverticulum or tract to the neuraxis. 4. Tracts or diverticula between intestine and neuraxis without defects in closure of spine or neuraxis.

The formation of neurenteric cysts evidently dates to the first three weeks of gestation when ectodermal and entodermal tissues are closely approximated. The cysts have been attributed to a persistent neurenteric duct, a transient open passage between the yolk sac and the neural groove through the primitive knot. However, the position of the neurenteric duct corresponds to the coccygeal region later in life (Bremer, 1952), which is inconsistent with the cervicothoracic localization of neurenteric cysts. The intimate contact between entodermal tissue and the notocord at the end of the third week of embryonal life is followed by separation of these structures and proliferation of the intervening mesodermal tissue; the latter organizes into segments from which the spinal column develops. Failure of separation of the entodermal tissue of the foregut from the notocord has been proposed as a mechanism in the formation of enteric cysts (Veeneklaas, 1952). That enteric cysts are formed during early embryogenesis by a disturbance of the interrelations between notocord, neural tube, entoderm and mesenchyma is fairly convincing; the attribution of a primary role to any of these structures and the cause-effect relationships remain a matter of conjecture.

Cystic Teratomas (Teratomatous Cysts). Cystic teratomas differ from neurenteric cysts in being true neoplasms. They contain disarrayed tissues belonging to all three germinal layers, at sites where these tissues normally do not occur. Teratomas may include tissue of the alimentary tract, but its contribution to the tumor mass is usually minor, and it lacks the orderly relations to the cyst wall found in enteric cysts. Twelve of the 19 cases of cystic spinal teratomas reviewed by Rewcastle and Francoeur (1962) were males and all but one were older than 2 years. Cystic teratomas may be found at any level of the spinal column but are commonly located dorsal to the cord. A symptomatology of intermittent cord compression has been stressed by Adams and Wegner (1947). The microscopic structure of these lesions is characterized by the random intermingling of various types of tissue. Teratomas may be associated with posterior spina bifida, particularly when occurring in the sacrococcygeal region.

Studies of the chromatin body (Bar body) at the nuclear membrane suggests that the nuclear sex of about one half of the teratomas in males is female. Hoefnagel *et al.* (1962) on examining several earlier reports on spinal teratomas observed chromatin positive (female) epithelial nuclei in teratomas of 2 males. Female sex chromatin bodies were also found in 2 of 4 male patients in a series of 6 spinal teratomas (Rewcastle and Francoeur, 1962). The reliability of nuclear sex chromatin as a guide to identifying the caryotype has been questioned however (Dayan, 1963), and there is reason to believe that the nuclear sex is not a reliable index of the chromosome complement of the cell.

Anterior Sacral Meningocele. Anterior sacral meningocele is an uncommon lesion. Reports on 67 published cases were tabulated by Thierry *et al.* (1969) and show a massive female preference, for 57 of 64. According to their survey, the disease usually becomes symptomatic during early adult life, only approximately 10 percent manifesting in early infancy. The lesions consist either of lateral sacral defects below the second sacral segment, with replacement of bone by fibrous tissue, or of median sacral or coccygeal defects which consistently spare the upper portions of the sacrum and the adjoining iliac wings. A sac containing herniated leptomeningeal and dural tissue protrudes through the defect, presenting as a mass in the abdominal cavity. Peritoneal adhesions may form at the surface of the sac; meningitis is a common complication. Pathologic descriptions of the lesions are rudimentary and refer to a wall composed of dura and arachnoid membrane; myelinated fibers may be found at the inner surface of the sac.

Anterior sacral meningocele is commonly associated with malformations of the genital tract, including uterus didelphys and duplication of the vagina and uterus; associated lipomas, teratomas or dermoid cysts have been observed.

Occult Intrasacral Meningocele. This lesion was described by Enderle (1932) and is rather rare—less than 20 cases having been reported in the literature (Kak *et al.*, 1972). Most are adults, and there is slight preponderance of females. The lesions consist of an abnormal caudal elongation of the spinal canal located entirely within the sacrum. A dermal sinus or a skin lesion may be associated; the main clinical symptoms are pain, bladder dysfunction or variable neurologic deficits. No detailed pathologic studies of the lesions seem to be available.

References

Adams, R. D., Wegner, W.: Congenital cysts of the spinal meninges as a cause of intermittent compression of the spinal cord. Arch. Neurol. Psychiat. (Chic.) 58: 57—69, 1947.

Bale, P. M.: A congenital intraspinal gastroenterogenous cyst in diastematomyelia. J. Neurol. Neurosurg. Psychiat. 36: 1011—1017, 1973.

Bremer, J. L.: Dorsal intestinal fistula: accessory neurenteric canal: diastematomyelia. Arch. Path. 54: 132—138, 1952.

Brun, A., Saldeen, T.: Intraspinal enterogenous cyst. Acta path. microbiol. scand. 73: 191—194, 1968.

Cameron, A. H.: Malformations of the neurospinal axis, urogenital tract and foregut in spina bifida attributable to disturbances of the balstomere. J. Path. Bact. 73: 213—221, 1957.

Dayan, A. D.: Nuclear sex of testicular teratoma. Brit J. Cancer 17: 46—49, 1963.

Dorsey, J. F., Tabrisky, J.: Intraspinal and mediastinal foregut cyst compressing the spinal cord. J. Neurosurg. 24: 562—567, 1966.

Enderle, C.: Meningocele intrasacrale occulto (rivelato con la mielografia). Riv. Neurol. 5: 418—423, 1932.

Feller, A., Sternberg, H.: Zur Kenntnis der Fehlbildungen der Wirbelsäule. Virchows Arch. path. Anat. 272: 613—640, 1929.

Guillery, H.: Eine in die Wirbelsäule eingewachsene mediastinale Zyste (Vorderdarmzyste). Zbl. allg. Path. 69: 49—53, 1937.

Harriman, D. G.: An intraspinal enterogenous cyst. J. Path. Bact. 75: 413—419, 1958.

Hoefnagel, D., Benirschke, K., Quarte, J.: Teratomatous cysts within the vertebral canal. J. Neurol. Neurosurg. Psychiat. 25: 159—164, 1962.

Kak, V. K., Chugh, K. S., Sodhi, J. S.: Occult intrasacral meningocele. Neurochirurgia 15: 148—152, 1972.

Klump, T. E.: Neurenteric cyst in the cervical spinal canal of a 10-week-old boy. Case report. J. Neurosurg. 35: 472—476, 1971.

Knight, G., Griffiths, T., Williams, I.: Gastrocytoma of spinal cord. Brit. J. Surg. 42: 635—638, 1955.

Korff, H.: Über ein Darmstück in einer Wirbelspalte als Ausdruck einer unvollkommenen neurenterischen Verbindung. Virchows Arch. 299: 190—202, 1937.

Millis, R. R., Holmes, A. E.: Enterogenous cyst of the spinal cord with associated intestinal reduplication, vertebral anomalies, and a dorsal dermal sinus. Case report. J. Neurosurg. 38: 73—77, 1973.

Nemeth, K.: Enterogene Cyste des Rückenmarkes. Zbl. allg. Path. 108: 196—200, 1965.

Puusepp, M.: Variété rare de tératome sous-dural de la région cervicale (intestinome). Rev. Neurol. 62, 879—886, 1934.

Rhaney, K., Barclay, G. P. T.: Enterogenous cysts and congenital diverticula of the alimentary canal with abnormalities of the vertebral column and spinal cord. J. Path. Bact. 77: 457—471, 1959.

Rewcastle, N., Francoeur, J.: Teratomatous cysts in the spinal canal. Arch. Neurol. (Chic.) 11: 91—100, 1962.

Scoville, W. B., Manlapaz, J. S., Otis, R. D., Cabieses, F.: Intraspinal enterogenous cyst. J. Neurosurg. 20: 704—706, 1963.

Thierry, A., Archimbaud, J.-P., Fischer, G., Freidel, M., Mansuy, L.: La méningocèle sacrée antérieure. Revue de la litérature et présentation d'un cas. Neurochirurgie 15: 389—412, 1969.

Veeneklaas, G. M. H.: Pathogenesis of intrathoracic gastrogenic cysts. J. Dis. Child. 83: 500—507, 1952.

Yamashita, J., Maloney, A. F. J., Harris, P.: Intradural spinal bronchiogenic cyst. Case report. J. Neurosurg. 39: 240—245, 1973.

27. Disturbances in the Bulk Growth of Nervous Tissue

Diseases affecting the bulk growth of the nervous system may be negative, resulting in a deficit in the formation of neural parenchyma, that is micrencephaly, or positive, resulting in a surplus, or megalencephaly.

Micrencephaly. It is important to retain the distinction between micrencephaly and microcephaly, terms which are often erroneously used interchangeably. Microcephaly designate smallness of the cranial vault without specifying its cause. It may be induced either by a primary hypoplasia of the brain, or by scarred, cavitated, or atrophic lesions including such defects as multilocular cystic encephalopathy, periventricular infarcts, ulegyria, postinfectious encephalopathies, hydranencephaly, progressive sclerosing cortical atrophy, metabolic processes and others. A primary hypoplasia of the brain occurs with such malformations as agyria, pachygyria and arhinencephaly, all of which are associated with abnormally low brain weight. The cerebral hypoplasia associated with these malformations may be considered micrencephaly, at least in a general sense. It is more practical, however, to restrict the usage of this term for those instances in which subnormal size of brain, or of the cerebral hemispheres, respectively, is the dominant or the sole pathologic alteration. These cases constitute true micrencephaly, or "microcephalia vera", using Giacomini's (1885) terminology.

The clinical manifestations of micrencephaly consist of smallness of the cranial vault disproportional to the size of the face, a thickened scalp and thickened bones of the cranial vault. The scalp may be deeply folded (cutis verticis gyrata), but this condition is known to occur with many other disease processes as well (Polan and Butterworth, 1953). Micrencephaly is associated with intellectual impairment, which, if of slight degree, permits social adjustment, but more commonly results in imbecility or idiocy. Epileptic convulsions may occur but are not a consistent feature. Life expectancy is usually reduced by intercurrent diseases, although survival to advanced age is possible. Micrencephaly may occur sporadic or in families (Jakob, 1936; Hanhart, 1958), and, in the latter instances, appears to be transmitted by an autosomal recessive gene. Much of the genetic information, however, refers merely to clinical data on microcephaly rather to instances for which the types of cerebral lesions are documented (Böök *et al.*, 1953; Komai *et al.*, 1955; Koch, 1959; Kloepfer *et al.*, 1964). While many of these families may indeed represent true micrencephaly, one must also consider the fact that acquired cerebral vascular lesions causing microcephaly may occur in sibs (Davies and Kirman, 1932) or in twins (Chapter 11); ulegyria in watershed distribution, for example, which is accepted as an acquired circulatory lesion, was observed in microcephalic cousins and was attributed to a recessive inheritance (Sylvester, 1959). Microcephaly occurs also as a component of a great number of dysgenetic syndromes, too varied to be listed here, most of which lack proper identification of the type of cerebral lesion.

The morbid anatomy of micrencephaly is characterized by small cerebral hemispheres, which, in extreme cases, present as rudimentary appendages of the brain stem containing a few gyri. There may be less severe or absent affection of the cerebellar hemispheres which appear disproportionately large. A simplified convolutional pattern is seen in the cerebral cortex, the individual gyri being normal in size or somewhat coarsened. Sectioning of the brain discloses that the reduction in its size is mostly due to hypoplasia of the cortex and white matter, while the size of the basal ganglia may be normal and has even been reported as being above normal. Minor anomalies in cortical architecture (Chapter 29) are found on microscopic examination, such as columnar arrangement of the nerve cells or an abnormal allocortical architecture (Robain and Lyon, 1972). The two epileptic sisters reported by Jacob (1936) showed nearly identical nodular heterotopias near the insular cortex. Cases in which more massive dysplasias prevail should be classified according to the prevalent lesion rather than as micrencephaly. Pachygyric brains, for example, characteristically have reduced weight (Chapter 29); the same is true for many instances of large heterotopias, as, for example, the micrencephalic cases described by Minkowski (1955). In the extremely small brain of 25 gm described by von Monakow (1926) the lesions were dominated by agenesis of the corpus callosum.

Micrencephaly can be induced experimentally by agents interfering with cell replication in the fetus. It was induced in rats by x-irradiation between the 14th and 18th day of gestation (Hicks, 1953, 1954). Autoradiographic studies after a single dose of 150 R on the 14th day of gestation indicate a 75 percent decrease of thymidine labelling during the first 5 hours after radiation and a subsequent depression lasting for 15 hours; the effect is less pronounced when radiation is applied on the 18th day (Wegner and Mecking, 1969). It has also been implied that neuroblasts are particularly radiosensitive during their migratory phase (Altman *et al.*, 1968). Damage, accordingly, is maximum when the agent is applied during the most vulnerable phase. The resultant pattern of damage varies with the period of gestation; 600 R given to 7-day-old rats, for example, induces a 61 percent deficit in cerebellar weight rather than in cerebral hemispheres (Dobbing *et al.*, 1970). Micrencephaly can also be induced by chemical interference with cell replication; a single injection of cycasine at the 14th to 15th day of pregnancy in rats results in a permanent reduction in hemispheric size that is not transmitted to the second generation (Spatz and Laqueur, 1968) and in reduction in cerebral DNA content (Matsumoto *et al.*, 1972). Injection of 5-azacytidine at the same phase of gestation causes a cortical neuronal deficit, with abnormal neuronal forms, but without other malformations (Langman and Shimada, 1971). Reduction in brain size and in total DNA may also be induced experimentally with ethylnitrosourea (Pfaffenroth *et al.*, 1974) or by long-term treatment with corticosterones during infancy (Howard, 1968). Hypophysectomy on the 4th to 5th day of life, on the other hand, is ineffective in reducing brain weight (Gregory and Diamond, 1968). These experiments show that micrencephaly with a permanent deficit of cells results from nonspecific interference with neuronal proliferation in the fetus. The inhibition of hemispheric growth is maximum if the agent is applied during maximum cell replication, while the same agent may be ineffective when applied after neuronal replication has subsided (Chapter 1). These experimental data are evidently relevant to the understanding of micrencephaly in man. Specifically, the micrencephaly induced by X-ray radiation in laboratory animals may be compared with the radiogenic microcephaly (Zappert, 1926; Goldstein, 1930) of infants that had been exposed to X-rays *in utero,* mostly prior to the fifth month of gestation, or with a microcephaly in survivors of atomic bomb radiation. The latter was induced by exposure prior to 26 weeks of gestation, in most instances before the 15th week (Wood *et al.*, 1967), and its frequency increased to reach 50 percent if the radiation dose exceeded 200 R (Blot and Miller, 1973). Microcephaly in these infants, however, is not necessarily the result of true micrencephaly, since a variety of other cerebral lesions may develop following *in utero* exposure to radiation.

Considerable attention has been paid in recent years to the effects of undernutrition and other environmental factors on cerebral development. Infants dying with severe malnutrition have been shown to have decreased brain weight (Brown, 1965). Experimental malnutrition in rat reduces brain weight and total cerebral DNA (Zamenhof *et al.*, 1971), as well as other constituents of the brain (Bass *et al.*, 1970); the cerebellum is affected preferentially (Neville and Chase, 1971). The damage of a brief period of malnutrition may be corrected upon return to normal diet (Winick *et al.*, 1968), but a persistent defect results from extended exposure (Bass *et al.*, 1970). On the basis of these and similar data it has been postulated that nutritional growth retardation may induce true micrencephaly (Dobbing and Sands, 1971). However, the magnitude of the cerebral changes induced by experimental malnutrition under carefully controlled conditions is generally well within the range of variation in brain weight accepted as normal in a human autopsy material. Some of this variation may conceivably be due to nutritional factors but it is doubtful whether these are the most important ones; there is no substantial evidence to indicate that the severely sub-normal brain weight of human micrencephaly can be explained on the basis of nutritional or environmental deprivation.

Megalencephaly. The term megalencephaly was introduced by Fletcher (1900) to designate a true hyperplasia of the brain. The term, however, has also been applied to a variety of heterogeneous disease processes which have in common that they cause an increased bulk of brain tissue. In a number of reports published prior to 1940 megalencephaly was attributed to diffuse glial overgrowth; these can be reclassified as instances of increase in brain weight due to diffusely infiltrating well differentiated astrocytomas or other gliomas. Other nonneoplastic or subneoplastic disorders involving abnormal cell proliferation, such as tuberous sclerosis, may also result in increased brain weight, as does the accumulation of abnormal metabolites in storage disease, particularly in gangliosidosis. When applied to this group of disease processes, the term megalencephaly refers to a symptom rather than to a disease entity. The usage of the term megalencephaly for describing a disease process should be reserved to those instances in which there is a true hyperplasia, or overproduction of cerebral parenchyma. The morbid anatomy of megalencephaly varies as the disease may affect portions or all of the brain, may be bilateral or unilateral, accompanied by various degrees of disorganization in tissue architecture, or by hyperplasia of other parts of the body. These aspects of the disease are found in various combinations which overlap to the extent that definition of subtypes becomes arbitrary.

An abnormally heavy brain which is well proportioned in all its parts and without microscopic alterations is the most common type of megalencephaly (de Lange, 1932; Wilson, 1933; Apley and Symons, 1947). The small number of reported cases is not representative of the frequency of this form of the disease as most go unrecorded. Megalencephaly of this type is often an occasional finding at autopsy in adults. A perusal of the clinical and social history discloses average ways of life without evidence of exceptional capacities. For some, however, intellectual performance may be above or below normal. Jakob (1927) tabulated abnormally heavy brains for 50 gifted subjects and for 39 that were mentally subnormal. Megalencephaly may manifest in infancy by an abnormally large head, which may grow faster than normal, without any specific type of cranial disfigurement; some infants have convulsions, but this is not a common feature. Occurrence of megalencephaly has been observed as an autosomal recessive trait (De Myer, 1972); it was described in association with achondroplasia (Dennis *et al.*, 1961) and with visceral lipomatosis and angiomatosis (Bannayan, 1971).

The pathologic definition of megalencephaly is essentially that of the upper range of normalcy of human brain weight. Blinkov and Glezer (1968) tabulated the mean values from 13 investigations; among these, the smallest averages were 1296 gm for man and 1170 gm for woman and the highest 1445 and 1325 gm respectively. Pearl (1905) reports an average coefficient of variation of 8.25 percent for mean brain weights ranging from 1220 to 1389 gm. In practice, therefore, an adult brain weight above 1600 gm should be considered megalencephaly, provided that all CSF was carefully drained, and that an increase in weight from edema, infiltrating or space-occupying lesions was excluded. Escourolle and Poirier (1973) define megalencephaly as above 1800 gm, which, needless to say, greatly reduces its incidence. These brains show an increased volume and individual gyri may appear more bulky. All portions of the cerebrum are diffusely enlarged, commonly in proportion to each other; in some instances certain portions of the brain, *e.g.*, the cerebellum, are disproportionately enlarged. The cut surfaces of the brain discloses ventricles of normal size. Cortical thickness and volume of white matter are usually increased; the corpus callosum may be thicker than normal, but an abnormally thin corpus callosum has been described as well. No significant alterations are found on microscopic examination of the cortex. Data on cell size are conflicting; an increase was reported by Peter and

Schluter (1972) but none was found by de Lange (1932). There may be other minor anomalies in megalencephalic brains, such as small heterotopias (de Lange, 1932) or syringomyelia in the cervical cord (Dyggve and Tygstrup, 1964).

Unilateral megalencephaly is much less common than diffuse enlargement of the entire brain, but it is more often reported because the manifestations are usually more striking. Many case reports pertain to infants or children, but adult cases have also been observed. In some the enlargement may affect the entire half of the brain, including hemispheres, brain stem and cerebellum, as if two brains of different sizes had been joined in the midline (Hallervorden, 1923). Others show enlargement of one cerebral hemisphere only, the brain stem and cerebellum being symmetrical. A corresponding enlargement of the cranium is evident. The affected cerebral hemisphere bulges with an abnormal surface pattern of an increased number of broadened and coarse gyri (Webster, 1908; Laurence, 1964). This gyral pattern resembles that of pachygyria or polymicrogyria and was reported under these terms, though without documentation of the characteristic microscopic architecture of a pachygyric or polymicrogyric cortex. The cut brain reveals a unilateral diffuse thickening of the cortex with an excessive piling up of gray matter which may reach the extent of obliterating gyri and sulci. The available microscopic reports are rudimentary and describe disorganized masses of gray matter without specific laminar organization (Laurence, 1964). Other instances show a lesser degree of derangement in cortical architecture, which consists of more widely spaced neurons, some showing abnormal orientation (Gross and Uiberrak, 1955). Bignami *et al.* (1968) measured a three-fold increase in the volume of nuclei and a six-fold increase in that of nucleoli and a 30 percent increase in DNA in the enlarged hemisphere, compared with the normal contralateral hemisphere. Some instances show nodular heterotopias of gray matter in the enlarged hemisphere; these were rather massive in a case illustrated by Norman (1969) and inconspicuous in that of Gross and Uiberrak (1955). Although these concurrences are rare, they are of particular interest as they imply that nodular heterotopias may result not only from hindrance of migration of neuroblasts, but perhaps also from their overproduction.

Unilateral megalencephaly may occur as the only lesion (Laurence, 1964), or it may coexist with overgrowth of the face (Gross and Uiberrak, 1955), or the hair of the scalp, the upper or lower extremities, or the entire body half (Webster, 1908; Hallervorden, 1923; Rugel, 1946). The overgrowth of body and brain is always homolateral, in distinction to the crossed pattern of disturbances in growth on a neurogenic basis. Unilateral megalencephaly has accordingly been considered a forme fruste of hemihypertrophy (Ward and Lerner, 1947).

The pathogenesis of megalencephaly is not clear. There is no evident relation to endocrine disturbances of growth, or to cerebral gigantism, a disease attributed to a hypothalamic disturbance which manifests with advanced height and weight for age, accelerated skeletal maturation, nonprogressive mental retardation, and physical features resembling acromegaly in children (Stephenson *et al.*, 1968; Schelling-Dürst, 1974). The available data on megalencephaly seem more consistent with an initial overproduction of cells than with an abnormality in the growth of a normal number of cells; no convincing evidence has been presented to indicate that the affected neurons are other than diploid. Spectrophotometric measurements in a 6-month-old megalencephalic girl studied by the present author yielded negative results in this regard. The causes of the disease are probably to be

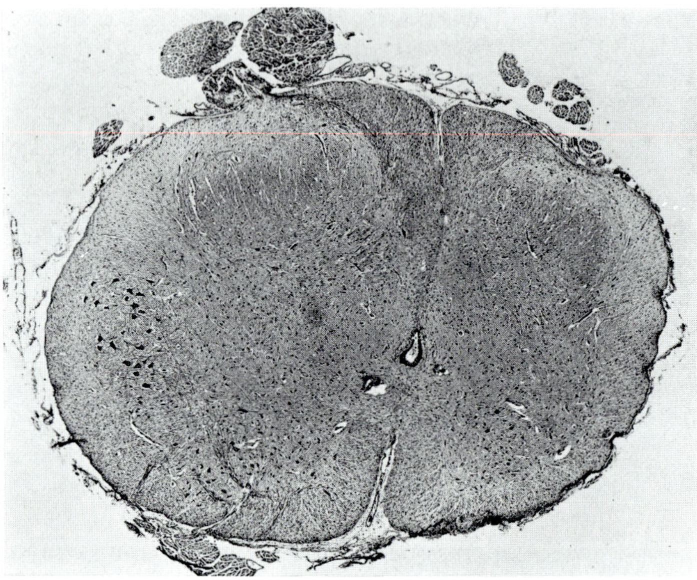

Fig. 84. Hemihypoplasia of the lumbosacral spinal cord (see text); Bodian ×14

sought in disturbances in the regulation of cell proliferation. It has been shown that various neuronal systems in the fetus undergo an initial overproduction of neurons, followed by elimination of those unable to establish their definite connections. Accordingly, a surplus of neurons, or nervous parenchyma, respectively, may result from either redundant formation or subnormal rate of neuronal decay. No method for inducing megalencephaly in experimental animals has been devised. Induction of increased weight and DNA content of the brain by injection of growth hormones into pregnant rats (Zamenhof *et al.*, 1966) is inconsistent with later reports (Diamond *et al.*, 1969) and could not be reproduced in the present author's laboratory.

An apparently neoplastic or subneoplastic diffuse hypertrophy of one cerebral hemisphere has been observed in a few infants (Davis and Nelson, 1961; Dom and Brucher, 1969; Townsend *et al.*, 1975, case 2, 3). The enlarged hemisphere showed glial proliferation and irregularly arranged large misshapen neurons involving cortex as well as basal ganglia with atrophy of corticospinal tract. The lesions were interpreted as ganglioglioma, forme fruste of tuberous sclerosis, or lesions comparable to diffuse hypertrophy of the cerebellar cortex (Chapter 31).

Anomalies in the Bulk Growth of Spinal Cord. Hyperplasia, or overgrowth, of the spinal cord was observed in association with the lesions of spina bifida, and the interpretation of this phenomenon has figured prominently in the theories on pathogenesis of dysraphic lesions (Chapter 24). There appear to be no other reports on local hypo- or hyperplasia of the spinal cord, or on the degree of its involvement in micrencephaly or megalencephaly. A case of hemihypoplasia of the cord may be presented here (Fig. 84). The 2-day-old boy had been born prematurely at a weight of 1740 gm, the first child after one previous abortus. The short postnatal course was complicated by hemorrhagic hypovolumenic shock from cord avulsion, respiratory distress and terminal anuria. There were many anomalies including clubfoot, being more severe on the left side, hypoplasia of the left femur and tibia, shortening of the limb with atrophy of musculature and contracture of the left knee. The sacrum and coccygeum were deficient on the left. Other abnormalities included facies with epicanthal folds and small palpebral fissures, a triangular mouth and asymmetric ears suggestive of Potters syndrome. The karyotype was normal. Autopsy disclosed absence of left kidney and polycystic change with double ureter on the right, accessory ribs, imperforate anus and single umbilical artery. The lumbosacral cord was asymmetric, being smaller on the left side with corresponding reduction in the calibers of dorsal and ventral roots and of the left lumbosacral plexus. On microscopic examination the number of motor neurons on the left side was about 25 percent that on the right side, gray and white matter being reduced in proportion, though without local deformities or scarring. The gray matter of the thoracic cord was symmetric, but the dorsal tracts were only half normal size on the left, the median fissure being off the midline; myelination was normal. Several recent hemorrhagic infarcts were found in the cerebral hemispheres, but there were no other malformations.

References

Altman, J., Anderson, W. J., Wright, K. A.: Differential radiosensitivity of stationary and migratory primitive cells in the brains of infant rats. Exp. Neurol. 22: 52—74, 1968.

Apley, J., Symons, M.: Megalencephaly: a report of 2 cases. Arch. Dis. Child. 22: 172—174, 1947.

Bannayan, G. A.: Lipomatosis, angiomatosis and macrencephalia. Arch. Path. 92: 1—5, 1971.

Bass, N. H., Netsky, M. G., Young, E.: Effect of neonatal malnutrition on developing cerebrum. I. Microchemical and histologic study of cellular differentiation in the rat. Arch. Neurol. (Chic.) 23: 289—302, 1970.

— — — Effect of neonatal malnutrition on developing cerebrum. II. Microchemical and histologic study of myelin formation in the rat. Arch. Neurol. (Chic.) 23: 303—313, 1970.

Bignami, A., Palladini, G., Zappella, M.: Unilateral megalencephaly with nerve cell hypertrophy. An anatomical and quantitative histochemical study. Brain Res. 9: 103—114, 1968.

Blinkov, S. M., Glezer, I. I.: The Human Brain in Figures and Tables. A Quantitative Handbook. New York: Plenum Press 1968.

Blot, W. L., Miller, R. W.: Mental retardation following in utero exposure to the atomic bombs of Hiroshima and Nagasaki. Radiology 106: 617—620, 1973.

Böök, J. A., Schut, J. W., Reed, S. C.: A clinical and genetical study of microcephaly. Amer. J. ment. Defic. 57: 637—660, 1953.

Brown, R. E.: Decreased brain weight in malnutrition and its implications. E. Afr. med. J. 42: 584—595, 1965.

Davies, H., Kirman, B.: Microcephaly. Arch. Dis. Child. 37: 623—627, 1962.

Davis, R. L., Nelson, E.: Unilateral ganglioglioma in a tuberosclerotic brain. J. Neuropath. exp. Neurol. 20: 571—581, 1961.

de Lange, C.: Über Megalencephalie. Acta Psychiat. Neurol. 7: 955—980, 1932.

De Myer, W.: Megalencephaly in children. Clinical syndromes, genetic patterns, and differential diagnosis from other causes of megalocephaly. Neurology (Minneap.) 22: 634—643, 1972.

Dennis, J. P., Rosenberg, H. S., Alvord, E. C., Jr.: Megalencephaly, internal hydrocephalus and other neurological aspects of achondroplasia. Brain 84: 427—445, 1961.

Diamond, M. C., Johnson, R. E., Ingham, C., Stone, B.: Lack of direct effect of hypophysectomy and growth hormone on postnatal rat brain morphology. Exp. Neurol. 23: 51—57, 1969.

Dobbing, J., Hopewell, J. W., Lynch, A., Sands, J.: Vulnerability of developing brain: I. Some lasting effects of X-irradiation. Exp. Neurol. 28: 442—449, 1970.

— Sands, J.: Vulnerability of developing brain. IX. The effect of nutritional growth retardation on the timing of the brain growth-spurt. Biol. Neonat. 19: 363—378, 1971.

Dom, R., Brucher, J. M.: Hamartoblastome (gangliocytome diffus) unilatéral de l'écorce cérébrale. Rev. Neurol. 120: 307—318, 1969.

Dyggve, H., Tygstrup, I.: Megalencephaly. Develop. Med. Child. Neurol. 6: 581—584, 1964.

Escourolle, R., Poirier, J.: Manual of Basic Neuropathology (Rubinstein, L. J., translator). Philadelphia: Saunders 1973.

Fletcher, H. M.: A case of megalencephaly. Path. Soc. London 51: 230—232, 1900.

Giacomini, C.: Contributo allo studio della microcefalia. Arch. Psych. (Torino) 6: 63—81, 1885.

Goldstein, L.: Radiogenic microcephaly. Arch. Neurol. Psychiat. 24: 102—115, 1930.

Gregory, K. M., Diamond, M. C.: Effects of early hypophysectomy on brain morphogenesis in the rat. Exp. Neurol. 20: 394—402, 1968.

Gross, H., Uiberrak, B.: Klinisch-anatomische Befunde bei Hemimegalencephalie. Virchows Arch. path. Anat. 327: 577—589, 1955.

Hallervorden, J.: Angeborene Hemihypertrophie der linken Körperhälfte einschließlich des Gehirns. Zbl. Neurol. Psychiat. 33: 518—519, 1923.

Hanhart, E.: Über einfache Rezessivität bei Mikrocephalia vera, spuria et combinata. Acta Genet. Med. (Roma) 7: 445—520, 1958.

Hicks, S. P.: Developmental malformations produced by radiation: a time table of their development. Amer. J. Roentgenol. 69: 272—293, 1953.

— Mechanism of radiation anencephaly, anophthalmia and pituitary anomalies. Arch. Path. 57: 363—378, 1954.

Howard, E.: Reductions in size and total DNA of cerebrum and cerebellum in adult mice after corticosterone treatment in infancy. Exp. Neurol. 22: 191—208, 1968.

Jacob, H.: Eine Gruppe familiärer Micro- und Mikrencephalie. Z. ges. Neurol. Psychiat. 156: 633—645, 1936.

Jakob, A.: Anatomie und Histologie des Großhirns. Leipzig-Wien: Franz Deuticke 1927.

Kloepfer, H. W., Platou, R. V., Hanschew, J.: Manifestation of recessive gene for microcephaly in a population isolate. J. Génét. hum. 13: 52—59, 1964.

Koch, G.: Genetics of microcephaly in man. Acta Genet. Med. (Roma) 8: 75—85, 1959.

Komai, T., Kishimoto, K., Ozaki, Y.: Genetic study of microcephaly based on Japanese material. Amer. J. hum. Genet. 7: 51—65, 1955.

Langman, J., Shimada, M.: Cerebral cortex of the mouse after prenatal chemical insult. Amer. J. Anat. 132: 355—374, 1971.

Laurence, K. M.: A case of unilateral megalencephaly. Develop. Med. Child. Neurol. 6: 585—590, 1964.

Matsumoto, H., Spatz, M., Laqueur, G. L.: Quantitative changes with age in the DNA content of methylazoxymethanol-induced microencephalic rat brain. J. Neurochem. 19: 297—306, 1972.

Minkowski, M.: Sur les altérations de l'écorce cérébrale dans quelques cas de microcéphalie. Schweiz. Arch. Neurol. Psychiat. 76: 110—173, 1955.

Monakow, C. v.: Biologisches und Morphogenetisches über die Mikrocephalia vera. Schweiz. Arch. Neurol. Psychiat. 12: 1—39, 1926.

Neville, H. E., Chase, H. P.: Undernutrition and cerebellar development. Exp. Neurol. 33: 485—497, 1971.

Norman, R. M.: Malformations of the nervous system, birth injury and diseases of early life. I. Prenatal malformations. In: Greenfield's Neuropathology, Chapter 6, pp. 324—440. London: Arnold 1969.

Pearl, T.: Biometrical studies in man. Variation and correlation in brain weights. Biometrica 4: 13—104, 1905.

Peter, K., Schluter, K.: Über Megalencephalie als Grundlage der Idiotie. Z. ges. Neurol. Psychiat. 108: 21—40, 1927.

Pfaffenroth, M. J., Das, G. D., McAllister, J. P.: Teratologic effects of ethylnitrosourea on brain development in rats. Teratology 9: 305—316, 1974.

Polan, D., Butterworth, T.: Cutis verticis gyrata. Amer. J. ment. Defic. 57: 613—631, 1953.

Robain, O., Lyon, G.: Les micrencéphalies familiales par malformation cérébrale. Etude anatomoclinique. Acta neuropath. (Berl.) 20: 96—109, 1972.

Rugel, S. J.: Congenital hemihypertrophy. Amer. J. Dis. Child. 71: 530—536, 1946.

Schelling-Dürst, V.: Makrozephaler Großwuchs. Klin. Pädiat. 186: 97—106, 1974.

Spatz, M., Laqueur, G. L.: Transplacental chemical induction of microencephaly in two strains of rats. I. (34404). Soc. exp. Biol. Med. 129: 705—710, 1968.

Stephenson, J. N., Mellinger, R. C., Manson, M.: Cerebral gigantism. Pediatrics 41: 130—138, 1968.

Sylvester, P. E.: Cerebral atrophy in microcephalic cousins. Arch. Dis. Child. 34: 325—330, 1959.

Townsend, J. J., Nielsen, S. L., Malamud, N.: Unilateral megalencephaly: hamartoma or neoplasm. Neurology 25: 448—453, 1975.

Ward, J., Lerner, H. H.: Review of subject of congenital hemihypertrophy and complete case report. J. Pediat. 31: 403—414, 1947.

Webster, J. H. D.: A case of unilateral cerebral hyperplasia, which coexists with "acromegaly" of the feet, and a slight degree of unilateral gigantism. J. Path. Bact. 12: 306—321, 1908.

Wegner, G., Mecking, H.: Autoradiographische Untersuchungen der DNS-Neubildung in Gehirnanlagen nach einmaliger Röntgenbestrahlung später Embryonal- und Fetalstadien der Ratte. Z. ges. exp. Med. 149: 2—12, 1969.

Wilson, K. A. S.: Megalencephaly. J. Neurol. Psychopath. 14: 193—216, 1934.

Winick, M., Fish, I., Ross, P.: Cellular recovery in rat tissues after a brief period of neonatal malnutrition. J. Nutr. 95: 623—626, 1968.

Wood, J. W., Johnson, K. G., Omori, Y.: In utero exposure to the Hiroshima atomic bomb. Pediatrics 39: 385—392, 1967.

Zamenhof, Z., Mosley, J., Schuller, E.: Stimulation of the proliferation of cortical neurons by prenatal treatment with growth hormone. Science 152: 1396—1397, 1966.

— van Marthens, E., Grauel, L.: DNA (cell number) in neonatal brain: Second generation (F_2) alteration by maternal (F_0) dietary protein restriction. Science 172: 850—850, 1971.

— — Margolis, F. L.: DNA (cell number) and protein in neonatal brain: Alteration by maternal dietary protein restriction. Science 160: 322—323, 1968.

Zappert, J.: Über röntgenogene foetale Mikrozephalie. Arch. Kinderheilk. 80: 34—50, 1926.

28. Dysplasias of Cerebral Hemispheric Organization

Arhinencephaly, Holoprosencephaly, Olfactory Aplasia. The facial deformities associated with holoprosencephaly are—as those of anencephaly—obvious and unmistakable, and early descriptions go back to the medieval literature (Frutiger, 1969). The first reports on the morbid anatomy were published during the nineteenth century, but the classification and identification of the characteristic morphologic features of these lesions is based on the comprehensive treatise of Kundrat (1882). A considerable number of reports on cyclopia and arhinencephaly in man and domesticated animals were published during the first half of this century and were reviewed by Köhn (1952). More recently, series of cases were studied by Yakovlev (1959), De Myer *et al.* (1964), Robain and Gorce (1972), and Jellinger and Gross (1973).

Kundrat (1882) recognized aplasia of the olfactory bulbs and tracts as the most consistent denominator of this group of deformities and coined the term "arhinencephaly". This designation has been criticized repeatedly as a misnomer because aplasia of the olfactory bulbs and tracts does not involve aplasia of other cerebral representations of the rhinencephalon (Stewart, 1939; Carrier *et al.*, 1974). The criticism is valid in terms of the contemporary definition and usage of the word rhinencephalon. However, the central connections of the olfactory system were unknown at the time of Kundrat's studies, and the term rhinencephalon was used for the olfactory bulbs and tracts to emphasize that they were portions of the brain rather than being peripheral nerves. Kundrat also suggested that the term arhinencephaly signifies a malformation of the cerebral hemispheres of which olfactory aplasia is only a part. The terms holotelencephaly (Yakovlev, 1959) or holoprosencephaly (De Myer *et al.*, 1964) were proposed as substitutes for arhinencephaly, and the latter is widely accepted. Yet, holoprosencephaly falls short as a proper designation for this entire group of malformations, and it is even less appropriate than arhinencephaly when applied to brains showing only aplasia of the olfactory bulbs and tracts. In the present text the shortened term "olfactory aplasia" is used to describe aplasia of the olfactory bulbs and tracts and of their immediate cerebral terminations; the term holoprosencephaly is used for the entire complex of hemispheric deformities which typically associate with olfactory aplasia. Arhinencephaly is used as a generic term for the entire class of malformations.

Olfactory aplasia has been confused in the literature with absence of the olfactory bulbs in hydranencephaly or in anencephaly. Both processes may involve absence of the olfactory bulbs and a nonperforation of the lamina cribrosa. However, absence of olfactory bulbs in hydranencephaly is due to and is part of the extensive hemispheric cavitation; in anencephaly it is not a primary factor in the disorganization of nervous tissue and in the hypoplasia or absence of cranial bones. Neither of these diseases involve a specific primary nonformation of the olfactory bulbs, and their biologic behavior differs on many points from arhinencephaly.

Clinical Features. The craniocerebral deformities of holoprosencephaly are often found in stillborn infants and in infants surviving with poikilothermia, spasticity, apneic spells, and motor and mental retardation. The prognosis as to life or potential development depends on the severity of the cerebral malformation, and herein lies the importance of the clinical recognition of the type of cerebral dysplasia. Most cases occur sporadic, but Hintz *et al.* (1968) and Khan *et al.* (1970), who also cite earlier observations, report occurrences in families. The type of lesion may vary within the same family, ranging from cyclopia to lesser deformities (Klopstock, 1921). There is no sex preference. Frutiger (1969) estimates the frequency of holoprosencephaly as 1 per 13,000 births. Olfactory aplasia with minimal or without other cerebral malformations represents the mildest degree of arhinencephaly. It may be observed as an incidental finding at autopsy in clinically unremarkable patients; anosmia may have been the only clinical symptom in some, but others had exhibited various degrees of mental subnormality.

Chromosome analysis shows that many cases of holoprosencephaly are manifestations of 13–15 trisomy. Arhinencephaly was found in 25 of 35 infants with 13–15 trisomy (Warkany *et al.*, 1966). Generally, 13–15 trisomy is likely if holoprosencephaly is associated with multiple visceral malformations, while chromosomal anomalies are more often absent if holoprosencephaly is the only lesion (De Myer *et al.*, 1964). This rule, however, has its exceptions (Chapter 33) as holoprosencephaly may occur in the absence of chromosome anomalies, and, conversely, 13–15 trisomy may occur without holoprosencephaly. Holoprosencephaly is also observed in chromosome anomalies other than the 13–15 trisomy, as in a ring chromosome in the 13–15 group (Bain and Gauld, 1963), a short arm of chromosome 18 (Nitowsky *et al.*, 1966; Gorlin *et al.*, 1968), or chromosomal mosaicism (Cohen, 1966). The available data are insufficient for determining the percentage of holoprosencephalies caused by chromosome anomalies. Excrescences of the nuclei of leukocytes were observed in 8 of 10 cases (Kakulas and Rosman, 1965), but this criterion was found to have no practical value for diagnosing trisomy (Fine *et al.*, 1965).

The cerebral deformities of holoprosencephaly coexist with typical facial and cranial malformations, and the extent of one is usually proportionate to that of the other. Hence, it was suggested that the cerebral deformities can be predicted from the facial features (De Myer *et al.*, 1964), but the correlation has not been found to be of sufficient reliability (Patel *et al.*, 1972). Various subclassifications of the facial deformities were reviewed by Frutiger (1969); they are, essentially, modifications of the scheme proposed by Kundrat (1882). Cyclopia is the most severe degree of facial deformity, involving fusion of the orbits which contain one or two closely approximated or partially fused eyeballs; a small proboscis projects from the forehead above the orbits. A lesser deformity is characterized by separated, though closely approximated, orbits (hypotelorism), with microphthalmia and narrowed eyelids. The nose is flattened and replaced by a proboscis having single or paired nostrils (ethmocephaly). In cebocephaly there are two eyes and two orbits, but the area between the eyes is flattened and has one or two nostrils, resembling the facial features of the cebus monkey from which the name derives. There is, however, variation in the usage and definition of the terms used for subclassification. Still lesser deformities show normal formation of orbits and nose, but there are various types of cleft lips and cleft palate. Trigonocephaly consists of a sharply pointed forehead, usually in the absence of facial deformities. Visceral deformities in holoprosencephaly include polydactyly, cardiac anomalies and others (Chapter 33).

Morbid Anatomy. The base of the skull is shortened and narrowed in its frontal portion and the crista Galli and lamina cribrosa are generally

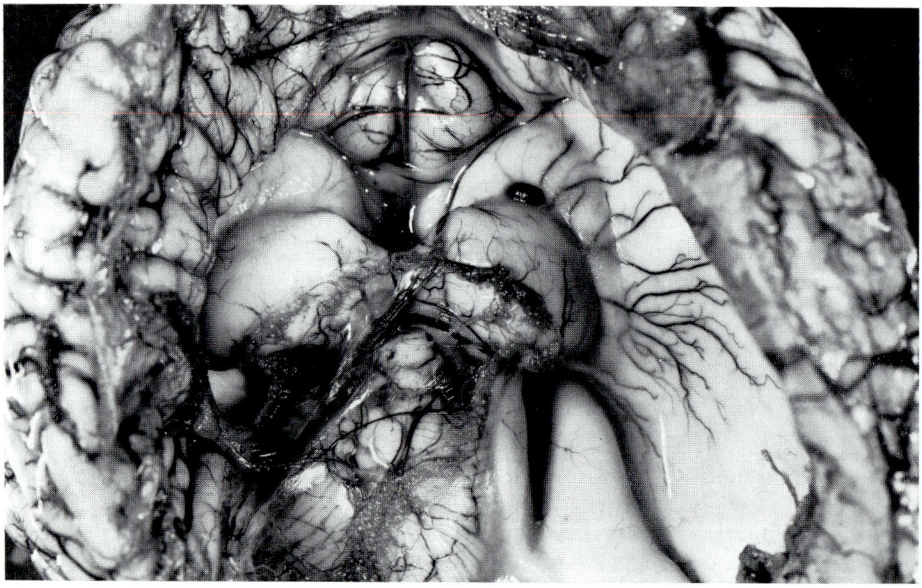

Fig. 85. Holoprosencephaly; view from occipital of the partially fused basal ganglia and the unpaired ventricular cavity

absent. With the more severe degrees of deformity there is hypoplasia or absence of other bones forming the nasal cavities or total absence of the latter. The frontal bones show approximation of their centers, with synostosis, or one single median anlage. In trigonocephaly the suture of frontal bones is pointed. The sella turcica may be absent or shallow. There is no falx or superior sagittal sinus except for rudiments in the occipital portion; the tentorium is present and often has an elevated insertion.

The most severe type of cerebral deformity in holoprosencephaly consists of an abnormally small brain, which may weigh less than 100 gms. The cerebral hemispheres are fused into one single mass (alobar holoprosencephaly). This mass is tilted frontally like a shield and no interhemispheric fissure is seen at its convexity. Viewed from occipital the mass is horseshoe shaped and has a large median opening leading into a common ventricle (Fig. 85). The rim of this opening is fringed by an arch of white matter which, in turn, is encompassed by cortical gyri stretching across the midline.

The opening of the common ventricle is covered with leptomeninges which are continuous with the membranous roof of the third ventricle (Kundrat, 1882). These membranes are often distended to form a large cyst which occupies the space between the hemispheres and the caudally displaced tentorium and cerebellum; the roof of the third ventricle forms the apex of the cyst and abuts the cranial vault. Choroid plexus is found in the wall of the cyst; the pineal gland is often absent. Generally, the size of this cyst increases with the degree of hemispheric deformity and hypoplasia. The cyst

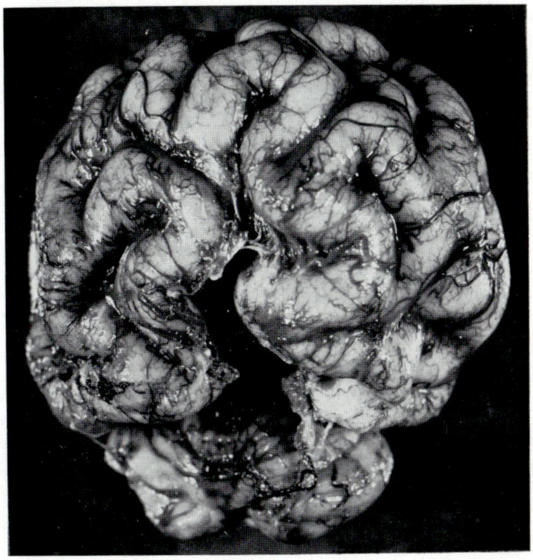

Fig. 86. Holoprosencephaly; coarse gyri traverse the midline in front of an opening leading into the common ventricle

is often disrupted upon removal of the brain, and the fixed specimens merely show a wide separation of the rudimentary hemispheric mass from the cerebellum. In some instances the cystic tissue appears to be without communication with the rest of the CSF spaces.

The frontal surface of the fused hemispheres is smooth or is covered with gyri of approximately normal size, though running in a disorderly manner, often traversing from one side to the other (Figs. 86, 87, 89). Studies of the cytoarchitecture of the cortex (Yakovlev, 1959) showed that the cortex bordering the opening of the common ventricle has the cytoarchitecture of Ammon's horn, presubiculum, and of the areas entorhinalis and prepyriformis (Fig. 88). The area gigantocellularis is situated anterior to the allocortex and projects along the midline; cortex having the cellular architecture of neocortex is found in small symmetrical areas of the anterior portions of the holosphere. Hence, the cortical anomaly may be classified as an extreme degree of neocortical hypoplasia. The cortex is supplied by bilateral middle cerebral arteries, while the anterior cerebral artery may be single. Hypo-

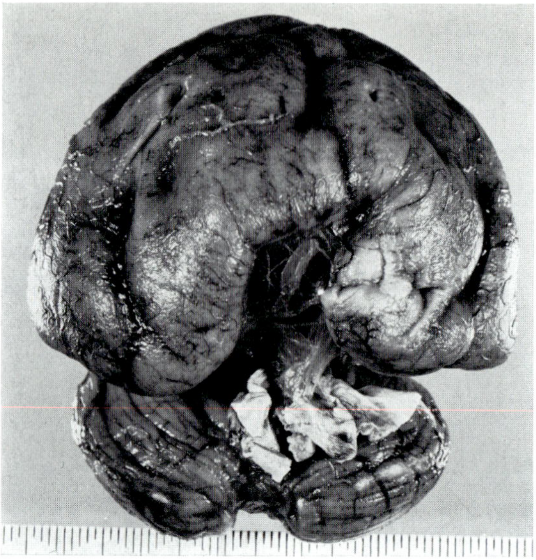

Fig. 87. Holoprosencephaly and pachygyria

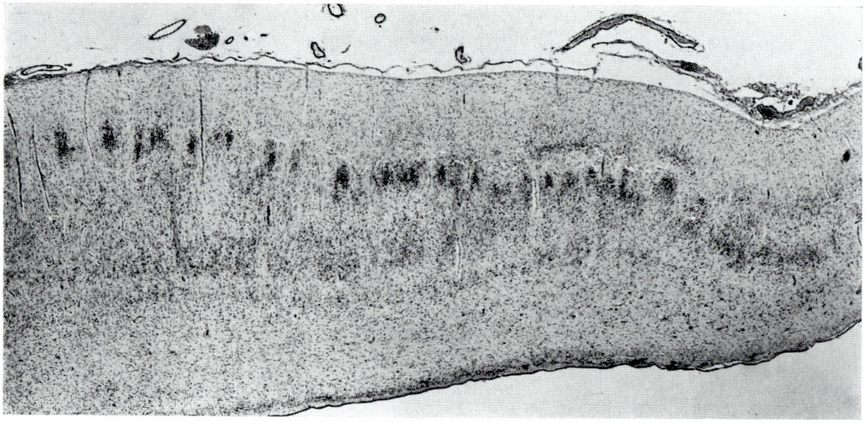

Fig. 88. Holoprosencephaly. The cortex bordering the common ventricular opening shows the laminar architecture characteristic of entorhinal or pyriforme areas; cresyl violet ×7

plasia of optic nerves corresponds to the degree of eye deformity. In cyclopia a single optic nerve may arise from a domed protrusion at the diencephalon, and there may be a single cerebral peduncle.

Sectioning of the brain shows a large single ventricle, without midline structures, bounded by a thin, smooth layer of white matter covered with ependyma. The degree of differentiation of the basal ganglia varies. The corpus striatum may be absent in severely malformed brains. The thalamus is usually identifiable but may be fused in the midline, particularly in its basal portion, with obliteration of most of the third ventricle. The common lateral ventricles communicate with the cranial orifice of the aqueduct by way of the cystic upper portion of the third ventricle. Brain stem and cerebellum are usually not severely deformed. Mammillary bodies may be fused.

Less severe degrees of holoprosencephaly show variable separation of the hemispheres by an interhemispheric fissure, and there is less reduction in brain weight (Fig. 89). If the interhemispheric fissure is incomplete, it is always better developed in the occipital portion of the brain. The fissure may extend as a short cleft into the hemispheric mass, or the hemispheres

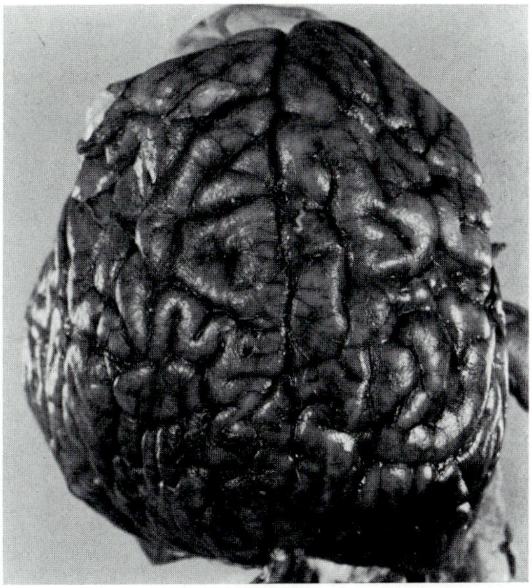

Fig. 89. An unusual variant of holoprosencephaly in which hemispheric fusion was more pronounced occipital where gyri cross the midline, while the sagittal fissure had formed frontally. The lesion was associated with aplasia of the fourth ventricle (Fig. 107). Only other anomaly was persistent ductus arterious. Hemispheric distension is only slight due to early surgical shunting

may form two V-shaped lobes joined at their frontal portions. Still lesser deformities show an interhemispheric fissure along the entire midline, but sectioning of the brain discloses that the cerebral cortex is uninterrupted in the depth of the fissure and extends in continuity from one hemisphere to the other. The brain may show hypoplasia of the frontal lobes, being pointed in its anterior portion similar to the brains of lower mammals; this deformity may coexist with trigonocephaly.

Each of these anomalies in hemispheric cleavage is typically associated with aplasia of the olfactory bulbs and tracts; very rarely is there unilateral hypoplasia. There is variance, however, in regard to the presence of olfactory epithelium and nerve fibers in the nasal mucosa (Köhn, 1952). Olfactory aplasia may occur as a minimum lesion in the absence of other hemispheric deformities (Fig. 90). These instances are sometimes said to be rare, but it is more likely that many go unnoticed, and nearly all go unrecorded. In these cases there is absence of the olfactory bulbs, the tracts, the trigone, and the anterior perforated area; Ammon's horn, fornix and limbic system are intact (Stewart, 1939). Sclerosis of the Ammon's horn may occur as a secondary change in epileptic patients. There may be various other anomalies of hemispheric development; for example, hypoplasia of the corpus callosum and high brain weight (1,506 gm) were found in Stewart's (1939) case.

Dissection of the basis of the skull in holoprosencephaly often discloses absence of the anterior pituitary lobe, and in these instances hypoplasia of

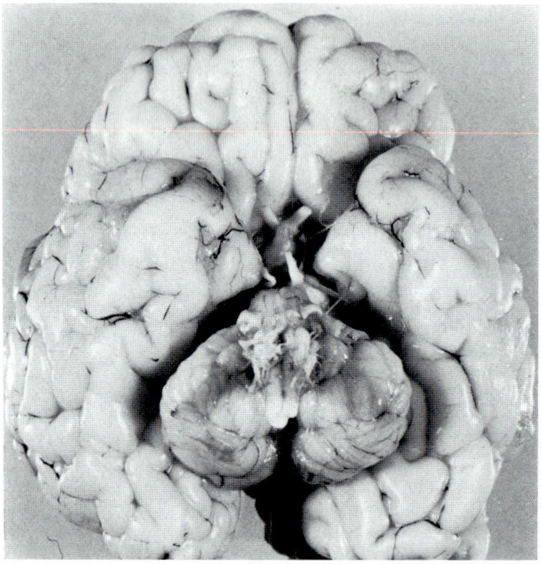

Fig. 90. Olfactory aplasia as the only lesion in a newborn

the adrenal glands and of the thyroid may also be found (Edmonds, 1950; Haworth *et al.*, 1961); corresponding endocrine anomalies may be documented during the patient's life (Hintz *et al.*, 1968).

Pathogenesis. Holoprosencephaly is generally attributed to a severe impairment of the development of the cranial end of the neural tube, including absence of formation of the olfactory buds and of the cleavage of the prosencephalon into paired optic and cerebral vesicles. Yakovlev (1959) distinguished these disturbances of cleavage from those of migration of neuroblasts causing cortical dysplasias and from those of fusion of the neural plate causing dysraphic states. Holoprosencephaly dates to early embryogenesis, that is the fourth to sixth week of gestation during which cleavage of hemispheric vesicles develops. One may also assume that holoprosencephaly develops later than anencephaly, or dysraphic lesions in general, since closure of the neural tube antedates the outgrowth of paired vesicles. An undetermined percentage of cases of holoprosencephaly are accounted for by chromosomal anomalies. The overlap with agenesis of the corpus callosum is discussed below. Etiology of the others is obscure; it is questionable whether a single factor accounts for all. Maternal diabetes has been observed in several instances (Dekaban and Magee, 1958; Dekaban, 1959; Yakovlev, 1959), and toxoplasmosis and syphilis have been implicated though without direct evidence. There is no precise documentation of the dating of etiologic factors during gestation in man except that Gross and Jellinger (1969) briefly mention an infant with holoprosencephaly born after attempted abortion between the 50th and 60th day after the first day of the last menstruation. Holoprosencephaly can be induced experimentally, for example, in the fish heteroclitus by exposure at early embryonic stages to elevated magnesium (Stockard, 1909; Lewis, 1909) and in the zebra fish by exposure to nitrogen (Ingalls and Murakami, 1962). Sheep feeding on veratrum californicum during the second and third week after conception also develop cyclopia in their offspring (Binns *et al.*, 1962). Rogers (1963) tabulates 93 references on studies on experimental induction of cyclopia. Cyclopia also occurs as a genetic anomaly in a strain of guinea pigs (Wright, 1960).

Fronto-Nasal Dysplasia (Median Cleft Face Syndrome). The facial changes observed in this syndrome may be considered opposite in nature to those in holoprosencephaly. They consist of an abnormal separation of the eyes (hypertelorism) associated with a broadened root of the nose and lack of formation of a nasal tip. There are variable degrees of a median facial cleft affecting nose, lip and palate, and cranial bones, and the scalp shows a V-shaped prolongation of hairs into the forehead. Contrary to holoprosencephaly there is usually no impairment of intellect. The syndrome has been reviewed recently by De Myer (1967) and Sedano *et al.* (1970) who offer different systems of subclassification of the facial deformities. A mild hypertelorism also is a frequent feature in infants with the Arnold-Chiari malformation and in frontal encephaloceles.

The majority of reports on fronto-nasal dysplasia is clinical, and neuropathologic reports are scanty and inconsistent. Among the findings reported are frontal meningoceles, agenesis of corpus callosum, occult encephaloceles, frontal lipomas, dermoids or teratomas (De Myer, 1967, references).

Agenesis of Corpus Callosum. Agenesis, or aplasia, of the corpus callosum was described by Reil (1812) and remained an incidental observation at autopsy, either unsuspected or in mentally abnormal patients, until the foundations for the clinical recognition of the defect were laid by Davidoff and Dyke (1934). Pneumencephalograms show marked separation of the ventricles and angular dorsal extension of the lateral ventricle, referred to as bat-wing shape, which may be associated with a concave mesial profile of the ventricle; the occipital portion of the lateral ventricles is dilated and the enlarged third ventricle shows an unusual dorsal extension. Less common radiologic findings are elongation of the interventricular foramina, a radial arrangement of sulci at the roof of the third ventricle and other anomalies in ventricular shape or size. Recognition of the disease ante mortem stimulated interest in its clinical features; Carpenter and Druckemiller (1953) could review clinical data for 43 cases diagnosed by encephalography, and increasingly larger series of cases were reported subsequently. Unterharnscheidt *et al.* (1968) reviewed 179 cases.

Agenesis of corpus callosum was found in 45 of 6,450 encephalograms (0.7 percent) by Grogono (1968); a much lower actual frequency must be assumed as cases subjected to encephalography are evidently preselected. There is no indication of a sex preference. Most instances occur sporadic, but Naiman and Frazer (1955) described occurrence in sisters, and Menkes

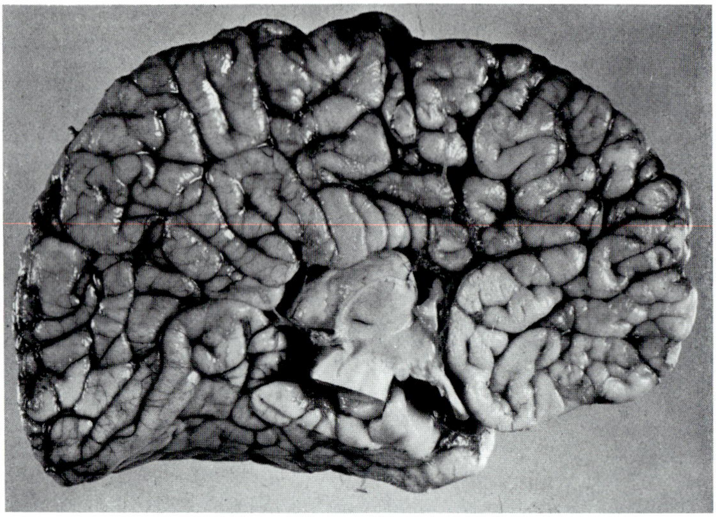

Fig. 91. Absence of cingular gyrus and radial arrangement of interhemispheric gyri in agenesis of the corpus callosum

et al. (1964) reported agenesis as a sex-linked recessive trait. Agenesis of the corpus callosum may occur in the absence of any clinical manifestations; indeed, a remarkable degree of compensation for the defect may be found on behavioral testing (Ettlinger *et al.*, 1974). Symptoms develop before the age of 20 for a majority of patients; in Grogono's (1968) series of 45 children epilepsy was found in 20, hydrocephalus in 16 and mental retardation in 18. The symptoms, however, are in all probability not the result of the callosal defect, but rather those of the associated malformations which are common and varied. Hemiatrophy, spina bifida, facial deformities, ocular deformities and microcephaly have been observed, and there may be congenital heart disease and other visceral anomalies. A syndrome of agenesis of the corpus callosum, chorioretinopathy and infantile spasms was observed in girls (Aicardi *et al.*, 1969; Renier *et al.*, 1973) but has not been documented thus far as a pathologic entity.

The morbid anatomy of agenesis of the corpus callosum was reviewed by Baker and Graves (1933), Marburg (1949), and Loeser and Alvord (1968). The defect may be complete or partial. In partial agenesis the rostrum and genu are usually intact while splenium and variable portions of the body are absent. The rostrum may be reduced to a small commissure of a hook-shaped profile. Exposure of the interhemispheric surface reveals an abnormal gyral pattern, with absence of the cingular gyrus, the gyri extending perpendicular to the roof of the third ventricle (Fig. 91). In partial agenesis of the corpus callosum the cingular gyrus is usually discernible frontally where there is a corpus callosum. The abnormal gyral pattern is probably an adaptation of gyral architecture to the callosal defect, although it has also been interpreted as agenesis of the limbic system; there is, however, no

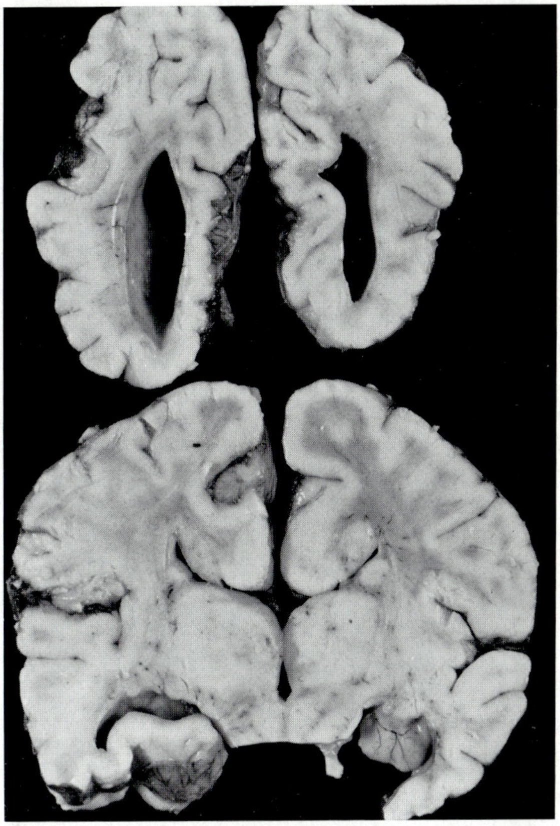

Fig. 92. Agenesis of the corpus callosum with characteristic "bat wing" ventricular shape and enlargement of the occipital horns

selective reduction in the volume of interhemispheric cortex. Coronal sections of the cerebral hemispheres demonstrate ventricles with pointed upper corners bounded in the midline by a membranous roof and, farther laterally, by short rudimentary stumps of white matter (Fig. 92). The median surface of these stumps is smooth, rounded or pointed and covered with leptomeninges. These stumps are formed by fibers projecting in a fronto-occipital direction (longitudinal callosal bundle), as first observed by Onufwrowicz (1887) and later described in detail by Probst (1901) after whom the bundle is commonly named. Probst proposed that the bundle derives from the deviated fibers that normally cross in the corpus callosum, an interpretation supported by studies in mice with hereditary agenesis of corpus callosum (King, 1936);

alternate interpretations have also been discussed. The volume of Probst's bundle is usually less than the normal volume of fibers in the corpus callosum, and it varies from case to case, the bundle being very small in some instances. The fibers are myelinated if the infants have reached the appropriate age. The occipital horns of the lateral ventricles are commonly much larger than the remainder of the ventricular system and may show a striking bulbous distention. This enlargement is not the result of hydrocephalus from increased pressure, though its causes are not clear; absence of the psalterium has been

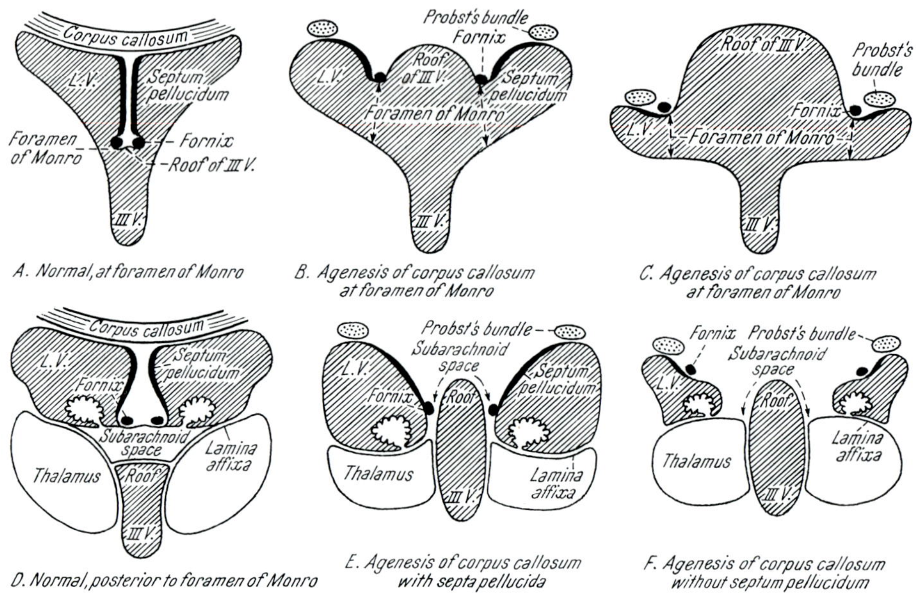

Fig. 93. Schematic presentation of the form of ventricles in agenesis of corpus callosum (Courtesy Loeser and Alvord, Brain 91 : 553, 1968)

implicated, but this explanation is not convincing when considering the volume of fibers crossing in the psalterium. Selective distention of the occipital horns should always prompt close examination of the corpus callosum; some instances with large occipital horns and a very thin splenium may perhaps be interpreted as *forms fruste* of agenesis of the corpus callosum.

The relationship of the septum pellucidum, fornix, and membranous roof of the third ventricle to the ventricular cavity is of particular interest (Fig. 93). The septum pellucidum may appear to be absent while, in fact, its two leaves are separated and project laterally from the fornices to Probst's bundles, forming a membranous roof of the lateral ventricles. The roof of the third ventricle is distended and bulges upward between the abnormally separated occipital horns of the lateral ventricles. Frontally, the roof of the third ventricle attaches to the fornices and bulges between them. The upward extension of the third ventricle displaces the fornices laterally and they descend in close approximation to Probst's bundle. The fornices are usually not malformed, except that the hippocampal commissure (the psalterium) between the occipital portions of the fornices is missing. There are no consistent anomalies of the hippocampal gyri. The extent of involvement of the anterior commissure varies from intact to absent in instances of complete agenesis of the corpus callosum. The posterior commissure is always intact.

Agenesis of the corpus callosum may be found coexistent with a great variety of malformations or with other fetal lesions, including heterotopias,

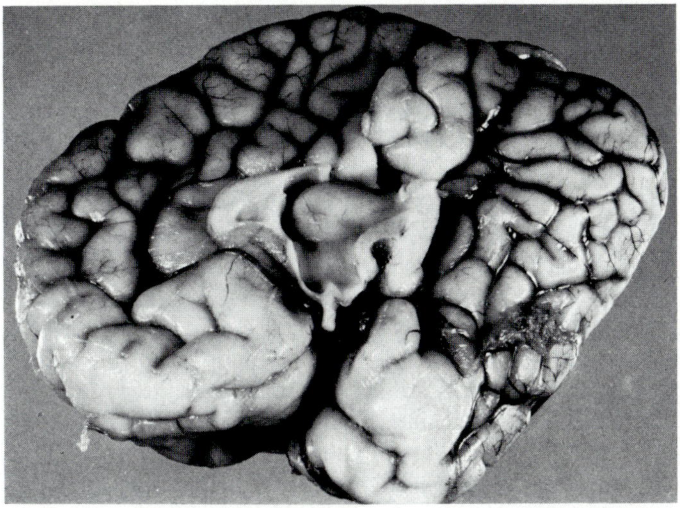

Fig. 94. Combination of olfactory aplasia with partial agenesis of the corpus callosum. This infant had an unbalanced translocation 4–15. It also suffered from multiple congenital anomalies including hypoplasia of ascending aorta and valve, of mitral valve, septal defect, persistent ductus arteriosus and left superior vena cava, syndactyly, microphthalmia, epicanthal folds and high palate

the Dandy-Walker malformation, anomalies in cerebral cortical architecture, polymicrogyria, porencephaly or hydrocephalus. Agenesis of the corpus callosum may concur with lipomas in the interhemispheric fissure, as reviewed by List *et al.* (1946). No interhemispheric lipomas are found in the vast majority of cases of agenesis of corpus callosum; on the other hand, callosal defects are relatively common in the presence of interhemispheric lipomas. Discussion on the pathogenesis of these lesions has centered on whether the lipoma interferes with the normal development of the corpus callosum, or whether both lesions are concurrent malformations.

Agenesis of the corpus callosum and arhinencephaly generally present as morphologically and clinicopathologically distinct types of malformations. There is, inherently, no corpus callosum nor septum pellucidum with the complete fusion of the cerebral hemispheres in holoprosencephaly, and some of these cases have falsely entered the literature as reports on agenesis of the corpus callosum. If fusion of the hemispheres involves only their frontal portion, the splenium may be rudimentary. These severe defects usually are associated with a deficiency of the fornix, which generally is intact in agenesis of corpus callosum. For a small group of cases, however, the two types of lesions overlap in such a way that classification as one or the other type of malformation becomes a matter of subjective preference. These cases present with simple olfactory aplasia in the absence of hemispheric maldevelopment except for complete or partial agenesis of the corpus callosum. The features of the latter are typical, showing a hook-shaped profile of the reduced corpus callosum, radial arrangement of interhemispheric gyri and, often, a hypoplastic anterior commissure (Fig. 94). Hegner (1965) gave a description of a case of this type, and Jellinger and Gross (1973) mention others. The present author's preference goes toward listing these cases as two coexistent malformations. The combination of the characteristic features of olfactory aplasia and agenesis of corpus callosum in a given case implies that these two types of malformations are teratogenetically closely related.

It may also be mentioned at this point that large porencephalic defects in the cerebral hemispheres may be associated with extreme atrophy of the corresponding segments of the corpus callosum, either from direct destruction or from secondary atrophy. Such residual lesions need to be distinguished from true agenesis of the corpus callosum.

The pathogenesis of agenesis of the corpus callosum was reviewed in detail by Loeser and Alvord (1968). The corpus callosum forms within the commissural plate, a local thickening of the lamina terminalis which is the most frontal boundary of the neural tube in the midline. The commissural plate is well formed at 41 days gestation; it consists of an area poor in neuroblasts which serves as a pathway for the crossing of fibers from one hemispheric vesicle into the other. The fibers destined to form the anterior commissure develop in the commissural plate, in close proximity to those forming the corpus callosum at an embryonal age of 78 days. Later on, these fibers become separated by the formation of a small cavity from which the cavum septi pellucidi develops. The subsequent growth of the corpus callosum occurs mainly after the 4th month and displaces and disperses the fornix, the psalterium, the insertion of the choroid plexus and the diencephalic-telencephalic junction in an occipital direction. The presence of malformations in these widely dispersed structures, accordingly, can be traced to their common origin within the commissural plate. No specific etiology of agenesis of the corpus callosum has been implicated in man, nor is there a precise timing of the disturbance except from inferences from normal embryonic development. Sporadic occurrence of agenesis of corpus callosum has been observed in horses, calves, cats, monkeys, goats, and lambs (Innes and Saunders, 1962, references). Callosal defects with Probst's bundle were observed as a hereditary defect in mice (King, 1936) and were induced in mice and rats by X-irradiation between the 11th and 21st day of gestation (Hicks, 1953).

Cysts of the Septum Pellucidum. A cavum septi pellucidi is a normal, consistent feature of the newborn brain (Chapter 1). It is typically located between the descending crura of the fornices and extends for variable distances in an occipital direction. A second cavum was described by Verga in 1851 in the posterior portion of the septum pellucidum, between the psalterium and the splenium. Dandy (1931) translated portions of Verga's text and reviewed it in its historical perspective. The cavum Vergae and the cavum septi pellucidi may form two separate, noncommunicating cavities; more often, there is broad communication of the cavum Vergae and the cavum septi pellucidi, forming one single space extending through the entire length of the septum pellucidum. The term cavum Vergae, therefore, is often loosely applied to describe an occipital extension of the cavum septi pellucidi.

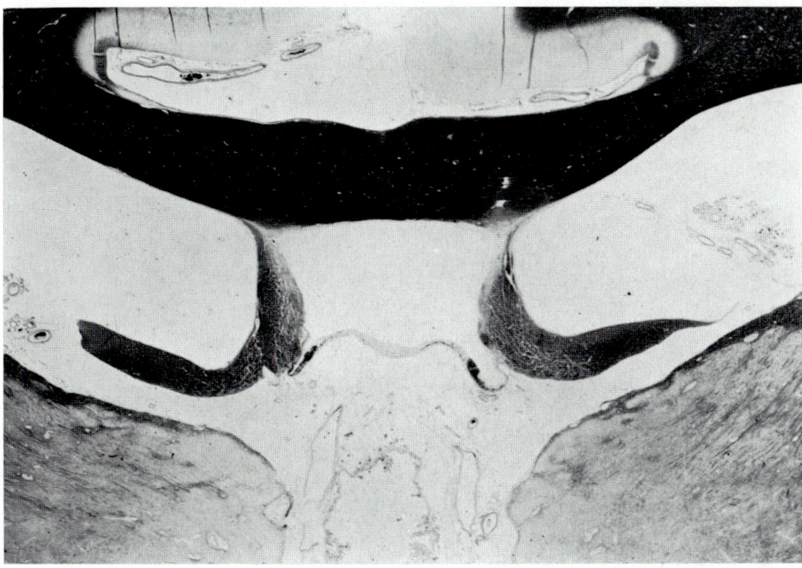

Fig. 95. A large cavum Vergae extends underneath the splenium; rudimentary bundles of the hippocampal commissure (psalterium) are seen in the ventral membranaceous wall of the cavum; myelin stain ×7

Schwidde (1952) found it at autopsy in 2 percent of adults, but his report errs in regard to the frequency in infants. The cavum does not possess an ependymal lining in infants, but it may be lined with low cuboidal cells in adults, presumably from metaplasia of superficial glia cells (Wolf and Bamford, 1935). The adult cavum often communicates with the lateral ventricles.

Neither a cavum septi pellucidi nor a cavum Vergae can be considered abnormal or dysplastic. However, instances of an exceptionally large cavum Vergae may present as midline cysts between displaced lateral ventricles having a much smaller lumen than the midline cyst (Fig. 96). The fornices are widely separated throughout their course, and the leaves of the septum pellucidum are closely approximated to the surfaces of the caudate nuclei. There may be associated absence of the hippocampal commissure (psalterium) (Fig. 95) or an abnormally thin corpus callosum. Anomalies of this type have been described by Dandy (1931); they may be considered extreme variants of normal development or, perhaps, minimal lesions or *formes fruste* of the

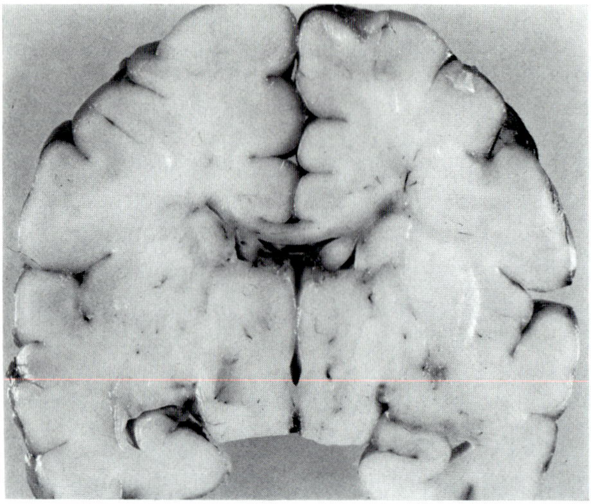

Fig. 96. An exceptionally large cavum Vergae results in lateral displacement of fornices and very small lateral ventricles

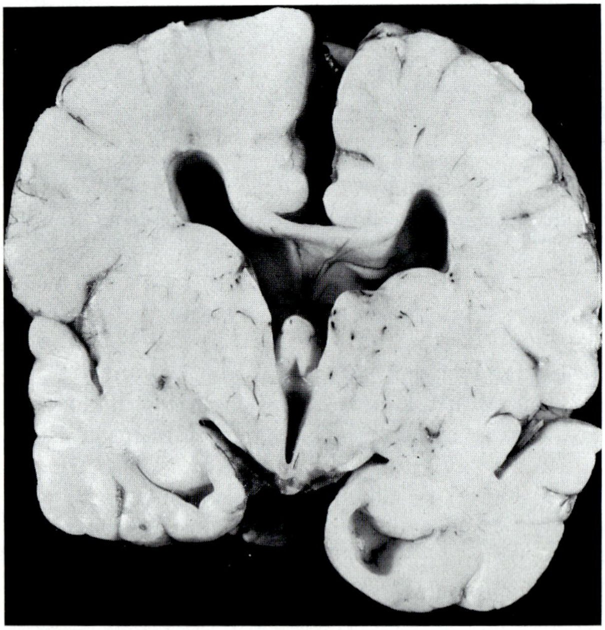

Fig. 97. Absence of the septum pellucidum as the only anomaly in a newborn

same type of disturbance which produces, in more severe degrees, agenesis of the corpus callosum. Within these limitations, abnormally large midline cysts may be considered anomalies in the development of the septum pellucidum.

Absence of the Septum Pellucidum. Instances of complete absence of the septum pellucidum, with or without other cerebral lesions, have been described sporadically as "agenesis of the septum pellucidum", usually in brains with markedly distended ventricles (Dolgopol, 1938). de Morsier (1956) suggested that they occur as a syndrome with optic nerve malformations, and Gross and Hoff (1959) reviewed a number of cases, many of which were considered secondary involution of the septum pellucidum. This group of cases presents with difficulties in interpretation as the septum pellucidum is rather susceptible to atrophy upon stretching or to destruction. Fenestration of the septum pellucidum is a characteristic feature of long-standing hydrocephalus, and its destruction may occur secondary to neonatal leptomeningitis or in porencephaly. Absence of the septum is also a characteristic feature of holoprosencephaly or it may be simulated by agenesis of the corpus callosum as described above. It is likely that these lesions, or secondary changes, account for most of the instances of "agenesis of the septum pellucidum" reported in the literature. Occasional observations on complete absence of the septum pellucidum without other cerebral lesions are curiosities without known clinical significance (Fig. 97).

References

Aicardi, J., Chevrie, J. J., Rousselie, F.: Le syndrome: spasmes en flexion, agénésie calleuse, anomalies choriorétiniennes. Arch. franç. Pédiat. 26: 1103—1120, 1969.

Bain, A. D., Gauld, I. K.: Multiple congenital abnormalities associated with ring chromosome. Lancet 2: 304—305, 1963.

Baker, R. C., Graves, G. O.: Partial agenesis of the corpus callosum. Arch. Neurol. Psychiat. 29: 1054—1065, 1933.

Binns, W., James, L. F., Shupe, J. L., Tacker, E. J.: Cyclopian-type malformation in lambs. Arch. environm. Hlth (Chic.) 5: 106—108, 1962.

Carpenter, M. B., Druckemiller, W. H.: Agenesis of the corpus callosum during life. Arch. Neurol. Psychiat. 69: 305—322, 1953.

Carrier, H., Bethenod, M., Gilly, J., *et al.*: A propos d'un cas d'arhinencéphalie simple. Ann. Pediat. 21: 96—100, 1974.

Cohen, M. M.: Chromosomal mosaicism associated with a case of cyclopia. J. Pediat. 69: 793—798, 1966.

Dandy, W. E.: Congenital cerebral cysts of the cavum septi pellucidi (fifth ventricle) and cavum Vergae (sixth ventricle). Arch. Neurol. Psychiat. (Chic.) 25: 44—66, 1931.

Davidoff, L. M., Dyke, C. G.: Agenesis of the corpus callosum. Its diagnosis by encephalography. Amer. J. Roentgenol. 32: 1—10, 1934.

Dekaban, A. S.: Arhinencephaly in an infant born to a diabetic mother. J. Neuropath. exp. Neurol. 18: 620—626, 1959.

— Magee, K. R.: Occurrence of neurologic abnormalities in infants of diabetic mothers. Neurology (Minneap.) 8: 193—200, 1958.

de Morsier, G.: Agénésie du septum lucidum avec malformation du tractus optique. La dysplasie septo-optique. Schweiz. Arch. Neurol. Psychiat. 77: 267—292, 1956.

De Myer, W.: The median cleft face syndrome. Neurology (Minneap.) 17: 961—971, 1967.

— Zeman, W., Palmer, C. G.: The face predicts the brain: diagnostic significance of median facial anomalies for holoprosencephaly (arhinencephaly). Pediatrics 34: 256—263, 1964.

Dolgopol, V. B.: Absence of the septum pellucidum as the only anomaly in the brain. Arch. Neurol. Psychiat. (Chic.) 40: 1244—1248, 1938.

Edmonds, H. W.: Pituitary, adrenal and thyroid in cyclopia. Arch. Path. 50: 727—735, 1950.

Ettlinger, G., Blakemore, C. B., Milner, A. D., Wilson, M. J.: Agenesis of the corpus callosum: A further behavioural investigation. Brain 97: 225—234. 1974.

Fine, R. N., Wang, M., Heath, C.: Nuclear projections of neutrophils in the 13—15 trisomy. Pediatrics 35: 712—714, 1965.

Frutiger, P.: Zur Frage der Arhinencephalie. Acta anat. (Basel) 73: 410—430, 1969.

Gorlin, R. J., Yunis, J., Anderson, V. E.: Short arm deletion of chromosome 18 in cebocephaly. Amer. J. Dis. Child. 115: 473—476, 1968.

Grogono, J. L.: Children with agenesis of the corpus callosum. Develop. Med. Child. Neurol. 10: 613—616, 1968.

Gross, H., Hoff, H.: Sur les malformations ventriculaires dépendantes des dysgénésies commissurales. In: Malformations congénitales du Cerveau (Heuyer, Feld, and Gruner, eds.), pp. 329—351. Paris: Masson 1959.

— Jellinger, K.: Morphologische Aspekte zerebraler Mißbildungen. Häufigkeit und diagnostische Probleme im Rahmen kindlicher Hirnschäden. Wien. Z. Nervenheilk. 27: 9—37, 1969.

Haworth, J. C., Medovy, H., Lewis, A. J.: Cebocephaly with endocrine dysgenesis. J. Pediat. 59: 726—733, 1961.

Hegner, B.: Klinisch-anatomischer Beitrag zur Frage gekoppelter Mißbildungen nach Varicelleninfektion. Acta anat. 60: 422—442, 1965.

Hicks, S. P.: Developmental malformations produced by radiation. Amer. J. Roentgenol. 69: 272—293, 1953.

Hintz, R. L., Menking, M., Sotos, J. F.: Familial holoprosencephaly with endocrine dysgenesis. J. Pediat. 72: 81—87, 1968.

Ingalls, T. H., Murakami, V.: Cyclopia, ectromelia and other monstrosities in zebra fish. Arch. environm. Hlth (Chic.) 5: 114—121, 1962.

Innes, J. R. M., Saunders, L. Z.: Comparative Neuropathology. New York: Academic Press 1962.

Jellinger, K., Gross, H.: Holoprosencephalie und Arhinencephalie. In: Current Topics in Neuropathology (Jellinger, K., ed.), pp. 62—71. Wien: Facultas 1973.

Kakulas, B. A., Rosman, N. P.: 13–15 trisomy in 8 cases of arhinencephaly. Lancet 2: 717—718, 1965.

Khan, M., Rozdilsky, R., Gerrard, J. W.: Familial holoprosencephaly. Develop. Med. Child. Neurol. 12: 71—76, 1970.

King, L. S.: Hereditary defects of the corpus callosum in the mouse. J. comp. Neurol. 64: 337—363, 1936.

Klopstock, A.: Familiäres Vorkommen von Cyklopie und Arhinencephalie. Mschr. Geburtsh. Gynäk. 56: 59—71, 1921.

Köhn, K.: Über die Arhinenzephalie. Abl. allg. Path. 88: 246—258, 1952.

Kundrat, H.: Arhinencephalie als typische Art von Mißbildung. Graz: Leuschner and Lubensky 1882.

Lewis, W. H.: The experimental production of cyclopia in the fish embryo (Fundulus heteroclitus). Anat. Rec. 3: 175—181, 1909.

List, C. F., Holt, J. F., Everett, M.: Lipoma of the corpus callosum. A clinicopathologic study. Amer. J. Roentgenol. 55: 125—134, 1946.

Loeser, J. D., Alvord, E. C.: Clinicopathological correlations in agenesis of the corpus callosum. Neurology (Minneap.) 18: 745—756, 1968.

— — Agenesis of the corpus callosum. Brain 91: 553—570, 1968.

Marburg, O.: So-called agenesia of the corpus callosum (callosal defect). Arch. Neurol. Psychiat. 61: 297—312, 1949.

Menkes, J. H., Philippart, M., Clark, D. B.: Hereditary partial agenesis of corpus callosum. Arch. Neurol. (Chic.) 11: 198—208, 1964.

Naiman, J., Frazer, F. C.: Agenesis of the corpus callosum. Arch. Neurol. Psychiat. 74: 182—185, 1955.

Nitowsky, H. M., Sindharananda, N., Konigsberg, U. R., Weinberg, T.: Partial 18 monosomy in the cyclops malformation. Pediatrics 37: 260—269, 1966.
Onufwrowicz, W.: Das balkenlose Mikrocephalengehirn Hoffmann. Arch. Psychiat. 18: 305—328, 1887.
Patel, H., Dolman, C. L., Byrne, M. A.: Holoprosencephaly with median cleft lip. Clinical, pathological, and echoencephalographic study. Amer. J. Dis. Child. 124: 217—221, 1972.
Probst, M.: Über den Bau des vollständig balkenlosen Großhirns sowie über Mikrogyrie und Heterotopie der grauen Substanz. Arch. Psychiat. 34: 709—786, 1901.
Reil, J. C.: Mangel des mittleren und freien Teils des Balkens im Menschengehirn. Arch. Physiol. 11: 341—344, 1812.
Renier, W., Gabreels, F., Mol, L., Korten, J.: Agenesis of the corpus callosum, chorioretinopathy and infantile spasms (Aicardi syndrome). Psychiat. Neurol. Neurochir. 76: 39—45, 1973.
Robain, O., Gorce, F.: Arhinencephalie. Etude clinique, anatomique et étiologique de 13 cas. Arch. franç. Pédiat. 29: 861—879, 1972.
Rogers, K. T.: Experimental production of perfect cyclopia in the chick by means of LiCl with a survey of the literature on cyclopia produced experimentally by various means. Develop. Biol. 8: 129—150, 1963.
Schwidde, J. T.: Incidence of cavum septi pellucidi and cavum Vergae in 1,032 human brains. Arch. Neurol. Psychiat. (Chic.) 67: 625—632, 1952.
Sedano, H. O., Cohen, M. M., Jirasok, J., Gorlin, R. J.: Frontonasal dysplasia. Pediatrics 76: 906—913, 1970.
Stewart, R. M.: Arhinencephaly. J. Neurol. Psychiat. (Chic.) 2: 303—312, 1939.
Stockard, C. R.: The artificial production of one-eyed monsters and other defects, which occur in nature, by the use of chemicals. Anat. Rec. 3: 167—173, 1909.
Unterharnscheidt, F., Jachnik, D., Gott, H.: Der Balkenmangel. Berlin-Heidelberg-New York: Springer 1968.
Warkany, J., Passarge, E., Smith, L. B.: Congenital malformations in autosomal trisomy syndromes. Amer. J. Dis. Child. 112: 502—517, 1966.
Wolf, A., Bamford, T. E.: Cavum septi pellucidi and cavum Vergae. Bull. Neurol. Inst. New York 4: 294—309, 1935.
Wright, S.: The genetics of vital characters of the guinea pig. J. cell. comp. Physiol. (Philadelphia) 56: 123—151, 1960.
Yakovlev, P. I.: Pathoarchitectonic studies of cerebral malformations. J. Neuropath. exp. Neurol. 18: 22—55, 1959.

29. Dysplasias of Cerebral Cortex

The lesions described in this chapter result from anomalous cortical development dating to the fetal period. Only those sufficiently severe to impede survival are commonly observed in infants or children; many others are survived with various degrees of functional impairment and are found at autopsy in adults. During the nineteenth century dysplasias of the cerebral cortex were generally not distinguished from residual lesions due to loss of parenchyma and scarring. The first step in this direction was taken by Bresler (1899) who differentiated the cortical scarring of ulegyria from the cortical maldevelopment of polymicrogyria, which he called "microgyria". The term microgyria had been used earlier for small gyri of any type; this practice carried on for at least a decade after Bresler's report and, sporadically, into the more recent literature. There is some overlap in the usage of the names given to various specific types of cortical dysplasias, but this reflects mainly individual semantics rather than disagreement about the basic features and identity of the lesions.

Agyria (Lissencephaly) and Pachygyria. The term agyria is preferable to lissencephaly. The latter was introduced by Owen (1868) to distinguish the flat „lissencephalic" surface of the brains of lower mammalian species and of fetuses from the folded surface of "gyrencephalic" brains. The term was later applied to malformed brains lacking gyri. Agyria differs from pachygyria (macrogyria) only in the severity of the lesions: Agyria, or lissencephaly, implies absence of gyri; pachygyria, a reduced number of coarse, broadened and shallow gyri with less than normal folding of the cortex. Both types of lesions may coexist in different portions of the same brain, so that the classification of a given case may become a matter of subjective judgement. Some authors use agyria and pachygyria synonymously, but it seems advantageous to retain the distinction as the severity of clinical manifestations tends to be in proportion to the degree of morphologic derangement; also, it is incongruous to refer to a brain with coarse gyri as being agyric or lissencephalic. Pachygyria needs to be distinguished from the laminar subcortical heterotopias—described later in this chapter—in which the gyral pattern and the laminar architecture of the cortex are normal.

Clinical features of agyria, reviewed by Miller (1963) and by Daube and Chou (1966), consist of microcephaly, decerebrate posture and severe motor retardation. The infants are unresponsive to environment, commonly suffer from recurrent infections and fail to thrive. Epileptic seizures develop nearly always before the age of 1 year, and most of the infants die before they reach 2 years, although survival to 6 years has been observed with nearly total agyria (Münchoff and Noetzel, 1965). Cardiac or ocular anomalies may be associated with the cerebral changes. Patients with pachygyria have a better prognosis in terms of life span, but they are always severely retarded and epilepsy is common. Agyria and pachygyria are infrequent, and most instances occur sporadic; occurrence of agyria in siblings has been observed (Miller, 1963).

The morbid anatomy of agyria and pachygyria has been described in numerous publications, particularly in the concise report of Crome (1956) that also reviews the early literature. The infants are always microcephalic, with a small misshapen skull and thickened bones. The brain weight is below normal. The hemispheric surface, is, in cases of agyria, completely smooth, lacking primary fissures. The neocortex is typically affected, but normal gyration and normal laminar architecture may be found in the hippocampus, the adjoining temporal cortex and the limbic cortex. Gross inspection of pachygyric brains discloses a few coarse, broad gyri separated by shallow sulci (Fig. 98). The surface features of pachygyria may be rather similar to those of polymicrogyria, and the two types of lesions have been confused in the literature although their microscopic organization is distinctive. Agyric and pachygyric cortices are much thicker than normal. The volume of white matter is reduced, with a resultant reversal of the normal proportions of gray and white matter. The claustrum and capsula extrema are consistently absent, but putamen and pallidum show only minor anomalies or none at all; the thalamic architecture is blurred. The cerebral ventricles are enlarged, but the degree of enlargement varies.

The microscopic architecture of agyric or pachygyric cortex is always abnormal, most commonly in the form of a four-layered cortex consisting of: 1. A molecular layer. 2. A relatively thin superficial layer of nerve cells which may be unusually large and are oriented perpendicular to the cortical surface. 3. A tangential plexus of myelinated fibers containing few neuronal elements. 4. A thick cell layer in which the neurons often lack orderly arrangement and merge with the sparse underlying white matter. In young infants, before the onset of myelin formation, the tangential fiber plexus

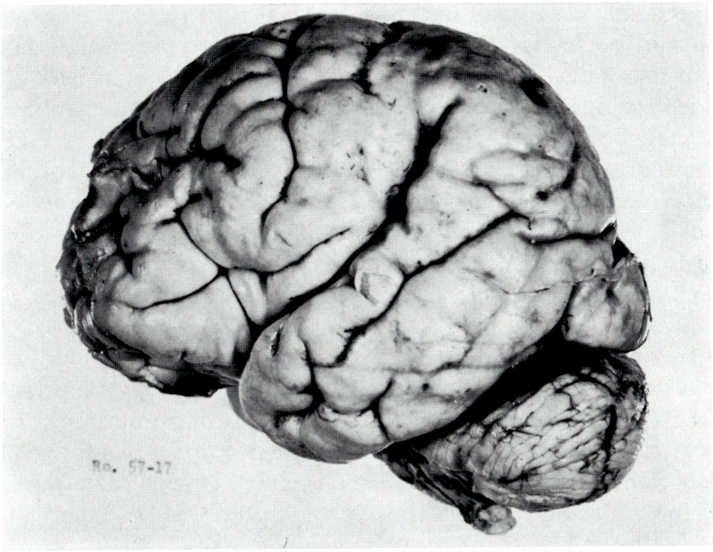

Fig. 98. Pachygyria (courtesy of Dr. Lindenberg)

may not be discernible, and the superficial and deep cell layers form a single broad band of gray matter. In older infants there may be further subdivision of the deep cell layer by several strata of myelinated fibers (Münchoff and Noetzel, 1965). The juncture between pachygyric cortex and adjacent normal neocortex shows blending of the upper cell layers of pachygyric cortex with the neocortex. The deep cell layer of the pachygyric cortex does not fuse with the neocortex; it forms a subcortical mass of gray matter. This feature differs from the behavior of the deep cell layer in polymicrogyric cortex which fuses with the adjacent normal cortex.

Agyria of the cerebral cortex commonly coexists with heterotopias of the inferior olivary nuclei of the medulla oblongata (Chapter 32). Malformations of the cerebellar dentate nucleus are less common and occur in the form of redundant gyration and heterotopic masses of neurons which may be of dentate or Purkinje cell origin. Ectopia of granule cells in the molecular layer of the cerebellar cortex (Chapter 31) may coexist, as well as other dysplasias of cerebellar cortical architecture. The pyramids are hypoplastic, corresponding to the degree of cortical derangement.

The most plausible concept of the pathogenesis of agyria is that of an arrest of the migration of neuroblasts on their path from the periventricular matrix to the cortical surface (Bielschowsky, 1923). This interpretation is consistent with the high degree of similarity between the malformations and the neuronal migration patterns seen in fetal brains. The establishment of laminar cortical architecture from successive waves of neuroblasts migrating from the periventricular matrix is reviewed in Chapter 1. Hanaway *et al.* (1968) proposed that the neurons in the second phase of migration, destined to form the superficial cortical layers, are unable to pass beyond the first wave, so that the large cortical neurons normally forming the deep layers remain superficial. The coexistence of agyria with olivary heterotopias and with ectopia of cerebellar granule cells suggests that neuroblast migration is disturbed in many other portions of the brain. There is also reason to assume that a relatively specific type of interference with the migration of neuroblasts has taken place, rather than nonspecific tissue damage: Pachygyria is usually not found in association with cavitated defects as is polymicrogyria. Experimental damage to neuroblasts, *e.g.*, by radiation, is known to induce death of cells without arresting migration. Repeated chemical insults with a cytidine analogue in mice resulted in reduced cortical cell numbers and abnormal shapes of neurons without altering migration patterns or cortical architecture (Langman and Shimada, 1971).

The developmental derangement responsible for agyria evidently occurs earlier in gestation than that responsible for polymicrogyria which dates to approximately the fifth month. The earlier development of agyria is indicated particularly by its association with olivary heterotopias (Chapter 32); it may also coexist with other malformations of early embryonic determination, such as with agenesis of the corpus callosum (Josephy, 1944). Hence, the lesions probably date to the first trimester of pregnancy.

Heterotopic Gray Matter in Cerebral Hemispheres. Subcortical masses of heterotopic gray matter do not represent dysplasias of cerebral cortex in a strict sense; yet, it is appropriate to consider them in this chapter as they derive from the same pool of cells from which the cortex forms. Two types of heterotopias, the laminar and the nodular, can be distinguished (Jakob, 1936).

The laminar type of heterotopia, or diffuse symmetrical heterotopia, is closely related to pachygyria. Few instances of this lesion have been reported. This may be due, at least in part, to problems in classification. Indeed, the report of Matell (1893) is widely quoted as the first description of pachygyria, although the case showed laminar heterotopia with normal cortical gyration and was identified as such by the author. The difference between the two types of lesions may be defined as follows: In laminar heterotopias the heterotopic tissue is separated from the cortex by a thick layer of white matter, and the cortex shows normal or subnormal gyration and normal laminar architecture. In pachygyria there is only a thin layer of tangential fibers between the superficial and the deep layers of gray matter, and the cell layers combine to form a cortex of distinctly abnormal architecture. The two cases illustrated by Wiest and Hallervorden (1958) are typical examples of either type of lesion.

Laminar heterotopias present as bilateral, symmetrical ribbons of gray matter in the centrum semiovale, situated between cortex and ventricular walls, and separated from both by well developed layers of white matter. The heterotopic tissue presents as solid sheets of gray matter, or it may be split into innumerable elongate islands (Fig. 99), with their axes radiating toward the hemispheric surface. The cerebral cortex usually has normal thickness; the gyral pattern may be completely normal, or there may be slight reduction in the number of gyri. Microscopic examination discloses a normal six-layered cortex, and the tangential fibers at the line of Gennari

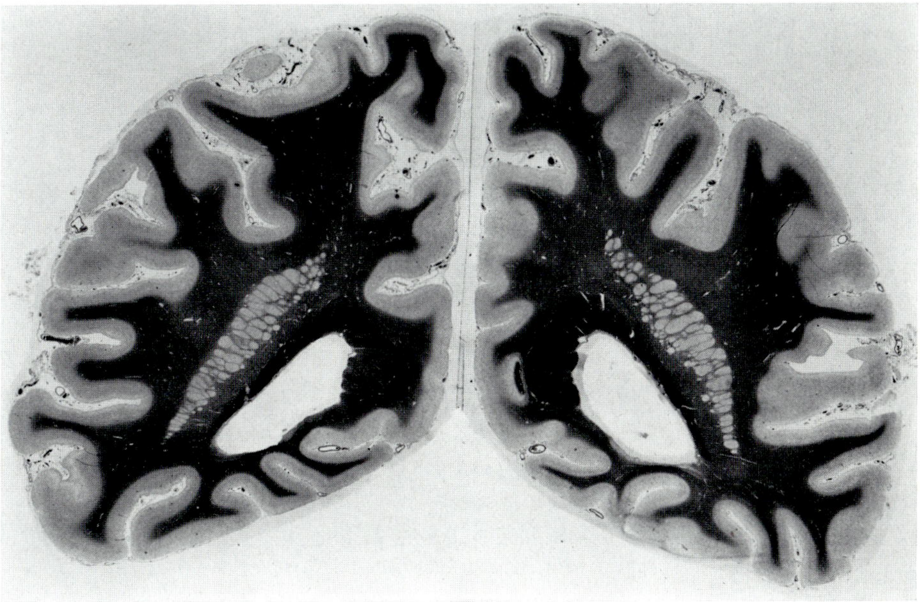

Fig. 99. Symmetric laminar heterotopias; there is normal architecture and gyration of the cerebral cortex

are fully developed. A few instances have been described having features transitional between laminar heterotopia and pachygyria; in these the gyri were unusually shallow. The case 4 of Jakob (1936) showed deeply situated masses of heterotopic gray matter combined with a malformed four-layered cortex of the type found in pachygyria. In a later report Jakob (1938) lists cases of laminar heterotopias and cases of agyria and pachygyria.

It is reasonable to assume that laminar heterotopia, pachygyria and agyria are different degrees in severity of basically the same type of lesion. Distinguishing between laminar heterotopia and pachygyria avoids the confusion of referring to a brain with normal gyration and normal laminar architecture as being pachygyric. There are few clinical data on laminar heterotopias; the lesions are often found in adults requiring institutional care because of mental retardation and epilepsy; they are not inconsistent with social adaptation, however, as, for example, in the subject shown in Fig. 99, who had worked as a truck driver.

The second type of heterotopias, the nodular, consists of conglomerate masses of gray matter in proximity of the ventricular walls (Fig. 100), most often at the corners of the lateral ventricles or the ventrolateral circumferences of the temporal horns. Early descriptions were given by Meschede (1864, 1866) and Virchow (1867), who quote still earlier reports. Nodular heterotopia is more common than laminar heterotopia and numerous descriptions are found in the literature. The heterotopic gray matter forms rounded or irregular, often tightly clustered nodules separated from each other by

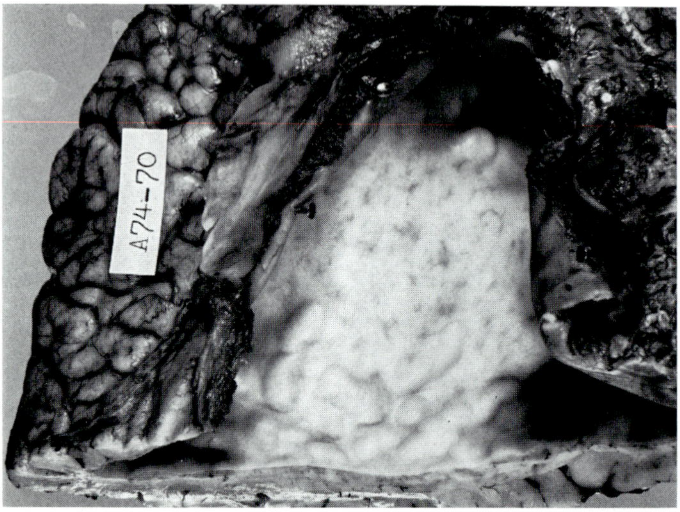

Fig. 100. Nodular heterotopias protrude from the hydrocephalic ventricular walls of an infant with Arnold-Chiari malformation

thin layers of myelinated fibers. Microscopic examination discloses neurons and glial tissue lacking a consistent architecture, although rudimentary layering may be evident.

Nodular heterotopias may occur alone, or in association with cortical malformations, particularly with micropolygyria (Crome, 1952); they may coexist with agenesis of the corpus callosum (Kirschbaum, 1947) and other malformations. The brain weight is often reduced, but nodular heterotopias have also been observed in megalencephaly (Chapter 27). The degree of mental impairment and disability varies; severe retardation and epilepsy are less consistent than for pachygyria or for laminar heterotopias. Riggs *et al.* (1956) produced subcortical heterotopias in rat brain by X-irradiation 5 to 9 days prior to birth.

Scattering of single neuronal perikarya throughout the white matter may be considered a minimal degree of heterotopia. It is, to some extent, a normal feature in infants, occurring particularly in the immediately subcortical white matter, where there is deep scattering of neurons from the sixth cortical layer. An unusually large number of neurons scattering throughout the deeper portions of white matter, may be found in developmentally disturbed brains, but the change is not specific for any given type of lesion, nor are there consistent symptoms. It should be considered persistence of a fetal trait rather than a specific malformation or disorder of neuronal migration.

Polymicrogyria. Gross descriptions of cases highly suggestive of polymicrogyria are found in the literature of the nineteenth century, *e.g.*, Binswanger (1882). The characteristic microscopic features of the lesions were described by, among others, Bielschowsky (1915), Crome (1952), and Dekaban (1965). The now widely accepted term polymicrogyria was introduced by Bielschowsky (1915) and is much preferable to either microgyria or status verrucosus; the derivation of the latter term is discussed in the next section of this chapter.

Patients with polymicrogyria show various degrees of functional impairment, depending on the extent and localization of the lesions. Small patches of polymicrogyria are sometimes found incidentally at autopsy in the absence of history of neurologic deficit or epilepsy. Extensive polymicrogyria covering the entire cortical surface, or bordering porencephalic defects, is observed in retarded patients with neurologic impairment.

Gross inspection of the cortical surface often does not give the impression of an increase in the number of gyri. Rather, there may be fewer and coarser gyri having an irregular surface of numerous smooth protrusions in an embossed pattern that has been compared to morocco leather. This feature may be mistaken for pachygyria, as in the case reported as lissencephaly by Walker (1942). The full extent of the lesion may also be concealed if the abnormal cortex is situated preferentially within the sulci. The cut surface shows abnormal thickening of the cortex, due to the piling upon each other of numerous small gyri having fused surfaces. Polymicrogyria may cover the entire hemispheric surface, either unilateral or bilateral, or may occur in irregular patches which often correspond to the territories of major cerebral arteries, most frequently the middle cerebral artery. Porencephalic or hydranencephalic defects are frequently fringed by zones of polymicrogyria. Reduction in brain weight varies with the extent of polymicrogyria and associated lesions. Polymicrogyria in the cerebral cortex may occur in association with nodular heterotopias in the white matter (Crome, 1952) or with "polymicrogyria" of the cerebellar cortex (Chapter 31).

The polymicrogyric cortex is characterized by: 1. An abnormal arrangement of cell layers and intracortical fiber plexus, and 2. an excessive folding of all or the upper layers and absence of separation of individual gyri due to fusion of their surfaces. The most typical pattern is a four-layered cortex displaying: 1. a molecular layer, 2. an upper dense cell layer, 3. an intermediate layer of low cell density containing a horizontal plexus of myelinated fibers, and 4. a deep cell layer which borders white matter. The cortical nerve cells may be smaller than normal, with persistence of immature forms. An abnormal concentration of myelinated tangential fibers may be seen in the superficial portion of the molecular layer (Fig. 101). The combined thickness of all four layers is less than that of normal cortex. On occasion the four-layered architecture may be seen in gyri of normal configuration, particularly at the zone of transition between polymicrogyric and normal cortex.

Typically, however, the four-layered architecture coexists with abnormal cortical folding. The folding may affect only the superficial cell layer, the deep cell layer remaining straight and parallel to the cortical surface. More severe folding involves both cell layers alike. A still more severe degree of derangement consists of a rudimentary two-layered cortex consisting of a molecular

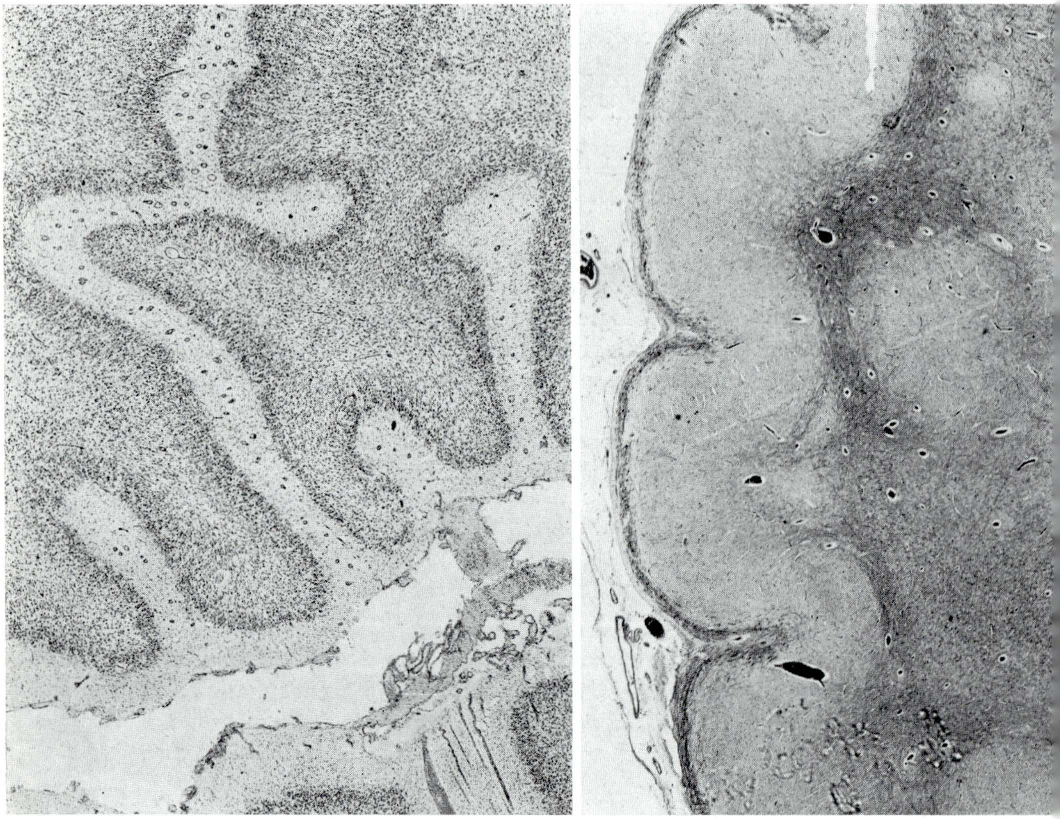

Fig. 101. Polymicrogyria. Left: fusion of molecular layers; large vessels mark the seams of fused gyri; cresyl violet ×16. Right: there is an anomalous subpial plexus of myelinated fibers; myelin stain ×16

layer and a single cell layer. Microscopic sections of this type of cortex may show, because of its extensive folding and contorsion, irregular profiles, nests or islands of nerve cells disseminated among irregular zones of neuropil representing the fused molecular layers.

The leptomeninges may show abnormal vascularity consistent with persistent fetal leptomeningeal vascularization (Chapter 34), and aggregates of large sinusoid vessels may mark the seams at which the molecular layers are fused. The vascular supply of the cortex has been described as being anomalous, in that the deep cortical layers derive their vessels from the white matter, the upper layers from the meninges (Bertrand and Gruner, 1955).

It is doubtful, however, whether this is sufficient reason for assuming that the lesions are induced by a primary derangement of vascular development.

The boundary between the polymicrogyric cortex and the adjacent normal neocortex is usually abrupt; in this zone the superficial layer of the polymicrogyric cortex can be seen to blend with the second and third neocortical

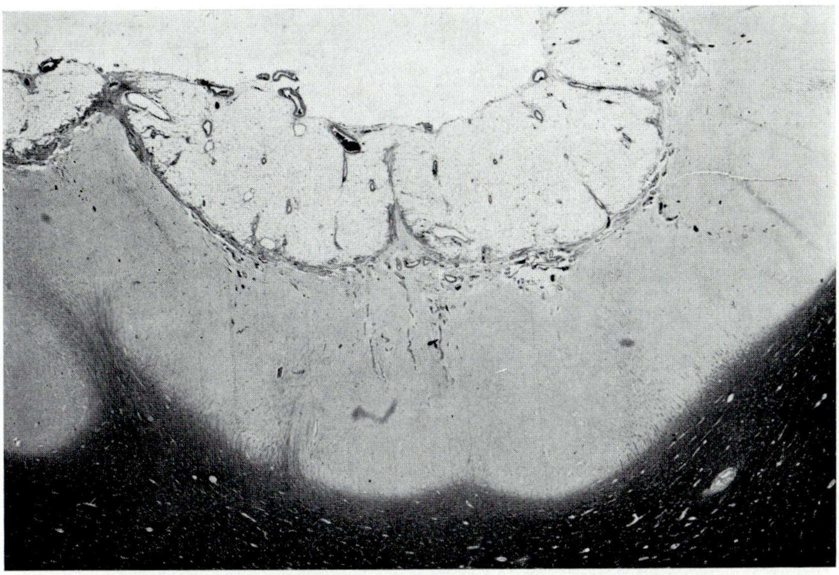

Fig. 102. Meningeal lipomatosis overlies a thickned, polymicrogyric cortex; ×6.5

layers, the deep cell layer with the fifth neocortical layer. The layer of tangential fibers tapers off and disappears near the level of the fourth neocortical layer (Rabinowitsch, 1933; Scherer, 1935; Jakob, 1940; Crome, 1952), differing from pachygyria where the deep cell layer forms a separate mass that does not unite with the normal cortex (Crome, 1956).

Rare instances of polymicrogyria are associated with leptomeningeal lipomatosis. The case reported by Scherer (1935) had a palm-sized leptomeningeal lipoma covering an area of polymicrogyria. The adipose tissue was encompassed by dense collagen connective tissue, with fibrous tissue obliterating subarachnoid space; there was an increased number of blood vessels, some with intima proliferation. The superficial portions of the polymicrogyric cortex were mineralized. Similar observations were reported by Demus (1967) and Dragojević *et al.* (1973). A case without cortical mineralization is illustrated in Fig. 102. The combination of lipoma and polymicrogyria is reminiscent of the association of lipomas with other malformations such as agenesis of corpus callosum or various forms of spina bifida.

Polymicrogyria dates to a developmental disturbance near the 5th or before the 6th month of gestation. The dating is based on the onset of cortical gyration during this period, and it is verified by a few recorded dated lesions. Hallervorden (1944) reported a 1-year-old infant born after an attempted suicide with gas at the 5th month of pregnancy, having extensive polymicrogyria associated with cavitated hemispheric defects and necrotic lesions in the basal ganglia. An infant born with hydranencephaly following accidental intoxication with household gas at the 24th week of gestation also showed polymicrogyria in the residual cortex (Bankl and Jellinger, 1967). An early stage of unilateral polymicrogyria centering on the Sylvian region in a 27-week-fetus was described by Richman *et al.* (1974). Two similar cases from

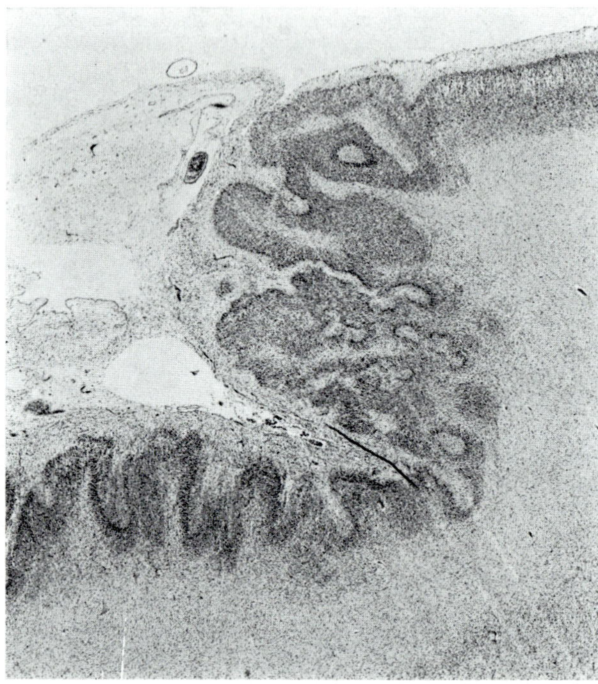

Fig. 103. Polymicrogyria in the formative stage in a fetus of 24 weeks gestation; same case as in Fig. 37

the present author's material, born at 24 and 32 weeks gestation, respectively, show that the abnormal undulation of the polymicrogyric cortex commences before there is formation of sulci in the normal cortex (Fig. 103). They also demonstrate an imbalance in cell populations between superficial and deep layers. Conceivably, the first wave of neuronal migration, forming the deep layer, became damaged, while the undamaged second wave of migration formed a disproportionately dense and undulating upper cell layer.

Polymicrogyria has been attributed to disturbances of neuronal migration; however, the disturbance affects the arrangement of cells within the cortex to a greater degree than it does their migration to the cortex. It has been proposed that the excessive folding of the cortex results from an imbalance in the growth rates of the supra- and infragranular layers due to differences in the numbers of their cells (de Leon, 1972) or from the postmigratory, selective destruction of layers (Richman *et al.*, 1974). A four-layered cortex is a persistent trait in the entorhinal cortex and other allocortical areas (Bielschowsky and Rose, 1929), and its presence in polymicrogyria may be considered a throwback into a more primitive pattern of cortical organization. The disturbances causing polymicrogyria appear to be local and nonspecific, as shown by its common occurrence adjacent to porencephalic defects and by its association with lesions caused by intrauterine infections such as toxoplasmosis or cytomegalovirus (Chapters 11, 16).

Nodular Cortical Dysplasia. Nodular cortical dysplasia is a circumscript, isolated cortical deformity that is sometimes confused with polymicrogyria because of an overlapping usage of the terms brain warts, status verrucosus and polymicrogyria. This terminology can be traced to an article by Ranke (1910) containing one of the first microscopic descriptions of polymicrogyria. The author called polymicrogyria "status verrucosus deformis" and distinguished it from "status verrucosus simplex" which he described as innumerable semicircular protrusions of uniform size at the cortical surface. Each protrusion was formed by an outward bulge of the molecular layer and the upper portion of the cell layers, and it was separated from the next bulge by a sharp indentation. The interpretation of this alteration has been highly controversial; it has been considered a normal aspect of fetal cortical development between the 4th and 6th month of gestation by some, a pathologic lesion by others. What Ranke illustrated as status verrucosus simplex is almost certainly a preparative artefact resulting from the obsolete practice of supporting fetal brains during fixation in a bag of gauze. The term status verrucosus without additional qualification has since been used to designate either polymicrogyria or nodular cortical dysplasia.

The most comprehensive account of nodular cortical dysplasia was given by Morel and Wildi (1952) who referred to this lesion as dysgénésie nodulaire disséminée de l'encorce frontale. Jakob (1940) had described it earlier under the name brain warts, and still earlier accounts were published by Simon (1868), Otto (1887), and Bundschuh (1913). Jakob observed the lesions in 11 of 50 examined brains, and Morel and Wildi in 25 patients aged 21 to 91. The distribution between sexes was even and there were no clinical symptoms, nor was there any consistent relationship to underlying disease processes.

Nodular cortical dysplasia is evident upon stripping the leptomeninges off the cortex, revealing small rounded protrusions of gray matter, 1 to 2 mm in diameter, situated at the crown or the lateral extent of gyri, rarely in the sulci. There are usually two to three lesions per brain, but up to sixteen have been counted. They are most commonly found in the frontal lobe, near the operculum or at the orbital surface. Microscopic sections through the center of the nodule show a bundle of radial myelinated fibers projecting into the upper cortical layers, where they split in the form of a fountainhead and radiate into the adjacent cortex. The bundle corresponds to a zone of low cell density with irregularly disposed neurons. The upper cortical layers bulge and their architecture is disorganized, but there is no corresponding indentation in the lower surface of the cortex. The molecular layer is thin at the apex of the node and contains a dense plexus of tangential fibers and aggregates of bipolar tangential cells. A large, thin-walled artery runs upward through the axis of the nodule and branches in the upper layers. The cortex bordering the nodule is normal. Jakob (1940) observed this type of lesion in a 7-month-old infant with the Arnold-Chiari malformation; it formed a vertical streak without nerve cells covered with piled-up cells in the molecular layer.

In none of the above reports was nodular cortical dysplasia associated with polymicrogyria. The association of these lesions in one instance (Grcevic and Robert, 1960) is insufficient reason to assume that the two disease processes are related. Their morphologic similarity is only superficial, and they differ in topographic distribution, types of occurrence and clinicopathologic correlations.

Leptomeningeal Glioneuronal Heterotopias. Microscopic protrusions or nests of disorganized glial tissue in the leptomeninges are relatively common in malformed brains (*e.g.*, holoprosencephaly, agenesis of corpus callosum, dysraphic states, etc.) or in brains with cavitated lesions dating to the developmental period (*e.g.*, hydranencephaly, porencephaly, fetal infections). They are uncommon in otherwise normal brains. Leptomeningeal heterotopias consist of microscopic, irregularly shaped nodules or of sheets composed mainly of astrocytic glial tissue of rather irregular architecture; neurons are occasionally included either scattered or in groups. There may be ependyma, or even choroid plexus in the heterotopic tissue (Popoff and Feigin, 1969). Brun (1965) tabulated 18 reports on leptomeningeal heterotopias, and these were found in association with a variety of cerebral disease processes. He speculated on the possibility that glioneuronal heterotopias develop from the superficial granular layer of the cerebral cortex (Chapter 1). Other interpretations include an excessive proliferative response of the cerebral surface upon a variety of irritative processes in the subarachnoid space, or the leptomeningeal implantation of undifferentiated cells shed into the CNS from destructive lesions elsewhere in the brain. Heterotopia of skeletal muscle in the leptomeninges is extremely rare (Hoffman and Rorke, 1971).

Leptomeningeal glioneuronal heterotopias differ from nodular cortical dysplasia in being smaller, of less regular shape, and in the absence of disorganization of cortical architecture. They also need to be distinguished from the so-called brain hernias forming upon chronic increase in intracranial pressure. In the latter nodular protrusions of molecular layer and pia mater herniate into lacunar erosions of the cranial bones, particularly at the base of the skull.

Persistence of Horizontal Cells of Cajal. The horizontal cells of Cajal (1891, 1911) or of Retzius (1893, 1894) are spindle shaped or triangular neurons in the molecular layer projecting numerous short processes and two bipolar axons parallel to the cortical surface within the molecular layer. They are the only pluri-axonal neurons known. The horizontal cells are a normal aspect of cortical architecture during late gestation, but they diminish greatly in density or disappear completely after birth. Persistence of horizontal cells has been described in various cerebral disease processes and should be interpreted as a nonspecific fetal trait of little significance; it is a rather consistent component of nodular cortical dysplasia.

The case described by Rebeiz *et al.* (1968) under the name "dystopic cortical myelinogenesis" may be considered in this category. A severely retarded 11-year-old girl showed numerous bundles of myelinated fibers projecting at random through the upper three cortical layers. The fibers probably arose from small and large abnormally situated neurons, and there was general paucity of neurons and disturbance in cortical architecture.

Columnar Arrangement of Nerve Cells. Arrangement of nerves in columns which project in register perpendicular to the cortical surface is a typical feature of the fetal cortex. The columns tend to be narrow, tightly spaced and separated by zones of low cell density formed by bundles of fibers. This arrangement is known to persist in the normal adult cortex (von Bonin and Mehler, 1971) though becoming much less conspicuous than in the fetal cortex. A striking columnar arrangement of cells is sometimes observed in malformed adult brains and it has been described as a microscopic feature in subnormal brains, for example in Down syndrome. However, the pattern is neither specific nor diagnostic of a given disease; it should be considered a persistent fetal trait.

Abnormal Laminar Architecture. The laminar architecture characteristic of the entorhinal or pyriforme cortex is sometimes observed in malformed brains, particularly in holoprosencephaly or encephaloceles. This architecture consists of a thick molecular layer and segmentation of the superficial cell layer into roughly spherical aggregates of neurons separated by zones of low cell density. There is a continuous deep layer of nerve cells. Occurrence of this cortical pattern at sites where archicortex is not normally present may be considered a throwback into a primitive pattern of cortical organization. This interpretation, however, needs to be tempered with caution. An abnormal cortical architecture in holoprosencephaly, for example, results from severe hypoplasia of the neocortex, due to which the allocortical areas are disproportionally large and abnormally situated. Hence the seemingly abnormal cortical architecture may result from redistribution of cortical regions rather than from a true neocortical malformation.

Focal Dysplasia of the Cerebral Cortex in Epilepsy. Anomalies in cortical architecture were described by Taylor *et al.* (1971) in the brains of 10 patients, 8 men and 2 women, suffering from intractable epilepsy. No changes were discernible with the naked eye. Microscopic alterations consisted of local disruptions of cortical architecture, with an excess of large aberrant cells scattered throughout all cortical layers except the molecular. Most of these cells were neurons, but large abnormal cells of undetermined origin were also observed. The abnormal neurons occupied sharply delineated cortical segments, rarely more than 2 cm in length, or they formed foci in the depth of the sulci. The thickness of the cortex was normal or slightly increased. The similarity between these lesions and tuberous sclerosis was pointed out, but there were none of the cutaneous or somatic stigmata, no evidence of other lesions, absence of familial occurrence and late onset of symptoms. The structure of the lesions also differed from tuberous sclerosis in that they were single, did not form nodular masses and showed no anomalous glial hyperplasia.

Abnormal Gyration of Malformed Brains. Hydrocephalic distension of the cerebral hemispheres in early infancy is often accompanied with an anomalous cortical architecture characterized by an abundance of relatively small, irregularly disposed gyri. These have normal architecture on microscopic examination. The anomalous gyration is often seen with the Arnold-Chiari malformation, but it is not specific of the latter, occurring with infantile hydrocephalus of other causes as well. When found with the Arnold-Chiari malformation, the anomalous cortical gyration is often referred to as microgyria or polymicrogyria, with the implication that both the brain stem deformity and the anomalous cortical architecture are component of a complex malformation affecting the entire brain. The usage of the term polymicrogyria in this context is incorrect and misleading as the laminar architecture of the cortex is normal in contrast to the severe and specific type of derangement found in polymicrogyria. The anomalous gyration of hydrocephalic brains may be explained as the result of distension of the growing cortex (Chapter 21) or as a minor derangement of general cortical growth. Other anomalies in the gross arrangement of gyri are found with a variety of hemispheric lesions: they may be considered adaptations to an existing defect, *e.g.*, the radial arrangement of gyri at a porencephaly or with aplasia of the corpus callosum, as relative discrete gyral anomalies, *e.g.*, in 17–18 trisomy, or as manifestation of general hemisperic disfigurement as in holoprosencephaly or in some instances of megalencephaly.

Cerebro-Hepato-Renal Syndrome of Zellweger. Although there is reason to believe that the cerebro-hepato-renal syndrome is a disease of intermediary energy metabolism, it is described in the present chapter because cerebral cortical dysplasias are a prominent part of its neuropathology. Cerebral changes, nonetheless, have not been found for all the recorded cases. The syndrome was described by Bowen *et al.* (1964) for two siblings, one of them documented by autopsy findings. The authors also reported two sibs from another family, whom they considered similar to the first set although they lacked hepatic and renal changes and their brains showed agenesis of the corpus callosum. The essential features of the cerebro-hepato-renal syndrome as defined by subsequent observations (Passarge and McAdams, 1967; and others) are: marked generalized hypotonia and weakness, depressed reflexes, hepatic enlargement with fibrosis and hemosiderosis, multiple renal cortical cysts, patchy calcification in joint cartilages, and a cranio-facial deformity characterized by high forehead and hypertelorism, high arched palate, abnormal ear helices and other deformities. Other malformations are congenital cataract or glaucoma, congenital cardiac anomalies and minor skeletal anomalies.

The syndrome is apparent soon after birth; the infants fail to thrive and often die within the first week, or else during the first year. Seizures are common. The disease occurs in families, suggestive of an autosomal recessive inheritance affecting both sexes.

The brain may have greater than normal weight, in contrast to the micrencephaly usually seen in pachygyric brains. Its external surface shows anomalies in gyral pattern with plump, broadened gyri suggestive of pachygyria as well as of microgyria. The medullary olives protrude very little. Early microscopic descriptions refer to anomalous cortical architecture, heterotopic neurons and plump configuration of inferior olivary nuclei (Passarge and McAdams, 1967; Jan *et al.*, 1970). Detailed histologic studies of one brain were reported by Volpe and Adams (1972) and show a remarkable coexistence of different types of developmental anomalies, all consistent with a generalized disturbance of neuronal migration. Disturbances in cortical architecture affected mostly the neocortex which showed typical pachygyria for some regions, typical polymicrogyria for others; there was also displacement of neurons into the subcortical white matter. No changes were seen in the basal ganglia except for absence of the claustrum. The cerebellum showed subcortical aggregates of heterotopic Purkinje cells as well as disorganization of cortical architecture in the nodulus. The inferior olivary nucleus was smaller than normal and had a plump configuration lacking its normal undulating profile; a similar configuration was seen in the cerebellar dentate nucleus; there was fasciculation of the corticospinal tract.

Several other changes have been reported, in particular a sudanophilic leukodystrophy (Passarge and McAdams, 1967). However, the reported degree of myelination is not inconsistent with age; furthermore, the deposition of lipids in astrocytes in the absence of macrophages is consistent with diffuse fatty change of white matter (Chapter 5). No evidence of leukodystrophy was found by later authors. Subependymal cysts were also seen in several cases but are most likely residual to periventricular infarcts (Chapter 4). It is of interest to compare the cerebral changes of the cerebro-hepato-renal syndrome with the two siblings described by Norman *et al.* (1962); one of these had pachygyria with a sudanophilic leukodystrophy and, also, hepatomegaly, extraordinary large ears and a high and arched palate; there were, however, no renal abnormalities and the patient lived with spasticity to the age of 18 months.

Early considerations of pathogenesis were based on increased serum levels of iron and iron deposition in various tissue. Recent electron microscopic studies demonstrated striking defects in two organelles; there were no peroxisomes in liver and kidney and abnormal mitochondria were found in fibrous astrocytes and hepatocytes (Goldfischer *et al.*, 1973; Moore *et al.*, 1973). The data suggest a defect in mitochondrial oxydation, probably at the level of nonheme iron protein.

References

Bankl, H., Jellinger, J.: Zentralnervöse Schäden nach fetaler Kohlenoxydvergiftung. Beitr. path. Anat. 135: 350—376, 1967.

Bertrand, I., Gruner, J.: The status verrucosus of the cerebral cortex. J. Neuropath. exp. Neurol. 14: 331—347, 1955.

Bielschowsky, M.: Über Mikrogyrie. J. Psychol. Neurol. 22: 1—47, 1916.

— Über die Oberflächengestaltung des Großhirnmantels bei Pachygyrie, Mikrogyrie und bei normaler Hirnentwicklung. J. Psychol. Neurol. 30: 29—76, 1923.

Bielschowsky, M., Rose, M.: Über die Pathoarchitektonik der micro- und pachygyren Rinde und ihre Beziehungen zur Morphologie normaler Rindengebiete. J. Psychol. Neurol. 38: 42—46, 1929.

Binswanger, O.: Über eine Mißbildung des Gehirns. Virchows Arch. 87: 427—476, 1882.

Bowen, P., Lee, C. S. N., Zellweger, H., Lindenberg, R.: A familial syndrome of multiple congenital defects. Bull. Hopkins Hosp. 114: 402—414, 1964.

Bresler, J.: Klinische und pathologisch-anatomische Beiträge zur Microgyrie. Arch. Psychiat. 31: 566—573, 1899.

Brun, A.: Marginal glioneural heterotopias of the central nervous system. Acta path. microbiol. scand. 65: 221—233, 1965.

Bundschuh, E.: Über warzige Hyperplasien des normal gefurchten Hirns bei einem Fall von Syringomyelie. Beitr. path. Anat. 55: 91—116, 1913.

Cajal, R. S.: Sur la structure de l'écorce cérébrale de quelques mammifères. La cellule 7: 123—176, 1891.

— Histologie du Système Nerveux, 1911. Volume II, translated into French (Azoulay, L.), 1955. Consejo Superior de Investigaciones Cientificas, Instituto Ramon Y Cajal, Madrid.

Crome, L.: Microgyria. J. Path. Bact. 64: 479—495, 1952.

— Pachygyria. J. Path. Bact. 71: 335—352, 1956.

Daube, J., Chou, S. M.: Lissencephaly: Two cases. Neurology (Minneap.) 16: 179—191, 1966.

Dekaban, A.: Large defects in cerebral hemispheres associated with cortical dysgenesis. J. Neuropath. exp. Neurol. 24: 512—530, 1965.

de Leon, G. A.: Observations on cerebral and cerebellar microgyria. Acta neuropath. 20: 278—287, 1972.

Demus, H.: Neue Gesichtspunkte zur Entstehung der pialen Lipome. Arch. Psychiat. Nervenkr. 209: 426—442, 1967.

Dragojević, S., Mehraein, P., Bock, H. J.: Beobachtung eines Lipoms der Temporalregion mit Rindenmißbildung und Epilepsie. Klinisch-pathologische Studie. Arch. Psychiat. Nervenkr. 217: 335—342, 1973.

Goldfischer, S., Moore, C. L., Johnson, A. B., *et al.*: Peroxisomal and mitochondrial defects in the cerebro-hepato-renal syndrome. Science 182: 62—64, 1973.

Grcevic, N., Robert, F.: Verrucose dysplasia of the cerebral cortex. J. Neuropath. exp. Neurol. 20: 399—411, 1960.

Hallervorden, J.: Über eine Kohlenoxydvergiftung im Fetalleben mit Entwicklungsstörung der Hirnrinde. Allg. Z. Psychiat. 123: 289—298, 1944.

Hanaway, J., Lee, S. I., Netsky, M. G.: Pachygyria: relation of findings to modern embryologic concepts. Neurology (Minneap.) 18: 791—799, 1968.

Hoffman, S., Rorke, L. B.: On finding striated muscle in the brain. J. Neurol. Neurosurg. Psychiat. 34: 761—764, 1971.

Jakob, H.: Genetisch verschiedene Gruppen entwicklungsgestörter Gehirne. Z. ges. Neurol. Psychiat. 155: 1—39, 1936.

— Genetisch verschiedene Gruppen entwicklungsgestörter Gehirne. Z. ges. Neurol. Psychiat. 160: 615—648, 1938.

— Die feinere Oberflächengestaltung der Hirnwindungen; die Hirnwarzenbildung und die Micropolygyrie. Z. ges. Neurol. Psychiat. 170: 68—84, 1940.

Jan, J. E., Hardwick, D. F., Lowry, R. B., McCormick, A. Q.: Cerebro-hepato-renal syndrome of Zellweger. Amer. J. Dis. Child. 119: 274—277, 1970.

Josephy, H.: Congenital agyria and defect of corpus callosum. J. Neuropath. exp. Neurol. 3: 63—68, 1944.

Kirschbaum, W.: Agenesis of the corpus callosum and associated malformations. J. Neuropath. exp. Neurol. 6: 78—94, 1947.

Langman, J., Shimada, M.: Cerebral cortex of the mouse after prenatal chemical insult. Amer. J. Anat. 132: 355—374, 1971.

Matell, M.: Ein Fall von Heterotopie der grauen Substanz in den beiden Hemispheren des Großhirns. Arch. Psychiat. Nervenkr. 25: 124—136, 1893.

Meschede, F.: Über Neubildung grauer Hirnsubstanz in den Wandungen der Seiten-Ventrikel und über eine bisher nicht beschriebene, durch Hyperplasie grauer Corticalstubstanz bedingte Structur-Anomalie der Hirnrinde. Psychiat. u. Psychisch. Gerichtl. Med. 21: 481—505, 1864.

— Ein neuer Fall von abnormen Einlagerungen grauer Hirnsubstanz innerhalb der Medullarsubstanz des großen Gehirns. Virchows Arch. 37: 567—570, 1866.

Miller, J. Q.: Lissencephaly in 2 siblings. Neurology (Minneap.) 13: 481—850, 1963.

Moore, C. L., Valsamis, M. P., Johnson, A. B., *et al.*: Cerebro-hepato-renal syndrome: A defect in oxidative metabolism. J. Neuropath. exp. Neurol. 32: 166—166, 1973.

Morel, F., Wildi, E.: Dysgénésie nodulaire disseminée de l'encorce frontale. Rev. Neurol. 87: 251—270, 1952.

Münchoff, C., Noetzel, H.: Über eine nahezu totale Agyrie bei einem 6 Jahre alt gewordenen Knaben. Acta Neuropath. 4: 469—475, 1965.

Norman, R. M., Tingey, A. H., Valentine, J. C., Danby, T. A.: Sudanophil leucodystrophy in a pachygyric brain. J. Neurol. Neurosurg. Psychiat. 25: 363—369, 1962.

Otto, B.: Hyperplasie der Hirnrinde und kleine Geschwülste an der Oberfläche der Windungen. Virchows Arch. 110: 81—94, 1887.

Owen, R.: On the Anatomy of Vertebrates, Vol. 3. London: Longmans, Green 1868.

Passarge, E., McAdams, A. J.: Cerebro-hepato-renal syndrome. J. Pediat. 71: 691—702, 1967.

Popoff, N., Feigin, I.: Heterotopic central nervous tissue pervading subarachnoid space. J. Neuropath. exp. Neurol. 23: 177—178, 1964.

Rabinowitsch, A.: Cytoarchitektonik in einem Fall von Mikrogyrie. Z. ges. Neurol. Psychiat. 144: 653—656, 1933.

Ranke, O.: Beiträge zur Kenntnis der normalen und pathologischen Hirnrindenbildung. Beitr. path. Anat. 47: 51—125, 1910.

Rebeiz, J. J., Wolf, P. A., Adams, R. D.: Dystopic cortical myelinogenesis ("driftwood cortex"). A hitherto unrecognized form of developmental anomaly of the cerebrum of man. Acta Neuropath. 11: 237—256, 1968.

Retzius, G.: Die Cajal'schen Zellen der Großhirnrinde beim Menschen und bei Säugetieren. Biol. Untersuch. N.F. 5: 1, 1893.

— Weitere Beiträge zur Kenntniss der Cajal'schen Zellen der Großhirnrinde des Menschen. Biol. Untersuch. N.F. 6: 29, 1894.

Richman, D. P., Stewart, R. M., Caviness, V. S., Jr.: Cerebral microgyria in a 27-week fetus. An architectonic and topographic analysis. J. Neuropath. exp. Neurol. 33: 374—384, 1974.

Riggs, H. E., McGrath, J. J., Schwarz, H. P.: Malformation of the adult brain (albino rat) resulting from prenatal irradiation. J. Neuropath. exp. Neurol. 15: 432—446, 1956.

Scherer, E.: Über die pialen Lipome des Gehirns. Z. ges. Neurol. Psychiat. 154: 45—61, 1935.

Simon, T.: Über Neubildung von Gehirnsubstanz in Form von Geschwülsten an der Oberfläche der Windungen. Virchows Arch. 58: 310—316, 1868.

Taylor, D. C., Falconer, M. A., Bruton, C. J., Corsellis, J. A. N.: Focal dysplasia of the cerebral cortex in epilepsy. J. Neurol. Neurosurg. Psychiat. 34: 369—387, 1971.

Virchow, R.: Heterotopie der grauen Substanz. Virchows Arch. 38: 138—142, 1867.

Volpe, J. J., Adams, R. D.: Cerebro-hepato-renal syndrome of Zellweger: An inherited disorder of neuronal migration. Acta neuropath. (Berl.) 20: 175—198, 1972.

von Bonin, G., Mehler, W. R.: On columnar arrangement of nerve cells in cerebral cortex. Brain Res. 21: 1—9, 1971.

Walker, A. E.: Lissencephaly. Arch. Neurol. Psychiat. 48: 13—29, 1942.

Wiest, W. D., Hallervorden, J.: Migrationshemmungen im Groß- und Kleinhirn. Dtsch. Z. Nervenheilk. 178: 224—238, 1958.

30. Dysplasia of Cerebellar Hemispheric Organization

This chapter covers atresia of the cerebellar foramina, the Dandy-Walker malformation and cerebellar aplasia, and includes notes on aspects of cerebellar development pertinent to the understanding of these lesions. Dysplasias affecting primarily the architecture of the cerebellar cortex are described in the next chapter.

Atresia of Cerebellar Foramina. Atresia of cerebellar foramina and the Dandy-Walker malformation were considered one and the same disease process in the older literature, but later studies showed that atresia of cerebellar foramina is neither a consistent nor a characteristic feature of the Dandy-Walker malformation and may occur without evident relationship to the latter. In this text, therefore, atresia of cerebellar foramina and the Dandy-Walker malformation are dealt with as separate entities.

A few comments on the normal anatomy and development of cerebellar foramina may be of help in interpreting pathologic changes. The cerebral ventricles communicate with the subarachnoid space by means of the foramina of Luschka, situated in the lateral recesses of the fourth ventricle, and the foramen of Magendie, situated in the middle of its membranous roof. The patency of the foramina of Luschka is evident on gross inspection of the brain stem by the exposed tufts of choroid plexus lateral to the ponto-medullary junction. There has been considerable controversy as to whether a foramen of Magendie exists, which can be traced to generalizations based upon species-specific findings. A comparative study of 27 vertebrate species demonstrated foramina of Luschka for all, but many had no midline foramen (Cammermeyer, 1971). The latter was absent in cat, dog, goat, rabbit, mouse, rat and others and present in guinea pig and several primate species. The average size of the foramen of Magendie in 118 human brains was 16 mm^2; a very small foramen was found in 3 percent and none in only one instance (Barr, 1948).

The foramen of Magendie forms during fetal life from a dehiscence of tissue developing at the apex of an outpouching of the caudal portion of the membranous roof of the fourth ventricle. Blake (1900) found the midline foramen and the foramina of Luschka patent by 130th and 120th days respectively, and Wilson (1936) demonstrated patency of the midline foramen at the 5th fetal month. Considerably earlier formation of the foramen was reported by Brocklehurst (1969), who found it in several 12-week-old embryos and demonstrated its patency from the redistribution of india ink injected into the lateral ventricle.

Atresia of one or two of the three cerebellar foramina is an occasional incidental finding at autopsy. Atresia of the foramen of Magendie consists of a nonperforated, membranous roof of the fourth ventricle. Atretic foramina of Luschka form deep pouches lateral to the ponto-medullary junction walled by a thin membrane of ependyma-lined glia tissue; the choroid plexus is concealed on outside inspection of the brain stem.

Partial atresia of the cerebellar foramina is of no pathologic significance. Each of the three cerebellar foramina is large enough to allow undisturbed drainage of CSF from the ventricles. The lateral and third ventricles can be drained normally if the aqueduct has a minimum caliber of 1 mm^2; the additional volume of CSF produced in the fourth ventricle can hardly require a drainage opening more than twice that size, which is still much less than the normal caliber of each of the three cerebellar foramina. Hence, the significance of stenosis or partial atresia of cerebellar foramina should not be overrated.

Complete atresia of cerebellar foramina is found in some instances of the Dandy-Walker malformation. It also occurs in cases where the characteristic triad of the latter (malformation of vermis, membranous cyst, and elevated torcular) is absent. Cases of the latter type have not commanded the same attention as the Dandy-Walker malformation and their relatively sparse descriptions in the literature are probably not representative of their true frequency (Benda, 1954, case 1; Holland and Graham, 1958; Gardner *et al.*, 1960; Amacher and Page, 1971).

Atresia of cerebellar foramina results in obstructive hydrocephalus, with dilation of the entire ventricular system. The roof of the fourth ventricle is expanded uniformly in all directions; the vermis is stretched but has no defects and is not rotated anteriorly, and there is no cystic expansion of the posterior roof of the fourth ventricle. The foramina of Luschka and Magendie are sealed off by membranes which may be distended into pouches. These may be inconspicuous as they collapse upon removal of the brain, but they bulge if, in the resected hind brain, the aqueduct is covered with a finger and the cerebellum compressed. Microscopic examination of the membranes shows a layer of glial tissue usually covered with ependyma. The presence of the glial membrane distinguishes atresia of foramina from obstructive hydrocephalus due to fibrosis of the subarachnoid space in the basal cysterns.

Atresia of cerebellar foramina may be attributed to their primary nonformation or to secondary occlusion, but it may be difficult to determine which of these mechanisms was operative. Some cases show evidence of active or past ventriculitis, suggesting the possibility of acquired occlusion by reactive gliosis of the foramina; such occlusion is possibly facilitated if the foramina are small or not fully developed in the first place. For example, a 31-year-old man showed atresia of both foramina of Luschka; the foramen of Magendie was not identified and a pigmented cyst was located over the roof of the fourth ventricle (Holland and Graham, 1958). It is unlikely that all the lesions found in this case were the result of primary atresia. Benda (1954, case 1) described a twin to a dead embryo, in whom atresia of the foramina was associated with marked granular ependymitis. In the autopsy case of Vuia (1973) the paraflocculus was asymmetrically enlarged in a child having foraminal atresia; the interpretation of this case as a specific syndrome is debatable.

The Dandy-Walker Malformation. Dandy and Blackfan (1914) attributed enormous cystic dilation of the fourth ventricle and anterior displacement of the vermis in an infant to primary atresia of the cerebellar foramina. The entity became well defined through the report of three cases and the review of the literature by Taggart and Walker (1942). Benda (1954) suggested the now widely accepted name of Dandy-Walker malformation, but he emphasized that atresia of the cerebellar foramina is not an essential feature. Gibson (1955) reviewed 24 cases and added detailed morphologic descriptions of two of his own. The frequency of the various features of the Dandy-Walker malformation were studied on hand of 9 cases by D'Agostino *et al.* (1963) and, particularly, in the series of 28 cases of Hart *et al.* (1972).

The patients present with signs of hydrocephalus early in life, though usually of lesser degree than in the Arnold-Chiari deformity. Contrary to the latter, the vast majority of patients lives beyond the first year without the benefit of surgical shunting, and many occurrences in juveniles or adults are on record. The skull is enlarged with a characteristic prominent bulging of the occiput; neurologic signs also refer to the posterior fossa and include cranial nerve palsies, nystagmus and trunkal ataxia. Radiologic examination shows thinning and bulging of the bone of the considerably enlarged posterior fossa and a bone impression that marks an elevated position of the torcular (Walker, 1944). The lateral sinuses are displaced upward, forming an inverted Y at their juncture with the sagittal sinus. There is an even distribution between sexes.

Pathologic examination discloses hydrocephalic distension of the lateral ventricles, varying from extreme to barely detectable. The greatly enlarged posterior fossa shows the characteristic triad of a malformed vermis, a large membranous cyst formed by the distended roof of the fourth ventricle, and an upward displacement of the lateral sinuses, falx and torcular. The vermis is absent in approximately one-fourth of the cases; in others it is rotated anteriorly and may be adherent to the tentorium. Hypoplasia or absence of lobes in the vermis is most marked in its posterior portion which merges with the cyst wall, being extended into a flat tongue of nonfoliated or malformed cerebellar cortex and a thin sheet of white matter. The deformity of the vermis is documented best in median sagittal sections. The roof of the fourth ventricle posterior to the vermis consists almost entirely of a thin translucent membrane which is attached laterally to the cerebellar hemispheres and tonsils and caudally to the medulla oblongata. The membrane readily disrupts on removal of the brain, affording a view of the broadened floor of the fourth ventricle (Fig. 104). Its anterior and lateral walls are formed by the smooth-surfaced white matter of the vermis and cerebellar hemispheres (Fig. 105). The choroid plexus is found in the lateral recesses, from where it continues along the caudal insertion of the membrane at the medulla oblongata, and not at its normal position at the posterior aspect of the vermis. Microscopic examination of the cyst wall discloses an outer layer of connective tissue continuous with the leptomeninges and an inner layer of glio-ependymal tissue. Heterotopias or cortical malformations may be seen in the adjacent cerebellar tissue. The patency of cerebellar foramina varies: All or some were open in 5 of the 6 cases of D'Agostino *et al.* (1963), and only 5 of 21 cases of Hart *et al.* (1972) had all foramina closed.

The Dandy-Walker malformation is frequently associated with cerebral or systemic malformations, for example in two-thirds of the cases of Hart *et al.* (1972). There may be agenesis of the corpus callosum, malformation and heterotopia of the inferior olivary nucleus (Hanaway and Netsky, 1971; also, Chapter 32) and heterotopia and disorganization in cerebellar cortical architecture (Taggart and Walker, 1942). Disturbances in cortical architecture, stenosis of aqueduct, lipomas, harmatomas, absence of corticospinal tract,

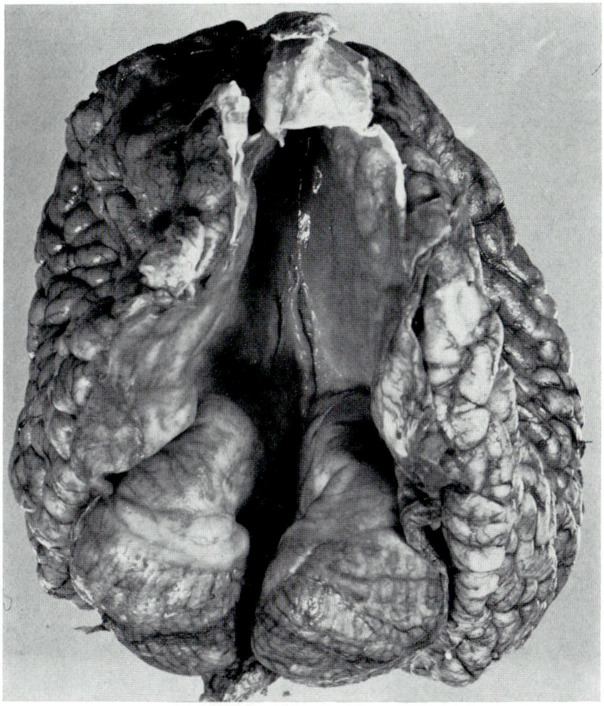

Fig. 104. Dandy-Walker malformation; the cyst communicates broadly with the fourth ventricle by subtotal absence of the vermis; portions of the anterior vermis are discernible in the form of strings of tissue running vertically in the depth of the cyst cavity

syringomyelia and others have also been seen. Systemic anomalies include polydactylism, syndactylism, cleft palate, Klippel-Feil syndrome, Cornelia de Lange syndrome and sixth lumbar vertebra syndrome.

Several other deformities of vermis and fourth ventricle need to be considered in the differential diagnosis of the Dandy-Walker malformation; the latter term should be reserved for lesions exhibiting the triad of malformation of vermis, cystic roof of the fourth ventricle and elevated tentorium. This definition separates these cases from those of atresia of cerebellar foramina described above. The Arnold-Chiari (Cleland-Chiari) deformity (Chapter 25) differs from the Dandy-Walker malformation in that the posterior fossa is small, the torcular low, the fourth ventricle compressed and entirely bounded by cerebellar tissue, and the vermis herniated into the foramen magnum. Retrocerebellar arachnoid or glio-ependymal cysts

(Chapter 20) may resemble the Dandy-Walker malformation in their midline location, lateral displacement of cerebellar hemispheres and elevation of the torcular. However, arachnoid cysts override the vermis and displace it downward; the cavity of the cyst, therefore, is bounded by leptomeninges rather than by an excessively enlarged fourth ventricle, and disruption of the arachnoid cyst exposes the displaced and compressed vermis and hemispheres rather

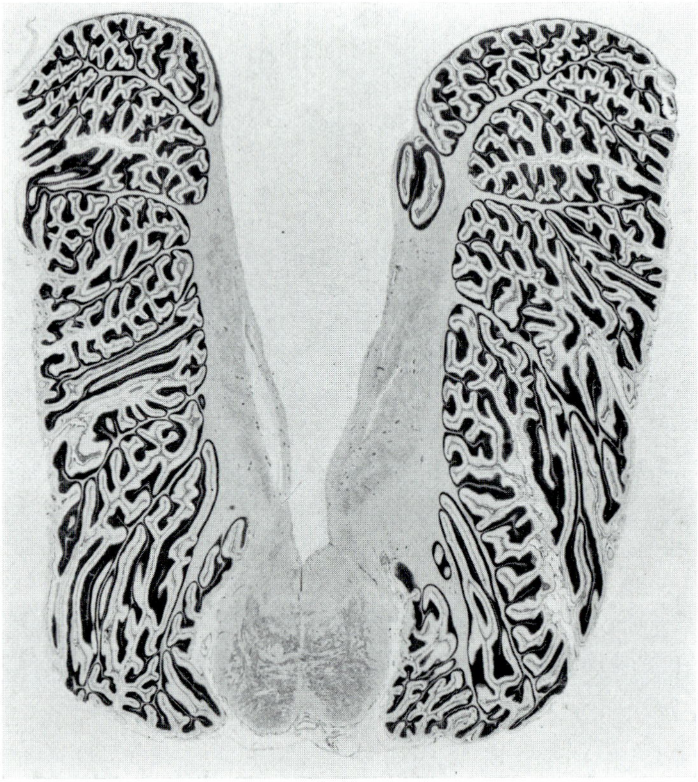

Fig. 105. Aplasia of the vermis in the Dandy-Walker malformation; cresyl violet

than the floor of the fourth ventricle. The lobulated outline of arachnoid cysts has been considered characteristic on radiologic examination (Haller *et al.*, 1971). A retrocerebellar arachnoid cyst in a 64-year-old woman reported by Gardner *et al.* (1972) had caused an elevated tentorium and herniation of the cerebellum into the foramen magnum; the floor of the cyst was formed by the vermis. The authors misinterpreted the case as a combination of the Arnold-Chiari and Dandy-Walker malformation.

An insight into the pathogenetic factors involved in the Dandy-Walker malformation was obtained through studies of a very similar malformation causing hydrocephalus in the house mouse (Brodal *et al.*, 1944; Bonnevie and Brodal, 1946). The following structures may be distinguished during early embryogenesis in the membranous roof of the fourth ventricle of the mouse.

A thickened portion in the middle of the roof, which contains the choroid plexus, is connected anteriorly with the cerebellar anlage by the anterior membranous area, and posteriorly with the medulla by the posterior membranous area. The roof of the embryonal human fourth ventricle is essentially similar (Brocklehurst, 1969). The anterior membranous area normally disappears during early fetal development, whereby the choroid plexus becomes attached to the vermis; thereafter, the foramen of Magendie forms by perforation of the posterior membranous area. In the hydrocephalic mouse, there is no involution of the anterior membranous area, which persists and expands, interposing itself between the vermis and choroid plexus, similar to the membrane in the human Dandy-Walker malformation. It is unlikely that the anterior membranous area expands because of nonopening of the cerebellar foramina since it normally disappears before the foramina open. Hence, the most convincing explanation of the Dandy-Walker malformation is a developmental arrest in the hindbrain, with persistence of the anterior membranous area, and other arrests of development including nonopening of the cerebellar foramina and hindrance of migration of neuroblasts to the inferior olivary nuclei. The elevated position of the tentorium and torcular may also be interpreted as an arrest of development, because the location of the straight sinus during early embryogenesis is at the vertex, migrating subsequently into its deep occipital position (Streeter, 1915). The descent of the sinus may be hindered by an arrest of development, or it may be interfered with mechanically by the cystic enlargement of the fourth ventricle. These considerations, as well as the teratogenetic determination period of other associated cerebral malformations, indicate that the origin of the Dandy-Walker malformation dates before the 3rd fetal month. Occurrences in siblings suggest that a genetic factor may be involved in some cases (Benda, 1954; D'Agostino *et al.,* 1963).

Cerebellar Aplasia. Understanding of the lesions of cerebellar aplasia (agenesis) is helped by a few comments on the initial stages of cerebellar development (Larsell, 1947). The primitive cerebellar anlage forms from proliferation of originally paired centers in the rhombic lip which fuse in the midline along the cerebellar commissure situated anterior to the choroid plexus in the membranous roof of the fourth ventricle (embryos of 27 mm length). The first subdivision of the cerebellar anlage is formed by the flocculo-nodular fissure which separates the flocculi of the hemispheres and the nodule of the vermis from the rest of the cerebellum; hence, these portions are sometimes referred to as archicerebellum. The next subdivision of the cerebellar anlage occurs in the 78 mm embryo by formation of the so-called fissura prima which corresponds in the adult cerebellum to the fissure between the culmen and declive of the vermis. The portion of the vermis and cerebellar hemispheres anterior to the fissura prima is generally referred to as anterior lobe of the cerebellum, and that portion between fissura prima and nodulus and flocculus as the posterior lobe. The main fissures and subdivisions of the anterior and posterior lobes of the vermis are demarcated in the 120 mm embryo. The posterior lobe undergoes greatest growth in mammals, receiving the influx of pontocerebellar fibers. Generally, the growth of the vermis antedates that of the cerebellar hemispheres. Accordingly, the flocculi of the hemispheres and the entire vermis are often referred to as paleocerebellum, the remainder of the hemispheres as neocerebellum.

These developmental principles have been applied to the classification of cerebellar aplasias. Defects of the vermis are referred to as paleocerebellar aplasia, those of the hemispheres as neocerebellar aplasia. If aplasia of the vermis is partial, its caudal portion, posterior to the fissura prima, is consistently involved. The features of paleo- and neocerebellar aplasia may combine, however, and the validity of this system of classification is not beyond question. Some cases of cerebellar aplasia seem to correspond more closely to aplasias of the anterior or of the posterior cerebellar lobes, rather than of the paleo- or neocerebellum. Complete agenesis of the cerebellum (Sternberg, 1912) appears to be extremely rare. The usage of the term aplasia is somewhat loose when applied to the cerebellum; it is not restricted to a primary nonformation but includes also lesions from damage to the cerebellar anlage at an early embryonal stage.

There is considerable variance in the clinical manifestations of cerebellar aplasia. The lesions have been observed in patients of normal intelligence having no neurologic abnormalities, but the majority showed signs of incoordination, difficulties or inability to walk, and mental deficiency. Hydrocephalus is not a common feature. Most reported cases are sporadic, but familiar occurrence has been observed (De Haene, 1955). Aplasia of the vermis in four sibs was described by Joubert *et al.* (1969), who also noticed a syndrome of episodic hyperpnea alternating with apnea, abnormal eye movements, ataxia and psychomotor retardation; these authors also tabulated 16 reports on agenesis of the vermis, ranging in age from 2 days to 70 years. Aplasia of the vermis was also described in litter-mates Boston bull terriers (Dow, 1940). Cerebellar aplasia is usually not associated with disorganization or focal lesions in the cerebral hemispheres, although the latter are usually smaller than normal.

Aplasia of the vermis causes a disproportionately small cerebellum which shows a midline defect bridged by a translucent membrane which may contain choroid plexus. Aplasia of the vermis may be complete or partial, and the caudal portion of the vermis is usually involved in the latter. The nuclei fastigii are absent and involvement of roof nuclei is more severe than that of the dentate nuclei.

A rare and interesting type of aplasia of the vermis was described by Obersteiner (1916) and Gross and Hoff (1959); the superior vermis was absent and the cerebellar hemispheres were fused in the midline, their dentate nuclei forming a single mass bridging the midline; there were no paleocerebellar nuclei. The authors considered the lesion synraphic rather than dysraphic.

Neocerebellar aplasia (Brun, 1917; Vogt and Astwazaturow, 1897; Scherer, 1933; and others) is characterized by a small rudimentary vermis and extreme smallness or absence of the cerebellar hemispheres except for persistence of the flocculi. Hemispheric defects may coexist with agenesis of the inferior vermis (Rubinstein and Freeman, 1940), thus combining features of neo- and paleocerebellar aplasia. Sectioning of the cerebellum

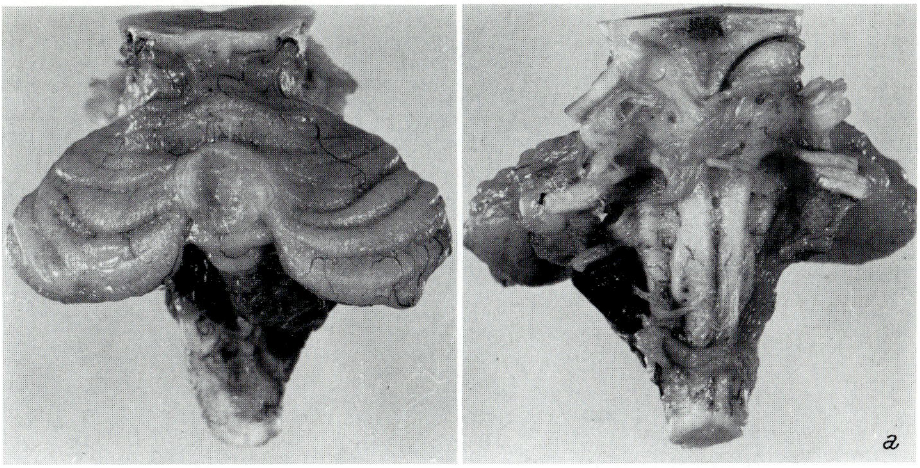

Fig. 106 a. Neocerebellar hypoplasia in an infant born at 35 weeks gestation

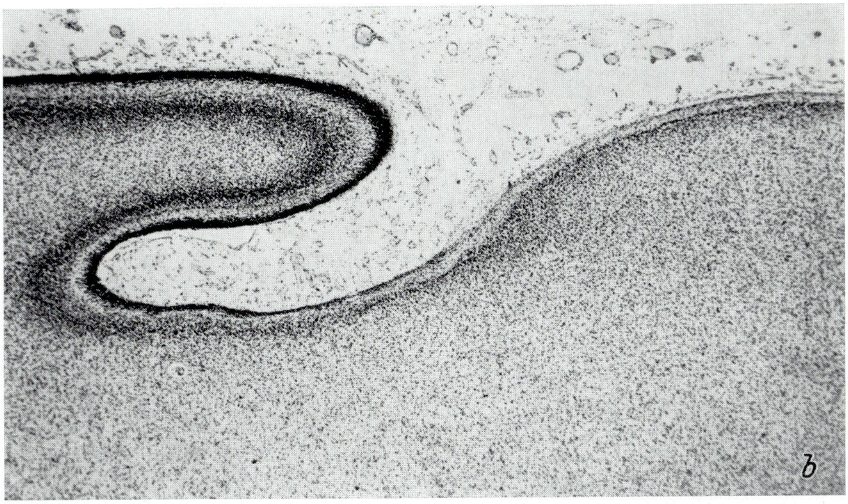

Fig. 106 b. Same case: Transition between the normally developed cortex of the vermis (left) and the hemispheric surface (right) which is almost totally devoid of neurons; cresyl violet ×32

discloses large cortical defects, usually bilateral and roughly symmetrical, in which fibrotic white matter abutts the surface. The defects are fringed by normal cerebellar cortex, but the zone of transition may show atrophy of the cortex, shrunken gyri, heterotopic tissue, or disorganization of cortical architecture. In other instances the cortex is not completely absent, but is poorly developed having fewer than normal gyri. The dentate nucleus is more affected than the cerebellar roof nuclei; it may be absent altogether, or its architecture may be disorganized. In several instances the nucleus was broken up into a chain of separate islands of gray matter (Brun, 1917;

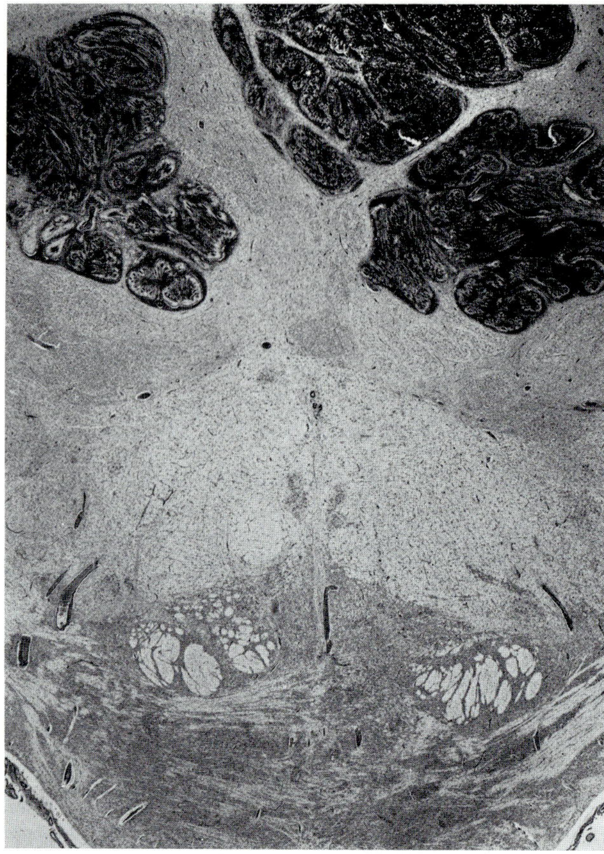

Fig. 107. Aplasia of the fourth ventricle, which is replaced with masses of heterotopic tissue simulating cerebellar cortex as well as cerebellar nuclei. A few ependymal tubuli form the only ventricular remnant. The cerebral hemispheres of this case are shown in Fig. 89; cresyl violet ×6.5

Biemond, 1955), a change which Brun interpreted as persistence of features seen in this nucleus during early embryogenesis.

Changes of the inferior olivary nuclei commonly coexist with aplasia of the vermis or the hemispheres; absence of olivary changes, as in the case of Vogt and Astwazaturow (1897), is less common. Dysplastic olivary nuclei show a coarse profile lacking the normal undulations; the nucleus is often hook-shaped and narrowed in its dorsal portion, and nerve cells may be regionally absent. Other nuclear groups of the brain stem may be hypoplastic or absent, such as, particularly, a severe hypoplasia of the pontine gray matter in instances of neocerebellar aplasia (Brun, 1917; Scherer, 1933; Rubinstein and Freeman, 1940; Biemond, 1955). Absence of the vestibular complex and of dorsal spinal tract nuclei was also recorded (Lyssenkow, 1931; Martin, 1950). Aplasia of the cerebellum may coexist with malformations of the cerebral hemispheres including agenesis of corpus callosum and arhinencephaly. The neocerebellar aplasia shown in Fig. 106 was found in a 2-day-old boy, born at 35 weeks gestation; he was third to one miscarriage and one sib who had died at the age of 5 days. Brain weight was 200 gm. The small cerebellum showed only a few coarse gyri in the hemispheres and a normal appearing vermis. The pons was hypoplastic and the olives flat. Microscopic examination disclosed much of the hemispheric surface devoid of neurons or laminar architecture, glial tissue abutting the meninges; the transition to the intact portions of cortex was gradual. There was subtotal absence of neurons from the pontine gray matter and marked reduction in the inferior olivary nucleus which had a plump configuration. A band of gliotic tissue replaced the dentate nuclei. An unusual case in which arhinencephaly was associated with cerebellar hypoplasia, atresia of the fourth ventricle and massive heterotopias is shown in Fig. 107.

The types of cerebellar aplasia described above should be distinguished from the cerebellar lesions that often accompany occipital encephaloceles. Indeed, some of the most severe cerebellar defects are found in this association (Fig. 108), accounting for some instances of so-called cerebellar agenesis. Evrard and Caviness (1974) give a description of cerebellar cortical disorganization and olivary changes in an infant with occipital encephalocele.

Several disease entities need to be considered in the differential diagnosis of cerebellar aplasia. Aplasia of the vermis is a component of the Dandy-Walker malformation. Indeed, numerous instances of the latter were reported under the title of aplasia of the vermis, particularly in the continental literature, where the term Dandy-Walker malformation was slow in acceptance. The aplasia of the vermis of the Dandy-Walker malformation is associated with cystic dilation of the fourth ventricle and elevated tentorium and torcular, lesions that are absent in cerebellar aplasia. Aplasia of the vermis has also been classified as "dysraphia of the cerebellum", but the relationship between aplasia of vermis and neocerebellar aplasia (which clearly is not a dysraphic lesion) is much more intimate than that between aplasia of vermis and dysraphic lesions. The only overlap, in this regard, is the absence or severe deformity of the cerebellum found in association with occipital encephaloceles. However, the cerebellar lesion in these cases is only a component of a larger deformity. The same applies to absence of the cerebellum with anencephaly or hydranencephaly if these extend into the posterior fossa; the case of complete cerebellar aplasia described by Priestley (1920), for example, is an instance of hydranencephaly. Differential diagnostic difficulties may arise from isolated cavities in the cerebellum caused by circulatory disturbances or other unknown factors during late gestation or in the early postnatal period. These defects are usually irregular in shape, lacking symmetry, and show no correspondence to the fetal patterns of cerebellar development. The lesions also differ from cerebellar aplasia in that there is usually no correspondence between the affection of the cortex and of the appropriate groups of cerebellar nuclei.

Neocerebellar aplasia differs, in principle, from aplasia of the cerebellar granular layer (Chapter 31); the former results from changes in the cerebellar anlage at an early fetal age and involves all neuronal components of the

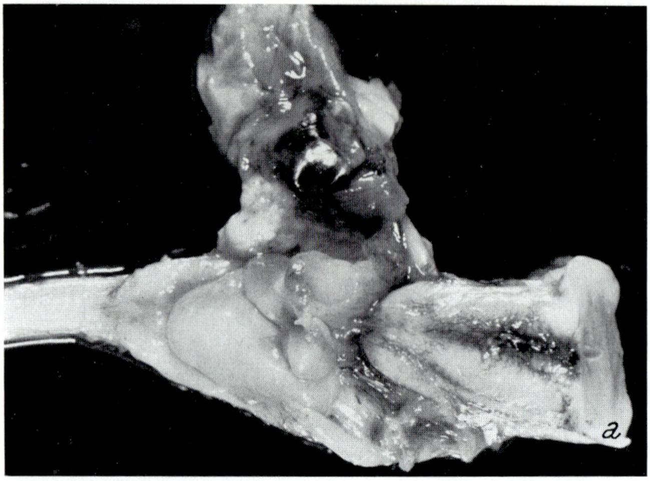

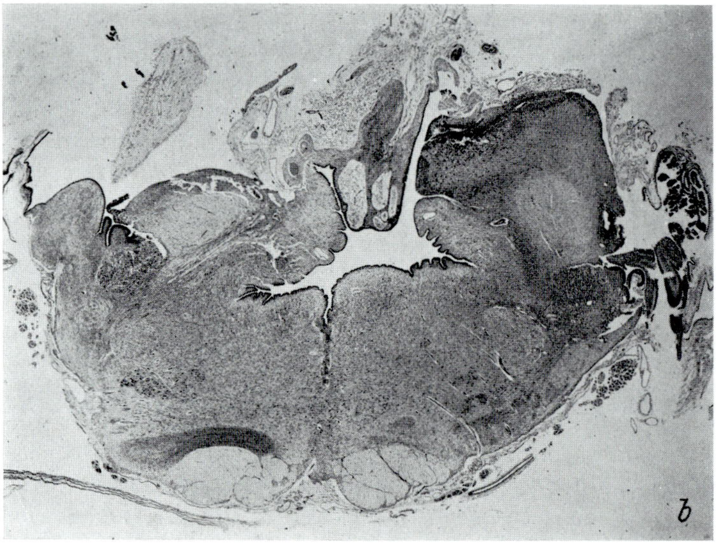

Fig. 108. A: Subtotal cerebellar aplasia in an infant with occipital encephalocele. B: Medulla oblongata of same case; minimal residua of cerebellar tissue and anomalous pyramidal tracts

cortex, while the latter is due to late fetal damage to the superficial granular layer. The formation of gyri is well advanced at this time; they may shrink to extreme atrophy upon damage to the outer granular layer, but they will not be aplastic as in cerebellar aplasia.

The hypoplasia of the pontine gray matter in cases of neocerebellar aplasia may resemble the severe atrophy of the pons developing upon ponto-subicular neuronal necrosis (Chapter 7); indeed, the attribution of some cases reported as neocerebellar aplasia to either of these two diseases is in doubt. Lesions in the Ammon's horn and absence of gyral aplasia in the cerebellum are consistent with residual lesions of ponto-subicular neuron necrosis.

References

Amacher, A. L., Page, L. K.: Hydrocephalus due to membranous obstruction of the fourth ventricle. J. Neurosurg. 35: 672—676, 1971.

Barr, M. L.: Observations on the foramen of Magendie in a series of human brains. Brain 71: 281—289, 1948.

Benda, C. E.: The Dandy-Walker syndrome or the so-called atresia of the foramen of Magendie. J. Neuropath. exp. Neurol. 13: 14—29, 1954.

Biemond, A.: Hypoplasia ponto-neocerebellaris, with malformation of the dentate nucleus. Fol. Psychiat. Neurol. Neurochir. Neerland. 58: 2—7, 1955.

Blake, J. A.: The roof and lateral recesses of the fourth ventricle considered morphologically and embryologically. J. comp. Neurol. 10: 79—108, 1900.

Bonnevie, K., Brodal, A.: Hereditary hydrocephalus in the house mouse. IV. The development of the cerebellar anomalies during fetal life. Skr. Norske Vidensk. Akad. I Mat. Nat. Kl. 4: 1—60, 1946.

Brocklehurst, C.: The development of the human cerebrospinal fluid pathway with particular reference to the roof of the fourth ventricle. J. Anat. 105: 467—475, 1969.

Brodal, A., Bonnevie, K., Harkmark, W.: Hereditary hydrocephalus in the house mouse. II. The anomalies of the cerebellum: Partial defective development of the vermis. Skr. Norske Vidensk. Akad. I Mat. Nat. Kl. 8: 1—42, 1944.

Brun, R.: Zur Kenntnis der Bildungsfehler des Kleinhirns. Schweiz Arch. Neurol. Psychiat. 1: 61—123, 1917; 2: 48—105; 3: 13—88, 1918.

Cammermeyer, J.: Median and caudal apertures in the roof of the fourth ventricle in rodents and primates. J. comp. Neurol. 141: 499—512, 1971.

D'Agostino, A. N., Kernohan, J. W., Brown, J. R.: Dandy-Walker syndrome. J. Neuropath. exp. Neurol. 22: 450—471, 1963.

Dandy, W. E., Blackfan, V. D.: Internal hydrocephalus. Amer. J. Dis. Child. 8: 406—482, 1914.

De Haene, A.: Agénésie partielle du vermis du cervelet à caractère familial. Acta neurol. psychiat. belg. 55: 622—628, 1955.

Dow, R. S.: Partial agenesis of cerebellum in dogs. J. comp. Neurol. 72: 569—586, 1940.

Evrard, P., Caviness, V. S., Jr.: Extensive developmental defect of the cerebellum associated with posterior fossa ventriculocele. J. Neuropath. exp. Neurol. 33: 385—399, 1974.

Gardner, W. J., McCormack, L. J., Dohn, D. F.: Embryonal atresia of the fourth ventricle. J. Neurosurg. 17: 226—237, 1960.

— Smith, J. L., Padget, D. H.: The relationship of Arnold-Chiari and Dandy-Walker malformations. J. Neurosurg. 36: 481—486, 1972.

Gibson, J. B.: Congenital hydrocephalus due to atresia of the foramen of Magendie. J. Neuropath. exp. Neurol. 14: 244—262, 1955.

Gross, H., Hoff, H.: Sur les dysraphies cranio-encéphaliques. In: Malformations Congénitales du cerveau (Heuyer, G., Feld, M., Gruner, J., eds.), pp. 287—296. Paris: Masson & Cie 1959.

Haller, J. S., Wolpert, S. M., Rabe, E. F., Hills, J. R.: Cystic lesions of the posterior fossa in infants: A comparison of the clinical, radiological and pathological findings in Dandy-Walker syndrome and extra-axial cysts. Neurology (Minneap.) 21: 494—506, 1971.

Hanaway, J., Netsky, M. G.: Heterotopias of the inferior olive: Relation to Dandy-Walker malformation and correlation with experimental data. J. Neuropath. exp. Neurol. 30: 380—389, 1971.

Hart, M. N., Malamud, N., Ellis, W. G.: The Dandy-Walker syndrome: A clinicopathological study based on 28 cases. Neurology (Minneap.) 22: 771—780, 1972.

Holland, H. G., Graham, W. L.: Congenital atresia of the foramen of Luschka and Magendie with hydrocephalus. J. Neurosurg. 15: 688—794, 1958.

Joubert, M., Eisenring, J.-J., Robb, J. P., Andermann, F.: Familial agenesis of the cerebellar vermis: A syndrome of episodic hyperpnea, abnormal eye movements, ataxia, and retardation. Neurology (Minneap.) 19: 813—825, 1969.

Larsell, O.: The development of the cerebellum in man in relation to its comparative anatomy. J. comp. Neurol. 87: 85—129, 1947.

Lyssenkow, N. K.: Über Aplasia palaeocerebellaris. Virchows Arch. path. Anat. 280: 611—625, 1931.

Martin, F.: Über eine vestibulo-cerebellare Entwicklungshemmung im Rahmen ausgedehnter osteo-neuraler Dysgenesien. Acta psychiat. neurol. scand. 25: 207—222; 415—421, 1950.

Obersteiner, H.: Ein Kleinhirn ohne Wurm. Arb. neurol. Inst. Wien 21: 124—136, 1916.

Priestley, D. P.: Complete absence of the cerebellum. Lancet II: 1302—1302, 1920.

Rubinstein, H. S., Freeman, W.: Cerebellar agenesis. J. nerv. ment. Dis. 92: 489—502, 1940.

Scherer, H. J.: Beiträge zur pathologischen Anatomie des Kleinhirnes III. Genuine Kleinhirnatrophien. Z. ges. Neurol. Psychiat. 145: 335—405, 1933.

Sternberg, C.: Über einen vollständigen Defekt des Kleinhirns. Verh. dtsch. path. Ges. 15: 353—359, 1912.

Streeter, G. L.: The development of the venous sinuses of the dura mater in the human embryo. Amer. J. Anat. 18: 145—178, 1915.

Taggart, T. K., Walker, A. E.: Congenital atresia of the foramina of Luschka of Magendie. Arch. Neurol. Psychiat. 48: 583—612, 1942.

Vogt, H., Astwazaturow, M.: Über angeborene Kleinhirnerkrankungen mit Beiträgen zur Entwicklungsgeschichte des Kleinhirns. Arch. Psychiat. 49: 75—203, 1897.

Vuia, O.: Malformation of the paraflocculus and atresia of the foramina of Magendie and Luschka in a child. Psychiat. Neurol. Neurochir. 76: 261—266, 1973.

Walker, A. E.: A case of congenital atresia of the foramina of Luschka and Magendie. J. Neuropath. exp. Neurol. 3: 368—373, 1944.

Wilson, J. T.: On the nature and mode of origin of the foramen of Magendie. J. Anat. 71: 423—429, 1936.

31. Dysplasias of Cerebellar Cortex

The following remarks amplify the basic aspects of normal cerebellar cortical development described in Chapter 1 and may help the understanding of developmental derangements in cortical architecture. Labelling with tritiated thymidine has shown that the Purkinje cells and the cells of the cerebellar nuclei originate from the division of precursors in the rhombic lip much earlier than the granule cells, basket cells and stellate cells which derive from the division of cells in the superficial granular layer of the cortex. Altman (1969) and Das and Nornes (1972) determined the time of origin of various other types of cortical neurons and added data on regional variation in maturation. In the rat, the Purkinje cells form on the 15th and 16th day of gestation, the interstitial nerve cells on the 15th through 18th day, the marginal cells on the 16th day and the Golgi cells on the 17th through 19th day. Cells intermediate between Golgi and granule cells arise on the 21st day. The earliest stock of granule cells, basket cells and stellate cells appears near birth in the nodulus and flocculus. In other portions of the cerebellar cortex the formation of these cells occurs entirely during the postnatal period. Regional differences in maturation are superimposed on this general schedule of cell types. The lingula and the nodule of the vermis mature before the tuber, the clive and culmen, and all show earlier maturation in the depth of the fissures than at the top of the sulci. The maturation of the cerebellar hemispheric cortex is, for most portions, later than that of the vermis (Altman, 1969). The growth and development of the superficial granular layer seems to be involved in some way in the growth in cortical surface area as well as growth of gyri. The cells of the superficial granular layer proliferate in 2-day-old mice at a 38 percent greater rate at the crowns of gyri than in the depth of sulci (Mareš and Lodin, 1970); also, experimental destruction of the superficial granule layer retards surface growth of the cerebellum, inducing excessive crowding of Purkinje cells.

The origin of the neuronal populations of the cerebellar cortex, in summary, occurs at different phases of development at different anatomical sites. The pathologic disturbances of these rather complicated processes may be grouped, for the benefit of classification, into two major types. The first type involves disturbances in the migration of cells from the rhombic lip and in their arrangement after reaching their definite sites. Heterotopias and focal dysplasias of cortical architecture belong into this category; the lesions affect the distribution of Purkinje cells as well as other cortical components. The second type of disturbance occurs much later in development and results from interference with the formation of cells in the superficial granular layer or with their descent toward the deeper portions of the cortex. The lesions develop after the Purkinje cells have reached their definite sites and affect mainly the formation of the cerebellar granular layer. Disturbances of this type develop almost entirely during the postnatal period in rat; the corresponding developmental phase in man begins late in gestation and continues through the first 9 months of postnatal life. This postnatal continuation of developmental processes obscures the difference between a true dysplasia (that is a lesion produced by an abnormal course of development) and a residual defect (that is a lesion whose features are determined only by the patterns of damage and repair).

The clarification of disturbances affecting the superficial granular layer of the cerebellum was made possible through the systematic analysis of experimental damage to this layer by X-radiation, the autoradiographic technique of thymidine labelling, and electron microscopy. Based on these data, granule layer aplasia and granule cell heterotopia can be recognized as true dysplasias and are, accordingly, described in the present chapter rather than in Chapter 7 on perinatal cortical damage.

Minor Dysplasias in Newborns. Minor anomalies in the distribution or the architecture of gray matter are rather frequent in the cerebellum of newborns and were found in as many as 84 percent of 147 normal infants (Rorke *et al.*, 1968). These authors distinguished four types of anomalies: 1. Clusters of matrix cells in the dentate nucleus (32 percent); 2. small compact groups of large nerve cells near the dentate nucleus (58 percent); 3. heterotopic portions of cortex in the white matter having a normal, layered architecture (3 percent); 4. local dysplasias of the cortex (heterotaxias) consisting of poorly organized mixed cell nests (14 percent). Only the matrix nests (1) and the heterotopias (3) were found at significantly higher frequency in infants with trisomies than in normal infants.

The frequency of these minor anomalies is not representative of that of major malformations found in the cerebellum later in life. The nests of matrix cells in the dentate nucleus (1) undergo involution after the 9th month (Chapter 1) and do not result in permanent dysplasias. The nests of large neurons near the dentate nucleus (2) are usually quite small and contain only a few cells per section; it is not clear whether they undergo involution, or whether they are too small to be found without scrutiny in the adult cerebellum. These cell nests, nonetheless, as well as the heterotopias of the cerebellar cortex (3), differ only in size from the larger heterotopias in malformed brains. The focal cortical dysplasias (4) are reviewed below.

Heterotopias. Large heterotopias of cerebellar gray matter, discernible with the naked eye, appear to have been described first by Meschede (1872) who observed abnormal aggregates of gray matter in the cerebellar white matter of 3 subjects. The clinical manifestations of cerebellar heterotopias vary, and probably depend more on other associated cerebral lesions than on the heterotopias themselves. Sizable cerebellar heterotopias may be found incidentally at autopsy in patients who had no history of neurologic disturbance. Heterotopias also occur in association with various types of cerebellar dysplasias and have been described with the Dandy-Walker malformation, cerebellar aplasia, or the Arnold-Chiari deformity. Their occurrence with each of these diseases has been overemphasized as evidence of a generalized disturbance of cerebellar development, but heterotopias are nonspecific and are not consistently associated with any particular type of cerebellar dysplasia. An increased frequency of comparatively large cerebellar heterotopias, and large matrix nests, are found in 13–15 trisomy (Chapter 33).

Heterotopias occur more frequently in the cerebellar hemispheres than in the vermis; they are rounded or they form irregular clusters or sheets of gray matter in the subcortical white matter (Fig. 109). Two types are distinguishable on microscopic examination: The first type consists exclusively of large neurons having rounded cell bodies and a sizeable amount of cytoplasm. The cells are arranged in scattered groups within a loosely textured neuropil; they are most likely Purkinje cells, but their distinction from neurons of the cerebellar nuclei is often difficult. The second type of heterotopias contains Purkinje cells along with other components of the cerebellar cortex, including granular and molecular layer. If this type is found in infants less than one year old, there is also matrix tissue of the superficial granular layer. Well organized heterotopias of this type form segments of cortex having no continuity with the rest of the cerebellar cortex and being abnormal only in their localization. Less well organized heterotopias show an irregular scrambling and intermingling of the various components of cerebellar cortex. The large neurons evidently emit long axons but it is not clear whether they are capable of connecting with other cells. At times they seem to terminate in axonal swellings within or near the heterotopia.

Focal Cortical Dysplasias (Cerebellar Polymicrogyria). The nomenclature on focal dysplasias of the cerebellar cortical architecture is confusing and often misleading. Brun (1917) proposed the term "heterotaxia" for disturbances for which cortical tissue is found at its normal site, its components, however, being arranged in an irregular "perverted" distribution. The term heterotaxia has not gained wide acceptance; it became customary, instead, to describe cerebellar cortical dysplasias with names that had been coined to describe cerebral cortical dysplasias. The practice is of doubtful merit as cerebral and cerebellar lesions are not strictly comparable. The term polymicrogyria has gained wide acceptance in denoting focal dysplasias in cerebellar cortical architecture, although it is a misnomer as these lesions show neither excessive folding nor abnormally small gyri. The terms pachygyria and agyria were used for describing an unusually smooth surface, but do not refer to a specific type of disturbance in cerebellar cortical architecture.

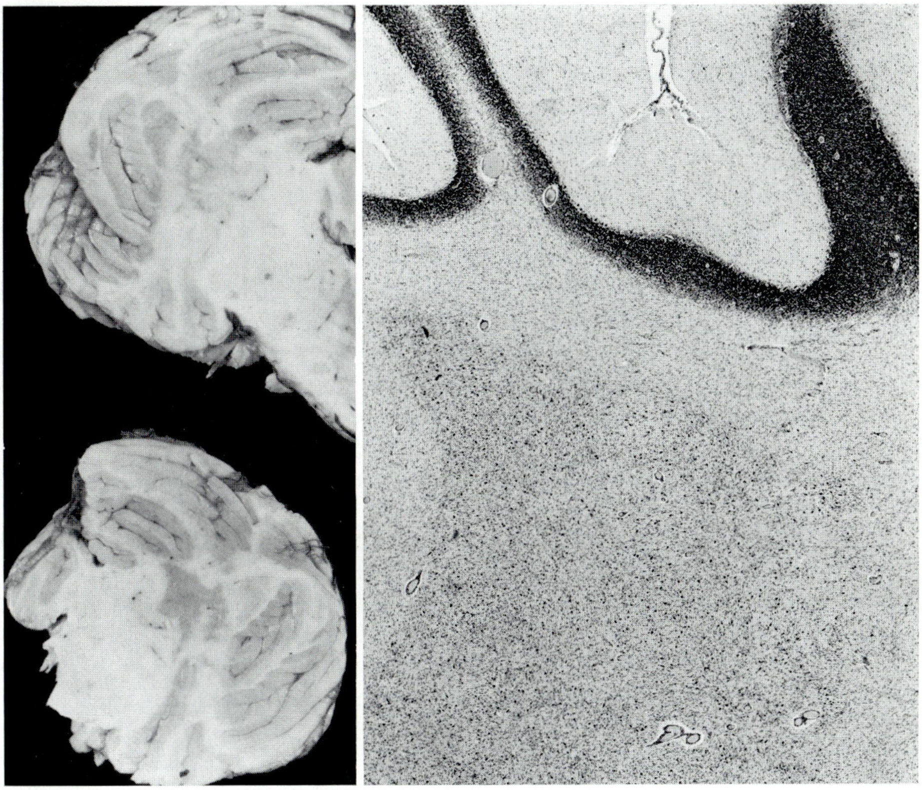

Fig. 109. Subcortical cerebellar heterotopia consisting of widely scattered large neurons consistent with Purkinje cells, or neurons of the cerebellar nuclei. Incidental finding in an asymptomatic patient; cresyl violet ×7

Focal dysplasias of cortical architecture are a relatively frequent finding in the cerebellum of newborn infants. These minor anomalies are usually observed at the basal portions and at margins of the cerebellar cortex, that is particularly in the nodulus, flocculus, tonsils, in the lingula at the medullary velum, and at the borders of cortex and cerebellar peduncles. At all these sites one may find foci of abrupt disorganization in cortical architecture, with islands of superficial granular layer, molecular layer, and granular layer dispersed at random and disalignment of the Purkinje cells. Although these dysplastic zones are relatively small, they tend to be rather conspicuous in young infants due to the cellularity of their superficial granular layer. When the same regions are studied in adults, one finds minor disorganizations in cortical architecture, with disalignment of Purkinje cells and irregular disposition of the granular layer. Since focal dysplasias are common in the nodulus, they are often seen in the herniated cerebellar vermis in the Arnold-Chiari malformation, and they have been unduly emphasized as evidence of abnormal cerebellar development. The majority of the small focal cortical dysplasias at the margins of cerebellar cortex are developmental variants of no consequence. The cerebellar cortical dysplasias in malformed brains described as heterotaxias by Brun (1917) were, generally, of this type, and Brun mentions in a footnote that he found the same type of lesion in serial sections of the brain of a normal 16-day-old child that he used as a laboratory standard.

The lesions commonly reported as micropolygyria of the cerebellar cortex have essentially the same microscopic structure as the small foci of dysplasia in the marginal portions of the cerebellar cortex (Fig. 110). The so-called micropolygyrias are much larger, however, and they affect any portion of the cerebellar cortex, unilateral or bilateral, or they occupy large portions of the hemispheric surface. They are sharply delineated from the adjacent normal cortex, and gliosis, scarring or atrophy are absent. The cortex is thicker than normal, and the dysplasia is made up of interlacing nests of granular and molecular layers; Purkinje cells are disposed mostly at the boundaries of these layers. There is no evidence of excessive cortical folding or of selective destruction of certain neuronal components of the cortex. The cortical surface may appear abnormally smooth where dysplastic tissue is exposed.

Focal dysplasia of the cerebellar cortex may occur as the sole lesion, or coexist with a variety of other cerebral malformations, particularly with polymicrogyria of the cerebral cortex, especially often in cases in whom intrauterine infective processes were documented or suspected (Chapter 16).

Diffuse Hypertrophy of Cerebellar Cortex. These lesions are included here for completeness of reference although they have not been observed in children and their classification as dysplasias is debatable. The first report on diffuse hypertrophy of cerebellar cortex is that of Lhermitte and Duclos (1920), and the subsequent literature consists almost entirely of single case reports. Hallervorden (1959) listed 21 cases; Cook *et al.* (1962), who introduced the name "diffuse hypertrophy of the cerebellum", found 26. The lesions have been reported earlier under a great variety of names such as Purkinjeoma, gangliocytoma, gangliocytoma amyelinicum diffusum, myelinated neurocytoma or gangliocytoma dysplasticum. The disease produces increased intracranial pressure; its average course lasts from one to a few years, but extremes range from 4 months to 30 years; males are affected with greater frequency.

There is a circumscribed enlargement of one portion of a cerebellar hemisphere, which may extend into the vermis or, occasionally, into the contralateral hemisphere. The enlarged portion shows a fairly sharp boundary with the adjacent normal cortex. The gyri in the enlarged portion are broadened and firm to the touch. On cross section there is continuity between normal cortex and cortex in the lesion, but in the latter the gyri are coarsened and the cortex is much thicker than normal. Microscopic examination discloses

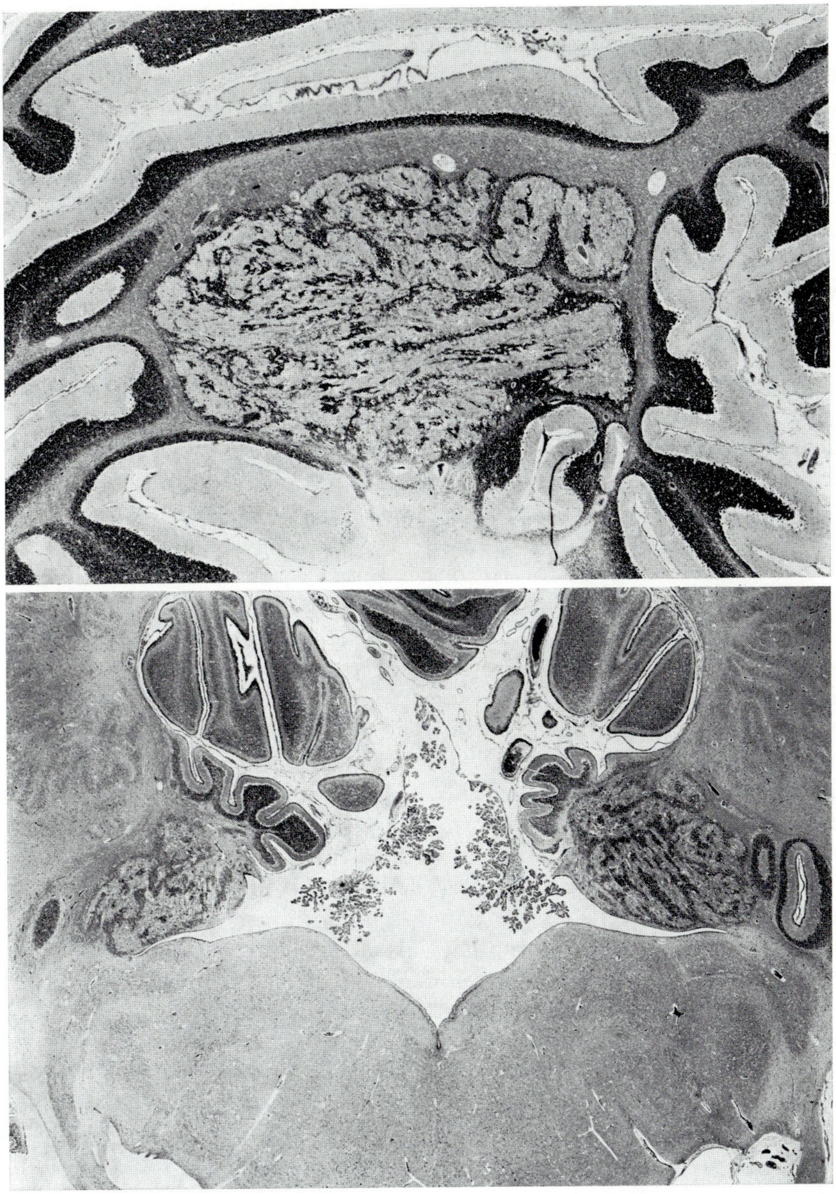

Fig. 110. Focal dysplasia of cerebellar cortex, often referred to as polymicrogyria. Top: an isolated dysplasia in the hemispheric cortex; H & E ×11.5. Bottom: unusually large, symmetric foci of dysplasia in the paraflocculi; H & E ×7

a thick layer of abnormal nerve cells underneath the molecular layer, replacing the granular layer. Some of these cells are of the size and configuration of Purkinje cells, but many are somewhat smaller, though still larger than granule cells. The folia of white matter entering the abnormal gyri are thinner than normal and contain only a few myelinated fibers, or, occasionally, none at all. The molecular layer is often thicker than normal and receives myelinated fibers which radiate from the abnormal cell population toward the cortical surface. There may be mineral deposits in the tissue and in the walls of the blood vessels. The abnormal cortex blends with the adjacent normal cortex; at the junction the layer of abnormally large cells can be seen to override the granular layer. A detailed account of the microscopic features of these lesions was given by Hallervorden (1959).

Diffuse hypertrophy of the cerebellar cortex has been considered neoplastic on the basis of the increase in cerebellar volume, increase in intracranial pressure and the progressive course of the disease. The lesions are exceptional, however, in the faithful production of a regular though distinctly abnormal cortical architecture, with emission of abnormal fiber plexus into the molecular layer. They differ from gangliocytomas in that they are entirely neuronal and do not involve abnormal proliferation of the glia tissue.

Lesions of Experimental Damage to the Superficial Granular Layer. Granular layer aplasia has been known for a long time. Yet, only recently have experimental data led to the understanding of its pathogenesis and its derivation from damage to the superficial granular layer. The data were obtained from systematic studies of the effects of X-radiation on the developing cerebellum, combined with radioautographic and electron microscopic methods. These are of such importance for the understanding of human pathology that they are reviewed here as an introduction to the description of the lesions found in human brains. The most comprehensive and cohesive series of experiments was performed by Altman and coworkers, whose numerous reports form the basis of the following paragraphs.

The outer granular layer may be destroyed subtotally by application of 200 R X-rays during the first 5 days of life; necrosis of granule cells, with reduced width of the outer granular layer, develops within 24 to 48 hours. However, even near total destruction of the layer is followed by complete or subtotal restitution within 4 days. Due to this prodigious power of regeneration, a completely normal cerebellum may be found after the rats have grown up (Altman *et al.*, 1969). Permanent elimination of the superficial granular layer necessitates repetition of damage over an extended period. If radiation is applied from birth through the 13th day, the formation of basket, stellate and granule cells is essentially prevented, except for the nodulus and uvula which mature earlier. The main neuronal component of the damaged cortex are the Purkinje cells, which are tightly crowded because of arrested cortical surface growth, and which have a tendency to scatter into the molecular layer. Anomalies in the growth and alignment of the dendrites are also seen. If the damage is started on the 4th postnatal day and continued through the 13th day, the Purkinje cells are initially aligned in a monolayer, but they become disaligned later and develop distortions of their dendritic arborization as their crowding does not permit normal expansion. Abnormal synaptic contacts with normally not affiliated fibers are seen with the electron microscope (Altman and Anderson, 1973). This type of lesion has all the features of granular layer aplasia in man.

The lesions are substantially modified if the outer granular layer is permitted to regenerate after being damaged by daily radiation for several days; the critical factor is not the age at which damage is started, but that when it is discontinued. Incomplete or delayed regeneration of the superficial granular layer results in ectopia of granule cells and in reorientation of parallel fibers (Altman, 1973). The ectopic granule cells are fixed in the lower portion of the molecular layer, in which they form a lamina of increased cell density, the cells either being diffusely scattered or clustered. The distance of this abnormal cell layer from the cortical surface varies regionally; generally, it is situated the closer to the cortical surface the later the damage is discontinued. This phenomenon was explained by Ebels (1972) and Altman (1973) as a disturbance of the coordination between the descent of granule cells from the cortical surface and the ascent of the afferent mossy fibers. It was postulated that the mossy fibers grow into the molecular layer if the descent of granule cells is delayed, and that the descent of these cells becomes arrested when they reach contact with mossy fibers. Accordingly, the ectopic cells become fixed the nearer to the cortical surface the greater the delay is in their descent.

Animals with granule cell ectopia also exhibit an alteration in the fiber texture of the molecular layer, described as "reorientation of parallel fibers". This change consists of an abnormal layer of tightly packed fibers located in the superficial portion of the molecular layer; the abnormal layer is sharply separated from the inner portion of the molecular layer, even in electron micrographs. Its fine structure consists of tightly packed neurites rather than of glial fibers. These neurites do not run parallel to the axis of gyri, as the so-called parallel fibers normally do. The abnormal superficial layer of fibers may be associated with a characteristic stunting in the growth of Purkinje cell dendrites, which do not enter the abnormal layer and appear like cut-off at its lower border. These types of changes, granule cell ectopia and reorientation of superficial fibers, are also seen in human pathology.

The experiments reviewed above pertain to lesions produced by variation in the age when X-ray radiation is applied, a technique developed by Hicks (1950). Similar changes can be induced by postnatal X-irradiation in puppies (Phemister *et al.*, 1969). The lesions may be duplicated with other agents damaging the dividing cells of the outer granular layer with similar selectivity. The capacity of the superficial granular layer to restore after a single episode of damage can also be seen after postnatal treatment of rats with 5-fluorodeoxyuridine, an agent that interferes with DNA synthesis, or with the aglycone of cycasine, a known teratogenic agent, or with cyclophosphamide (Hirano *et al.*, 1969; Shimada and Langman, 1970; Nathanson *et al.*, 1969). All these agents can induce aplasia of the granular layer and granule cell ectopia. An entirely different type of agent, which is of great potential significance in human pathology, is intrauterine infection with rat virus or panleukopenia virus; these infections induce granular layer aplasia in cats, rats, and ferrets (Kilham and Margolis, 1966; Margolis *et al.*, 1966). The viruses have special affinity for the dividing cells of, among other tissues, the superficial granular layer; nuclear inclusions may be found in the latter. Infection with tamiami virus also induces granule cell ectopia (Gilden *et al.*, 1971). A hereditary disturbance of the superficial granular layer appears to be present in the staggerer mutant of the mouse (Sidman *et al.*, 1962).

Granular Layer Aplasia (Primary Degeneration of the Granular Layer). The first report of this type of cerebellar cortical lesion was published for a litter of cats by Herringham and Andrew (1888); another extremely similar litter was described by Jelgersma (1917). Occurrence of a granular layer aplasia in man is not linked to a single specific etiology. It may occur in the absence of recognized general disease processes as the sole cerebral lesion. These patients show disturbances in coordination and, rather consistently, severe retardation of intellectual development. The symptoms are present from early childhood and remain stationary; epileptic convulsions are not a characteristic feature. The disease is rare and is observed in sporadic cases (Ule, 1952) or in siblings (Norman, 1940; Jervis, 1950). Granular layer aplasia was also described in an infant that had been subjected to radium irradiation during the 5th to 6th month of gestation (Van Bogaert and Rademecker, 1955): Aplasia of the granular layer affected the cerebellar hemispheres; the Purkinje cells had persisted and were displaced into the molecular layer; the vermis was spared. This interesting case is probably the closest approximation between human pathology and the experimental lesions described above.

Inspection of the brain in cases of granular layer aplasia usually discloses no disorganization of the cerebral hemispheres, although the brain weight is reduced, often in excess of the loss accounted for by the cerebellar atrophy. The normal gyral pattern of the cerebral hemispheres is in sharp contrast to the severe atrophy of the cerebellar cortex. The atrophy affects vermis as well as hemispheres, although the damage may be less severe in vermis, tonsils and flocculi. The shrunken cerebellar cortex is whitish, sclerotic, and firm to the touch, and the diminuted atrophic gyri are readily discernible on the cortical surface. Microscopic examination discloses marked thinning of the cortex, in which the layer of Purkinje cells is the predominant if not the sole neuronal component. The bodies of these cells appear to be unusually large in comparison to the diminuted gyri. The cells may be packed abnormally thight, but their density is subject to variation. Cells are often disaligned and some are dislocated into the superficial portions of the molecular layer *. The latter is much thinner than normal and the granular layer is subtotally or completely devoid of granule cells. The damage in the white matter is surprisingly slight. Myelinated white matter extends into the atrophic gyri, and myelinated fibers are found immediately underneath the

* To be distinguished from the occasional displacement of a single Purkinje cell into the molecular or the granular layer, a change that can be seen on scrutiny in almost every cerebellum.

Purkinje layer. There may be marked gliosis throughout the cortex, which has been interpreted as evidence of scarring, but the increase in glial density will also result from the shrinkage of tissue alone, after the neuronal population has disappeared. The dentate and olivary nuclei may be normal or may show loss of neurons.

Deformities in the shape and ramification of the dendritic trees of Purkinje cells consist of asymmetry or of rudimentary development of branchings. Local swellings of dendrites are called "asteroid bodies" and consist of local pools of dendritic cytoplasm from which numerous thin anomalous dendrites radiate in all directions. These pools can be seen with conventional stains as angulated aggregates of cytoplasm in the molecular layer; demonstration of their relationship to deformed Purkinje dendrites requires silver impregnation. "Cactus shaped" or other bizarre dendritic deformities are also seen. The dendritic deformities are not specific for granular layer aplasia and occur in other types of cerebellar lesions dating to the developmental period. Dendritic deformities have been observed, on occasion, in damaged adult cerebellar cortex, but their occurrence in abundance, particularly in the form of typical asteroid bodies, seems to be fairly characteristic of infantile cerebellar damage. Asteroid bodies are most likely to develop upon damage during the period of maximum growth of the Purkinje dendrites, that is between the 36th month of gestation and the 8th postnatal month (Chapter 1).

Axonal swellings of Purkinje cells are commonly referred to as torpedoes. They occur in the proximity of the cell body and are always situated within the granular layer. Their shape is irregular, drop shaped, or fusiform. Torpedoes are nonspecific manifestations of cerebellar cortical damage and develop in adults as well as in infants.

The description of granular layer aplasia given above refers to instances in which it is found as the only or, at least, the dominant lesion. However, aplasia of the granular layer occurs also as a component of the cerebral changes of many infantile metabolic diseases. A typical example is GM_2 gangliosidosis (Chapter 36) in which the atrophic cerebellum may show a preferential loss of the granule cells with persistence of Purkinje cells (Bielschowsky, 1920), as well as granule cell ectopia and reorientation of superficial fibers in the molecular layer. The changes may be less specific from the start, or the pattern of granular layer aplasia may become obliterated upon destruction of the Purkinje cell population. Granular layer aplasia may also be found in a variety of other metabolic diseases such as metachromatic leukodystrophy (Chapter 38), mannosidosis (Chapter 35), Pelizaeus-Merzbacher disease and related conditions (Chapter 41), or as a syndrome with congenital thrombocytopenia (Chapter 46), attesting to the nonspecific nature of etiologic factors.

Ectopia of Granule Cells and Reorientation of Superficial Fiber Plexus. The experimental production of this type of lesions is described earlier in this chapter. They have received comparatively little attention in human pathology. The first report of granule cell ectopia was apparently published by Deganello and Spangaro, and their illustrations were reprinted by Vogt and Astwazaturow (1912), showing separation of the molecular layer into two laminae, the lower having increased cell density. Bielschowsky (1913, 1920) noticed increased cell density in the lower portion of the cerebellar molecular layer in cases of amaurotic idiocy, and they described a stratum of densely packed fibers at the surface of the molecular layer; however, the latter has often been interpreted as superficial gliosis (Westphal, 1917). The association of increased cell density in the lower portion of the molecular layer and reorientation of superficial fibers was described by the present author (1964) as a distinctive type of cerebellar cortical degeneration (arrested cerebellar development) in 6 cases.

Ectopia of granule cells is usually a component of aplasia or of hypoplasia of the internal granular layer, and the gross appearance of the cerebellum is similar for both. In ectopia of granule cells there is an increased cell density in the lower portion of the molecular layer which contains numerous small round nuclei in random distribution or in local aggregates. The zone of increased cell density is usually sharply separated from the upper portion of the molecular layer in which cell density is normal.

Ectopia of granule cells without other changes in the cerebellar cortex has also been observed coexistent with pachygyria of the cerebral cortex, probably as a manifestation of a widespread derangement of neuronal migration. Crome (1956) described this change in terms of an increased cell density of the lower portion of the molecular layer in a pachygyric patient, and Wiest and Hallervorden (1958) illustrated lenticular islands of granule cells, their long axes parallel to the cortical surface, in one case of pachygyria and one of diffuse laminar heterotopia (Chapter 29). Using silver impregnations, a few ectopic granule cells may be found in the cerebellar cortex of normal laboratory animals (Sosa *et al.*, 1971).

Ectopia of granule cells in the depth of the molecular layer usually coexists with reorientation of fiber plexus at the surface of the molecular layer, except for the cases in whom it is associated with pachygyria. In reorientation of superficial fibers the texture of the molecular layer permits distinction of two sharply separated zones: The lower zone shows the characteristic criss-crossing of fibers and cell processes running perpendicular as well as parallel to the cortical surface, while the superficial zone is almost entirely devoid of perpendicular elements, containing tightly packed fibers running parallel to the cortical surface (Fig. 111). The boundary between these two zones runs parallel to the cortical surface, but its distance from the cortical surface varies, usually being greater in the depth of sulci than at the crown of gyri, a feature consistent with the different speed of maturation of gyri and sulci (Altman, 1969). Silver impregnations of the dendritic arborizations of the Purkinje cells show the dendrites restricted sharply to the lower zone, and terminating, as if cut off, at the border of the superficial fiber layer. When stained with various enzyme histochemical methods, the superficial layer of parallel fiber lacks succinate dehydrogenase, cytochrome oxydase and NAD-diaphorase, but it contains increased activities of nonspecific cholinesterase and acetyl cholinesterase (Friede, 1964). The latter is consistent with the occurrence of neurites in the fiber plexus. In experimental studies, formation of the superficial fiber plexus has been attributed to reorientation of parallel fibers. However, as Ule (1952)

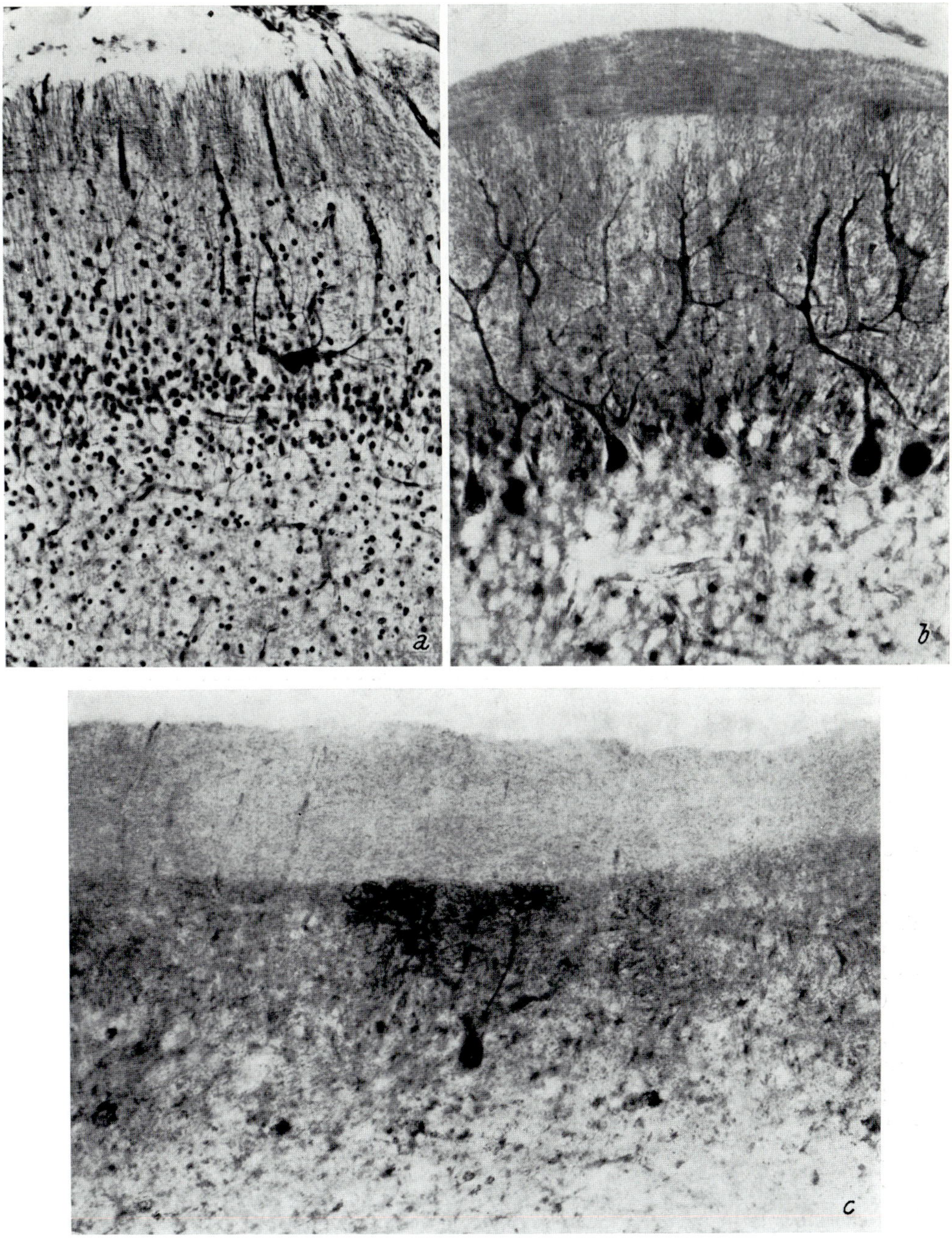

Fig. 111. Ectopia of granule cells and reorientation of superficial fiber plexus. A: Bodian stain shows ectopic granule cells in the lower portion of the molecular layer and aplasia of granular layer; ×100. B: Sharp separation of layers is evident with the histochemical reaction for lactate dehydrogenase; ×100. C: Cutoff of Purkinje dendrites at the interface of the layers is shown with the reaction for NAD-diaphorase; ×90

has pointed out, there is considerable ambiguity in the usage of the terms tangential and parallel fibers, as well as in their alleged origin. In summary, ectopia of granule cells and formation of a superficial fiber plexus in the molecular layer may be considered variants of granular layer aplasia resulting from abortive regeneration of the superficial granular layer following prolonged damage.

References

Altman, J.: Autoradiographic and histological studies of postnatal neurogenesis. III. Dating the time of production and onset of differentiation of cerebellar microneurons in rats. J. comp. Neurol. 136: 269—293, 1969.

— Experimental reorganization of the cerebellar cortex. III. Regeneration of the external germinal layer and granule cell ectopia. J. comp. Neurol. 149: 153—180, 1973.

— Experimental reorganization of the cerebellar cortex. IV. Parallel fiber reorientation following regeneration of the external germinal layer. J. comp. Neurol. 149: 181—192, 1973.

— Anderson, W. J.: Experimental reorganization of the cerebellar cortex. II. Effects of elimination of most microneurons with prolonged X-irradiation started at four days. J. comp. Neurol. 149: 123—152, 1973.

— — Wright, K. A.: Reconstitution of the external granular layer of the cerebellar cortex in infant rats after low-level X-irradiation. Anat. Rec. 163: 453—472, 1969.

Bielschowsky, M.: Über spätinfantile familiäre amaurotische Idiotie mit Kleinhirnsymptomen. Dtsch. Z. Nervenheilk. 50: 7—29, 1913.

— Zur Histopathologie und Pathogenese der amaurotischen Idiotie mit besonderer Berücksichtigung der zerebellären Veränderungen. J. Psychol. Neurol. 26: 123—244, 1920.

Brun, A.: Zur Kenntnis der Bildungsfehler des Kleinhirns. Schweiz. Arch. Neurol. Psychiat. 1: 61—123; 2: 48—105; 3: 13—88, 1917/18.

Cook, T., Holt, S., Yates, P. O.: Diffuse hypertrophy of the cerebellum. J. Neurol. Neurosurg. Psychiat. 25: 218—221, 1962.

Crome, L.: Pachygyria. J. Path. Bact. 71: 335—352, 1956.

Das, G. D., Nornes, H. O.: Neurogenesis in the cerebellum of the rat: An autoradiographic study. Z. Anat. Entwickl.-Gesch. 138: 155—165, 1972.

Deganello and Spangaro: Cited from Vogt and Astwazaturow.

Ebels, E. J.: Studies on ectopic granule cells in the cerebellar cortex—with a hypothesis as to their aetiology and pathogenesis. Acta neuropath. (Berl.) 21: 117—127, 1972.

Friede, R. L.: Arrested cerebellar development: a type of cerebellar degeneration in amaurotic idiocy. J. Neurol. Neurosurg. Psychiat. 27: 41—45, 1964.

— Further clinical and histochemical data on arrested cerebellar development. Neurology (Minneap.) 14: 1054—1057, 1964.

Gilden, D. H., Friedman, H. M., Nathanson, N.: Tamiami virus induced cerebellar heterotopia. J. Neuropath. exp. Neurol. 33: 29—41, 1974.

Hallervorden, J.: Über die Harmartome (Ganglioneurome) des Kleinhirns. Dtsch. Z. Nervenheilk. 179: 531—563, 1959.

Herndon, R. M., Margolis, G., Kilham, L.: The synaptic organization of the malformed cerebellum induced by perinatal infection with the feline panleukopenia virus (PLV). I. Elements forming the cerebellar glomeruli. J. Neuropath. exp. Neurol. 30: 196—205, 1971.

Herringham, W. P., Andrews, F. W.: Two cases of cerebellar disease in cats, with staggering. St. Barth. Hosp. Rep. 24: 241, 1888.

Hicks, S. P.: Acute necrosis and malformation of developing mammalian brain caused by X-ray. Proc. Soc. exp. Biol. Med. 75: 458—489, 1950.

Hirano, I., Shibuya, C., Hayashi, K.: Induction of a cerebellar disorder with cycasin in newborn mice and hamsters. Proc. Soc. exp. Biol. Med. 131: 593—669, 1969.

Jelgersma, G.: Drei Fälle von Cerebellar-Atrophie bei der Katze; nebst Bemerkungen über das cerebro-cerebellare Verbindungssystem. J. Psychol. Neurol. (Lpz.) 23: 105—134, 1917.

Jervis, G. A.: Early familial cerebellar degeneration. J. nerv. ment. Dis. 111: 398—407, 1950.
Kilham, L., Margolis, G.: Viral etiology of spontaneous ataxia of cats. Amer. J. Path. 48: 991—1011, 1966.
— — Spontaneous hepatitis and cerebellar "hypoplasia" in suckling rats due to congenital infections with rat virus. Amer. J. Path. 49: 457—475, 1966.
Lhermitte, J., Duclos, P.: Sur un ganglioneurome diffus du cortex du cervelet. Bull. Assoc. franç. Cancer 9: 99—107, 1920.
Mareš, V., Lodin, Z.: The cellular kinetics of the developing mouse cerebellum. II. The function of the external granular layer in the process of gyrifaction. Brain Res. 23: 343—352, 1970.
Margolis, G., Kilham, L., Johnson, R. H.: The paraviruses and replicating cells. Insights into the pathogenesis of cerebellar hypoplasia. Lab. Invest. 17: 465—475, 1966.
Meschede, F.: Heterotopie grauer Hirnsubstanz im Markstamme der Hemisphären des kleinen Gehirns. Drei Beobachtungen. Virchows Arch. 56: 82—96, 1872.
Nathanson, N., Cole, G. A., van der Loos, H.: Heterotopic cerebellar granule cells following administration of cyclophosphamide to suckling rats. Brain Res. 15: 532—536, 1969.
Norman, R. M.: Primary degeneration of the granular layer of the cerebellum: An unusual form of familial cerebellar atrophy occurring in early life. Brain 63: 365—379, 1940.
Phemister, R. D., Shirely, J. N., Young, S.: The effects of gamma irradiation on the postnatally developing canine cerebellar cortex. J. Neuropath. exp. Neurol. 28: 119—127, 1969.
Rorke, L. B., Fogelson, M. H., Riggs, H. E.: Cerebellar heterotopia in infancy. Develop. Med. Child. Neurol. 10: 644—650, 1968.
Shimada, M., Langman, J.: Repair of the external granular layer of the hamster cerebellum after prenatal and postnatal administration of methylazoxymethanol. Teratology 3: 119—134, 1970.
Sidman, R. L., Lane, P. W., Dickie, M. M.: Staggerer, a new mutation in the mouse affecting the cerebellum. Science 137: 610—612, 1962.
Sosa, J. M., Palacios, E., de Sosa, M. S.: Heterotopic cerebellar granule cells inside the plexiform layer. Acta Anat. 80: 91—98, 1971.
Ule, G.: Kleinhirnrindenatrophie vom Körnertyp. Dtsch. Z. Nervenheilk. 168: 195—226, 1952.
van Bogaert, L., Radermecker, M. A.: Une dysgénésie cérébelleuse chez un enfant du radium. Rev. Neurol. (Paris) 93: 65—82, 1955.
Vogt, H., Astwazaturow, M.: Über angeborene Kleinhirnerkrankungen mit Beiträgen zur Entwicklungsgeschichte des Kleinhirns. Arch. Psychiat. Nervenkr. 49: 75—203, 1912.
Westphal, A.: Beitrag zur Lehre von der amaurotischen Idiotie. Arch. Psychiat. Nervenkr. 58: 248—283, 1917.
Wiest, W. D.: Hallervorden, J.: Migrationshemmungen im Groß- und Kleinhirn. Dtsch. Z. Nervenheilk. 178: 224—238, 1958.

32. Dysplasias of Brain Stem and Spinal Cord

Congenital Facial- and Ophthalmoplegia. Infants afflicted by this uncommon disease exhibit a peculiar facies from birth, characterized by drooping corners of the mouth in association with variable manifestations of ophthalmoplegia. A review of 61 cases by Henderson (1939) showed facial dysplasia in all, abducens palsy in 45, external ophthalmoplegia in 15, ptosis in 6, lingual paresis in 18 and trigeminal paresis in 4; other abnormalities were club foot (19), brachial malformations (13), pectoral muscle defects (8), and mental deficiency (6).

There are only few autopsy reports in the literature (Heubner, 1900; Rainy and Fowler, 1903; Spatz and Ullrich, 1931). The lesions are characterized by hypoplasia or absence of the affected nuclear groups and their nerve roots; the persisting nerve cells may be abnormally small or heterotopic. The nuclear territories are shrunken, but the residual neurons are uniformly distributed without the focal gaps that suggest dropping out of cells. Glial proliferation and scar formation are absent. Sensory nuclei are spared; the dorsal longitudinal fascicle was found intact by Spatz and Ullrich but missing by Heubner. The lesions tend to be bilateral and symmetrical, though unilateral hypoplasia of the facial nucleus was observed by Richter (1960). Pitner *et al.* (1965) present a case in which they found subtotal unilateral absence of the inferior olivary nucleus and hemihypoplasia of the cerebellum, its peduncles and the dentate nucleus. The facial nerve nuclei were intact, but severe hypoplasia was found in the facial muscles. The authors suggest in their comprehensive discussion that the syndrome, similar to arthrogryphosis, may be either neurogenic or myogenic.

The changes of hypotensive brain stem necrosis (Chapter 9) need to be considered in the differential diagnosis of this disease, particularly as some of the patients have a record of difficult birth, such as for the case reported by Möbius (1888), after whom the syndrome is often named. These two disease processes differ in clinical course and in the type of lesion: Congenital facial- and ophthalmoplegia is characterized by stationary cranial nerve defects from birth and by atrophy of the nuclei without scarring; hypotensive brain stem necrosis develops after cardiac arrest and shows scarring of cranial nerve nuclei, particularly in their central portion, and is often associated with more widespread neuronal loss in other portions of the brain.

Dysplasias of the Inferior Olivary Nuclei. Dysplasias of the inferior olivary nuclei occur in association with other cerebral malformations; there does not appear to be any satisfactory documentation of their occurrence in the absence of the latter. Two general categories of dysplasias may be distinguished—the heterotopias, and the dysplasias affecting the structure of the nucleus itself. The clinical features of these lesions are dominated by the associated malformations.

Heterotopias of the inferior olivary nuclei typically occur in association with agyria or pachygyria (Chapter 29) but not with polymicrogyria; they have also been observed with the Dandy-Walker malformation (Chapter 30). The lesions consist of single or multiple, irregularly shaped islands of gray matter, commonly found along a line extending from the inferior olivary nucleus to the lateral edge of the fourth ventricle near the corpus restiforme. Heterotopic islands are found less frequently closer to the midline near the hypoglossal rootlets (Fig. 112). The heterotopias vary from microscopic to fairly large masses of gray matter, which are identified as belonging to the inferior olivary nucleus by their mimicking its characteristic convoluted pattern; the size of the nerve cells and their arrangement within a generous amount of neuropil without myelinated fibers is also reminiscent of the olivary nucleus. The heterotopias are sharply outlined by a layer of encompassing myelinated fibers at their immediate surface.

Olivary heterotopias are generally considered the results of arrest of migration of neuroblasts from the matrix tissue to their permanent destination. The neurons of the inferior olivary nucleus originate from the rhombic lip (His, 1891; Essick, 1912), from where they migrate in a ventromedial direction. Ellenberger *et al.* (1969) reviewed the various usages of the term rhombic lip and concluded that it should be used to designate the lateral extension of the actively proliferating neuroepithelium at the dorsal surface of the brain stem, at least when used for rodents. Their radioautographic studies with tritiated thymidine show that most olivary neurons originate

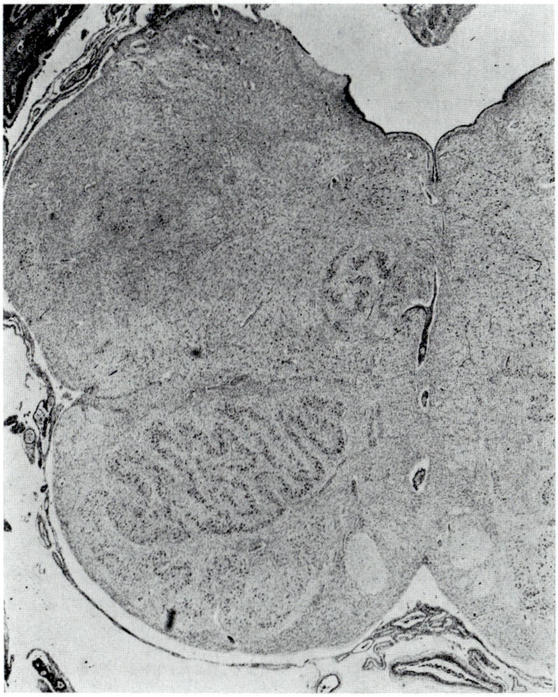

Fig. 112. Anomalous architecture of inferior olivary nucleus and heterotopia of same (underneath the hypoglossal nucleus) in a pachygyric brain; cresyl violet ×9.5

from the lateral portion of the neural plate (rhombic lip); a smaller portion originates closer to the midline, explaining the occasional olivary heterotopias in the medial portion of the medulla oblongata. Formation of olivary neurons in mice occurs on the 10th day of gestation (Table 1); in rats, on the 14th and 15th day, the olivary nucleus being well formed by the 21st day (Ellenberger *et al.*, 1969). The corresponding developmental period in man has not been established with the same precision, but the migration of neuroblasts to the olivary nucleus has been observed in fetuses of 20 mm to 143 mm length (Essick, 1912), that is mostly before the 3rd month of pregnancy. Formation of olivary heterotopias, therefore, dates to the first trimester of pregnancy.

Dysplasias of the inferior olivary nucleus occur with cerebellar aplasia and with 17–18 trisomy. The latter are characterized by a thickening of the dorsal portion of the nucleus with obliteration of its undulating profile (Chapter 33). The dysplasia in cerebellar agenesis varies; the nucleus may show a simplified structure resembling a hook or a "C"; its dorsal portion is usually thinner than normal and there may be regional loss of neurons, indicating superseding processes of transneuronal degeneration. Atrophy and gliosis of the inferior olivary nucleus also develops secondary to acquired cerebellar lesions from transneuronal degeneration, but these lesions do not represent developmental dysplasias in a strict sense. A dysplastic olivary nucleus is also seen in Zellweger's syndrome (Chapter 29).

Nonspecific Deformities of Brain Stem. Disorganization of the architecture of the brain stem, with gross distortions in anatomy and with aplasia or disorganization of nuclei and fiber tracts, is observed with occipital encephalocele. It also occurs with anencephaly or hydranencephaly provided these lesions extend into the posterior fossa. These changes are secondary to the massive deformities of the cerebral or cerebellar hemispheres; no specific or characteristic pattern of disorganization has emerged, except for anomalies in the crossing of corticospinal tracts.

Anomalies of Corticospinal Tracts. Four types of anomalies of corticospinal tract relate to the developmental period: 1. Variations in the course of the tract, 2. aplasia, 3. degeneration, and 4. hypertrophy. Only the first two lesions are dysplasias in a strict sense; however, the difference between aplasia and degeneration is often only in the severity and in the timing of the corresponding hemispheric lesions.

The most common anomalies in the course of the corticospinal tract consist of incomplete or absent crossing (Fig. 113). Absent decussation without cerebral malformations is rare (Verhaart and Kramer, 1952) and is probably an extreme degree of incomplete crossing. In incomplete crossing a majority of the fibers descends in the ventral corticospinal tract which is much larger than normal; only a small portion of the fibers crosses into the lateral corticospinal tract which normally receives more than 90 percent of the descending fibers. Incomplete crossing may occur unilateral; in these instances there is an increase in the volume of the white matter on one side of the cord, which contains both the uncrossed fibers from the homolateral hemisphere and the crossed fibers from the contralateral hemisphere; the other half of the cord is correspondingly reduced in volume. These dysplasias are uncommon, though not extremely rare, and were illustrated by Obersteiner (1912) and Crosby (1962). Anomalies in the crossing of corticospinal tract often occur in infants with encephaloceles (Verhaart and Kramer, 1952) or with other types of malformations, although they may escape detection being overshadowed by the other, more conspicuous lesions.

An anomalous descent of the corticospinal tract at the periphery of the cord, at the very surface of the lateral tracts, is rare. This anomaly was described by Verhaart and Kramer (1952) in an infant with encephalocele and was associated with an abnormally high crossing of the tracts in the brain stem. Another, less important anomaly occasionally seen in newborns is an exaggerated fasciculation at the level of the pyramids, where the tract may appear separated into numerous round to oval bundles by intervening

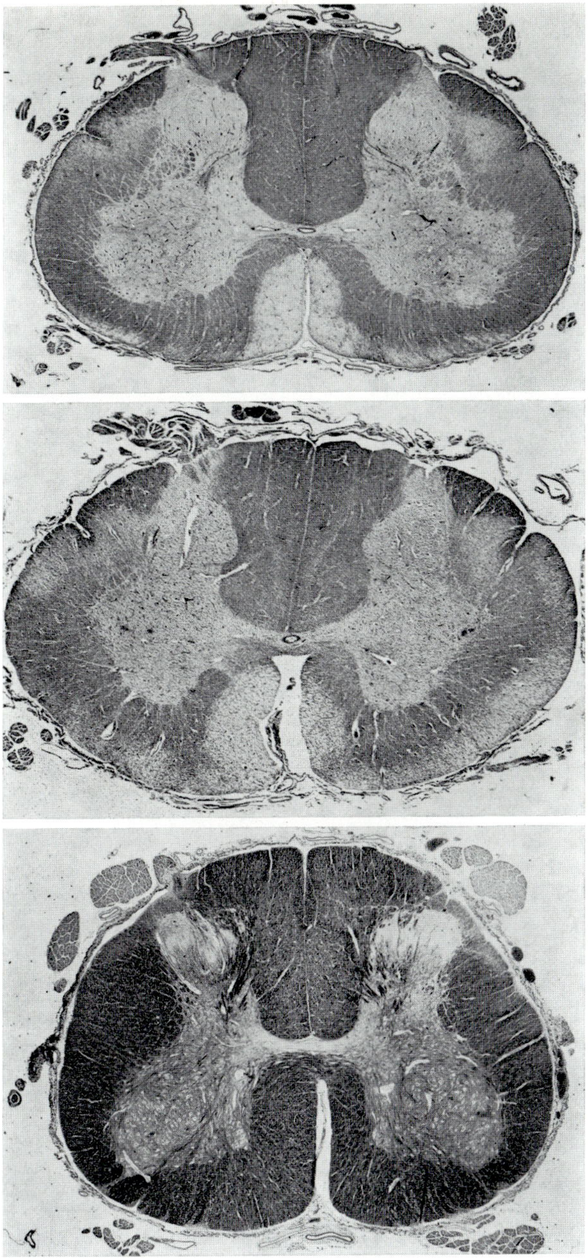

Fig. 113. Anomalous crossing of corticospinal tracts. Top: Newborn infant; a large portion of the tracts descends uncrossed; the tracts are readily discernible because of their absent myelination; ×14.5. Middle: Newborn; incomplete crossing and anomalous descent of the tract at the lateral surface of the cord; ×12. Bottom: Unilateral crossing of the tract in an adult; the anomaly is here evident only from the asymmetric volume of white matter as the tracts are fully myelinated; ×7

strands of glia tissue (Fig. 114). Asymmetric distribution of fiber bundles may also be seen in malformed brains at the pontine level, where the fibers traverse the islands of pontine gray matter.

There is no convincing evidence that anomalous crossing of the corticospinal tract is of clinical significance. False localizing signs may be expected only for discrete spinal lesions since the abnormal fibers do in all probability cross over near the level of their termination, similar to the behavior of the normal ventral corticospinal tract. False localizing signs have been alledged

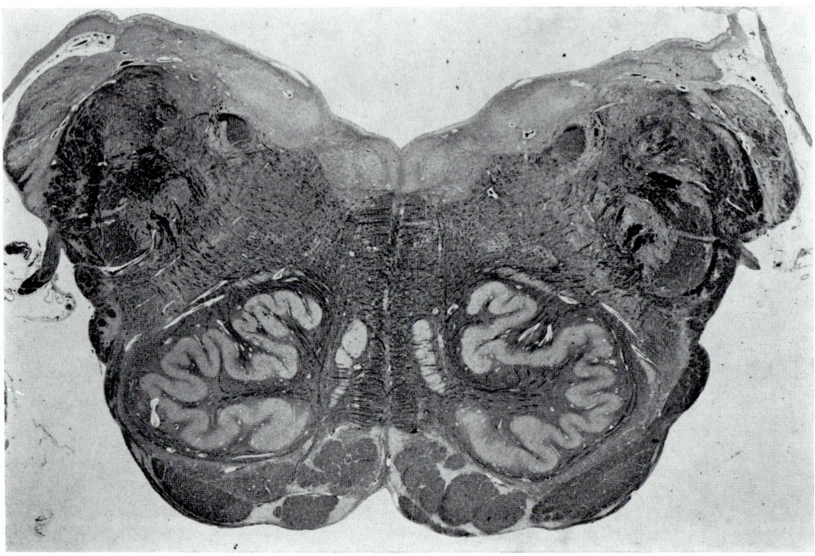

Fig. 114. Separation of corticospinal tract into fascicles; ×6.5

(Zenner, 1898), but in this case the extent of neoplastic invasion of the cerebral hemispheres by a tumor, probably a glioblastoma, had not been examined.

Aplasia of the corticospinal tract is observed with cortical defects or with profound hemispheric or cortical disorganization. It is a consistent feature in anencephaly and in holoprosencephaly; it also occurs in many instances of porencephaly and hydranencephaly. Aplasia of the corticospinal tract induces a closer spacing of the pontine islands of gray matter (Fig. 74). In the medulla there is absence of the pyramids and the olivary nuclei are approximated directly underneath the ventral surface of the medulla. They are covered with a layer of marginal glia of normal thickness, and there is no evidence of increased cell density or glial scarring. The cross-section of the spinal cord shows a characteristic change in configuration, caused by the predominance of the normal sized dorsal tracts, due to which the dorsal horns are rotated latero-ventrally, the lateral and ventral fiber tracts being very small. There are no discrete zones of absence of fibers. An abnormal sulcus may be seen at the lateral surfaces of the cord.

Aplasia may blend with degeneration if the lesions occur during the period of outgrowth of corticospinal fibers. If the hemispheric lesions form during the 5th or 6th fetal month, the spinal cord may show relatively small, hypoplastic tracts. Lesions occurring at a later stage induce degeneration of the tract; there is a normal configuration of the cross-section of the spinal cord, and the degenerated corticospinal tracts stand out as pale nonmyelinated areas in the lateral tracts (Halsey *et al.*, 1971).

Hypertrophy of the corticospinal tract is an uncommon anomaly, of which less than 20 cases have been reported. The earlier literature was reviewed by van der Bruggen (1930), Verhaart (1947, 1950) added four cases, and newer reports were published by Balthasar and Schlagenhauff (1965) and Scales and Collins (1972). Hypertrophy of the corticospinal tract is unilateral in the majority of cases; the contralateral tract is absent or severely atrophic, and there are cerebral lesions dating to infancy or early childhood. An exception are the three cases reported by Anton (1922), in whom hypertrophy of the corticospinal tract coexisted with extensive cerebellar defects. These cases, however, are described only briefly, without any specific documentation, and one of them had anomalous crossing of the corticospinal tract.

Unilateral hypertrophy of the tract is manifest by its exceptional bulk, whereby the homolateral inferior olivary nucleus is displaced dorsally; the hypertrophic tract may extend across the midline, bulging into the territory of the atrophic contralateral tract. Counts of the number of fibers in the hypertrophic pyramid gave conflicting results: van der Bruggen (1930) reported an increased number of myelinated fibers; in Verhaart's (1950) counts there was little or no increase in the number of fibers, but there were more of the thicker fibers; Scales and Collins (1972), in contrast, report an increase in the number of thin fibers. Interpretation of these data is difficult as they were obtained with different preparative techniques, and as hypertrophy may involve either a change in the number of fibers or one in their caliber, or both. The available data imply that hypertrophy of the corticospinal tract develops in the growing brain as a compensatory adaptive phenomenon caused by deficiency of the contralateral tract; hence, the term hypertrophy is preferable to that of hyperplasia.

Congenital Insensitivity to Pain. Developmental disturbances of centripetal fiber systems are rare. Congenital insensitivity to pain is a case in question; the interpretation of this disease hinges on whether patients actually lack the ability to perceive pain or exhibit an abnormal indifference to pain. Autopsy reports disclosed no abnormalities in the spinal cord or elsewhere in the central system (Baxter and Olszewski, 1960; Magee, 1963). Changes were recorded in a 12-year-old child, one of two brothers with a life-long history of insensitivity to pain, defective temperature sensation and absence of sweating (Swanson *et al.*, 1965). There was an absence of small neurons in the spinal ganglia which showed only tightly packed large neurons; the small fibers in the dorsal roots were also missing, and Lissauer's tract in the cord was absent. The clinical manifestations of congenital insensitivity to pain overlap to some extent with those of dysautonomia in that signs of autonomic dysfunction occur for both (Trush, 1973). The morphologic classification of these rare processes is still in emergence.

Familial Dysautonomia (Riley-Day Syndrome). Changes in ascending spinal tracts appear to be a consistent feature in familial dysautonomia, an autosomal recessive disturbance affecting patients of jewish extraction. Symptoms develop at an early age, including decreased lacrimation, transient skin blotching, instability of temperature control, hyperhidrosis, and fluctuations in blood pressure with postural hypotension and hypertensive episodes, indif-

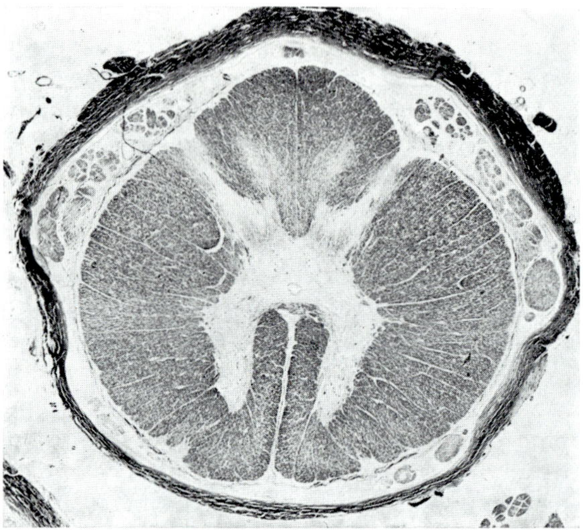

Fig. 115. Dysautonomia. Klüver Barrera; ×8

ference to pain and other symptoms. Only a small number of cases were studied at autopsy. A variety of lesions was reported initially, such as a defect in thalamus, ill-defined changes in the reticular formation of the medulla oblongata and vacuolation of neurons in the autonomic nervous system; no changes were found in others. Degeneration of tracts in the spinal cord was reported by Brown *et al.* (1964) and Fogelson *et al.* (1967) and appears to emerge as the most characteristic central manifestation of the disease (Sohn and Levine, 1974). It consists of sparsity of myelinated fibers in the dorsal roots and a symmetric degeneration of the bundle of Schutz (fasciculus interfascicularis) in the dorsal spinal tracts (Fig. 115). The neurons of autonomic ganglia are hypoplastic, and a paucity of nonmyelinated fibers was found in biopsies of sural nerve (Pearson *et al.*, 1974).

Aplasia of Dorsal Spinal Tracts. The present author observed what appears to be a unique case of aplasia of the dorsal spinal tracts. The 3-day-old boy had been born at term by cesarean section to a white mother. There were 3 normal girls, one miscarriage, and one brother who had been areflexic and floppy and had died at 1 week. No chromosomal anomalies had been found in this infant, and no autopsy was performed. The present pregnancy was complicated by first trimester bleeding. The infant was born severely hypotonic and areflexic; suck, gag, and Moro reflexes were absent. The ears were low-set with poor cartilage, the mandible hypoplastic and the palate arched; the abdomen was distended from hepatosplenomegaly. Spontaneous movements were normal. The infant had to be tube-fed and died on the 3rd day from massive pulmonary hemorrhage. No gross anomalies were noticed on inspection of the central nervous system. Microscopic examination of the spinal cord disclosed an extreme degree of hypoplasia of the dorsal tracts (tractus gracilis and cuneatus) which were presented by a tiny wedge

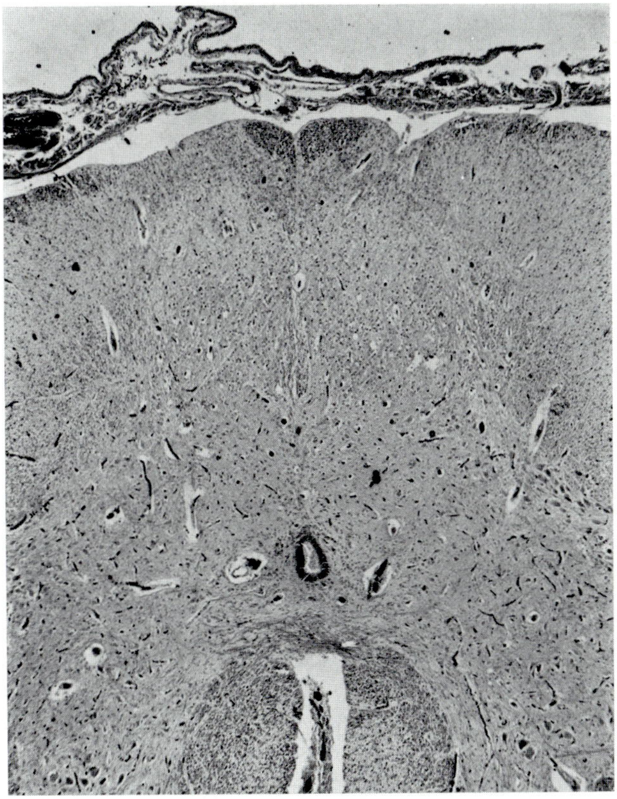

Fig. 116. Aplasia of dorsal tracts. Only minute bundles of myelinated fibers are seen at the dorsal surface of the cord; the dorsal horns touch each other in the midline; ×44

of myelinated fibers running midline underneath the dorsal surface of the cord (Fig. 116). The dorsal horns were lifted up, nearly touching each other at the midline. No nucleus dorsalis (Clarke's column) was seen in any segment of the cord; unfortunately, the spinal ganglia had not been removed for examination. Only thin vestiges of dorsal roots were seen at the surface of the cord, but ventral roots were normal. There were no anomalies in the gray matter of the ventral horns. The lateral and ventral tracts were myelinated except for the corticospinal tracts which could be seen in their normal positions at the median fissure and lateral to the dorsal horns. The cervicomedullary junction showed a broad area of scattered neurons caudal to the obex, presumably representing the nucleus gracilis and cuneatus, though lacking their typical configuration; there was poor delination of this mass of neurons caudally from the approximated dorsal horns of the cervical segments of the cord. No anomalous nuclear groupings were seen in the floor of the fourth ventricle cranial to the obex. The rest of the autopsy disclosed general retardation of muscular development.

Thalidomide-Induced Deformities. Despite the great number of infants born after 1959 with deformities of their extremities induced by medication of thalidomide during pregnancy, there are only a few autopsy observations and no specific changes in the spinal cord have been recorded. Hughes (1966) reports briefly that the brachial plexus was present and hypoplastic in several cases and the anterior horns showed a simplified configuration. Experimental data indicate that the lesions result from failure of differentiation of digits in the limb butt mesenchyma (Vickers, 1967).

Spinal Lesions in Arthrogryphosis Multiplex Congenita. The meaning of this term is "multiple congenital curved joints"; this well known deformity has also been referred to as multiple congenital articular rigidities, amyoplasia congenita, or myodystrophia fetalis deformans. It presents with congenital immobility of limbs with fixation of the thickened joints in various positions, the muscles being small. The large joints of arms and legs are commonly ankylosed in extension, the hands and wrists sharply flexed and the feet clubbed. Arthrogryphosis is not considered a specific disease process but, rather, a syndrome caused by a variety of underlying diseases affecting the skeletal muscles or their connective tissue, including instances of myopathy (Banker *et al.*, 1957), or nonprogressive congenital neuropathy (Yuiill and Lynch, 1974). Changes in the spinal cord were found in a number of cases, of which 11 were reviewed by Drachman and Banker (1961) who also presented a careful account of one of their own. Spinal changes consisted of paucity or subtotal loss of motor neurons, occasionally accompanied with neuronophagia. There was atrophy of the ventral roots and a reduction in the diameter of the cord. The skeletal muscles showed neurogenic (denervation) atrophy. Of particular interest in this disease is the bilateral loss of nerve cells from the trigeminal and ambiguus nuclei, as these changes possibly relate to the micrognathia, which often accompanies arthrogryphosis. Several later publications have not added to the already available information.

Arthrogryphosis associated with loss of motor neurons has been related tentatively to Werdnig-Hoffmann disease, but the relationship between the two disease processes is unlikely. The course of Werdnig-Hoffmann disease is characterized by relentless progression to death, whereas arthrogryphosis is fully developed at birth with no signs of progression. There is also some similarity between arthrogryphosis and congenital facial and ophthalmoplegia in terms of the involvement of cranial nerve nuclei or the presence of ankylotic joints; however, combination of these two disease processes has apparently not been observed.

Arthrogryphosis has also been observed with a variety of lesions in the cerebral hemispheres including tuberous sclerosis (Sandbank and Cohen, 1964), micropolygyria and heterotopias (Fowler, 1959). Arthrogryphosis in calves was associated with hydranencephaly in more than half of the cases (Whitten, 1957).

Congenital Absence of Abdominal Muscles. A diminution of the size and number of ventral horn motor neurons is found in the lower thoracic segments of the spinal cord in cases of congenital absence of abdominal muscles. The number of neurons is about half of normal, and no changes are seen in the lateral and posterior horns and in Clarke's column. The ventral roots are atrophic (Lichtenstein, 1939; Heffner, 1970).

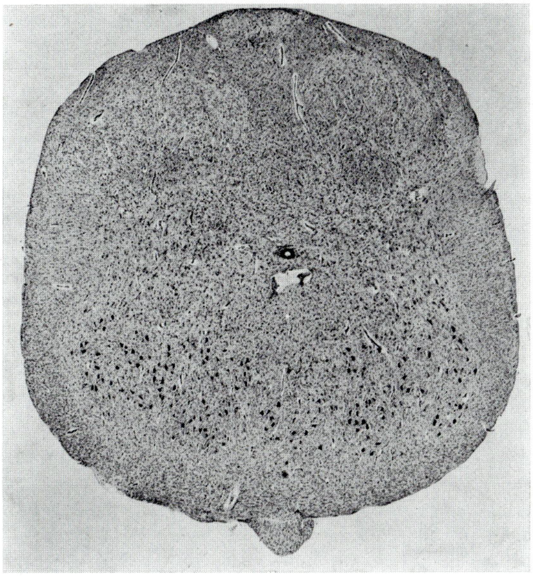

Fig. 117. Anomaly of the sacral cord in a case of sacral agenesis: fusion of ventral horns, anomalous gray matter dorsal in the midline, anomalous tract ventral in the midline; cresyl violet ×7

Sacral Agenesis. Sacral agenesis is an uncommon entity characterized by absence of the sacrum and coccyx, and apposition of the iliac wings which assume an almost vertical position. The pelvis is narrowed, and deformities of feet and urinary incontinence are common. The association of sacral agenesis with maternal diabetes has been stressed (Rusnak and Driscoll, 1965; Passarge and Lenz, 1966). Few descriptions of spinal cord lesions were found in the literature; Rusnak and Driscoll (1965) report a cleft-like central canal, hypoplastic sciatic nerves, and a variety of other nervous system or visceral malformations. Of two cases of sacral agenesis studied by the present author, one had a unique type of malformation of the sacral cord. There was absence of ventral and dorsal fissures and the gray matter of the ventral horns formed a continuous arc across the midline. An abnormal midline column of gray matter ran underneath the dorsal surface of the cord, and an abnormal midline tract on the ventral surface (Fig. 117). This infant also had cloacal, renal, ureteral and vesicular and anal agenesis, tracheoesophageal fistula and esophageal atresia. The other case had a strand of fibrous connective tissue fused with the tapering end of the cord and leading into the sacral defect; there was preterminal duplication of the central canal.

References

Anton, G.: Über Ersatz der Bewegungsleistungen beim Menschen und Entwicklungsstörungen des Kleinhirns. Zbl. Neurol. Psychiat. 30: 372—374, 1922.

Balthasar, K., Schlagenhauff, R.: Unilateral agenesis of pyramidal system. Proc. Vth Int. Cong. Neuropath., Zürich 1965. Excerpta Medica Foundation, Amsterdam, pp. 881—887.

Banker, B. Q., Victor, M., Adams, R. D.: Arthrogryphosis multiplex due to congenital muscular dystrophy. Brain 80: 319—334, 1957.

Baxter, D. W., Olszewski, J.: Congenital insensitivity to pain. Brain 83: 381—393, 1960.

Brown, W. J., Beachemin, J. A., Linde, L. M.: A neuropathological study of familial dysautonomia (Riley-Day syndrome) in siblings. J. Neurol. Neurosurg. Psychiat. 27: 131—139, 1964.

Crosby, E., Humphrey, T., Lauer, E. W.: Correlative Anatomy of the Nervous System. New York: Macmillan Co. 1962.

Dearborn, G.: Case of congenital general anesthesia. J. nerv. ment. Dis. 75: 612—615, 1932.

Drachman, D. B., Banker, B. Q.: Arthrogryphosis multiplex congenita. Arch. Neurol. (Chic.) 5: 77—93, 1961.

Ellenberger, C., Hanaway, J., Netsky, M. G.: Embryogenesis of the inferior olivary nucleus in the rat. J. comp. Neurol. 137: 71—87, 1969.

Essick, C. R.: The development of the nuclei pontis and the nucleus arcuatus in man. Amer. J. Anat. 13: 25—54, 1912.

Fogelson, M. H., Rorke, L. B., Kaye, R.: Spinal cord changes in familial dysautonomia. Arch. Neurol. (Chic.) 17: 103—108, 1967.

Fowler, M.: A case of arthrogryphosis multiplex congenita with lesions in the nervous system. Arch. Dis. Child. 34: 505—519, 1959.

Halsey, J. H., Jr., Allen, N., Chamberlin, H. R.: The morphogenesis of hydranencephaly. J. Neurol. Sci. 12: 187—218, 1971.

Heffner, R. R.: Syndrome of absent abdominal muscles. J. Neurol. Neurosurg. Psychiat. 33: 844—850, 1970.

Henderson, J. L.: The congenital facial diplegia syndrome: Clinical features, pathology, etiology. Brain 62: 381—403, 1939.

Heubner: Über angeborenen Kernmangel. Charité-Annalen 25: 211—243, 1900.

His, W.: Die Entwicklung des menschlichen Rautenhirns vom Ende des ersten bis zum Beginn des dritten Monats. Abh. Kön. Sächs. Ges. Wiss. 29: 1—74, 1891.

Hughes, J. T.: Pathology of the Spinal Cord. Chicago: Year Book Medical Publishers, Inc. 1966.

Lichtenstein, B. W.: Congenital absence of the abdominal musculature. Amer. J. Dis. Child. 58: 339—348, 1939.

Magee, K. R.: Congenital indifference to pain. Arch. Neurol. (Chic.) 9: 635—640, 1963.

Möbius, P. J.: Über angeborene doppelseitige Abducens-Facialis-Lähmung. Münch. med. Wschr. 35: 91—94, 108—111, 1888.

Obersteiner, H.: Anleitung zum Studium des Baues der nervösen Zentralorgane im gesunden und kranken Zustande. Leipzig-Wien: F. Deuticke 1912.

Passarge, E., Lenz, W.: Syndrome of caudal regression in infants of diabetic mothers. Pediatrics 37: 672—674, 1966.

Pearson, J., Axelrod, F., Dancis, J.: Current concepts of dysautonomia: Neuropathological defects. Ann. New York Acad. Sci. 228: 288—300, 1974.

Pitner, S. E., Edwards, J. E., McCormick, W. F.: Observations on the pathology of the Moebius syndrome. J. Neurol. Neurosurg. Psychiat. 28: 362—374, 1965.

Rainy, H., Fowler, J. S.: Congenital facial diplegia due to nuclear lesion. Rev. Neurol. Psychiat. 1: 149—155, 1903.

Richter, R. B.: Unilateral congenital hypoplasia of the facial nucleus. J. Neuropath. exp. Neurol. 19: 33—41, 1960.
Rusnak, S. L., Driscoll, S. G.: Congenital spinal anomalies in infants of diabetic mothers. Pediatrics 35: 989—995, 1965.
Sandbank, U., Cohen, L.: Arthrogryphosis multiplex congenita associated with tuberous sclerosis. J. Pediat. 64: 571—574, 1964.
Scales, D. A., Collins, G. H.: Cerebral degeneration with hypertrophy of the contralateral pyramid. Arch. Neurol. (Chic.) 26: 186—190, 1972.
Sohn, D., Levine, S.: Neuropathological changes in familial dysautonomia. J. Neuropath. exp. Neurol. 33: 195—195, 1974.
Spatz, H., Ullrich, O.: Klinischer und anatomischer Beitrag zu den angeborenen Beweglichkeitsdefekten im Hirnnervenbereich. Z. Kinderheilk. 51: 579—597, 1931.
Swanson, A. G., Buchan, G. C., Alvord, E. C.: Anatomic changes in congenital insensitivity to pain. Arch. Neurol. (Chic.) 12: 12—18, 1965.
Thrush, D. C.: Autonomic dysfunction in four patients with congenital insensitivity to pain. Brain 96: 591—600, 1973.
van der Bruggen, J.: Über Ersatz der Pyramidenbahnfunktion. Dtsch. Z. Nervenheilk. 113: 250—277, 1930.
Verhaart, W. J. C.: On thick and thin fibers in the pyramidal tract. Acta Psychiat. Neurol. 22: 271—281, 1947.
— Hypertrophy of pes penduncoli and pyramid as result of degeneration of contralateral corticofugal fiber tracts. J. comp. Neurol. 92: 1—15, 1950.
— Kramer, W.: The uncrossed pyramidal tract. Acta psychiat. neurol. scand. 27: 181—200, 1952.
Vickers, T. H.: Concerning the morphogenesis of thalidomide dysmyelia in rabbits. Brit. J. exp. Path. 48: 579—591, 1967.
Whitten, J. H.: Congenital abnormalities in calves. Arthrogryphosis and hydranencephaly. J. Path. Bact. 73: 375—387, 1957.
Yuiill, G. M., Lynch, P. G.: Congenital non-progressive peripheral neuropathy with arthrogryposis multiplex. J. Neurol. Neurosurg. Psychiat. 37: 316—323, 1974.
Zenner, P.: Ein Fall von Hirngeschwulst in der linken motorischen Sphäre, linksseitige Lähmung, Abwesenheit der Pyramidenkreuzung. Neurol. Zbl. 17: 202—203, 1898.

33. Dysplasias in Chromosome Disorders

The clinical expressions of anomalies of autosomes, which affect all body cells, are generally more severe than those of the sex chromosomes. Rather massive anomalies in the number of a sex chromosome, such as monosomy or polysomy, may be accompanied with comparatively slight derangements. Anomalies of that degree are incompatible with life for autosomes, and trisomy is the maximum degree of anomaly of one whole autosome in viable patients. Moreover, no whole chromosome anomalies have been observed for the larger autosomes (1–12), as these appear to be incompatible with life. The extent and severity of the malformations observed for trisomies of the chromosome groups 13–15, 17–18 and 21 decreases with the size of the chromosomes involved, probably reflecting the "dosage" of abnormal genetic information. The reviews of Eggen (1965), Joppich and Schulte (1968), and Warkany *et al.* (1966) may be consulted for general surveys. Malformations of the CNS have been observed with a great variety of chromosomal anomalies; the present chapter covers only the more common syndromes.

Down Syndrome (Mongolism). Down (1866) attempted classification of idiots by means of a system of ethnic characteristics. He distinguished a large group exhibiting mongoloid traits from the Caucasian, Ethiopian and Malai varieties. Down's interpretation of his findings was strongly influenced by the contemporary debate on the evolutionary theory; he thought that his observations demonstrated that ethnic characteristics can be subject to conversion, being an indication of the "unity of the human species". The term Down syndrome, therefore, is much preferable to that of mongolism. The syndrome afflicts approximately 1.4 per 1,000 newborns and the sex distribution is near even. Birth weight tends to be below normal after a slightly shortened gestation. The clinical features are characterized by incomplete Moro reflex, hypotonia of skeletal muscles and hyperextensibility of limbs. The facial profile is flat, the eyes showing an epicanthus, their lids being set in an oblique angle, and the ears being dysplastic. There is mental retardation. Bone anomalies include an arched palate, a dysplastic pelvis and middle phalanx of the fifth fingers. Dermal ridge patterns show a simian crease extending across the palm, but a triradius near the middle of the palm and digital loop patterns are more characteristic of this syndrome. Blood serotonin levels are below normal (Rosner *et al.*, 1965; Tu and Zellweger, 1965); however, this change manifests only after the 40th week of life, as normal or above normal serotonin levels are found during the first 25 weeks (Andersson *et al.*, 1973). Alterations of various serum enzymes have also been reported in trisomy 21; there is indication that these chemical changes are not present in the translocations. Down syndrome is frequently associated with various malformations. Approximately one half of 2,421 afflicted infants had congenital heart disease, duodenal obstruction, club foot, cataract, imperforate anus, syndactyly, cleft palate and congenital megalocolon, listed in order of decreasing frequency (Fabia and Drolette, 1970). There is an increased susceptibility to infection, but the disease is compatible with survival to adult age.

The relationship of Down syndrome to trisomy of the chromosome 21 was discovered in 1959 by Lejeune *et al.* and was rapidly confirmed by others, thus providing the main impetus for the development of chromosome analysis in human disease. Four types of chromosomal anomalies may be found in Down syndrome (Penrose, 1961): 1. Trisomy of the chromosome 21, which is found in approximately 90 percent of the infants with Down syndrome. A striking bimodal distribution of maternal ages corresponds to greatly different risks of affection of the next sibs; the risk is about 50-fold random for mothers less than 25 years, 5-fold random in the 25 to 34 years group and not distinctly above normal for mothers older than 35 (Carter and Evans, 1961). This bimodal distribution reflects the overlap between familiar occurrence at a young maternal age and an increase in the frequency of non-familiar occurrence with advanced maternal age. 2. Mosaic trisomies, in which a fraction of the cell population has normal chromosome sets, constitute approximately 2 percent of cases of Down syndrome and may be found with maternal or with paternal mosaic trisomy; the risk of affection of the next sib is higher in these instances. 3. Translocations, which may occur between chromosome 21 and a variety of other chromosomes, account for 1 to 5 percent of the instances of Down syndrome. Translocations account for 25 percent of the familiar occurrences of Down syndrome and occur with high frequency in infants of younger mothers. The risk varies with the type of chromosome involved in the translocation. 4. A variety of other rare chromosome findings may also be observed in Down syndrome.

The morbid anatomy of the central nervous system in Down syndrome is not sufficiently characteristic to permit its diagnosis in the absence of clinical or laboratory data. The brain weight is usually in the lower range of normal, near 1,000 gm, and the size of the cerebellum and brain stem may be reduced to a greater extent than the cerebral hemispheres (Davidoff, 1928). Measurements in 19 children gave an average reduction in total brain weight to 76 percent, and in the weights of brain stem and cerebellum to 66 percent, of normal (Crome *et al.*, 1966). The hemispheric surface shows a simplified convolutional pattern; the most consistent aberration, found in approximately half of the cases, is a narrow and straight superior temporal gyrus. A variety of other anomalies have been noticed, including a shortened occiput, a squareshaped configuration of the thalamus and others; such changes are minor and a matter of subjective evaluation. Microscopic examination discloses no characteristic structural alterations, although columnar arrangement of cells in the cortex, or a paucity of small neurons in the upper cortical layers, have been described (Davidoff, 1928). Measurements disclosed a reduction in cell density per volume of tissue and an increase in the volume of cell nuclei in the cerebral cortex, but these changes were confined to the visual area (Colon, 1972). Focal lesions described in brains of patients with Down syndrome include mineralization, gliosis and patchy demyelination of white matter, but these are evidently not characteristic of Down syndrome and reflect associated or intercurrent disease processes, including the often coexistent congenital cardiac disease (Meyer and Jones, 1939).

Patients afflicted with Down syndrome show a disposition to Alzheimer disease, which may develop at an early age, with typical manifestations of senile plaques and neurofibrillary alterations (Jervis, 1948; Solitare and Lamarche, 1966). The histopathology and fine structure of the changes are identical to those found in Alzheimer disease in adults (Ellis *et al.*, 1974). Down syndrome was found to be accompanied with an increased incidence of leukemia (Krivit and Good, 1957; and others). Rosner *et al.* (1972) on reviewing 276 recorded cases, 47 for newborns, drew attention to a leukemoid reaction from bone marrow dysfunction which mimicks acute myelocytic leukemia but disappears spontaneously over weeks or months.

Trisomy 17–18 (Trisomy E; Edwards Syndrome). Chromosome anomalies affecting the group E were described by Edwards *et al.* (1960) and are for the majority trisomies, although mosaicism has also been observed with a complete or abortive syndrome. The afflicted chromosome is thought to be number 18 by most authors. The frequency of trisomy 17–18 approximates 1 per 6,500 births (Taylor, 1967). The syndrome resembles Down syndrome in the distribution of maternal ages, showing two peaks, the nonfamiliar forms predominating at a higher maternal age; there is a 3 to 1 preference for females. Clinical features consist of low birth weight and poor postnatal growth and development. The cranium is dolichocephalic, with deep-seated ears and micrognathia. The hands have a characteristic flexion and overriding of fingers, the second digit overriding the third, and the fifth digit the fourth; the great toe is dorsoflexed. Various types of congenital heart disease, herniae, cutaneous hemangiomas and dysplasias of the digestive and urogenital tract are common; the papillary ridge pattern of fingers is characterized by three or more simple arches. Life expectancy is strikingly reduced, the chance of survival to the first month being 70 percent, to the first year 10 percent, and to the tenth year 1 percent (Weber *et al.*, 1964).

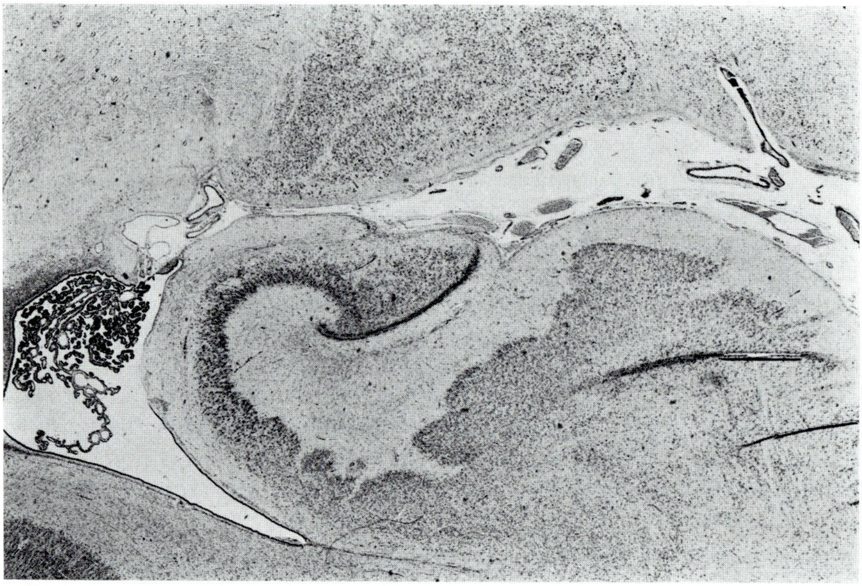

Fig. 118. Anomalous architecture of the Ammon's horn in 17–18 trisomy; cresyl violet ×8

Neuropathologic changes in trisomy 17–18 have been described by Sumi (1970) and Michaelson and Gilles (1972). The most consistent alterations are various anomalies in gyral and lobar patterns, dysplasias of hippocampus, lateral geniculate body and inferior olivary nuclei and hypoplastic basis pontis. The gyral anomalies include an excessive number of gyri, variations in the volume or discernibility of specific gyri including the superior temporal gyrus, gyrus rectus, and pre- and post-central gyri; there are also anomalies in the volume of temporal, parietal or occipital lobes. Dysplasias of the hippocampus consist of a small outward rotated fascia dentata, a hypercellular endplate and disproportions in the size of sectors of the Ammon's horn (Fig. 118). The lateral geniculate body shows disorganization including vertical layering of cells or a poor distinction of the magno- and parvocellular layers. The dorsal portion of the inferior olivary nucleus is thicker than normal, and the normal undulation of the nuclear profile is absent. There may also be other associated malformations including hypoplasia or absence of corpus callosum, heterotopias, and ectopic glial tissue in the leptomeninges. Earlier reports on the neuropathology of this syndrome are found in the literature (Passarge *et al.*, 1966), but these emphasize only the abnormal gyral patterns without describing the characteristic microscopic alterations. Nests of neuroblasts in the dentate nucleus or heterotopias in cerebellar white matter, dysplasias of the dentate nucleus, and focal disorganization of the gray matter had also received attention, but these are neither characteristic nor do they reach the extent observed in 13–15 trisomy. The matrix nests in the periventricular tissue of the cerebral hemispheres described by Terplan *et al.* (1970) are probably transient variations in the pattern of matrix involution.

Trisomy 13–15 (Trisomy D; Patau Syndrome). This group is less common than group E trisomy—1 per 4,600 births (Taylor, 1967)—and includes trisomy as well as mosaicism and translocations. The majority of afflicted infants is female, and they usually are born before term and small for gestation. There is microcephaly, occasionally with a cephalic skin defect, microphthalmia, deep-seated deformed ears, hare lip and cleft palate, and hemangiomata at the neck and dorsum of back. The extremities nearly always show polydactyly, a foot deformity described as rocker bottom feet, as well as other anomalies. Dermatoglyphics show an extremely distal axial triradius and a single transverse palmar crease. Congenital cardiac disease and defects of urogenital tract are common. Medium life expectancy is 101 $\pm$ 36 days (Taylor, 1967).

Neuropathologic manifestations of this syndrome are those of holoprosencephaly (arhinencephaly). Holoprosencephaly is usually a manifestation of 13–15 trisomy when occurring as a component of multiple malformations, but it has been observed in association with encephaloceles and extracerebral deformities in infants having normal chromosomes (Miller and Selden, 1967). Holoprosencephaly also occurs with chromosome lesions other than trisomy; holoprosencephaly and its clinicopathologic features are described in Chapter 28.

In addition to the deformities of cerebral hemispheres, massive heterotopias in the cerebellum were observed by Norman (1966) and Terplan *et al.* (1966). These consist of exceptionally large nests of matrix cells in the dentate nucleus, nests of heterotopic neurons in the subcortical white matter, dysplasias of the dentate nucleus, and focal disorganization of the cerebellar cortex, particular the vermis. Lesions of this general type are frequently seen in the brains of normal newborns (Chapter 31). However, they tend to be exceptionally large in 13–15 trisomy, and the matrix nests and cortical heterotopias may occur with higher frequency than in normal infants (Rorke *et al.*, 1968). Exceptionally large nests of matrix cells may also be found in the cochlear nucleus, where small nests occasionally occur in normal newborns (Chapter 1).

Sex Chromosome Anomalies. Mental deficiency is mentioned in many reports on sex chromosome anomalies; there is, however, considerable variation in degree, and instances of severe mental subnormality are less common than the mild degrees. No consistent pattern of cerebral dysplasia has emerged as yet. Megalencephaly (1,710 gm) and minor microscopic variations in cellular architecture were reported in a 12-year-old boy with XYY syndrome (Brun and Gustavson, 1972).

References

Andersson, H., Fallstrom, S. P., Lundborg, P., Roos, B.-E.: 5-hydroxy-indoleacetic acid in children with Down's syndrome. Acta paediat. scand. 62: 158—160, 1973.

Brun, A., Gustavson, K.-H.: Cerebral malformations in the XYY syndrome. Acta path. microbiol. scand. 80: 627—633, 1972.

Carter, C. O., Evans, K. A.: Risk of parents who have had one child with Down's syndrome. Lancet II: 785—787, 1961.

Colon, E. J.: The structure of the cerebral cortex in Down's syndrome. A quantitative analysis. Neuropädiatrie 3: 362—376, 1972.

Crome, L., Cowie, V., Slayer, E.: A statistical note on cerebellar and brain stem weight in mongolism. J. ment. Defic. Res. 10: 69—72, 1966.

Davidoff, L. M.: The brain in mongolian idiocy. Arch. Neurol. Psychiat. (Chic.) 20: 1229—1257, 1928.

Down, J. L. H.: Observation on an ethnic classification of idiots. Clin. Lect. Reports London Hosp. 3: 259—262, 1866.

Edwards, J. H., Harnden, A. H., Cameron, V., Crosse, V. M., Wolff, O. H.: A new trisomic syndrome. Lancet I: 787—789, 1960.

Eggen, R. R.: Chromosome Diagnostics in Clinical Medicine. Springfield, Ill.: Ch. C Thomas 1965.

Ellis, W. G., McCulloch, J. R., Corley, C. L.: Presenile dementia in Down's syndrome: Ultrastructural identity with Alzheimer's disease. Neurology (Minneap.) 24: 101—106, 1974.

Fabia, J., Drolette, M.: Malformations and leukemia in children with Down's syndrome. Pediatrics 45: 60—70, 1970.

Jervis, G. A.: Early senile dementia in mongoloid idiocy. Amer. J. Psychiat. 105: 102—106, 1948.

Joppich, G., Schulte, F. J.: Neurologie des Neugeborenen. Berlin-Heidelberg-New York: Springer 1968.

Krivit, W., Good, R. A.: Simultaneous occurrence of mongolism and leukemia. Report of a nationwide survey. Amer. J. Dis. Child. 94: 289—293, 1957.

Lejeune, J., Gauthier, M., Turpin, R.: Etude des chromosomes de neuf enfants mongoliens. C. R. Acad. Sci. (Paris) 248: 1721—1722, 1959.

Meyer, A., Jones, T. B.: Histological changes in the brain in mongolism. J. ment. Sc. 85: 206—221, 1939.

Michaelson, P. S., Gilles, F. H.: Central nervous system abnormalities in trisomy E (17–18) syndrome. J. Neurol. Sci. 15: 193—208, 1972.

Miller, J. Q., Selden, R. F.: Arhinencephaly, encephalocele, and 13–15 trisomy syndrome with normal chromosomes. Neurology (Minneap.) 17: 1087—1091, 1967.

Norman, R. M.: Neuropathological findings in trisomies 13–15 and 17–18 with special reference to the cerebellum. Develop. Med. Child. Neurol. 8: 170—177, 1966.

Passarge, E., True, C. W., Sueoka, W., Baumgartner, N. R., Keer, K. R.: Malformations of the central nervous system in trisomy 18 syndrome. Pediatrics 69: 771—778, 1966.

Patau, K., Smith, D. W., Therman, E., Inhorn, S. L., Wagner, H. P.: Multiple congenital anomaly caused by an extra autosome. Lancet I: 790—793, 1960.

Penrose, L. S.: Mongolism. Brit. med. Bull. 17: 184—189, 1961.

Rorke, L. B., Fogelson, M. H., Riggs, H. E.: Cerebellar heterotopia in infancy. Develop. Med. Child. Neurol. 10: 644—650, 1968.

Rosner, F., Lee, S. L.: (Acute Leukemia Group B). Down's syndrome and acute leukemia: myeloblastic or lymphoblastic? Report of forty-three cases and review of the literature. Amer. J. Med. 53: 203—218, 1972.

— Ong, B. H., Paine, R. S., Mahanand, D.: Blood-serotonin activity in trisomic and translocation Down's syndrome. Lancet I: 1191—1193, 1965.

Solitare, G. B., Lamarche, J. B.: Alzheimer's disease and senile dementia as seen in mongoloids: Neuropathological observations. Amer. J. ment. Defic. 70: 840—848, 1966.

Şumi, S. M.: Brain malformations in the trisomy 18 syndrome. Brain 93: 821—830, 1970,

Taylor, A. I.: Patau's, Edward and cri du chat syndromes: A tabulated summary of current findings. Develop. Med. Child. Neurol. 9: 78—86, 1967.

Terplan, K. L., Lopez, E. C., Robinson, H. B.: Histologic structural anomalies in the brain in trisomy 18 syndrome. Amer. J. Dis. Child. 119: 228—235, 1970.

— Sandberg, A. A., Aceto, T.: Structural anomalies in the cerebellum in association with trisomy. J.A.M.A. 197: 557—568, 1966.

Tu, J. B., Zellweger, H.: Blood-serotonin deficiency in Down's syndrome. Lancet II: 715—716, 1965.

Warkany, J., Passarge, E., Smith, L. B.: Congenital malformations in autosomal trisomy syndromes. Amer. J. Dis. Child. 112: 502—517, 1966.

Weber, W. W., Mamunes, P., Day, R., Miller, P.: Trisomy 17–18 (E): Studies in long term survival with report of two autopsied cases. Pediatrics 34: 533—541, 1964.

34. Dysplasias of Cerebral Vasculature

The subject matter covered below is restricted to the infantile manifestations of vascular dysplasias. The vascular anomalies forming a component of various phacomatoses are not covered despite their hereditary or developmental implications. The lesions of Sturge-Weber disease, Hippel-Lindau disease or ataxia telangiectatica are nearly always seen by the pathologist at higher ages.

Development of Cerebral Vasculature. A few comments on selected aspects of the development of vasculature may be of help in assessing possible teratogenetic determination periods of vascular malformations; a comprehensive survey was given by Kaplan and Ford (1966). Streeter (1915, 1918) distinguished five stages in the development of cerebral vascularization. The first stage, at a fetal age of approximately 24 days (3 mm embryonal length), is characterized by the formation of a primitive vascular plexus covering the surface of the brain, made up of vascular sprouts originating from the primordial vessels. Arteries, veins, and capillaries differentiate from this plexus during the second stage, at approximately 28 days (4 mm embryonal length); during this phase a deep sheet of capillaries, attached to the cerebral surface, separates from a superficial layer in which arteries and veins differentiate from the primitive vascular trunks. The third stage, which overlaps with the fourth, is ushered by the development of the cranium, concordant with which the vascular system cleaves into 3 distinct layers which supply the scalp, the dura and the pia mater. This process begins in the basal portions of the cranium in embryos 12 to 20 mm long, spreading from there to the convexity. The fourth stage begins in embryos approximately 18 mm in length and is characterized by a reorganization of the course and configuration of the cerebral vessels which adapt to the rapid changes in the shape and proportions of the major subdivisions of the brain. Arterial channels attain their definite arrangement earlier than venous channels. The basilar artery is formed by approximately 29 days and the differentiation of the main cerebral arteries begins by 32 days. The middle and anterior cerebral arteries are well advanced at 40 days, when the anterior communicating artery is still represented by a vascular plexus. Formation of the circle of Willis is completed by the 44th day, and all main arterial stems show adult type origins by 52 days (Padget, 1948). The venous drainage channels in the temporal region show a definite arrangement by 44 days; the superior sagittal sinus forms first in its frontal portion from the confluence of a venous plexus in the 54 mm embryo. The transverse sinus begins to form from the tentorial venous plexus in embryos 35 to 50 mm in length; initially it runs in a straight line with the internal jugular vein, migrating successively occipital to form a 90° angle. The primitive sinus rectus is not well developed until 80 mm fetal length, although the adult pattern of most sinuses and veins is reached by that stage. The last remnant of the embryonal venous plexus is represented by plexiform anastomoses of multiple channels at the confluence sinuum (Streeter, 1915). The fifth stage of vascular development is characterized by histologic changes in the walls of the vessels which begin to acquire the structural characteristics of adult arteries, veins, and sinus.

Arteriovenous Aneurysm of the Vein of Galen. The first description of this entity is commonly attributed to Steinheil (1895) although his case had an abnormal mass of vessels in the frontal lobe associated with dilation of the great vein of Galen. These features are more consistent with the dilation of vessels draining an arteriovenous malformation than with a true arteriovenous aneurysm of the great vein of Galen. A typical case of the latter was described by Wohak (1923) who, however, did not recognize the relation between the venous aneurysm and arterial shunting. The first comprehensive description of arteriovenous aneurysms of the vein of Galen were published by Jaeger *et al.* (1937) and Russell and Nevin (1940). Scattered case reports followed during the next decades; the rapid increase in the number of publications on this entity after 1960 indicates that it was underdiagnosed rather than truly rare. The essential features of the lesion consist of an aneurysmatic dilation of the great vein of Galen due to the direct shunting of major cerebral arteries into it. These features distinguish the lesion from the dilation of veins draining arteriovenous malformations, which may affect the vein of Galen if the malformation happens to be deep midline; they also distinguish the arteriovenous aneurysm of the vein of Galen from the shunting of arteries into cerebral sinus, or from diffuse angiodysplasia. The term arteriovenous aneurysm of the vein of Galen proposed by Hirano and Terry (1958) is most to the point and is preferable to arteriovenous fistula involving the vein of Galen, or aneurysm or varix of the vein of Galen. The literature was reviewed by Gomez *et al.* (1963) and Gold *et al.* (1964); Siqueira and Murray (1972) recently reviewed 75 cases, although not all of those quoted would fit the strict definition of the disease entity. Males predominated by 2 to 1 (65 percent).

The clinical course of ateriovenous aneurysm of the vein of Galen varies in relation to the age of the patient, probably in a direct relationship to the size of the shunt (Gomez *et al.*, 1963; Gold *et al.*, 1964). Manifestation in newborns and young infants is characterized by high output cardiac failure, as first recognized by Pollock and Laslett (1958). Cardiac failure in these infants is probably precipitated by the postnatal increase in cardiac output due to which the newborn heart is normally forced to work near capacity. The infants show an increased blood volume and an increase in cardiac output due to augmented stroke volume, which results in myocardial failure (Levine *et al.*, 1962). Without corrective surgery the majority dies within the first 2 weeks of life, most others during the first 5 months. Manifestation of the disease process in older infants and children is commonly by way of hydrocephalus, which occurs in about half of the cases. Its degree varies considerably; in some instances hydrocephalus is already present at birth, while it is late or slow in development in others. Hydrocephalus is caused by compression of the quadrigeminal plate and the aqueduct by the dilated vein of Galen, but the additional aggravating effect of increased venous pressure should not be ignored (Chapter 22). The most common symptoms in adolescents and adults are intracranial hemorrhages, neurologic deficits and seizures. Mental retardation or local neurologic signs may relate to secondary vasculo-occlusive cerebral lesions, or to the local compression of tissue by the aneurysm; the onset of symptoms may be relatively sudden.

The majority of reports on the disease is based on clinical and/or radiographic observations, but there are many descriptions of the morbid anatomy, including those of Russell and Nevin (1940), Hirano and Terry (1958), Pampus *et al.* (1960) and others. The main pathologic feature is a saccular dilation of the great vein of Galen which may present, if the blood is drained, as an oval or spherical, at times lobulated, cyst with thin smooth fibrous walls of grayish-white color. Its lumen communicates with the often dilated straight sinus and with the feeding vessels. The aneurysm may attain a size of several cms, compressing adjacent cerebral structures, particularly the quadrigeminal plate, with compression and displacement of the aqueduct. The carotids, vertebral and basilar arteries are often enlarged and are tortuous in some instances. The most common arterial shunting into the aneurysm is by way of the posterior cerebral arteries which may be branching or multiple. Next in frequency is a shunting of anterior cerebral arteries either alone or, more commonly, in combination with the posterior cerebral arteries (Fig. 119). Occasionally, shunting of the middle cerebral arteries can be demonstrated as well. The arteriovenous shunts occur commonly bilateral, rarely unilateral. The shunting arteries may show anomalies such as duplication, unilateral hypoplasia, or formation of anastomotic branches. The stem of the artery may dilate in the shape of a trumpet and enter the aneurysm directly, or it may dilate aneurysmatically before entering, or it may form a reticulum of intertwining vessels near the aneurysm. Microscopic examination of these arteries usually shows only minor changes, such as intima fibrosis or duplication of elastica (Pampus *et al.*, 1960). At the site of shunting there is a gradual transition between an arterial and a venous structure of the vascular wall with gradual thinning and loss of the internal elastic membrane and muscularis.

Complications occur in the form of acute or organized thrombi in the aneurysm or in the blood vessels connected to it. Mineralization of the wall of the aneurysm has been detected radiographically in 14 percent of cases, but always in juveniles or adults. The cerebral parenchyma is often completely free of gross or microscopic changes, particularly in newborns dying from cardiac failure. Yet, numerous instances of coexistent cerebral lesions have been described, presenting in the form of cavitated cortical infarcts (Gomez *et al.*, 1963), or as intraventricular hemorrhage from venous rupture, or as hemorrhagic infarcts of basal ganglia and corpus callosum (Hirano and Solomon, 1960), or as periventricular infarcts (Norman and Becker, 1974). The pathogenesis of the cerebral infarcts has not been specifically documented, but anoxia due to shunting or local compression of the tissue, heart failure, or phlebothrombosis have been implicated. Systemic lesions include cardio-

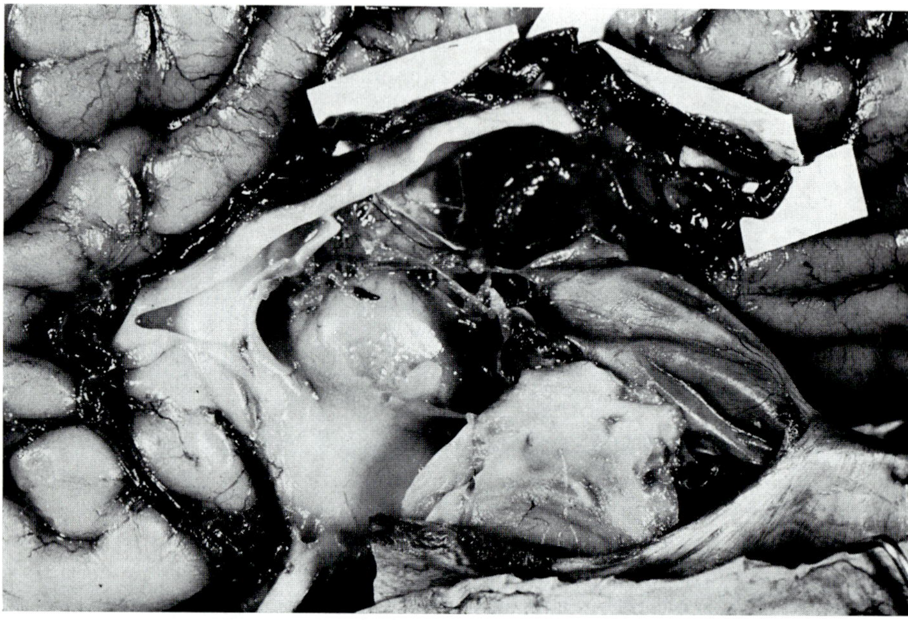

Fig. 119. Arteriovenous aneurysm of the great vein of Galen. The shunting of the distended anterior cerebral artery into the collapsed aneurysmal sac (right of center) is shown; middle and posterior cerebral arteries were shunted as well

megaly and hepatosplenomegaly. Anomalies of cardiac development are absent for the majority of cases, although transposition, septal defects, patent ductus arteriosus and anomalies of pulmonary drainage have been observed repeatedly (Hirano and Solomon, 1960; Levine *et al.*, 1962; Gomez *et al.*, 1963; Hernandez *et al.*, 1965; and others) and may compound the myocardial stress. Nearly all of the cases of aneurysm of the vein of Galen are sporadic, but a hereditary factor was implicated for an infant born to a family with hereditary hemorrhagic telangiectasia, the father having had an angioma removed from the spinal cord (Boynton and Morgan, 1973).

Shunting of Arteries into Intracranial Sinus. A small number of cases have been reported in whom abnormal shunting of cerebral arteries occurred into a dilated sinus rather than into the great vein of Galen. The morbid anatomy of these lesions differs sufficiently from those of aneurysm of the vein of Galen to consider them separately. Silverman *et al.* (1955) described two cases, one with gross communication of the middle and posterior cerebral arteries with the superior sagittal sinus, the other with a fistula between the middle cerebral artery and the sigmoid sinus; both were newborns who died from cardiac failure and both showed cavitated defects in the adjacent brain tissue. Litvak *et al.* (1960) described an 11-month-old girl with massive dilation of the sigmoid sinus, into which the middle and posterior cerebral arteries shunted, and a 15-year-old girl with massive dilation of the torcular, fed by a posterior communicating and a dilated left internal carotid artery.

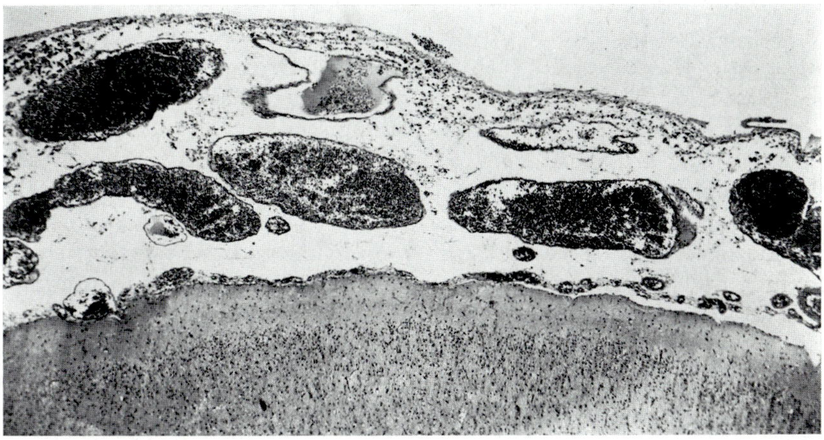

Fig. 120. Leptomeninges filled with distended thin-walled vessels in a case of diffuse meningeal angiodysplasia; H & E ×45

It is probable that the enormous dilation of the torcular in a 7-month-old boy described by Almeida and Pereira (1967) also belongs in this category, although the authors do not mention arterial shunting. Angiographic demonstration of 3 instances of this rare type of dysplasia were reported by Kosnik *et al.* (1974) with additional references.

Diffuse Meningocerebral Angiodysplasia. A small number of interesting cases have been published in whom the cerebral surface of newborns was covered entirely with an abundance of densely packed, dilated tortuous blood vessels (Fig. 120). The case described by Jellinger *et al.* (1966) is exemplary: The circle of Willis was replaced by a reticulum of vessels, which did not permit for the distinction between arteries and veins. The vein of Galen was excessively dilated. Microscopic examination revealed abrupt transitions between thick walled artery-like vessels and thin walled vessels having the characteristics of veins. Extensive destructive lesions in the cerebral hemispheres affecting cortex as well as white matter were associated with mineralization and with ectasia of small intracerebral vessels. The boy had also suffered from isthmus stenosis. These cerebral lesions were quite similar to those in the cyanotic boy described by Pollter (1954), in whom, also, numerous arteriovenous shunts were demonstrated microscopically; there was no cardiac malformation however. A newborn cyanotic boy without cardiac disease (Köhler, 1940) and a premature stillborn boy (Byrnes and Boellaard,

1958) also had angiodysplasia associated with extensive cortical and subcortical infarcts and mineralization; both cases had agenesis of the kidney as well and were considered by the authors to be infantile occurrences of Sturge-Weber disease. The case of Byrnes and Boellaard also had septal defect and patent ductus arteriosus. The changes in 3 newborns (Potter, 1948) were less severe than those described above, in that the angiodysplasia was entirely meningeal and neither parenchymal lesion nor hypervascularization was found in the brain tissue. The entire cerebral and cerebellar leptomeninges were crowded with tortuous vessels having the structure of capillaries and terminal veins. Myocardial hypertrophy was found in all 3 infants. Meningocerebral angiodysplasia was reported coexistent with arteriovenous aneurysm of the vein of Galen (Stehbens *et al.*, 1973), but the presence of angiodysplasia is not convincing from the supplied illustration.

Although this group of cases is quite small, and perhaps heterogeneous, it differs in many aspects from other types of lesions, as well as from arteriovenous malformations. In the cases of Jellinger *et al.* (1966) and Pollter (1954) extensive arteriovenous shunting evidently represented the key pathogenetic factors, and this anomaly should be searched for in the examination of new cases. Myocardial hypertrophy in Potter's (1948) cases is perhaps indicative of the presence of shunting. The classification of these cases as infantile Sturge-Weber disease is not acceptable as they lack cutaneous manifestations and glaucoma, and as the vascular dysplasia is bilateral. However, the case of Nellhaus *et al.* (1967), considered infantile Sturge-Weber disease with cutaneous angiomatosis and bilateral angiomatous, calcified lesions, illustrates the differential diagnostic difficulties. Residual lesions of cerebral phlebothrombosis (Chapter 13) also show cavitated infarcts associated with telangiectasia and dilation of residual vessels, but phlebothrombotic lesions are usually locally confined and do not show the same degree of vascular hyperplasia. Nonetheless, thrombic occlusion of many vessels in the white matter in the case of Byrnes and Boellaard (1958) indicates the need for a careful weighing of the cause-effect relationship.

The relationship between diffuse meningocerebral angiodysplasia in infants and a disease entity in adults described by Divry and van Bogaert (1946) as diffuse cerebromeningeal noncalcifying angiomatosis is not clear. Both processes may conceivably be the same disease, the less severe lesions manifesting later in life. Divry and van Bogaert originally thought that the angiomatosis in their cases was associated with a progressive sudanophilic leukodystrophy, and this interpretation was accepted in several subsequent case reports. However, a critical reappraisal of the lesions led to the rejection of the idea of a leukodystrophy (van Bogaert and Martin, 1971), and the sudanophilic changes in white matter and coexistent cortical necrosis were attributed to anoxia. Two sisters thought to be an infantile form of this disease were reported by Arseni *et al.* (1973). Two retarded adult sibs, in whom angiodysplasia was confined to the white matter, were described by Hori and Jacob (1972).

Persistent Fetal Meningeal Vascularization. Persistent fetal meningeal vascularization is a developmental trait, observed most commonly with dysraphic malformations. The gross and microscopic features of this type of vascular dysplasia were often described in the literature, but its significance was first recognized by Karch and Urich (1972). Persistence of a primitive fetal vascular pattern is characterized by abundant large sinusoid capillaries forming a dense vascular plexus in the leptomeninges abutting brain tissue (Fig. 121). This type of vascularization is characteristic of primitive nervous systems having no intrinsic capillary supply, and it persists to some degree after the capillaries have entered the parenchyma. It is a normal aspect

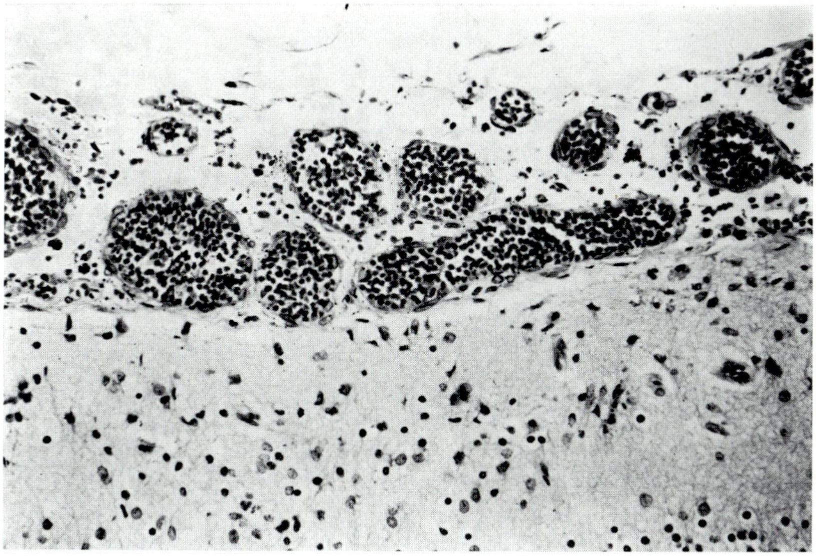

Fig. 121. Persistent fetal vascularization in tissue from an encephalocele: a plexus of sinusoid capillaries occupies the meninges in close contact with the brain surface; H & E ×115

of early embryogenesis, as well as a permanent feature of cerebrospinal vascularization in the lowest vertebrate species.

Persistent fetal meningeal vascularization is a rather conspicuous component of a variety of cerebral dysplasias, particularly the area cerebrovasculosa of anencephalics for which the crowded vessels usually dominate the lesion. The corresponding spinal lesion, the area medullovasculosa of myelomeningoceles, has similar structure. Persistent fetal vascularization also occurs with other dysplastic lesions, *e.g.*, encephaloceles, and it may be found throughout the leptomeninges for anatomically normal portions of the nervous system, *e.g.*, at the spinal cord of anencephalics (Chapter 23). Its occurrence is not limited to dysplasias: The residual tissue of acquired fetal encephaloclastic lesions, *e.g.*, membranous remnants of the hemispheres in hydranencephaly, may also show these changes. Persistent fetal vascularization has been interpreted as evidence of a concordance of a neuroectodermal and a mesodermal malformation, or as an independent angiomatous lesion (Zülch, 1956).

Persistent fetal meningeal vascularization is not a reliable index for dating lesions to the period of formation of the primitive fetal vascular plexus, as the pattern is known to persist beyond that period. Determinations of meningeal vascular density by counts of bifurcations per surface area showed that meningeal vascularity increases to a maximum at a fetal length of 33 cm; thereafter it decreased rapidly to less than one-third of that value in the 55 cm fetus, and to less than one half that value again in the 2-year-old child or adult (Pollter, 1956).

Involvement of Central Nervous System in Multiple Neonatal Angiomata. This rare disease entity was described by Ramdohr (1878) under the name

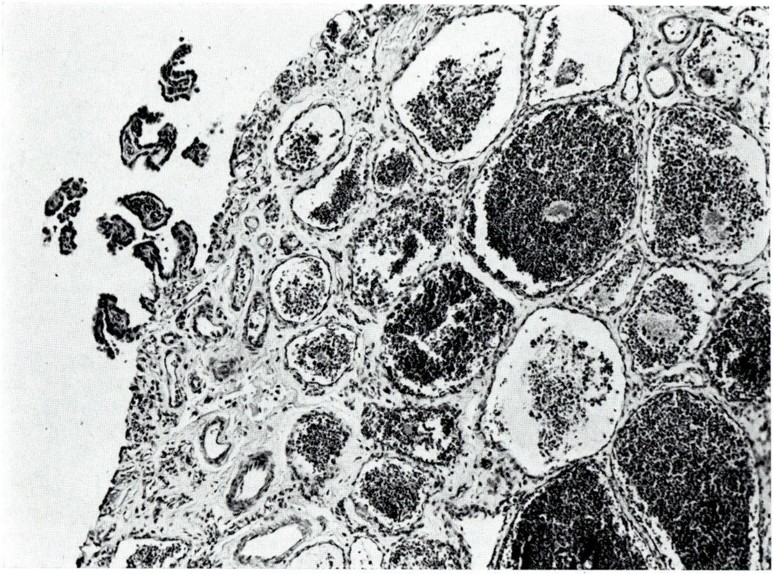

Fig. 122. Hemangioma of choroid plexus in a case of multiple neonatal hemangiomata; H & E ×85. (From the files of the Institute of Pathology: a case published by Cooper and Bolande, Pediatrics 35: 27, 1965)

of connatal multiple angiosarcoma. Holden and Alexander (1970) found only 6 cases in the literature and added 2 of their own. All the infants died during the first 6 months of life. The lesions consist of numerous circumscript, nonmalignant, angiomatous nodules in the skin and mucous membranes and in practically any of the parenchymatous organs, typically affecting 3 or more organ systems. Cerebral involvement had occurred in 6 of the 8 cases, with a random distribution of nodular masses up to several cms in diameter throughout the brain, brain stem, cerebellum and spinal cord; there was also involvement of the meninges, choroid plexus and peripheral nerves. Microscopic examination discloses angiomas composed of numerous thin-walled vessels lined by a single layer of flat endothelium and separated by variable amounts of loose connective tissue (Fig. 122). There is no evidence of malignancy. Three of the infants had evidence of heart failure indicative of extensive arteriovenous shunting; others were complicated by hydrocephalus or meningitis.

Arteriovenous Malformations. Arteriovenous malformations consist of focal convolutes of abnormal arteries and veins which contribute in variable proportions to the mass of the lesion. Arteriovenous shunting is common, with corresponding engorgement and dilation of the draining veins, resulting in a clinical triad of enlarged head, cranial bruit and cardiac failure (Long *et al.*, 1974). Deep midline arteriovenous malformations draining into the great vein of Galen may result in dilation of the latter, but the angiomatous character of the main lesion generally permits distinction between these cases and the arteriovenous aneurysms of the vein of Galen (Litvak *et al.*, 1960).

The majority of arteriovenous malformations becomes symptomatic during adult life, and only approximately 10 percent manifest in children. They are exceptionally rare in newborns, such as in a $7^1/_2$-month premature girl (Baird and Stitt, 1959) who had a mass of abnormal arteries and veins with interspaced neural tissue in the upper vermis fed by the left superior cerebellar artery. The main symptoms in a series of arteriovenous malformations in infants, 9 males and 4 females (Lagos and Riley, 1971), consisted of focal or general seizures or of subarachnoid bleeding; some showed cardiac failure from arteriovenous shunting. Subarachnoid hemorrhage below the age of 4 years is practically never caused by arteriovenous malformations, but the latter represent approximately one-third of the causes of hemorrhage in the age group of 15 to 19 years (Nishioka, 1966). At least some of the cryptic intracerebral hemorrhages in infants may be accounted for by a careful search for residual abnormal vessels at the edge of the hematoma, *e.g.*, in the 10-year-old girl reported by McDonald (1959).

The morbid anatomy of arteriovenous malformations in infants needs not to be described here in detail as it does not differ significantly from that of adults. The lesions may occur in any part of the brain, at its surface or in its depth. Enlarged feeding and draining vessels enter a more or less sharply defined conglomerate of abnormal vessels; these may show interspaced nervous tissue at the periphery, while abutting each other or being joined by fibrous tissue in the central portion of the lesion. Disorganization in the structure of the vascular wall is common, including reduplication, interruption or distortion of the internal elastic membrane of arteries, variation in the thickness of the media or muscularis, aneurysmatic dilation of vessels, and fibrosis of veins. Hemosiderin-laden macrophages and chronic inflammatory infiltrates may be seen in the adjacent brain tissue. The relative predominance of arterial and venous vessels in these malformations varies, and there are transitions between them and the local ectasias, varices, hyperplasias or abnormalities in the course and number of cerebral veins as, for example, for the venous abnormalities described by Dandy (1928).

References

Almeida, G. M., Pereira, W. C.: Hydrocephalus due to dilation of the dural sinuses. Case report. J. Neurosurg. 26: 267—269, 1967.

Arseni, C., Nereantiu, F., Nicolescu, P.: The infantile form of diffuse sclerosis with meningeal angiomatosis. Neurology (Minneap.) 23: 1297—1301, 1973.

Baird, W. F., Stitt, D. G.: Arteriovenous aneurysm of the cerebellum in a premature infant. Pediatrics 24: 455—457, 1959.

Boynton, R. C., Morgan, B. C.: Cerebral arteriovenous fistula with possible hereditary telangiectasia. Amer. J. Dis. Child. 125: 99—101, 1973.

Byrnes, A. L., Boellaard, J. W.: Renal agenesis and meningocerebral angiomatosis. Arch. Path. 66: 23—31, 1958.

Cooper, A. G., Bolande, R. P.: Multiple hemangiomas in an infant with cardiac hypertrophy. Pediatrics 35: 27—35, 1965.

Dandy, W.: Venous abnormalities and angiomas of the brain. Arch. Surg. (Chic.) 17: 715—793, 1928.

Divry, P., van Bogaert, L.: Une maladie familiale caractérisée par une angiomatose diffuse cortico méningée non calcificante et une démyelinisation progressive de la substance blanche. J. Neurol. Neurosurg. Psychiat. 9: 41—54, 1946.

Gold, A. P., Ransohoff, J., Carter, S.: Vein of Galen malformation. Acta neurol. scand. 40, Suppl. 11: 1—31, 1964.

Gomez, M. R., Whitten, C. F., Nolke, A., Bernstein, J., Meyer, J. S.: Aneurysmal malformation of the great vein of Galen causing heart failure in early infancy. Pediatrics 31: 400—411, 1963.

Hernandez, A., Schwartz, H. G., Goldring, D.: Cerebral arteriovenous fistulas and congenital heart disease. Pediatrics 66: 722—728, 1965.

Hirano, A., Solomon, S.: Arteriovenous aneurysm of the vein of Galen. Arch. Neurol. (Chic.) 3: 589—593, 1960.

— Terry, R. D.: Aneurysm of the vein of Galen. J. Neuropath. exp. Neurol. 17: 424—429, 1958.

Holden, K. R., Alexander, F.: Diffuse neonatal hemangiomatosis. Pediatrics 46: 411—421, 1970.

Hori, A., Jacob, H.: Diffuse Leukoangiomatosen bei erblichem Schwachsinn. Arch. Psychiat. Nervenkr. 216: 277—286, 1972.

Jaeger, R., Forbes, R. P., Dandy, W. E.: Bilateral congenital cerebral arteriovenous communicating aneurysm. Trans. Amer. Neurol. Ass. 63: 173—176, 1937.

Jellinger, K., Kucsko, L., Seitelberger, F.: Diffuse meningo-cerebrale Angiodysplasie mit hypoplasiogener Isthmusstenose bei einem Neugeborenen. Beitr. path. Anat. 133: 41—72, 1966.

Kaplan, H. A., Ford, D. H.: The Brain Vascular System. Amsterdam: Elsevier 1966.

Karch, S. B., Urich, H.: Occipital encephalocele: a morphological study. J. Neurol. Sci. 15: 89—112, 1972.

Köhler, U.: Sturge-Webersche Krankheit bei einer Frühgeburt. Zbl. allg. Path. 75: 81—85, 1940.

Kosnik, E. J., Hunt, W. E., Miller, C. A.: Dural arteriovenous malformations. J. Neurosurg. 40: 322—339, 1974.

Lagos, J. C., Riley, H. D.: Congenital intracranial vascular malformations in children. Arch. Dis. Child. 46: 285—290, 1971.

Levine, O. R., Jameson, A. G., Nelhaus, G., Gold, A. P.: Cardiac complications of cerebral arteriovenous fistula in infancy. Pediatrics 30: 563—575, 1962.

Litvak, J., Yahr, M., Ransohoff, J.: Aneurysm of the great vein of Galen and midline cerebral arteriovenous anomalies. J. Neurosurg. 17: 945—955, 1960.

Long, D. M., Seljeskog, E. L., Chou, S. N., French, L. A.: Giant arteriovenous malformations of infancy and childhood. J. Neurosurg. 40: 304—312, 1959.

McDonald, J.: Spontaneous intracerebral bleeding in children from cystic vascular hamartomas. J. Pediat. 55: 200, 1959.

Nellhaus, G., Haberland, C., Hill, B. J.: Sturge-Weber disease with bilateral intracranial calcifications at birth and unusual pathologic findings. Acta neurol. scand. 43: 314—347, 1967.

Nishioka, H.: Report of the cooperative study of intracranial aneurysms and subarachnoid hemorrhage. Section VII, Part 1. Evaluation of the conservative management of ruptured intracranial aneurysms. J. Neurosurg. 25: 574—592, 1966.

Norman, M. C., Becker, L. E.: Cerebral damage in neonates resulting from arteriovenous malformation of the vein of Galen. J. Neurol. Neurosurg. Psychiat. 37: 252—258, 1974.

Padget, D. H.: Development of cranial arteries in human embryo. Contr. Embryol. 32: 205—262, 1948.

Pampus, F., Gött, H., Kersting, G.: Das Aneurysma der Vena Galeni als Ursache des Hydrocephalus occlusus internus und apolektischer Blutungen im Säuglings-, Kindes- und Jugendalter. Neurochirurgia (Stuttg.) 3: 203—222, 1960.

Pollock, A. Q., Laslett, P. A.: Cerebral arteriovenous fistula producing cardiac failure in the newborn infant. J. Pediat. 53: 731—736, 1958.

Pollter, J.: Mißbildung der intracraniellen Gefäße beim Neugeborenen. Arch. Psychiat. Nervenkr. 192: 539—548, 1954.

— Untersuchungen an Blutgefäßen der Leptomeninx bei kongenitalen Herzfehlern mit Mischungscyanose. Virchows Arch. path. Anat. 329: 73—93, 1956.

Potter, E. L.: Diffuse angiectasis of the cerebral meninges in the newborn infant. Arch. Path. 46: 87—96, 1948.

Ramdohr, M.: Ein Fall von angeborenem multiplem Angiosarcom. Virchows Arch. path. Anat. 63: 459—460, 1878.

Russell, D. S., Nevin, S.: Aneurysm of the great vein of Galen causing internal hydrocephalus: report of two cases. J. Path. Bact. 51: 375—383, 1940.

Silverman, B. K., Breckx, T., Craig, J., Nadas, A. S.: Congestive failure in the newborn caused by cerebral A-V fistula. Amer. J. Dis. Child. 89: 539—543, 1955.

Siqueira, E. B., Murray, K. J.: Calcified aneurysms of the vein of Galen: report of a presumed case and review of the literature. Neurochirurgia (Stuttg.) 15: 106—112, 1972.

Stehbens, W. E., Sahgal, K. K., Nelson, L., Shaher, R. M.: Aneurysm of vein of Galen and diffuse meningeal angiectasia. Arch. Path. 95: 333—335, 1973.

Steinheil, S. O.: Über einen Fall von Varix aneurysmaticus im Bereich der Gehirngefäße. Inaug. Diss. Würzburg, 1895. Cited by Dandy, W. W.: Arteriovenous aneurysms of the brain. Arch. Surg. (Chic.) 17: 190—243, 1928.

Streeter, G.: The development of the venous sinuses of the dura mater in the human embryo. Amer. J. Anat. 18: 145—178, 1915.

— The developmental alterations of the vascular system of the brain of the human embryo. Contr. Embryol. 8: 5—38, 1918.

van Bogaert, L., Martin, J. J.: Analyse critique de la pathologie de l'angiomatose cérébroméningée diffuse non calcificante et de l'encéphalopathie de Binswanger. J. Neurol. Sci. 14: 301—314, 1971.

Wohak, H.: Ein Fall von Varix der Vena magna Galeni bei einem Neugeborenen. Virchows Arch. path. Anat. 242: 58—69, 1923.

Zülch, K. J.: Biologie und Pathologie der Hirngeschwülste. In: Handbuch der Neurochirurgie, Vol. 3, p. 564. Berlin-Göttingen-Heidelberg: Springer 1956.

Part 3. Metabolic Diseases

35. Diseases of Carbohydrate Metabolism

Glycogen Storage Diseases, General Comments and Classification. Two important principles which now pervade the entire field of heritable metabolic diseases originated in research on the etiology of glycogen storage diseases. The first principle, now generally applied to inherited metabolic disorders, derives from the proposal by Cori (1957) to classify types of glycogen storage diseases according to the deficient enzyme rather than in terms of organ involvement. The second principle grew out of chemical and electron microscopic studies on glycogen storage disease type II (acid maltase deficiency). Electron microscopic studies in this disease showed glycogen distributed in two forms, freely dispersed throughout the cytoplasm and enclosed in membrane-bounded vacuoles which were identified as lysosomes (Baudhuin *et al.*, 1964). As acid maltase is a lysosomal enzyme, it was concluded that an inability of the lysosomes to degrade glycogen after its inclusion into the organelle was the key feature of the disease process. The concept of lysosomal disability caused by deficiencies of specific lysosomal enzymes has proven extremely useful for the understanding of many other storage diseases.

An abstract review of the most important forms of glycogenoses is given in Table 5. Most are not associated with mental deficiency, nor are there distinct lesions in the central nervous system. Only for glycogenosis of type II is the deficient enzyme lysosomal, and the central nervous system is commonly affected. The systemic pathology of glycogenoses was reviewed by McAdams *et al.* (1974).

Type II Glycogenosis (Pompe Disease). Type II glycogen storage disease is caused by a deficiency of lysosomal acid maltase, a α-1-4-glucosidase (Hers, 1963). This enzyme is involved in one of the two alternative pathways of glycogen degradation. One pathway is phosphorolytic and requires two different enzymes for cleaving the 1–4 bonds of the straight chains and the 1–6 bonds of the branching points of the glycogen molecule; this pathway is active in the cytoplasmic sap and is not affected in type II glycogenosis. The other pathway is hydrolytic and takes place within lysosomes, acid maltase being capable of cleaving both types of linkages of the ramefied glycogen molecule. The end product of this pathway is glucose which diffuses into the cytoplasm across the lysosomal membrane. Deficiency of acid maltase disables the lysosomes in their capacity to degrade glycogen which accumulates and distends the lysosomes. There is hyperactivity of other lysosomal enzymes, as is characteristic of many other lysosomal storage diseases. The intralysosomal glycogen does not vary with fasting in the way the free glycogen does (Hug *et al.*, 1966) and appears to be more resistant to post-mortem lysis (Baudhuin *et al.*, 1964). This pathogenetic concept does account for the main features of the disease, but it has been criticized because it does not explain the accumulation of free glycogen in the cytoplasm.

Table 5. *Classification of Glycogenoses*

Designation			
Type I (v. Gierke)	Hepatic glucose-6-phosphatase	Liver, kidney	Enlargement of liver and kidney, stunting of growth, tendency to hypoglycemia and acidosis. Nuclear hyperglycogenosis
Type II (Pompe)	Lysosomal acid Maltase (α-1,4 glucosidase)	Generalized	Cardiomegaly, generalized muscular weakness, enlargement of tongue, hepatomegaly. Myopathy in the adult form
Type III (Forbes, Cori)	Debrancher enzyme (amylo-1,6-glucosidase)	Liver, heart muscle	Mild manifestations, hepatomegaly
Type IV (Andersen)	Brancher enzyme (amylo-1,4 $\rightarrow$ 1,6 transglucosidase)	Liver, probably other organs	Hepatomegaly and cirrhosis
Type V (McArdle)	Muscle phosphorylase	Muscle	Severe muscular pain, stiffness and weakness on slight excercise
Type VI (Hers)	Liver phosphorylase	Liver	Hepatomegaly, hypoglycemia, lipemia and acidosis

A number of additional types have been identified, but there is no consensus in the literature on their classification (compare Howell, 1972; McAdams *et al.*, 1974).

Glycogenosis type II causes the greatest degree of functional impairment in muscle tissue, involving heart as well as skeletal muscle, but the degree of involvement of each varies; in addition, glycogen storage is widespread throughout the body. The disease may manifest at any age, its symptoms varying with the age of onset. In the infantile form symptoms may be present from birth on, or they may manifest during the first month of life with cardiac enlargement and general muscular weakness without evidence of muscular atrophy. Enlargement of the tongue and a moderate and variable hepatomegaly are common. Death from cardiac failure often occurs before the age of 1 year is reached. Mental development is normal for many cases, but mental subnormality has been observed, and neurological signs, particularly of bulbar involvement, may develop during the course of the disease. As all other glycogenoses, type II is inherited autosomal recessive, and there is a slight but definite preponderance of males. The late infantile, juvenile or adult forms of the disease were recognized only after the deficiency of acid maltase was identified as the diagnostic feature; manifestations are those of a progressive muscular dystrophy (Hers and de Barsy, 1973, review).

Accumulation of glycogen in nervous tissue has often been described for Pompe disease, but most reports are brief and provide little detail. The extensive accounts by Crome *et al.* (1963) and Mancall *et al.* (1965) indicate, along with the rest of the data, a rather constant regional pattern of central nervous system involvement.

The consistency of the brain in glycogenosis type II has been recorded as being somewhat firm to the touch, but there are no other significant anomalies. No increase in cerebral weight has been recorded. Adequate fixation in alcohol or in other fixatives suitable for glycogen enhances the efficiency

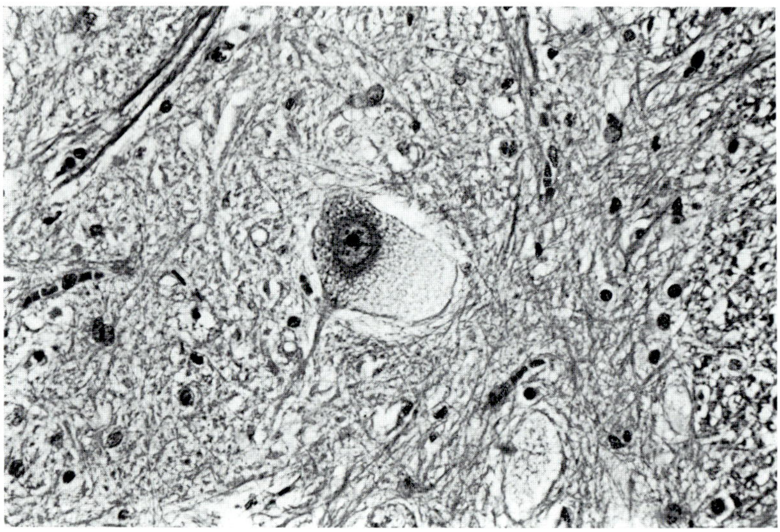

Fig. 123. Distension of a ventral horn motor neuron in Pompe disease; H & E ×275

of the microscopic demonstration of glycogen in nervous parenchyma. Maximum storage of glycogen is seen in the large neurons of spinal cord (Fig. 123), brain stem and cerebellar nuclei, particularly in the motor neurons of the anterior horns and cranial nerve nuclei, the spinal ganglia and the dentate nuclei. The cytoplasm of the cells is filled with fine glycogen granules and it may appear foamy or reticulated if the glycogen had been dissolved. The granules tend to crowd at the periphery of the cell and into the dendritic hillocks while the chromatin substance is preserved around the nucleus. With a moderate degree of glycogen storage the nucleus maintains its normal position, but it may become displaced peripherally when glycogen granules crowd the entire cytoplasm. Storage of glycogen within the nucleus itself is usually absent but is seen on occasion. There is much variance in the extent of glycogen storage from one cell to the other. In addition to excessive storage in the regions mentioned above, there is also marked storage of glycogen in Clarke's column, the brain stem reticular formation, the olives, and other brain stem nuclei, the pallidum and the substantia innominata. Relatively moderate storage is seen in the lateral thalamic and geniculate nuclei, and in the Ammon's horn except for Sommer's sector. The neurons of the cerebral cortex, of Sommer's sector of the Ammon's horn, the cerebellar Purkinje cells and granule cells, the amygdala and anterior medial and pulvinar portions of the thalamus show little or no storage (Martin *et al.*, 1973). A mild loss of neurons and a diffuse gliosis of white matter have been described, the latter being consistent with a decrease in myelin lipids (Crome *et al.*, 1963). Generally, however, the glycogen storage in glycogenosis is much less destructive to neurons than is the lipid storage in the various lipidoses, and the cerebellar atrophy found in many of the latter is absent for glycogen storage disease.

Aside from neurons, glycogen storage also occurs in other cells, mostly in astrocytes which may show their processes outlined by chains of glycogen granules, as seen particularly in the white matter. A subpial deposition of glycogen is probably accounted for by its accumulation in astrocytic footplates. A diffuse fine dusting of the tissue with glycogen granules had been erroneously considered extracellular before the electron microscope provided a better understanding of the fine structure of neuropil. Storage of glycogen also involves vascular endothelia, the ependyma and the epithelium of the choroid plexus. The profiles of myelin sheaths in peripheral nerves may be outlined with glycogen deposits, and there is also involvement of autonomic nervous system, as well as involvement of the retina (Toussaint and Danis, 1965). Chemical determinations of glycogen in brain tissue gave above normal values, and a greater increase in white than in gray matter has been observed.

Most studies on glycogenosis focussed on the storage of glycogen, but there is also evidence for the storage of an acidic mucosubstance in the tissue which differs from glycogen in being weakly periodic acid-Schiff positive, and staining metachromatic with toluene blue and azure blue and positive with alcian blue and dialyzed iron. This material is highly water soluble and may be lost from the tissue; loss during processing is prevented by fixation of specimens in dioxan and special processing techniques (Wolfe and Cohen, 1968, references). The occurrence of such non-glycogen polysaccharides in brain tissue was demonstrated by Schnabl (1965), who emphasized their high concentration in the astrocytes of white matter.

The most comprehensive accounts of the subcellular distribution of glycogen in nervous tissue in glycogenosis type II are those of Gambetti *et al.* (1971) and Martin *et al.* (1973). Their findings are consistent with those of other authors in revealing a distribution of glycogen similar to that in viscera as first described by Baudhuin *et al.* (1964): The glycogen occurs freely dispersed throughout the cytoplasm as well as enclosed in membrane-bound vacuoles. The amount of free glycogen varies somewhat, apparently depending on the degree of tissue preservation. Membrane-bounded vacuoles, tightly packed with glycogen granules, are seen in neurons, glia cells, vascular endothelia and the Schwann cells of peripheral nerves. Intranuclear deposition of glycogen is seen on occasion. An equivalent of the fine structural changes in glycogenosis type II has been found by Sandström *et al.* (1969) as an incidental observation in a clinically unremarkable cat.

Glycogenosis with Cerebral Storage of α-Glycogen. Electron micrographs of nervous tissue normally show glycogen only in the form of the so-called β-particles, roughly isodiametric granules of 150 to 300 Å, which have a somewhat irregular surface and a nodular substructure on high magnification. The β-particles are distributed at random throughout the cytoplasm. In hepatic tissue there is commonly aggregation of β-particles to larger, rosette shaped aggregates, the α-particles, which normally do not occur in brain.

Résibois-Grégoire and Dourov (1966) reported electron microscopic observations in a child with a progressive neurologic disorder who had died with amaurosis and quadruplegia at the age of 11 months. The only abnormalities found were in the central nervous system: Glia cells contained glycogen in its normal form of β-particles; whereas, neurons and their processes were crowded with α-particles, some of which had assumed giant proportions. Similar electron microscopic data were briefly reported by Hug and Schubert (1966) for a child with a progressive neurologic disease whose metabolic derangement had been studied extensively, showing increased hepatic glycogen and increased urinary excretion of catecholamines (Hug *et al.*, 1967). The classification of cerebral storage of α-glycogen is still obscure; no α-glycogen has been reported in brain tissue for glycogenosis type II.

Galactosemia. The enzyme catalyzing the exchange of α-galactose-1-phosphate with uridine-diphosphoglucose, forming α-glucose-1-phosphate and uridine-diphosphogalactose, is absent in galactosemic subjects with a consequent accumulation of galactose-1-phosphate (Schwarz *et al.*, 1956; Kalckar *et al.*, 1956). The disease presents in early infancy with vomiting and it may be accompanied with increased intracranial pressure (Huttenlocher *et al.*, 1970). It induces mental retardation. Hepatic cirrhosis, hepatomas and cataracts develop unless dietary regiment is started early.

Neuropathologic lesions in galactosemia were described for an 8-year-old boy by Crome (1962) and for a 25-year-old man by Haberland *et al.* (1971), being generally more severe in the latter. Both cases had micrencephaly with a diffuse gliosis of the white matter and advanced loss of cerebellar Purkinje cells. There were no changes in the cerebral cortex in Crome's case, except for a duplication of the pyramidal layer of the Ammon's horn. The other case had marked neuronal loss, patchy defects of myelin in the white matter and glial proliferation of Alzheimer type II. In addition, there was abnormal pigmentation and neuraxonal degeneration in the pallidum and the substantia nigra.

Aspartyl Glucosaminuria. The excretion of aspartyl glucosamine in the urine of two mentally retarded sibs was reported by Jenner and Pollitt (1967). The disease is found in mentally defective adolescents or young adults with a history of slow development. Manifestations include coarse facial features, deformities of the skull and spine, connective tissue alterations and mental retardation, more often with psychiatric symptoms and aggressive behavior than with neurologic signs. There is a variety of skin affectations and frequent infections; vacuolated lymphocytes are seen in the blood (Palo and Mattsson, 1970).

The neuropathology of this disease is still insufficiently documented; electron microscopic studies of brain bioptic material disclosed lysosomal anomalies in the neurons and glia cells consisting of enlargement and increase in the number of lysosomes with accumulation of lipid droplets in them (Arstila *et al.*, 1972).

Fucosidosis. Fucosidosis is due to a deficiency in lysosomal α-L-fucosidase, which results in the accumulation of fucose, water-soluble fucose-rich polysaccharides and sphingolipids in brain and liver. The deficiency of fucosidase is associated with hyperactivity of other lysosomal hydrolases. Only four cases had been recognized by 1973 (Van Hoof, 1973). The manifestations of the disease vary and symptoms may be similar to those in Hurler syndrome or to gangliosidosis or leukodystrophy. There is severe mental retardation which may be associated with spasticity and decerebrate rigidity, abundant sweating, thickened skin, recurrent infections, emaciation and cardiomegaly with myocarditis. Cytoplasmic vacuolization is found in lymphocytes. The disease leads to death in late infancy.

Neuropathologic examination of two cases revealed ubiquitous ballooning of nerve cells, some of which were filled with a finely granular, weakly basophilic material. There was widespread loss of neurons and deficiency of myelination in the cerebral white matter. Storage of abnormal material was seen in hepatic cells, skeletal muscle and dermis. Electron microscopic changes in brain tissue differed from the lamellar material found in Hurler syndrome or in gangliosidoses in that the cytoplasm of neurons was packed with small clear vacuoles containing a sparse floccular material; lamellar material was contained in the vacuoles only as an exception (Loeb *et al.*, 1969).

Mannosidosis. Mannosidosis is due to a deficiency of lysosomal mannosidase with a concurrent elevation of other lysosomal hydrolases. The enzyme deficiency causes an impaired glycoprotein metabolism with storage of oligosaccharides containing mannose and glucosamine. Only six cases have been recognized by 1973. The disease is probably of autosomal recessive inheritance. It is known to occur in angus cattle (Ockerman, 1973, review).

The clinical features of mannosidosis have certain similarities to Hurler syndrome, with a gargoyl-like face, psychomotor retardation, gibbus, abnormal bone structure, hepatosplenomegaly and vacuolized lymphocytes. Initial acceleration of growth is followed by stunting after the age of 2 years and there is agammaglobulinemia and episodes of ketoacidosis.

Neuropathologic changes in a 4½-year-old boy were reported by Kjellman *et al.* (1969). The slightly enlarged brain was abnormally firm, with cerebellar atrophy. The latter was of the granular layer type, but there was some reduction of Purkinje cells as well. There was ballooning of nerve cells throughout cerebral cortex, brain stem and cord, but involvement of the basal ganglia was sparse or absent. The ballooning of neurons was due to the accumulation of a highly water-soluble PAS positive material. The cerebral white matter was demyelinated with perivascular accumulation of lipophages.

Mucopolysaccharidoses (Glucosaminoglycan Storage Diseases). The mucopolysaccharidoses are a group of complex storage diseases affecting mainly bone and connective tissue, some in association with marked progressive mental retardation and morphologic alterations in the central nervous system.

The descriptions of the prototypes of two forms of the disease are usually credited to Hunter (1917) of Winnipeg, who reported its occurrence in two brothers, and to the report on two disproportioned nonrelated dwarfs by Gertrud Hurler (1919) of Munich. However, the customary attributions of priorities in the description of various types of mucopolysaccharidoses are often inconsistent with historical facts, as discussed in the comprehensive review of McKusick (1972), which sould be consulted for a detailed account of these diseases. The general classification of the mucopolysaccharidoses apart from the lipidoses is based on the findings of Brante (1952) who identified the abnormal material accumulating in the viscera in Hunter disease with a mucopolysaccharide. The ensuing concern with disturbances of the metabolism of mucopolysaccharides tended to over-shadow the fact, particularly pertinent to neuropathology, that there is also storage of lipids in the mucopolysaccharidoses.

The conventional approach in the identification of a storage disease is the isolation and chemical analysis of the abnormal material stored in the tissue, and then to deduce from its composition the affected chemical pathway and to identify its specific defects. This approach was not equally successful for the identification and classification of mucopolysaccharidoses because of the complexity of the substances stored in the tissue. Instead, the mucopolysaccharidoses were originally classified according to the mucopolysaccharide excreted in the urine, with additional consideration given to the genetics and the clinical features of the diseases. According to this widely accepted system, proposed by McKusick *et al.* (1965), the following types were distinguished: Type I, the Hurler syndrome, is associated with excretion of dermatan and heparan sulfates. Type II, the Hunter syndrome, excretes the same polysaccharides but differs in its sex-linked recessive inheritance; all other mucopolysaccharidoses are of autosomal recessive inheritance. Also, the course of type II is milder and corneal clouding is absent. Type III, the Sanfilippo syndrome, excretes heparan sulfate and is associated with mild somatic effects but severe mental retardation. Type IV, the Morquio syndrome, excretes keratan sulfate and affects the intellect only slightly while bone deformities are severe. Type V, the Scheie syndrome, excretes dermatan sulfate and heparan sulfate and shows generally mild manifestations without marked impairment of intellect. Type VI, the Maroteaux-Lamy syndrome, excretes dermatan sulfate and is associated with severe osseous or corneal changes, but no intellectual impairment. Several additional variants have been identified. The chemical nomenclature used in describing mucopolysaccharidoses has been subject to revisions; the following definitions may help in perusing the literature:

New Term	*Old Term*
Glucosaminoglycan	Mucopolysaccharide
Dermatan sulfate	Chondroitin sulfate B
Heparan sulfate	Heparitin sulfate
Keratan sulfate	Keratosulfate
Chondroitin-4-sulfate	Chondroitin sulfate A
Chondroitin-6-sulfate	Chondroitin sulfate C

Designation		Clinical features	Genetics	Excessive urinary MPS	Substance deficient
MPS I H	Hurler syndrome	Early clouding of cornea, grave manifestations, death usually before age 10	Homozygous for MPS I H gene	Dermatan sulfate Heparan sulfate	α-L-iduronidase (formerly called Hurler corrective factor)
MPS I S	Scheie syndrome	Stiff joints, cloudy cornea, aortic regurgitation, normal intelligence, ?normal life-span	Homozygosity for MPS I S gene	Dermatan sulfate Heparan sulfate	α-L-iduronidase
MPS I H/S	Hurler-Scheie compound	Phenotype intermediate between Hurler and Scheie	Genetic compound of MPS I H and I S genes	Dermatan sulfate Heparan sulfate	α-L-iduronidase
MPS II A	Hunter syndrome, severe	No clouding of cornea, milder course than in MPS I H but death usually before age 15 years	Hemizygous for X-linked gene	Dermatan sulfate Heparan sulfate	Hunter corrective factor
MPS II B	Hunter syndrome, mild	Survival to 30's to 50's, fair intelligence	Hemizygous for X-linked allele for mild form	Dermatan sulfate Heparan sulfate	Hunter corrective factor
MPS III A	Sanfilippo syndrome A	Identical phenotype:	Homozygous for Sanfilippo A gene	Heparan sulfate	Heparan sulfate sulfatase
MPS III B	Sanfilippo syndrome B	Mild somatic, severe central nervous system effects	Homozygous for Sanfilippo B (at different locus)	Heparan sulfate	N-acetyl-α-D-glucosaminidase
MPS IV	Morquio syndrome (probably more than one allelic form)	Severe bone changes of distinctive type, cloudy cornea, aortic regurgitation	Homozygous for Morquio gene	Keratan sulfate	Unknown
MPS V	Vacant				
MPS VI A	Maroteaux-Lamy syndrome, classic form	Severe osseous and corneal change, normal intellect	Homozygous for M-L gene	Dermatan sulfate	Maroteaux-Lamy corrective factor [2]
MPS VI B	Maroteaux-Lamy syndrome, mild form	Severe osseous and corneal change, normal intellect	Homozygous for allele at M-L locus	Dermatan sulfate	Maroteaux-Lamy corrective factor [2]
MPS VII	β-glucuronidase deficiency (more than one allelic form?)	Hepatosplenomegaly, dysostosis multiplex, white cell inclusions, mental retardation	Homozygous for mutant gene at β-glucuronidase locus	Dermatan sulfate	β-glucuronidase

[1] From McKusick, Victor A.: Heritable disorders of connective tissue, ed. 4. St. Louis: C. V. Mosby 1972.
[2] Probably arylsulfatase B (Fluharty *et al.*, Biochem. Biophys. Res. Com. 59: 455—461, 1971.

The basis for recent progress in the classification of mucopolysaccharidoses was the identification of corrective factors which prevent the metabolic derangement when added to fibroblast cultures obtained from patients affected by the various types of mucopolysaccharidoses (Neufeld and Cantz, 1973, review). This research paved the way for the further identification of the corrective factors with the enzymes that are deficient in the respective disease types. Identification of the missing enzymes revealed the need for an extensive reclassification of mucopolysaccharidoses. Some types, that had been thought to be different diseases were found to be caused by deficiency of the same enzyme: The Hurler and Scheie syndromes have a deficiency of α-L-iduronidase in common (Matalon *et al.*, 1971; Matalon and Dorfman, 1972). The Sanfilippo syndrome, on the other hand, was recognized to be phenotype caused by two different enzyme deficiencies, heparan sulfate sulfatase (Kresse and Neufeld, 1972; Kresse, 1973) and N-acetyl-α-d-glucosaminidase (O'Brien, 1972). McKusick (1972) reclassified mucopolysaccharidoses on the basis of these most recent developments (Table 6).

The clinical manifestations of the Hurler syndrome are to some extent representative of the entire group of mucopolysaccharidoses, although the presence or the extent of a given manifestation varies for the different types. The enlarged skull shows a flattening of the bridge of the nose and prominent supraorbital ridges, hypertelorism, thick everted lips, a protruding tongue, gingival hyperplasia and widely separated hypoplastic teeth, features expressed in the term "gargoylism". There is a stunting in growth, the neck being shortened and the thorax broad, and shortening and thickening of long bones. Fingers are short and stubby with limitation of motion. Limitation in the mobility of auditory ossicles causes hearing difficulties. Vertebral bodies are hypoplastic and ovoid with kyphosis of the spine which may become accentuated to gibbus formation which may cause compression of the spinal cord. Hair and skin are coarse; there are corneal opacities. The cytoplasm of circulating granulocytes, lymphocytes and monocytes contains the azurophilic granules described by Alder (1939) and Reilly (1941); on electron microscopic examination they consist of membrane-bound, clear vacuoles whose derivation from lysosomes is shown by their acid phosphatase activity (Belcher, 1972). Death often occurs from cardiac failure because of valvular deposits, coronary, endocardial or myocardial lesions.

Marked, progressive mental deterioration accompanies the anomalies of bone and connective tissue in the Hurler, Hunter, and Sanfilippo syndromes. The common denominator for the mental derangement may be a marked elevation of CSF mucopolysaccharides, heparatan sulfate being the predominant type; in Scheie syndrome, in which intelligence is not impaired, there are normal or only slightly elevated levels of CSF mucopolysaccharides (Dekaban and Constantopoulos, 1973). The coverage of the cerebral changes of these syndromes in the literature is uneven, but the available information suggests that the lesions are quite similar, safe for minor variations in the intensity and regional distribution, the significance of which has not been studied in sufficient detail.

On gross examination of the brain its consistency may be somewhat increased, or even rubbery, but there are usually no evident destructive or atrophic lesions of the cerebral cortex although the hemispheres may be enlarged and distended by obstructive hydrocephalus. The leptomeninges covering the hemispheric convexity as well as the basal cisterns are thickened and gelatinous and may, in extreme instances, increase in volume to the extent that the convolutional pattern of the cortex is completely obscured (Magee, 1950). The increase in the volume of connective tissue is also evident at the cut surface of the hemispheres where the perivascular spaces in the

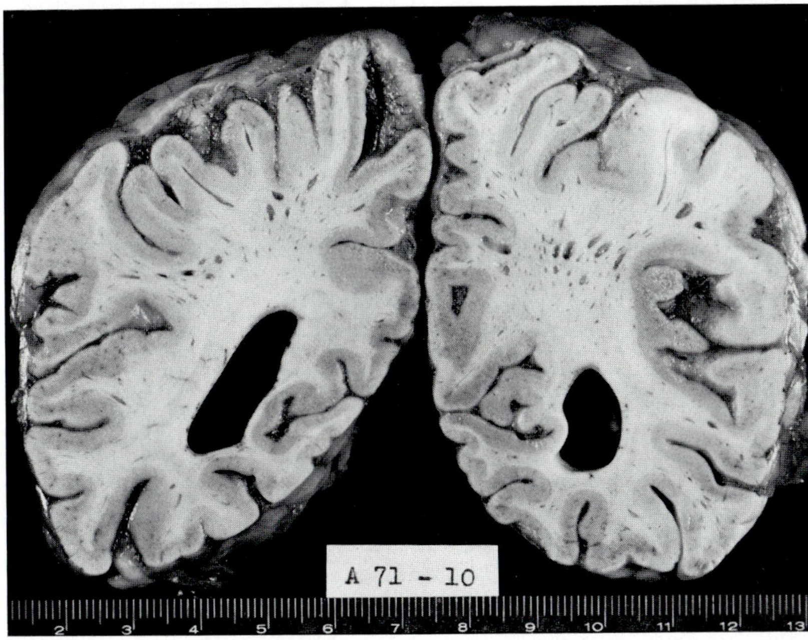

Fig. 124. Enlargement of perivascular spaces in Hurler disease

deep cerebral white matter are distended by an increase in the volume of the adventitia (Fig. 124); similar changes may be seen in the cerebellar white matter. When cut parallel to the axis of the long radiating vessels, the spaces form elongated cysts, up to several mm in diameter, with a central vessel. This characteristic alteration was emphasized first by Tuthill (1934) in her documentation of the pathology of one of the two cases described by Hurler, and later by Naidoo (1953) and many others.

Hydrocephalus with marked to excessive distension of the cerebral ventricles is a common feature of Hurler syndrome, and it, as well as the thickening of the skull and the increase in meningeal tissue, account for the characteristic enlargement of the head. The degree of ventricular distension is out of proportion to the mild or absent loss of parenchyma. Hydrocephalus is most likely caused by the obstruction of flow of CSF through the leptomeninges and several mechanisms may be operative in this disturbance: There may be meningeal fibrosis caused by an irritating effect of the stored material;

or the bulk of the accumulated polysaccharides may in itself impede the flow of CSF; or the dissolved mucopolysaccharides may alter the viscosity or osmolarity of the CSF, thereby slowing its flow through the meninges and hindering its reabsorption. The significance of these factors has not been compared in detail, but histologic examination of the leptomeninges usually discloses a reasonably wide mesh of subarachnoid trabecules, which appears to be more consistent with any of the two latter interpretations than with obstructive fibrosis.

The two dominant microscopic alterations in the mucopolysaccharidoses are an increase in the amounts of leptomeningeal and perivascular connective tissue and the storage of a lipidic, carbohydrate-containing substance in neurons. Microscopic examination of the distended perivascular spaces shows a considerable increase in the volume of adventitial tissue which forms a reticulum of fibroblasts with scattered collagen fibers (Fig. 125). There are wide meshes in this tissue which may contain scattered clusters of lipid-laden macrophages. The white matter encompassing the perivascular spaces shows, typically, no reduction in the density of myelinated fibers, but areas of focal demyelination may be seen on occasion (Jervis, 1950). The large empty lacunae in the basal ganglia described by Norman *et al.* (1959) are unusual, and they are somewhat reminiscent of the changes caused by postmortem gas formation. The leptomeninges are thickened and contain rather cellular arachnoid trabecules. This alteration is often described as an increase in leptomeningeal collagen tissue; however, there is much less deposition of collagen fibers than seen in instances of chronic adhesive meningitis and no actual evidence of scarring is found. Macrophages may be scattered throughout the leptomeninges.

Although the increase in leptomeningeal and adventitial tissue is evidently caused by the accumulation of mucopolysaccharides, there is usually no abnormal PAS staining of the tissue in specimens obtained by routine tissue processing. In specimens fixed in dioxane, however, an abundance of acid mucopolysaccharides may be demonstrated in the meninges (Wolfe *et al.*, 1964). The material stored in the meningeal connective tissue resembles, in this regard, that stored in the viscera in being more water soluble than that stored in neurons.

Microscopic changes in the nervous parenchyma consist of distended and ballooned neurons with deposition of lipidic carbohydrate-containing material in their cytoplasm (Fig. 125). Much of the abnormal material is extracted during routine processing and a foamy or reticular cytoplasm remains. The nucleus may be in its normal central position, or it may be displaced toward the periphery of the cell, depending on the degree of storage. The material deposited in the neurons is much less water soluble than that in meninges or viscera (Dawson, 1954; Bishton *et al.*, 1956) and stains, in frozen sections, pale reddish or orange with the various sudan reds, gray with sudan black, blue with nile blue, gray-black with Baker's stain, and gives a strong PAS reaction (Jervis, 1950); after embedding in paraffin, a weak, smudgy PAS staining remains. The lipidic nature of the material was recognized by Brante (1952) who identified it with gangliosides, an observation confirmed in many later studies, and also consistent with histochemical data (Diezel, 1954). There are differences in the chemical composition of the gangliosides stored in the mucopolysaccharidoses and those stored in the gangliosidoses (Gonatas and Gonatas, 1965; Ledeen *et al.*, 1965). Determinations of ganglioside patterns in gray and white matter showed a reduction of G_{T1} (G_1) and G_{T1D} (G_2) gangliosides

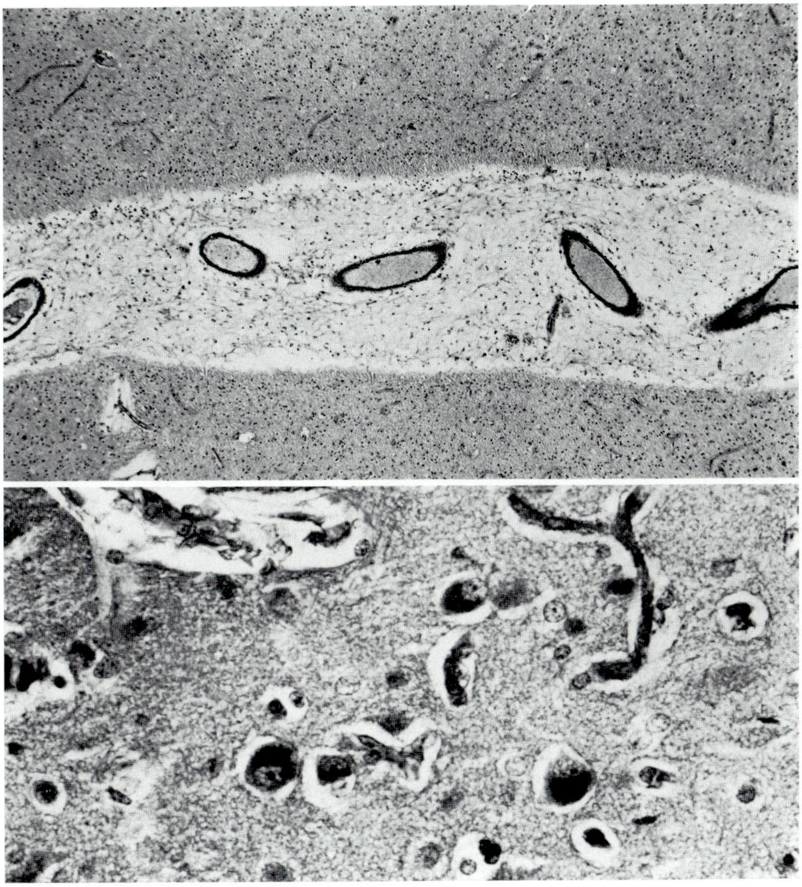

Fig. 125. Hurler disease. Top: Adventitial fibrosis; PAS ×45. Bottom: deposits of smudgy, PAS positive material in cortical neurons; ×350

in both; there was an elevation of G_{D3}, G_{M1}, G_{M2}, and G_{M3} (G_{3A}, G_4, G_5, and G_6) gangliosides in the gray matter and of G_{D1A} and G_{D3} (G_3 and G_{3A}) in the white (Roukema *et al.*, 1973). The significance of these subpatterns is still difficult to assess in view of the somewhat different alterations found by Dekaban and Patton (1971) for Hurler and Sanfilippo cases. The mucopolysaccharidoses and gangliosidoses also share subnormal activities of β-galactosidase; this enzyme is severely deficient in G_{M1}-gangliosidosis, and is reduced in Hurler and Hunter syndromes (Ockerman and Köhlin, 1968; Gerich, 1969). The reduction in the latter is less severe than the deficiency in

G_{M1}-gangliosidosis and is organ specific; it has been attributed to a secondary change caused by the storage of mucopolysaccharides. In view of the overlap in chemistry, it is not surprising that Hurler syndrome was classified in the first neuropathologic report as juvenile amaurotic idiocy (Tuthill, 1934), and that it was later called lipochondrodystrophy; also, neuropathologists have been inclined to classify it among the sphingolipidoses (Seitelberger, 1957).

Distension of neurons by storage tends to be widespread, particularly in the cerebral cortex and the basal ganglia; there is much variance in the extent of storage from one neuron to the other. Loss of nerve cells may ensue, but its degree as well as that of reactive gliosis usually is mild. Distension of nerve cells of brain stem nuclei, cerebellum and spinal cord tends to be less intense than in the cerebral hemispheres. The affection of the cerebellar cortex, in particular, does not approach the degree characteristic of gangliosidoses. Abnormal material may be found in the cytoplasm of Purkinje cells, along with focal distension of the proximal portions of their dendrites (Jervis, 1950; Bishton *et al.*, 1956), but the loss of Purkinje cells is moderate and there is no severe atrophy of the cerebellar cortex. Neuronal storage is also seen in the myenteric plexus (Green, 1948).

Electron microscopic examination of cerebral tissue in Hurler disease discloses the accumulation of several types of inclusions in the cytoplasm of neurons. The most characteristic ones are the so-called zebra bodies which are somewhat reminiscent of mitochondria in size and shape but possess a single unit membrane rather than a double membrane (Fig. 126). Zebra bodies are filled with regularly stacked transverse lamellae having a periodicity of 55 to 60 Å, separated, at intervals, by large clear spaces. They differ from the membranous cytoplasmic bodies of the gangliosidoses in that a concentric arrangement of lamellae is rarely seen. Zebra bodies may show transitions into other bodies composed partially or entirely of a fine granular material. Still different inclusions consist of sharply delineated clear vacuoles. Neurons contain all these inclusions whereas vascular endothelia contain also granular and vacuolar material (Aleu *et al.*, 1965; Uchimura *et al.*, 1965). Similar alterations in fine structure are also seen in the Sanfilippo syndrome, and the derivation of the abnormal cytosomes from lysosomes is demonstrated by their acid phosphatase activity (Wallace *et al.*, 1966).

The pituitary gland is consistently involved in the Hurler syndrome, with vacuolization of the adenohypophysial cells on light microscopic examination. Under the electron microscope the acidophils store mucopolysaccharides in the form of clear vacuoles; the basophils contain cytosomes similar to zebra bodies (Schochet *et al.*, 1974).

The neuropathologic data reviewed above refer to the Hurler, Hunter, and Sanfilippo varieties of the mucopolysaccharidoses in which affection of the central nervous system is marked. In the Morquio variant impairment of mentation is slight or absent; Gilles and Deuel (1971) found a regionally selective pattern of neuronal loss and intraneuronal storage of globules in a $4^{1}/_{4}$-year-old boy. The changes were most marked in the thalamus and in the resistant sector and endplate of the Ammon's horn and were only slight or scattered for other nuclear groups. The globular deposits in the cytoplasm

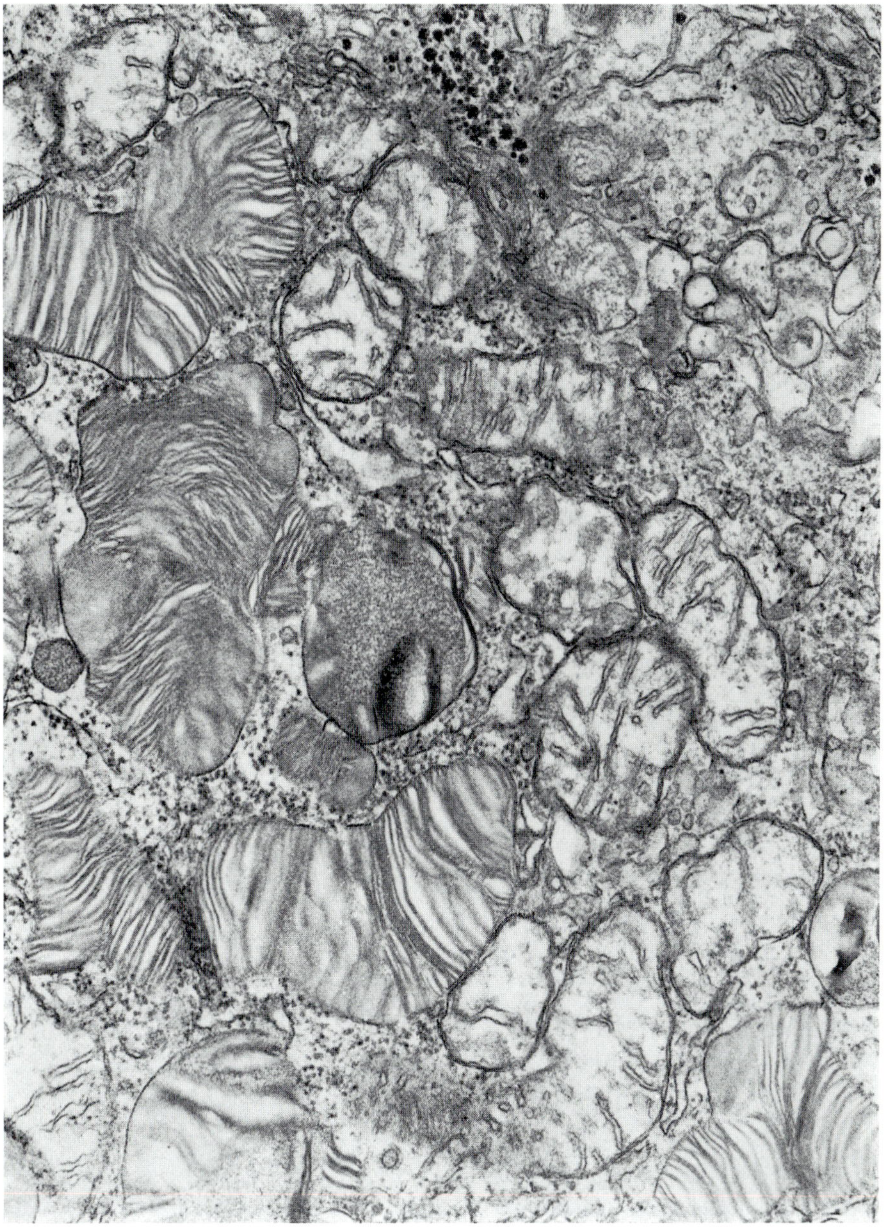

Fig. 126. Zebra bodies and mitochondria (courtesy Dr. Schochet)

of neurons were eosinophilic and stained weakly with various lipid stains and the PAS reaction. Their fine structure was similar to that of zebra bodies, but other deposits similar to lipofuscin were also observed.

Aside from the changes attributable to the metabolic disease, there is still another type of affectation of CNS in the mucopolysaccharidoses, that is from local compression due to bone anomalies of the spinal column or to subluxation of the odontoid process. Clinical manifestations of the cord compression were described for 8 patients with Morquio syndrome by Blaw and Langer (1969). The neuropathology of these secondary lesions has received relatively little attention, but flattening of the cervical cord and degeneration of lateral tracts in a case of Morquio syndrome was reported by Gilles and Deuel (1971).

General autopsy findings in mucopolysaccharidoses include hepatosplenomegaly with deposition of mucopolysaccharides in reticuloendothelial cells of liver, in the spleen, the myocardium, cardiac valves and arterial intima. There are irregularities in enchondral ossification with variations in size and shape of the diaphyses of the long bones, periosteal fibrosis and various degrees of fibrosis and lipid storage in marrow tissue.

References

Alder, A.: Über konstitutionell bedingte Granulationsveränderungen der Leucocyten. Dtsch. Arch. klin. Med. 183: 372—378, 1939.

Aleu, F. P., Terry, R. D., Zellweger, H.: Electron microscopy of two cerebral biopsies in gargoylism. J. Neuropath. exp. Neurol. 24: 304—317, 1965.

Arstila, A. U., Palo, J., Haltia, M., Riekkinen, P., Autio, S.: Aspartyl-glucosaminuria I: Fine structural studies on liver, kidney and brain. Acta neuropath. (Berl.) 20: 207—216, 1972.

Bach, G., Eisenberg, F., Jr., Cantz, M., Neufeld, E. F.: The defect in the Hunter syndrome: Deficiency of sulfoiduronate sulfatase. Proc. nat. Acad. Sci. (U.S.A.) 70: 2134—2138, 1973.

Baudhuin, P., Hers, H. G., Loeb, H.: An electron microscopic and biochemical study of type II glycogenosis. Lab. Invest. 13: 1139—1152, 1964.

Belcher, R. W.: Ultrastructure and cytochemistry of lymphocytes in the genetic mucopolysaccharidoses. Arch. Path. 93: 1—7, 1972.

Bishton, R. L., Norman, R. M., Tingey, A.: The pathology and chemistry of a case of gargoylism. J. clin. Path. 9: 305—315, 1956.

Blaw, M. E., Langer, L. O.: Spinal cord compression in Morquio-Brailsford's disease. J. Pediat. 74: 593—600, 1969.

Brante, G.: Gargoylism—a mucopolysaccharidosis. Scand. J. clin. Lab. Invest. 4: 43—46, 1952.

Cori, G. T.: Biochemical aspect of glycogen deposition disease. Mod. Probl. Paediat. 3: 344—358, 1957.

Crome, L.: A case of galactosemia with the pathological and neuropathological findings. Arch. Dis. Child. 37: 415—521, 1962.

— Cumings, J. N., Duckett, S.: Neuropathologic and neurochemical aspects of generalized glycogen storage disease. J. Neurol. Neurosurg. Psychiat. 26: 422—430, 1963.

Dawson, I. M. P.: The histology and histochemistry of gargoylism. J. Path. Bact. 67: 587—604, 1954.

Dekaban, A. S., Constantopoulos, G.: Mucopolysaccharidoses. Relation of elevated cerebral spinal fluid to mental retardation. Arch. Neurol. (Chic.) 28: 385—388, 1973.

— Patton, V.: Hurler's and Sanfilippo's variants of mucopolysaccharidosis. Arch. Path. (Chic.) 91: 434—443, 1971.

Diezel, P. B.: Histochemische Untersuchungen an primären Lipoidosen: Amaurotische Idiotie, Gargoylismus, Niemann-Picksche Krankheit, Gauchersche Krankheit, mit besonderer Berücksichtigung des Zentralnervensystems. Virchows Arch. 326: 89—118, 1954.

Durand, P., Barrone, C., Della Cella, G.: Fucosidosis. J. Pediat. 75: 665—674, 1969.

Gambetti, P., Di Mauro, S., Baker, L.: Nervous system in Pompe's disease. Ultrastructure and biochemistry. J. Neuropath. exp. Neurol. 30: 412—430, 1971.

Gerich, J. E.: Hunter's syndrome. Beta-galactosidase deficiency in skin. New Engl. J. Med. 280: 799—802, 1969.

Gilles, F. H., Deuel, R. K.: Neuronal cytoplasmic globules in the brain in Morquio's syndrome. Arch. Neurol. (Chic.) 25: 393—403, 1971.

Gonatas, N. K., Gonatas, J.: Ultrastructural and biochemical observations on a case of systemic late infantile lipidosis and its relationship to Tay-Sachs disease and gargoylism. J. Neuropath. exp. Neurol. 24: 318—340, 1965.

Green, M. A.: Gargoylism (lipochondrodystrophy). J. Neuropath. exp. Neurol. 7: 399—417, 1948.

Haberland, C., Perou, M., Brunngraber, E. G., Hof, H.: The neuropathology of galactosemia. A histopathological and biochemical study. J. Neuropath. exp. Neurol. 30: 431—447, 1971.

Hers, H. G.: α-glucosidase deficiency in generalized glycogen storage disease (Pompe's disease). Biochem. J. 86: 11—16, 1963.

— de Barsy, T.: Type II glycogenosis (acid maltase deficiency). In: Lysosomes and Storage Diseases (Hers, H. G., van Hoof, F., eds.), pp. 197—216. New York: Academic Press 1973.

Howell, R. R.: The glycogen storage diseases. In: The Metabolic Basis of Inherited Diseases (Stanbury, J. B., Wyngaarden, J. B., Fredricksen, D. S., eds.), Chapter VII. New York: McGraw-Hill 1972.

Hug, G., Garancis, J. C., Schubert, W. K., Kaplan, S.: Glycogen storage disease Types II, III, VIII, and IX. Amer. J. Dis. Child. 11: 457—474, 1966.

— Schubert, W. K.: Glycogenosis associated with degenerative disease of the brain: biochemical and electron microscopic findings. Clin. Res. 14: 441—441, 1966.

— — Chuck, G., Garancis, J. C.: Liver phosphorylase. Deactivation in a child with progressive brain disease, increased hepatic glycogen and increased urinary catecholamines. Amer. J. Med. 42: 139—145, 1967.

Hunter, C.: Rare disease in two brothers. Proc. Roy. Soc. Med. 10: 104—116, 1917.

Hurler, G.: Über einen Typ multipler Abartungen, vorwiegend am Skelettsystem. Z. Kinderheilk. 24: 220—234, 1919.

Huttenlocher, P. R., Hillman, R. E., Hsia, Y. E.: Pseudotumor cerebri in galactosemia. J. Pediat. 76: 902—905, 1970.

Jenner, F. A., Pollitt, R. J.: Large quantities of 2-acetamido-1(β^1-L-aspartamido)1,2-dideoxyglucose in the urine of mentally retarded siblings. Biochem. J. 103: 48—48, 1967.

Jervis, G. A.: Gargoylism (lipochondrodystrophy). Arch. Neurol. Psychiat. (Chic.) 63: 681—712, 1950.

Kalckar, H. M., Anderson, E. P., Isselbacher, K. J.: Galactosemia, a congenital defect in a nucleotide transferase. Biochem. Biophys. Acta 20: 262—268, 1956.

Kjellman, B., Gamstrop, I., Brun, A., Ockerman, P. A., Palmgren, B.: Mannosidosis: a clinical and histopathologic study. J. Pediat. 75: 366—373, 1969.

Kresse, H.: Mucopolysaccharidosis III A (Sanfilippo A disease): Deficiency of a heparin sulfamidase in skin fibroblasts and leukocytes. Biochem. biophys. Res. Commun. 54: 1111—1118, 1973.

— Neufeld, E. F.: The Sanfilippo A corrective factor. J. Biol. Chem. 247: 2164—2170, 1972.

Ledeen, R., Salsman, K., Gonatas, J., Tachavy, A.: Structure comparison of the major monosialogangliosides from brains of normal human gargoylism and late infantile systemic lipidosis. J. Neuropath. exp. Neurol. 24: 341—351, 1965.

Loeb, H., Tondeur, M., Résibois, A., Jonniaux, G., Van Hoof, F.: in: Proceedings of the Sixth Symposium of the Society of the Study of Inborn Errors of Metabolism (Allan, J. D., *et al.*, eds.), pp. 94—95. Edinburgh: Livingstone 1969.

McAdams, A. J., Hug, G., Bove, K. E.: Glycogen storage disease. Types I to X: Criteria for morphologic diagnosis. Human Path. 5: 463—488, 1974.

McKusick, V. A.: Heritable Disorders of Connective Tissue, Fourth edition. St. Louis: Mosby 1972.

— Kaplan, D., Wise, D., *et al.*: The genetic mucopolysaccharidoses. Medicine 44: 445—483, 1965.

Magee, K. R.: Leptomeningeal change associated with lipochondrodystrophy (gargoylism). Arch. Neurol. Psychiat. (Chic.) 63: 282—297, 1950.

Mancall, E. L., Aponte, G. E., Berry, R. G.: Pompe's disease (diffuse glycogenosis) with neuronal storage. J. Neuropath. exp. Neurol. 24: 85—96, 1965.

Martin, J. J., de Barsy, Th., Van Hoof, F., Palladini, G.: Pompe's disease: An inborn lysosomal disorder with storage of glycogen. A study of brain and striated muscle. Acta Neuropath. (Berl.) 23: 229—244, 1973.

Matalon, R., Cifonelli, J. A., Dorfman, A.: L-iduronidase in cultured human fibroblasts and liver. Biochem. biophys. Res. Commun. 42: 340—345, 1971.

— Dorfman, A.: Hurler's syndrome, an α-L-iduronidase deficiency. Biochem. biophys. Res. Commun. 47: 959—964, 1972.

Naidoo, P.: Gargoylism (Hurler's disease): A neuropathological report. J. ment. Sci. 99: 74—83, 1953.

Neufeld, E. F., Cantz, M.: The mucopolysaccharidoses studies in cell culture. In: Lysosomes and Storage Diseases (Hers, H. G., Van Hoof, F., eds.), pp. 262—275. New York: Academic Press 1973.

Norman, R. M., Urich, H., France, N. E.: Perivascular cavitation of the basal ganglia in gargoylism. J. ment. Sci. 105: 1070—1077, 1959.

O'Brien, J. S.: Sanfilippo syndrome: Profound deficiency of alpha-acetyl-glucosaminidase activity in organs and skin fibroblasts from type B patients. Proc. nat. Acad. Sci. 69: 1720—1722, 1972.

Ockerman, P. A.: Mannosidosis. In: Lysosomes and Storage Diseases (Hers, G. H., Van Hoof, F., eds.), Chapter 11. New York: Academic Press 1973.

— Köhlin, P.: Glycosidases in skin and plasma in Hunter syndrome. Acta paed. Scand. 57: 281—284, 1968.

Palo, J., Mattsson, K.: Eleven new cases of aspartylglucosaminuria. J. ment. Defic. Res. 14: 168—173, 1970.

Reilly, W. A.: The granules in the leucocytes in gargoylism. Amer. J. Dis. Child. 62: 489—491, 1941.

Résibois-Grégoire, A., Dourov, N.: Electron microscopic study of a case of cerebral glycogenosis. Acta neuropath. (Berl.) 6: 70—79, 1966.

Roukema, P. A., Oderkerk, C. H., van den Berg, G.: Gargoylism (mucopolysaccharidosis type II). Accumulation of glycosaminoglycans, gangliosides and glycoproteins and activity of some related glycolytic enzymes in liver, spleen and brain. Clin. Chim. Acta 44: 277—286, 1973.

Sandström, B., Westman, J., Öckerman, P. A.: Glycogenosis of the central nervous system in the cat. Acta neuropath. (Berl.) 14: 194—200, 1969.

Schnabl, R.: Über die Speicherung mucopolysaccharidartiger Substanzen im Gehirn bei generalisierter Glykogenose (Type II). Acta neuropath. (Berl.) 4: 646—658, 1965.

Schochet, S. S., Jr., McCormick, W. F., Halmi, N. S.: Pituitary gland in patients with Hurler syndrome. Arch. Path. (Chic.) 97: 96—99, 1974.

Schwarz, V., Golberg, L., Komrower, G. M., Holzel, A.: Some disturbances of erythrocyte metabolism in galactosemia. Biochem. J. 62: 34—40, 1956.

Seitelberger, F.: The position of gargoylism amongst the sphingolipidoses on the basis of the histochemistry of cellular storage substances. In: Cerebral lipidoses (Cumings, J. N., ed.), pp. 77—91. Springfield, Ill.: Ch. C Thomas 1957.

Toussaint, D., Danis, P.: Ocular histopathology in generalized glycogenosis (Pompe's disease). Arch. Ophthal. (Chic.) 73: 342—349, 1965.

Tuthill, C. R.: Juvenile amaurotic idiocy. Arch. Neurol. Psychiat. (Chic.) 32: 198—209, 1934.

Uchimura, Y., Toshima, Y., Sekeiya, T.: Zur elektronenmikroskopischen Pathomorphologie der Hirnrinde bei Gargoylismus. Acta neuropath. (Berl.) 4: 476—490, 1965.

Van Hoof, F.: Fucosidosis. In: Lysosomes and Storage Diseases (Hers, H. G., Van Hoof, F., eds.), Chapter 10. New York: Academic Press 1973.

Wallace, B. J., Kaplan, D., Adachi, M., Schneck, L., Volk, B. W.: Mucopolysaccharidosis type III. Morphologic and biochemical studies of two siblings with Sanfilippo syndrome. Arch. Path. (Chic.) 82: 462—473, 1966.

— Schneck, L., Kaplan, H., Volk, B.: Fine structure of the cerebellum of children with lipidoses. Arch. Path. (Chic.) 80: 466—486, 1965.

Wolfe, H. J., Blennerhasset, J. B., Young, G. F., Cohen, R. B.: Hurler's syndrome. A histochemical study. New techniques for localization of very water-soluble acid mucopolysaccharides. Amer. J. Path. 45: 1007—1027, 1964.

— Cohen, R. B.: Nonglycogen polysaccharide storage in glycogenosis type 2. Arch. Path. (Chic.) 86: 579—584, 1968.

36. Sphingolipidoses

The forms of sphingolipidoses described in the present chapter had in the past been classified into three disease entities: 1. Familial amaurotic idiocy was considered a lipid storage disease affecting the central nervous system only. 2. Gaucher and 3. Niemann-Pick diseases were thought to be generalized lipidoses with predominant visceral involvement. Amaurotic idiocy was subclassified according to its age of onset, as proposed by Vogt (1909) and amplified by later investigators: There was a congenital form (Norman-Wood), an infantile form (Tay-Sachs), a late infantile form (Bielschowsky-Jansky), a juvenile form (for which the subtypes Spielmeyer-Vogt, Batten-Mayou, and Sjögren had been proposed), and an adult form (Kufs). All these types were assumed to be manifestations of one and the same disease. Prior to the chemical identification of the lipids stored in these diseases (and even for some time thereafter), there was considerable controversy on whether amaurotic idiocy was indeed an entity or merely a variant of Niemann-Pick disease in which lipid storage is restricted to the nervous system.

The chemical characterization of infantile amaurotic idiocy in terms of the cerebral storage of gangliosides (Klenk, 1939, 1942) clearly distinguished it from Niemann-Pick disease for which the accumulation of sphingomyelin in viscera had been determined earlier (Klenk, 1935). Further studies on the chemistry of gangliosides led to a complete revision of the classification of the diseases that had been lumped under the designation "amaurotic idiocy". Most instances of infantile amaurotic idiocy are now identified as G_{M2}-gangliosidosis caused by deficient hexosaminidase activity, and three subtypes are presently distinguished: 1. A "classic" infantile form (Tay-Sachs disease) and 2. a juvenile form, both of which are caused by a deficiency of hexosaminidase A; and 3. total hexosaminidase deficiency (Sandhoff-Jatzkewitz disease), in which the hexosaminidases A and B are deficient. These G_{M2}-gangliosidoses differ from a second class of gangliosidoses which involve the storage of G_{M1}-ganglioside due to a deficiency of β-galactosidase; these cases had been reported as amaurotic idiocy with visceral involvement, neurovisceral lipidoses, or Landing disease. Turning to other sphingolipidoses, Niemann-Pick disease is characterized by the accumulation of spingomyelin as well as other lipids due to a deficiency of sphingomyelinase, at least in its infantile form; Gaucher disease consists of the accumulation of glucocerebrosides due to a deficiency of β-glucosidase. All the deficient enzymes are lysosomal and are involved in various steps in the degradation of sphingolipids (Fig. 127). As for other heritable metabolic diseases, heterozygous carriers may be detected from reduced enzyme activities in tissues or body fluids, as demonstrated for G_{M1}-gangliosidosis by Singer *et al.* (1972) or for G_{M2}-gangliosidosis by O'Brien *et al.* (1970). Pregnancies of high risk may be monitored by determination of enzyme activity in amnionic fluid or in cells grown therefrom (Milunski *et al.*, 1970).

The identification of ganglioside storage in the infantile and in some instances of the juvenile form of amaurotic idiocy rendered apparent that other forms, particularly the late infantile, juvenile and adult ones, could not be classified as gangliosidoses: there was neither significant storage of gangliosides nor corresponding enzyme deficiencies. Differences were also noted in the fine structure of the cytosomes accumulating in neurons. The chemical classification of these forms of "amaurotic idiocy" is still in evolution, and the available information does not permit to distinguish whether they are one single disease or a group of diseases causing similar lesions. The designations "juvenile lipidosis", "Batten disease", or "neuronal ceroid-lipofuscinosis" have been suggested to replace the term "amaurotic idiocy". The term "neuronal ceroid-lipofuscinosis", proposed by Zeman and Dyken (1969), is rapidly gaining acceptance (Chapter 37). It is advisable to discontinue the usage of "amaurotic idiocy" to designate nosologic entities, as its time-honored application to a group of heterogeneous diseases is obsolete, and as the term is semantically incorrect when applied to the entire group of diseases.

G_{M1}-Gangliosidosis. The abnormal accumulation of G_{M1} rather than of G_{M2}-ganglioside in a special form of infantile amaurotic idiocy was reported by Jatzkewitz and Sandhoff (1963). Landing *et al.* (1964) reviewed published cases that had been called pseudo-Hurler disease, generalized Tay-Sachs disease, or Tay-Sachs disease with visceral involvement (Norman *et al.*, 1959, 1964) and added a series of 8 cases of their own, 4 of whom were pairs of siblings. They recognized these cases as a nosologic entity which they called "neurovisceral lipidosis". Gonatas and Gonatas (1965) and Ledeen *et al.* (1965) demonstrated G_{M1}-ganglioside storage for a case whose similarity to Landing's series was soon realized. Chemical studies in a 9th patient of Landing's series concurrently disclosed storage of G_{M1}-gangliosides in brain and viscera (O'Brien *et al.*, 1965). A deficiency of lysosomal β-galactosidase activity was identified by Sacrez *et al.* (1967) and was confirmed by O'Brien (1969) and Sloan *et al.* (1969); the authors also demonstrated subnormal activity of this enzyme in heterozygose members of the sibship. G_{M1}-gangliosidosis was also found to occur in Friesean calves (Donelly, 1973).

G_{M1}-gangliosidosis occurs in two variants, an infantile form, and a late infantile or juvenile form (Derry *et al.*, 1968), but their distinction is not clear-cut and some cases may be considered intermediary. The two variants were initially attributed to deficiencies of different β-galactosidases, but later studies did not confirm a clear distinction of subtypes in terms of β-galactosidase pattern, nor was there a consistent correspondence between clinical course and biochemical criteria (Wolfe *et al.*, 1970; Suzuki *et al.*, 1971).

Many features of the infantile form of G_{M1}-gangliosidosis are intermediary between Hurler disease and G_{M2}-gangliosidosis, and there is overlap in their chemical manifestations. Hurler disease, an iduronidase deficiency (Chapter 35), is characterized by widespread storage of mucopolysaccharides, but it involves, also, storage of gangliosides. In G_{M1}-gangliosidosis the deposi-

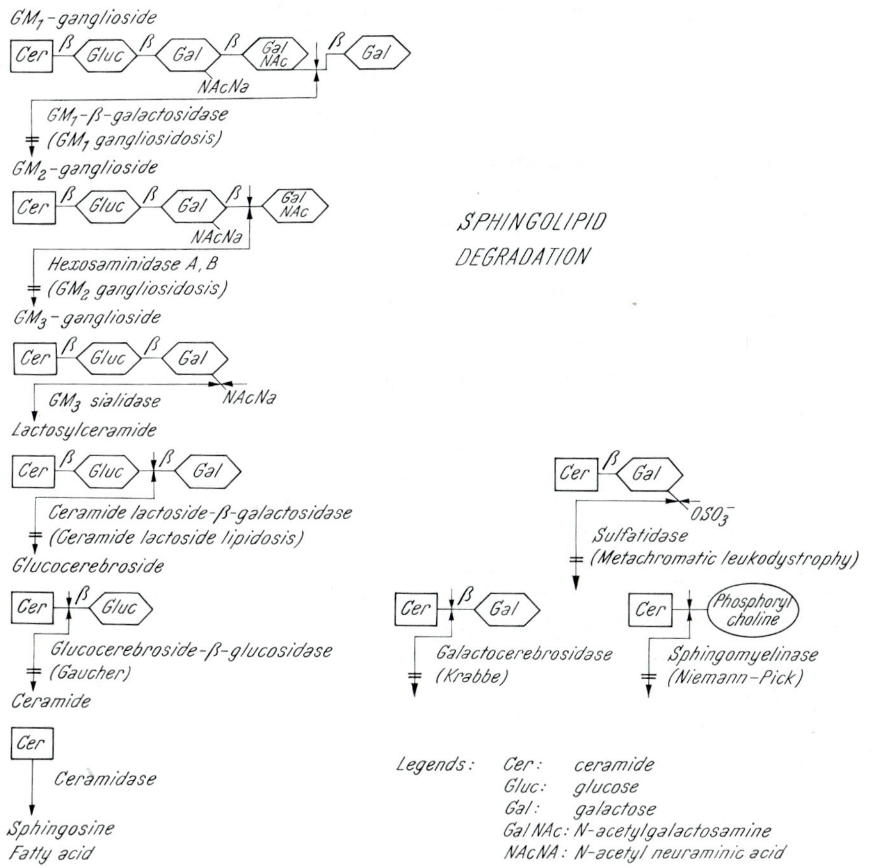

Fig. 127. Metabolic defects in sphingolipidoses

tion of gangliosides is greater and more widespread than in Hurler disease, but G_{M1}-gangliosidosis also involves a deposition of an excess of keratan sulfate-like mucopolysaccharides in the viscera (Suzuki *et al.*, 1969) due to impaired cleavage of galactose from mucopolysaccharides and from glycoproteins (MacBrinn *et al.*, 1969), as well as urinary excretion of keratan sulfate (Wolfe *et al.*, 1970). There is also overlap in enzymatic changes for the two diseases, in that the activity of galactosidase is reduced in Hurler disease, though variably in degree and in an organ specific pattern, whereas the deficiency of this enzyme in G_{M1}-gangliosidosis is universal and profound.

The overlap between G_{M1}- and G_{M2}-gangliosidoses consists of their virtually indistinguishable cerebral lesions as well as in terms of the variance in the extent of visceral involvement in the various subtypes. In spite of their overlapping manifestations, Hurler disease, G_{M1}- and G_{M2}-gangliosidoses are clearly different nosologic entities: No unequivocal transitional cases have been reported, nor has there been more than one of these diseases in any given sibship.

G_{M1}-gangliosidosis is of autosomal recessive inheritance without racial or sex preference. Its clinical manifestations vary considerably from patient to patient. The infantile form manifests soon after birth and is rapidly progressive, life expectancy rarely exceeding 2 years. This form shows greatest similarities with Hurler disease, including the characteristic facies, macroglossia, distension of the abdomen from hepatosplenomegaly and, sometimes, hirsutism. Bone anomalies similar to those in Hurler disease involve cranial enlargement, a shoe-shaped sella turcica, rarefication of the cortex, coarse trabeculation and deformities of the long bones which tend to taper distally, thickening of ribs and kyphosis of the spinal column associated with hypoplasia and beaking of vertebral bodies. There is vacuolization of circulating lymphocytes, but corneal opacity is seen only on exception. Neurologic manifestations consist of psychomotor regression, occasionally associated with convulsions. A cherry-red spot of the retina similar to that in infantile G_{M2}-gangliosidosis (Tay-Sachs disease) occurs in approximately one-half of the cases. Progressive neurologic deterioration leads to quadruparesis and, finally, to a state of complete disability with deafness, blindness and unresponsiveness to stimuli. The immediate cause of death is often from pulmonary involvement.

The delayed infantile, or juvenile, form of G_{M1}-gangliosidosis manifests toward the end of the first year and runs a more protracted course ranging between 3 and 10 years. Dominant features are psychomotor deterioration, seizures and a predilection for respiratory infection, the disease eventually leading to a decerebrate state. Bone anomalies and visceromegaly are minimal or absent. The onset of the disease may be as late as the 5th year (Lowden *et al.*, 1974).

G_{M2}-Gangliosidosis. The classical form of infantile amaurotic idiocy (Tay-Sachs disease) has been identified with the cerebral accumulation of G_{M2}-gangliosides (Svennerholm, 1962; Ledeen and Salsman, 1965) due to a deficient hexosaminidase A activity (Okada and O'Brien, 1969). Three variants of G_{M2}-gangliosidosis are presently recognized. In its most common form, the classic Tay-Sachs disease, there is a profound deficiency of hexosaminidase A while hexosaminidase B is unaffected or increased. A juvenile form (Bernheimer and Seitelberger, 1968) is caused by a less severe deficiency of hexosaminidase A. A third variant also manifests in early infancy but differs from Tay-Sachs disease in that both hexosaminidase A and B are deficient. This variant is referred to as total hexosaminidase deficiency, or Sandhoff-Jatzkewitz disease (Sandhoff *et al.*, 1968, 1971).

Infantile G_{M2}-gangliosidosis was first described by Tay (1881) of London, who observed the brownish-red discoloration of the macula and, later, the development of optic atrophy in an infant suffering from general weakness since the age of 3 weeks; he subsequently recorded similar ophthalmoscopic findings for 3 additional siblings. Sachs (1896) in his presidential address to the New York Neurologic Society summarized his experience with this disease, on which he had already reported 9 years earlier, and defined it as a distinct entity which he called "amaurotic family idiocy". He noted its rapid progressive fatal course and jewish predilection. Thousands of cases have been observed since these early reports.

Infantile G_{M2}-gangliosidosis is of autosomal recessive inheritance. It is the only type of gangliosidosis having a racial predilection, approximately 70 percent of the cases being jewish, mainly of Ashkenazi extraction, and 30 percent non-jewish. Symptoms usually manifest between 3 and 6 months of age, in spite of the fact that the enzyme deficiency and its tissue manifestations are already present at an early fetal stage. A startle reaction and extension response to sudden sharp sounds are characteristic early symptoms. Motor weakness becomes obvious after 6 months of age, and the infants may fail to learn to walk or become unable to do so. Motor and mental deterioration is rapid by the age of 1 year, leading to progressive deafness, blindness, convulsions and spasticity, the defects being fully developed at the age of 18 months. Death ensues in a state of decerebrate rigidity near the age of 3 years. A characteristic cherry red spot is seen in the macula of most but not all patients, and there is optic atrophy. Macrocephaly commonly develops upon survival beyond the first year. There are no connective tissue or bone changes as those in G_{M1}-gangliosidosis. Vacuolization of lymphocytes may be observed, but no characteristic cytosomes were found in the cytoplasm on electron microscopic examination (Lazarus *et al.*, 1967).

The variant of the disease characterized by total hexosaminidase deficiency (Sandhoff-Jatzkewitz disease) runs a similar course except for having no racial predilection. Its diagnosis is based on enzyme assays; there are also differences in the chemical composition of the stored material which, in addition to G_{M2}-ganglioside, includes elevated amounts of the asialoresidue of the ganglioside (trihexosyl ceramide), as well as globoside in liver, kidney and spleen (Sandhoff *et al.*, 1971; Suzuki *et al.*, 1971; Snyder *et al.*, 1972). The rapid increase in the number of reported cases of total hexosaminidase deficiency indicates that this variant is not as rare as originally thought; it may comprise a substantial fraction of the cases of Tay-Sachs disease without racial predilection.

The juvenile form of G_{M2}-gangliosidosis had been observed in only six instances when Brett *et al.* (1973) published their series of 8 cases. Its clinical manifestations start between 2 and 6 years, usually with neurologic disturbances including ataxia, loss of speech, progressive spasticity, athetoid posturing of extremities and minor seizures. A relentlessly progressive course leads to death between 5 and 15 years. Blindness develops late, and there is usually no cherry red spot in the retina; fundoscopic examination, however, may disclose optic atrophy or retinitis pigmentosa and an irregular, anomalous red spot with a halo of pallor has been observed (Brett *et al.*, 1973). None of the reported cases were jewish. The infantile form of the G_{M2}-gangliosidosis has been attributed to a partial deficiency of hexosaminidase A (Okada *et al.*, 1970; Suzuki and Suzuki, 1970), and the extent of accumulation of G_{M2}-gangliosides in the brain is less severe than in the infantile form (O'Brien, 1969; Suzuki *et al.*, 1970; Klibansky *et al.*, 1970; Menkes *et al.*, 1971). However, the series of Brett *et al.* (1973) showed no correlation between the degree of enzyme deficiency and clinical symptoms.

A G_{M2}-gangliosidosis remarkably similar to that in man occurs in the Siamese cat (Farrell *et al.*, 1973) and in the German short hair pointer; the lipidosis affecting the English setter, in contrast, has the features of neuronal ceroid-lipofuscinosis (Bernheimer and Karbe, 1970).

Cerebral Pathology of the Gangliosidoses. The following text on the neuropathology of the gangliosidoses is based mainly on Tay-Sachs disease, which has been studied in greatest depth. The coverage of the neuropathology of the other forms of gangliosidoses is still rather uneven, but no significant differences in microscopic, histochemical or electron microscopic features are apparent for the infantile forms of G_{M1}- and G_{M2}-gangliosidoses.

The volume changes in the brain tissue in infantile gangliosidosis are the product of two processes of opposite effects. Loss of nervous parenchyma causes cerebral atrophy and reduction in brain weight; whereas, an increase in tissue volume and weight is caused by the accumulation of abnormal material, possibly augmented by other, associated tissue changes. It is unlikely, however, that the latter include reactive gliosis, as is sometimes said, since equal or greater gliosis is commonly associated with tissue shrinkage in other diseases. Different stages of equilibrium between reduction and increase in tissue volume may be seen at different stages of the disease; furthermore, either process may characteristically prevail in certain portions of the brain. The cerebellum, for example, is usually not enlarged, as the atrophic process prevails, the shrunken cortex showing extremely narrow, firm gyri of a rather hard, rubbery consistency and ivory color. Atrophy is also evident in the optic nerves and tracts. The size of the cerebral hemispheres, in contrast, varies greatly, from atrophy to megalencephaly, and total brain weight may exceed normal adult brain weight by far. With enlargement of the brain, the cortical gyri may be excessively broadened and coarse, but there are no significant other anomalies in gyral pattern. The leptomeninges are clouded and fibrotic. The cut surface discloses abnormal firmness of the tissue and a diffuse discoloration of the hemispheric white matter which, in extreme cases, may be soft and gelatinous, tending to local subcortical cavitation. Ventricular distension varies with the extent of atrophic changes; the ventricles may be enlarged even if the brain weight is greater than normal.

Microscopic examination discloses universal distension of the neurons throughout brain and spinal cord, as first described by Schaffer (1905). The neuronal perikarya are enlarged and bulge to the degree of ballooning, due to the deposition of a fine granular, slightly eosinophilic material in their cytoplasm (Fig. 128). The nucleus is dislodged peripherally, bulging into the cell membrane, or into a dendritic hillock. The amounts of abnormal material are greatest in the perikaryon and diminish toward the dendrites; however, focal fusiform or ovoid distended dendrites or axons containing granular material similar to that in the cell body may occur. In cortical pyramidal

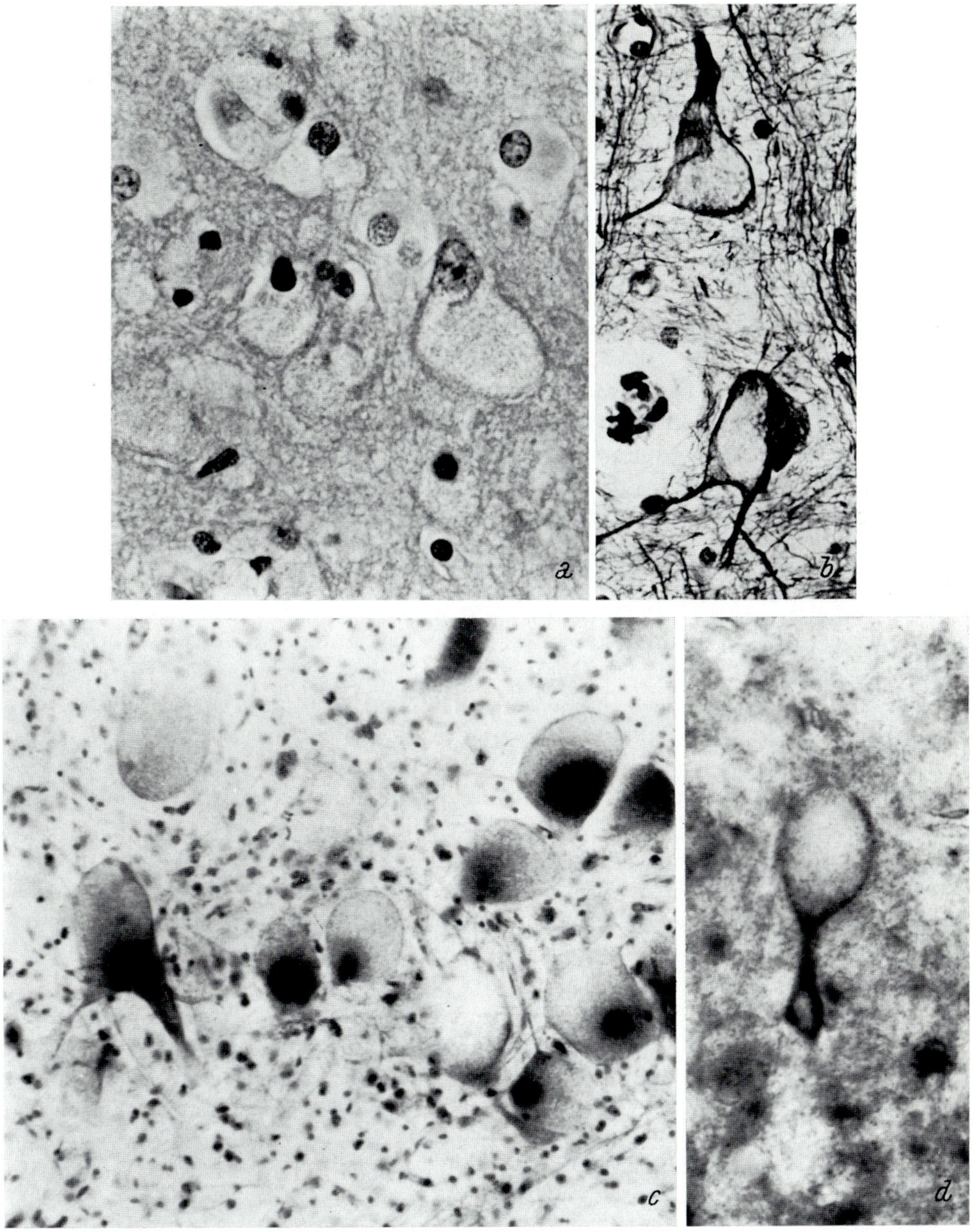

Fig. 128. Neuronal distension in G_{M2}-gangliosidosis (Tay-Sachs disease). A: H & E ×350. B: Bodian ×350. C: Displacement of acetylcholinesterase activity from perikarya; ×350. D: Distension of the apical dendrite of small cortical pyramidal cell; NAD-diaphorase ×300

cells the swellings involve either the axon or the apical dendrite, sparing the lateral dendrites, generally forming close to the origin of the processes from the perikaryon.

The granular material deposited in the neurons stains, in frozen sections, faintly with the various Sudan dyes, variable to bright pink with the PAS reaction and gray with myelin stains; it is resistant to osmication and is not double refractile (Diezel, 1954; Wolman, 1962). The material is readily extracted during routine tissue processing, leaving a foamy, faintly staining cytoplasm. The deposits in glia cells, in contrast, resist extraction, forming dense masses which stain brightly with the PAS reaction. Enzyme histochemical preparations for various oxydative and hydrolytic enzymes show them to be crowded out of the perikarya, except for acid phosphatase which has marked activity in the deposits (Lazarus *et al.*, 1962; Friede and Allen, 1964), consistent with their derivation from lysosomes.

Storage in distended neurons is seen throughout the central nervous system as well as in retina, autonomic ganglia and the myenteric plexus, but there may be regional variations in intensity. The cerebral cortex may show marked laminar or regional accentuation of neuronal changes, and devastation of cortical architecture may result from excessive loss of cells. The extent of storage and of loss of neurons in the Ammon's horn tends to be greatest in the resistant sector and the end plate, and it may also affect the fascia dentata; Sommer's sector, in comparison, is relatively resistant to the disease, a pattern inverse to that of anoxic damage (Scherer, 1932). Exceptionally severe loss of neurons is seen in the cerebellum. The granular layer may be affected to a greater degree than the Purkinje cells, presenting with a pattern of granular layer atrophy or its variant characterized by heterotopia of granule cells and reorientation of superficial fiber plexus (Chapter 31). The surviving Purkinje cells often show torpedoes in their axons and extensive dendritic swellings (asteroid bodies); storage of abnormal material is found in the swollen processes. Preservation of Purkinje cells is only relative, however, and complete depletion of the neuronal population may be observed in the end stages of the disease, when the greatly shrunken and gliotic gyri contain only a layer of proliferated Bermann-glia cells.

Whether the loss of neurons is caused by mechanical disruption of the cells or by metabolic dysfunction is a matter of conjecture, but the latter assumption appears more likely. Loss of neurons induces marked reactive gliosis, but the increase in the density of glial fibers in Holzer stains is usually not severe. Granular PAS positive deposits are seen in microglia cells as well as in astrocytes; their derivation from the uptake of material released by the decaying neurons or from a primary metabolic disturbance of the glia cells is discussed in the section on electron microscopy.

The white matter shows a diffuse reduction in the density of myelinated fibers, particularly in the centrum semiovale and in the cerebellar white matter, being least intense in many of the fiber tracts of brain stem and spinal cord. A subtotal to complete absence of myelin throughout the hemispheric white matter may be seen particularly in cases of long survival (Aronson *et al.*, 1955). Chemical studies demonstrate a progressive reduction in white matter lipids with the length of survival (Crocker, 1961), indicating a progressive destruction of myelin. The pathogenesis of the white matter changes in gangliosidoses is still controversial. Changes have been attributed to Wallerian degeneration, to a failure of myelination, or to a leukodystrophic process, and there is evidence for either of these interpretations. Wallerian degeneration is consistent with the progressive loss of cortical neurons and with the electron microscopic visualization of degenerating fibers in the white matter (Terry and Weiss, 1963), as well as with large amounts of esterified cholesterol in the tissue (Suzuki *et al.*, 1968). However, there often seems to be a disproportion between the severity of white matter changes and the extent of neuron loss, particularly when the intensity of these changes is compared with that in other lipidoses, *e.g.*, in ceroid-lipofuscinosis. The tendency to softening or local cavitation in the most severely affected portions of white matter, also, is inconsistent with Wallerian degeneration. A tract by tract comparison (Friede and Allen, 1964, references) of the degree of myelin deficit with the timing of normal myelination periods disclosed little or no changes in those tracts myelinating early, which seem rather resistant to the disease; tracts myelinating later showed evidence of active myelin breakdown, and those myelinating latest had no myelin at all. Similar observations were reported by Haberland and Brunngraber (1970) and Haberland *et al.* (1973). These authors and Crocker (1961) consider their chemical data inconsistent with simple Wallerian degeneration. There is also evidence that the white matter itself is involved in the storage of gangliosides (Suzuki *et al.*, 1969). There is doubt, therefore, that any of the pathogenetic mechanisms listed above can be considered critical to the exclusion of others. Loss of fibers from Wallerian degeneration undoubtedly occurs, but there may also be a coexistent inability of the diseased neurons to induce myelination of their axons, or a dysfunction of the sheath cells similar to that in metachromatic leukodystrophy in which a lipidosis causes predominantly leukodystrophic manifestations (Chapter 38).

The most characteristic electron microscopic alterations of the gangliosidoses are the membranous cytoplasmic bodies described by Terry and Korey (1960) and Terry and Weiss (1963). These are oval or rounded structures, approximately 1 μ in diameter, composed of densely packed, concentric, electron dense lipid membranes having a periodicity of approximately 50 to 60 Å (Fig. 129). The core of the bodies may contain finely granular amorphous material, as well as coarser granular deposits, vesicles or curved lamellar fragments, or there may be curved lamellae or stacks of parallel lamellae. The membranous cytoplasmic bodies of the gangliosidoses differ from the zebra bodies of the mucopolysaccharidoses mainly in the concentric rather than parallel orientation of the lamellae making up the body. Acid phosphatase activity may be demonstrated in membranous cytoplasmic bodies, which was thought to indicate that the bodies are derived from lysosomes (Wallace *et al.*, 1964). It has been stressed, on the other hand, that the outermost membrane of the bodies does not differ from the inner membranes, and that bodies of nearly identical structures may be created *in vitro*. The characteristic structure of membranous cytoplasmic bodies, thus, is not dependent on lysosomal activity. Isolation of cytosomes from brains with G_{M2}- or G_{M1}-gangliosidosis disclosed that roughly one-third of their dry weight is composed of gangliosides and an admixture of cholesterol, phosphatides and dry residue (Samuels *et al.*, 1963; Suzuki *et al.*, 1969). If gangliosides, cholesterol and phospholipids in molar ratios of 1 to 3 to 1 are incubated in an ionic medium, particles extremely similar to membranous cytoplasmic bodies can be created (Samuels *et al.*, 1964). Membranous cytoplasmic bodies also form in cultures of neural tissue exposed to a medium enriched with large amounts of gangliosides (Stern, 1972). Membranous cytoplasmic bodies are crowded, often in enormous numbers, in the cytoplasm of neurons where they displace the normal organelles without engaging in any consistent topographic relationship with them. Membranous cytoplasmic bodies are also found in the distended proximal axons and in the apical dendrites (Terry and Weiss, 1963) as well as in synapses (Gonatas *et al.*, 1968).

The fine structure of glia cells, mostly astrocytes, differs from that of neurons in that the deposits are mostly membrane bound, extremely pleomorphic forming dense lipid bodies with partial lamination or linear or circular densities. The different morphology of neuronal and glial cytosomes was attributed to the digestion by glia of lipids discharged from the neurons. However, the deposits in astrocytes were observed to form in close relation to and associated with changes in their mitochondria and the smooth endoplasmic reticulum, suggesting their derivation from a direct affliction of the astrocytes rather than from ingested material (Adachi *et al.*, 1971).

The structure of membranous cytoplasmic bodies is essentially the same in G_{M1}- and G_{M2}-gangliosidosis; electron microscopic data on total hexosaminidase deficiency disclose juxtaposition of membranous cytoplasmic bodies and zebra bodies (Vidailhet *et al.*, 1973; Juif *et al.*, 1973). Membranous cytoplasmic bodies, zebra bodies and lipofuscin granules were also observed in the juvenile form of G_{M2}-gangliosidosis (Volk *et al.*, 1969; Suzuki *et al.*, 1970; Menkes *et al.*, 1971), but these have a tendency to fuse and to form large confluent aggregates which may incorporate cytosomes of different structures; large amorphous deposits are also seen.

Information on the initial phases in the development of the cerebral lesions in G_{M2}-gangliosidosis was obtained from the examination of fetuses from therapeutic abortions, in which the diagnosis was confirmed from the absence of hexosaminidase activity in the fetal tissues (Adachi *et al.*, 1974). Abnormal inclusions were found as early as the 12th fetal week for the spinal cord and the 19th and 22nd week for the retina. They differ from the ones seen later in the disease in that amorphous and sparsely lamellar material accumulate first in cisterns of the endoplasmic reticulum, lacking acid phosphatase activity. Hence the abnormal material appears to form, initially, within the endoplasmic reticulum, and membranous cytoplasmic bodies evolve gradually after the 22nd week of gestation. Spinal ganglia have been suggested as samples of nervous tissue rich in neurons in which membranous cytoplasmic bodies may be found at 19 weeks of gestation (Cutz *et al.*, 1974). Of particular interest is that the development of cerebral and cerebellar cortices proceeds normally during the first 22 weeks of gestation (Adachi *et al.*, 1974).

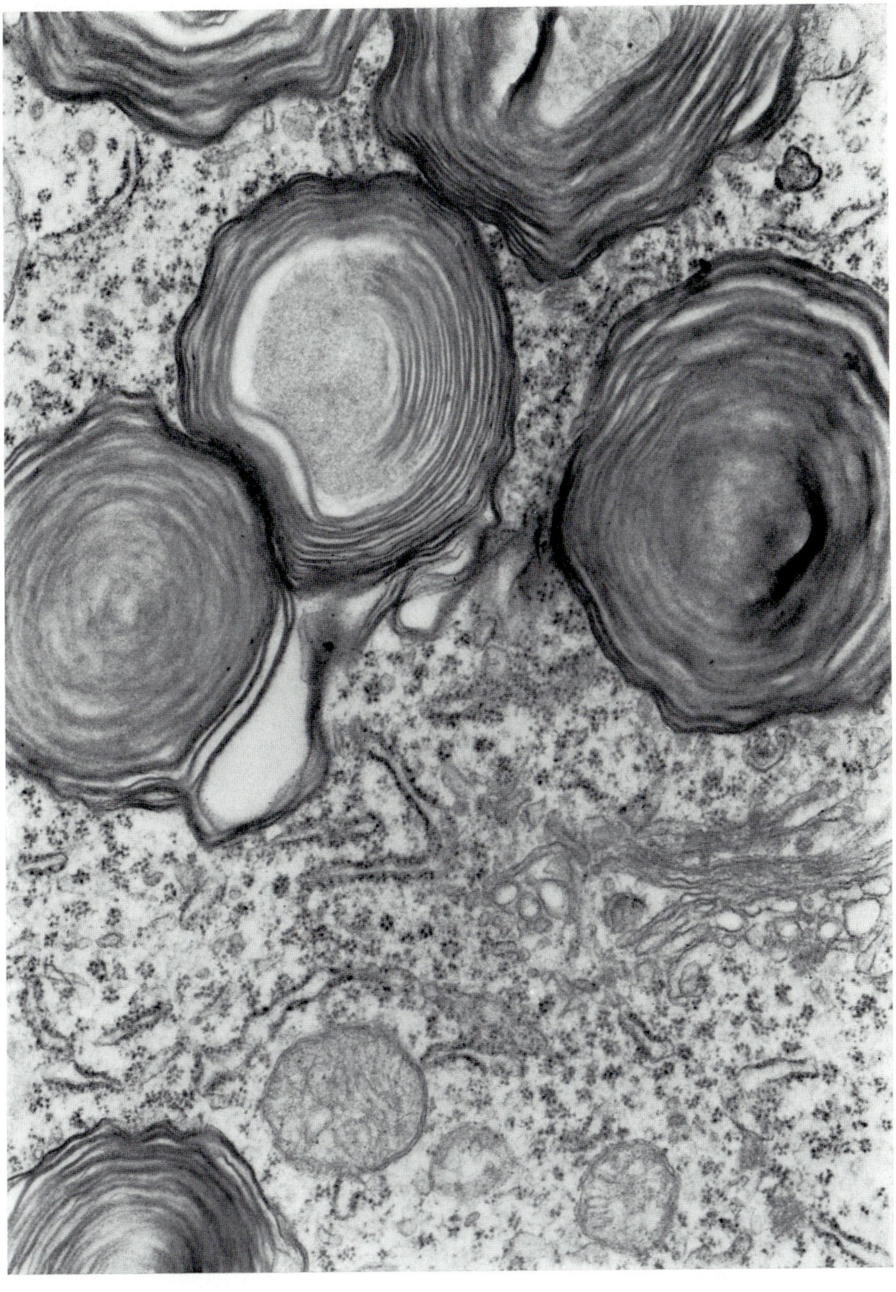

Fig. 129. Membranous cytoplasmic bodies, Tay-Sachs disease (courtesy Dr. Schochet)

The severe cerebellar and cerebral cortical damage in infants, therefore, must develop toward the end of gestation or during early postnatal life, when the development of these regions is particularly rapid. The visceral lesions of G_{M1}-gangliosidosis may also be seen at an early fetal age, including vacuolization of renal tubular epithelia and placental trophoblasts as well as zebra bodies in neurons (Lowden *et al.*, 1973).

Visceral Pathology of the Gangliosidoses. Although no evidence of visceral involvement is found in Tay-Sachs disease on light microscopic or histochemical examination, there is a definite increase in G_{M2}-gangliosides in the liver (Eeg-Olofson *et al.*, 1966), which is, indeed, of the same magnitude as that found in G_{M1}-gangliosidosis (Suzuki *et al.*, 1969), where it is associated with definite visceral lesions. Electron microscopic examination of hepatic cells in G_{M2}-gangliosidosis disclosed cytosomes similar to those found in the brain (Volk and Wallace, 1966).

Total hexosaminidase deficiency differs from the Tay-Sachs variant in that there are visceral lesions similar to those in G_{M1}-gangliosidosis though less severe. Hepatosplenomegaly is usually, though not always, absent, but lipid-laden histiocytes may be found in lung, spleen, lymph nodes, intestinal tract and bone marrow (Okada *et al.*, 1972). Vacuolization may be seen in the parenchymal cells of liver, kidney and pancreatic acini, and there may be luxol fast blue and Sudan positive granules in the cytoplasm of the cells of many organs. On electron microscopic examination there are membrane-bounded vacuoles containing a membranous material of greatly variable density, ranging from loosely coiled membranes to bodies intermediate between membranous cytoplasmic and zebra bodies (Dolman *et al.*, 1973).

Visceral lesions are widespread and pronounced in the juvenile form of G_{M1}-gangliosidosis and involve vacuolization of parenchymal cells as well as accumulation of histiocytes similar to those seen in Niemann-Pick disease, at least as far as their light microscopic structure and distribution are concerned (Landing *et al.*, 1964; Norman *et al.*, 1959, 1964). The histiocytes have small compact nuclei and a foamy, finely vacuolated cytoplasm containing a PAS positive material. They aggregate in the sinusoids of the liver, the spleen, lymph nodes, bone marrow, thymus, intestinal mucosa, and they may also involve the endo- and myocardium. Histiocytes may infiltrate the pulmonary alveoli in excessive numbers, becoming instrumental in the demise of the patients (Heyne *et al.*, 1972). The lesions in the parenchymal cells of various organs consist of large cytoplasmic vacuoles which differ from the fine foamy vacuolization characteristic of Niemann-Pick disease. Hepatic cells, pancreatic acini, the renal tubules and the excessively bulging glomerular epithelia are affected, as well as the thyroid, the pituitary and respiratory glands. The material stored in the viscera in G_{M1}-gangliosidosis differs from Niemann-Pick disease in being more readily soluble and in staining strongly positive with the PAS reaction; it also contains acidic groups that react with Alcian blue and Hale's dialyzed iron stain (Norman *et al.*, 1959).

Electron microscopic examination of the vacuolated parenchymal cells discloses large, membrane-bound vesicles containing a sparse floccular material; histiocytes contain membranous bodies (Themann *et al.*, 1970; Roels *et al.*, 1970; Severi *et al.*, 1971; Mihatsch *et al.*, 1973, references). Tubular inclusions, 210 Å, similar to those in Gaucher disease have been observed in visceral macrophages (Suzuki *et al.*, 1968).

The extent of visceral manifestations in the late form of G_{M1}-gangliosidosis varies considerably. There may be no changes whatever, or sparse histiocytes may be seen in spleen and liver (Patton and Dekaban, 1971). In other instances there are foam cells in bone marrow, lymphatic tissue and, less numerous, in spleen and liver, along with vacuolization of hepatic, renal tubular and glomerular cells similar in form but less severe in degree than those seen in infantile G_{M1}-gangliosidosis (Derry *et al.*, 1968).

Niemann-Pick Disease. The lipids accumulating in large amounts in the viscera and brain in the classical infantile form of Niemann-Pick disease were identified with sphingomyelin in the pioneering reports of Klenk (1934, 1935). There is storage of other lipids as well, including increases in lecithine and gangliosides; furthermore, the degree of cholesterol accumulation may overshadow that of sphingomyelin. The fatty acid composition of the sphingomyelin is subject to variation (Pilz and Jatzkewitz, 1964; Rouser *et al.*, 1965). After an exploration of sphingomyelin synthesis had failed to show anomalies (Crocker and Mays, 1961), the basic metabolic defect was identified as a deficiency in the enzymatic hydrolysis of sphingomyelin (Brady *et al.*, 1966). The enzyme deficiency, however, was found only for the infantile and the visceral forms of the disease (Schneider and Kennedy, 1967). Reduced sphingomyelinase activity is found in heterozygous carriers of the disease, and *in utero* diagnosis of fetal affliction is possible from deficient enzyme activity (Epstein *et al.*, 1971).

Four clinical types of Niemann-Pick disease were distinguished by Crocker (1961): Type A, the "classical" infantile and usually rapid progressive form; type B, characterized by severe visceral involvement without central nervous system changes; type C, of late onset takes a milder and prolonged course; type D, of still slower progression, found in a highly inbred group of costal Nova Scotia families. To these types, type E may be added for adult cases (Fredrickson and Sloan, 1972). The nosologic identity of these types as forms of one and the same disease, or as a group of disease entities, is not established, particularly concerning the last three types (Crocker and Farber, 1958).

The classical infantile form of Niemann-Pick disease manifests in early infancy with distension of the abdomen from hepatosplenomegaly, hepatic enlargement usually preceding splenic enlargement, and infiltration of lymph nodes; there is retardation of growth and a tendency to pulmonary infection. X-ray examination discloses pulmonary infiltrates; long bones show a widening of the medullary cavities and thinning of the cortex. Neurologic deterioration is similar to that in Tay-Sachs disease, with initial apathy progressing to idiocy; however, there is no hyperacusis, nor is there enlargement of the head. A cherry red spot in the retina is found for 25 to 50 percent of patients and may develop late, and the optic atrophy seen in Tay-Sachs disease is usually absent. Vacuolization of lymphocytes is seen in the blood, and abnormal cytosomes may be demonstrated in their cytoplasm with the electron microscope (Lazarus *et al.*, 1967). Changes in serum lipids have been observed, none consistent or diagnostic, and, in particular, there is no elevation in serum sphingomyelin levels. The disease usually leads to death within the first or second year, but it may take a somewhat prolonged course. Niemann-Pick disease is inherited in an autosomal recessive pattern; about one-half of the rapidly progressive cases are jewish, but no racial predilection is evident for the more moderate forms of the disease, except for its absence in negroes.

General pathologic findings consist of enlargement of lymphatic tissue, liver and spleen, the spleen showing a characteristic salmon pink color of the cut surface. Microscopically there is massive accumulation of foam cells, 15 to 90 μ in diameter, having central or eccentric, single or, occasionally, multiple nuclei, and a granular or finely vacuolated cytoplasm. The cytoplasm contains lipidic material most of which is readily extracted during routine tissue embedding, although a component of PAS- and Sudan-positive lipids persists. In frozen sections, the PAS reaction is weak or negative; a deep blue or black staining is obtained with the Smith-Dietrich reaction and a black or gray staining with Baker's method for phospholipids or with Sudan black, The material is osmophilic, not doubly refractile, and Sudan orange gives a faint staining.

Foam cells accumulate particularly in lymphatic and reticuloendothelial tissues; in the spleen they may displace most of the pulp, with resultant massive enlargement of the organ; similar infiltrates occupy the bone marrow, tonsils, thymus, and intestinal mucosa. Pulmonary alveoli may be filled with foam cells. Virtually every tissue of the body may be affected. Generally, liver and kidney are less severely affected than lymphatic tissues. The parenchymal cells, *e.g.*, in liver or pancreas, have a finely vacuolated, foamy cytoplasm which differs from the large vacuoles seen in G_{M1}-gangliosidosis (Norman *et al.*, 1959); excessive foamy change may result in complete obliteration of hepatic architecture. The histopathologic changes, including the neuronal lipid storage, may already be fully developed in the term fetus (Burne, 1953).

The brain in Niemann-Pick disease type A is usually reduced in size and weight, with shrunken gyri, and is remarkably firm to the touch. The cut surface shows a brownish atrophic cortex and comparatively well preserved white matter; there may be ventricular distension. Microscopic examination discloses widespread neuronal lipid storage with marked ballooning of cells similar to that seen in the gangliosidoses. Indeed, neither the cytologic changes of neurons nor their severity or regional distribution permit to distinguish the gangliosidoses from Niemann-Pick disease (Norman, 1970, review). Points in difference that have been emphasized are the presence of lipid deposits in vascular endothelia, arachnoid cells and choroid plexus epithelia in Niemann-Pick disease (Bielschowsky, 1928) and the consistently strong staining with the Smith-Dietrich and Baker stains; these reactions are more variable in the gangliosidoses (Wolman, 1962). The extent of cerebellar cortical atrophy varies, as it does in the gangliosidoses, but the type of granular layer atrophy with heterotopia of granule cells (Chapter 31) that is often seen in Tay-Sachs disease has not been noted for Niemann-Pick disease. Loss of Purkinje cells may be slight or absent in spite of the presence of massive lipid deposition in the layer of Bergmann-glia cells between the Purkinje cells. Myelin staining is moderately reduced in the cerebral white matter, but white matter lesions—if present at all—are usually much less severe than in the gangliosidoses and never reach the extent of massive leukodystrophic changes. Sparse collections of sudanophil granule cells in the white matter may indicate the presence of some myelin destruction. Chemical examination of cerebral tissue discloses a moderate increase in sphingomyelin and cholesterol (Crocker, 1961) as well as increases in the amounts of G_{M2}- and G_{M3}-gangliosides (Kamoshita *et al.*, 1964). The latter authors isolated the abnormal cytosomes and found them high in lipid content with little protein; 43 percent of their dry weight consisted of sphingomyelin, contrasting with an overall concentration of 9 percent in the gray matter. Peripheral nerves may show a neuropathy with cytoplasmic inclusions in Schwann cells having a dense poorly defined internal structure and occasional slightly curved parallel lines (Gumbinas *et al.*, 1975).

Information on the histopathology of the juvenile form of Niemann-Pick disease is still limited, but histopathologic changes in the reported cases were similar to those in the infantile form. Norman (1970) reports on the absence of lipid storage in choroid plexus, endothelia and meninges and on greater variation in neuronal involvement. The presence of a marked cerebellar atrophy has been emphasized (Norman *et al.*, 1967), but it does not appear to be a consistent feature. An unusual accumulation of lipopigments in pallidum and in the red zone of the substantia nigra, reminiscent of that in Hallervorden-Spatz disease, was observed by Martin *et al.* (1972) for a girl that survived to the age of 12 years. Chemical analyses of the brain of infantile cases show less, or even absent, increases in sphingomyelin (Crocker and Farber, 1958; Crocker, 1961; Cumings, 1962). Considerable variety is observed in the fine structure of the material accumulating in the various organs (Anzil, 1973, references). Visceral deposits contain coiled lamellar material of greatly variable density with an empty vacuolar core or with very loosely arranged lamellae (Tanaka *et al.*, 1963; Lynn and Terry, 1964; Wallace *et al.*, 1965; Volk and Wallace, 1966; and others). Cytosomes containing parallel or concentric aggregates of membranes occur in the circulating lymphocytes (Lazarus *et al.*, 1967). The neurons contain lamellar bodies resembling coarse, small membranous cytoplasmic or zebra bodies (Kamoshita *et al.*, 1969). There is, in addition, a variety of other deposits such as lipofuscin and cytosomes of variable texture, particularly in the juvenile form of the disease (Anzil *et al.*, 1973).

Storage of Ceramide Lactoside. The deposition of ceramide lactoside, monosialo ceramide lactoside and G_{M2}-ganglioside in the proportions of 10 : 2 : 3 was found in the brain of a 28-month-old child (Pilz *et al.*, 1966), who had earlier been reported as an atypical form of Niemann-Pick disease in which the neurons contain a PAS positive, metachromatic and Alcian blue-positive lipid suggestive of an acid glycolipid (Jørgensen *et al.*, 1964). The case reported by Jervis *et al.* (1962), in whom Rosenberg (1962) also found ceramide lactoside in the brain, appears to belong into the same category.

Gaucher Disease. Gaucher disease was the first lipid storage disease to be identified in terms of the chemical composition of the abnormal lipid. Lieb

(1924) of Graz found up to 10 percent of the splenic dry weight composed of a lipid thought to be kerasin; it was identified as principally glucocerebrosides (Halliday *et al.*, 1940; Klenk and Rennkamp, 1942), occurring tightly bound to protein (Uzman, 1951). After initial studies of glucocerebroside synthesis had shown no abnormalities (Trams and Brady, 1969), the metabolic defect was identified as a fault in the degradation of glucocerebrosides due to a deficiency of the enzyme cleaving glucose from cerebrosides (Brady *et al.*, 1965, 1966), which was later identified as an acid β-glucosidase (Ho *et al.*, 1972). Much of the glucocerebrosides accumulating in the spleen probably derive from the phagocytosis of erythrocytes in which globoside forms the major stromal lipid, consistent with an increase in splenic iron content also attributed to erythrophagocytosis (Lee *et al.*, 1967). However, nearly twice the normal plasma concentration of cerebrosides was found in splenectomized patients (Hillborg and Svennerholm, 1960).

Gaucher disease is of autosomal recessive inheritance, although a few sibships suggestive of a dominant inheritance have been reported (Hsia *et al.*, 1962). A jewish predilection has been noted for the adult cases, but is not evident for the rapidly progressive infantile form. Heterozygous carriers of the disease may be identified from reduced glucocerebrosidase activity (Ho *et al.*, 1972); also, prenatal diagnosis of the disease is possible from cells obtained by amniocentesis and grown in tissue culture.

An infantile, a juvenile and an adult form of Gaucher disease have been identified. The acute infantile form manifests with splenomegaly which often exceeds hepatomegaly in extent, infiltration of lymphatic tissue, mild hypochromic anemia, leukopenia and thrombocytopenia; no Gaucher cells or vacuolated lymphocytes are seen in the blood stream. The disease takes a rapid progressive course leading to death within two years. Neurologic signs are common and develop usually before the 6th month with apathy and retraction of the head leading to general stiffness. Symptoms referable to brain stem are common including strabismus, trismus, laryngospasm, dysphagia, spastic coughing, vomiting and profuse sweating. A cherry-red spot of the retina has never been recorded, and seizures are usually absent.

In the juvenile form hepato- and splenomegaly as well as bone involvement develop rapidly after the 2nd year of life, but the course of the disease is more protrated. Bone involvement produces a characteristic "Erlenmeyer flask" thinning of the cortex of the long bones. Neurologic manifestations are uncommon and usually do not manifest before the age of 6 years; they include mental retardation, rigidity, disorders of behavior, seizures and neurologic defects relating to the brain stem (Herrlin and Hillborg, 1962). The adult form of the disease advances only slowly, and organomegaly may be slight. Involvement of the central nervous system is absent.

The visceral pathology of Gaucher disease is characterized by the massing of Gaucher cells (Fig. 130) in the red pulp of the spleen, in lymph nodes, in bone marrow, and in the reticuloendothelial tissues in general, the massing being responsible for the organomegaly and erosion of bones. Gaucher cells present with strikingly enlarged, rounded bodies, 20 to 80 μ in diameter, and relatively small nuclei situated centrally or at the periphery of the cell;

multinucleated forms are common. The pale cytoplasm shows a characteristic texture of wrinkles and striations, particularly when stained with Mallory's aniline blue. The material deposited in the cytoplasm resists extraction during routine tissue embedding because of its strong protein binding; hence, the strong PAS reaction seen in frozen sections persists with variable intensity after paraffin embedding. There is a moderate autofluorescence, a weak staining with oil red O and Sudan black. Neither cholesterol nor lipofuscin can be demonstrated, and the Smith-Dietrich or Backer methods are negative. Enzyme histochemical stains show marked activity of acid phosphatase.

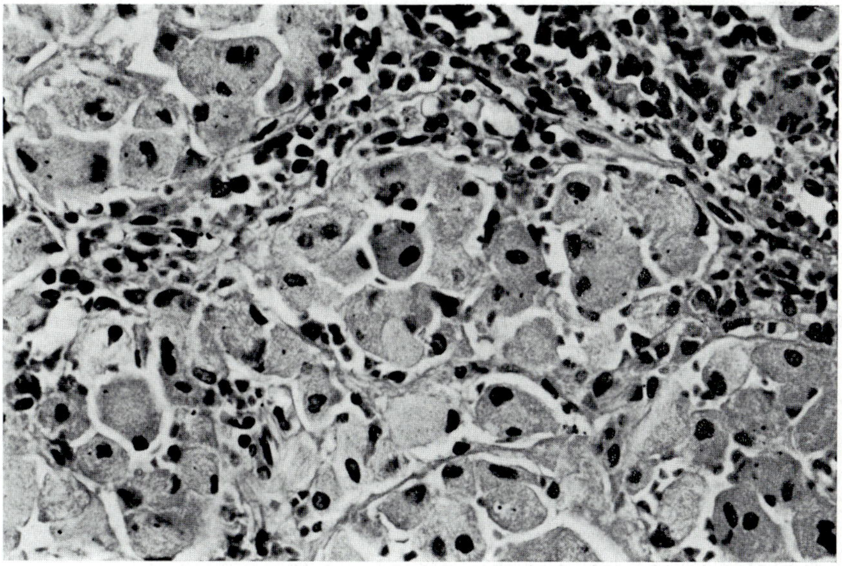

Fig. 130. Gaucher cells, spleen; H & E ×350

Neuropathologic changes are common features of the rapidly progressive infantile form and may affect mesodermal as well as neuroectodermal tissue structures. Affection of mesodermal tissue consists of the accumulation of typical Gaucher cells in the perivascular tissue spaces, as first described by Debré *et al.* (1951), varying from a few scattered cells to intense perivascular cuffing; cuffing may be the only change present in the brain (Seitelberger, 1964). Unusual manifestations are a secondary glial invasion of the Virchow-Robin space filled with Gaucher cells (Levine and Hoenig, 1972) or the occurrence of scattered Gaucher cells within the nervous parenchyma beyond the perivascular spaces (Banker *et al.*, 1962; Seitelberger, 1964).

The affection of the nervous parenchyma varies considerably in severity and distribution; it is unique among the lipidoses in that neuronal destruction is more pronounced than lipid storage, and that the former often occurs in the absence of evidence of the latter (Scherer, 1948; Norman *et al.*, 1956; Bérard-Badier *et al.*, 1962; Banker *et al.*, 1962; Seitelberger, 1964, references; Norman, 1970, review). Loss of neurons is usually widespread throughout cerebral and cerebellar hemispheres, brain stem and cord, and there may be accentuation of changes in certain nuclear groups, such as in the cerebral cortex where particularly the large cells of the deep layers are affected, in the basal ganglia and the pontine tegmentum; the dentate nucleus and adjoining white matter are affected with high frequency. There is, however, considerable variance from case to case, and no characteristic or consistent regional pattern of affection has emerged. Affection of the cerebellar cortex tends to be slight and patchy. Loss of neurons induces marked reactive gliosis, often in the form of neuronophagias or large focal areas of gliosis. Light microscopic evidence of abnormal lipid storage is absent in many cases; the neurons may be swollen having a loose, vacuolated cytoplasm in which, however, no abnormal material may be found with histochemical methods. For others, the neurons contain a PAS positive, metachromatic material, but the extent of accumulation usually does not account for the deformation and distension of the cells. The cerebral white matter is without characteristic changes.

Electron microscopic examination of neurons discloses membranous cytosomes similar to membranous cytoplasmic bodies or zebra bodies. The tubular structures characteristic of Gaucher cells are found only on exception (Adachi *et al.*, 1967; Hernandez and Bueno, 1973). Neurons also disclose degenerative alterations of the cytoplasm, mainly of the endoplasmic reticulum, occurring in the absence of abnormal cytosomes, which corroborates the light microscopic observations on a lack of relation between neural degeneration and lipid storage. No clear-cut chemical anomalies have been reported for brain tissue except for the juvenile case reported by Maloney and Cumings (1960), in whom an increase in glucocerebrosides as well as sphingomyelin was found; the case, however, is exceptional in presenting, histologically, with diffuse neuronal lipidosis. Svennerholm and Sourander (1966) found no elevation in cerebral cerebrosides, but the cerebrosides were chemically abnormal in having high glucose content, differing from their normally 100 percent galactose content.

The fine structure of the Gaucher cells in the viscera reveals membrane-bounded cytosomes containing 130 Å tubular units in a pale matrix, as first described by De Marsh and Kantz (1957) and later confirmed in many studies. Purified cerebroside obtained from normal tissue or from cases of Gaucher disease has a fine structure of tubular subunits which are nearly identical to those found in the cytosomes in Gaucher disease, lending credence to the concept that the tubular subunits are the substrate of abnormal cerebroside storage (Lee *et al.*, 1967; Lee, 1968). The cytoplasmic cytosomes containing the abnormal tubular structures can be identified with lysosomes by acid phosphatase activity in their matrix, which tends to decrease with the increase in the size of the cytosome (Hibbs, 1970). The fine structural changes have already developed to a considerable degree in the fetus, as shown by the presence of tubular as well as membranous cytosomes in the viscera of a 17-week fetus (Schneider *et al.*, 1972).

References

Adachi, M., Schneck, L., Volk, B. W.: Ultrastructural studies of eight cases of fetal Tay-Sachs disease. Lab. Invest. 30: 102—112, 1974.

— Torii, J., Karvounis, P. C., Volk, B. W.: Alterations of astrocytic organelles in various lipidoses and allied diseases. Acta neuropath. (Berl.) 18: 74—83, 1971.

— Wallace, B. J., Schneck, L., Volk, B. W.: Fine structure of the central nervous system in early infantile Gaucher's disease. Arch. Path. (Chic.) 83: 513—526, 1967.

Anzil, A. P., Blinzinger, K., Mehraein, P., Dozic, S.: Niemann-Pick disease type C: Case report with ultrastructural findings. Neuropädiatrie 4: 207—225, 1973.

Aronson, S. M., Volk, B. W., Epstein, N.: Morphologic evolution of amaurotic family idiocy. Amer. J. Path. 31: 609—631, 1955.

Banker, B. Q., Miller, J. Q., Crocker, A. C.: The cerebral pathology of infantile Gaucher's disease. In: Cerebral Sphingolipidoses (Aronson, S. M., Volk, B. W., eds.), pp. 73—99. New York: Academic Press 1962.

Bérard-Badier, M., Payan, H., Edgar, W. F.: Etude histologique du système nerveux central d'un cas de maladie de Gaucher dans une fratrie. Proc. 4th Int. Congr. Neuropath., Munich 3: 102—108, 1961.

Bernheimer, H., Karbe, E.: Morphologische und neurochemische Untersuchungen von 2 Formen der amaurotischen Idiotie des Hundes. Nachweis einer G_{M2}-Gangliosidose. Acta neuropath. (Berl.) 16: 243—261, 1970.

— Seitelberger, F.: Über das Verhalten der Ganglioside im Gehirn bei 2 Fällen von spätinfantiler amaurotischer Idiotie. Wien. klin. Wschr. 80: 163—164, 1968.

Bielschowsky, M.: Amaurotische Idiotie und lipoidzellige Splenohepatomegalie. J. Psychol. Neurol. (Lpz.) 36: 103—123, 1928.

Brady, R. O., Johnson, W. G., Uhlendorf, B. W.: Identification of heterozygous carriers of lipid storage diseases. Current status and clinical applications. Amer. J. Med. 51: 423—431, 1971.

— Kanfer, J. N., Bradley, R. M., Shapiro, D.: Demonstration of a deficiency of glucocerebroside-cleaving enzyme in Gaucher's disease. J. clin. Invest. 45: 1112—1115, 1966.

— — Mock, M. B., Fredrickson, D. S.: The metabolism of sphingomyelin. II. Evidence of an enzymatic deficiency in Niemann-Pick disease. Proc. nat. Acad. Sci. (U.S.A.) 55: 366—369, 1966.

— — Shapiro, D.: Metabolism of glucocerebrosides. II. Evidence of an enzymatic deficiency in Gaucher's disease. Biochem. biophys. Res. Commun. 18: 221—225, 1965.

Brett, E. M., Ellis, R. B., Haas, L., *et al.*: Late onset G_{M2}-gangliosidosis: clinical, pathological, and biochemical studies on 8 patients. Arch. Dis. Child. 48: 775—785, 1973.

Burne, J. C.: Niemann-Pick disease in a foetus. J. Path. Bact. 66: 473—477, 1953.

Crocker, A.: The cerebral defect in Tay-Sachs disease and Niemann-Pick disease. J. Neurochem. 7: 69—80, 1961.

Crocker, A. C., Farber, S.: Niemann-Pick disease: a review of eighteen patients. Medicine 37: 1—95, 1958.

Crocker, A., Mays, V. B.: Sphingomyelin synthesis in Niemann-Pick disease. Amer. J. clin. Nutr. 9: 63—67, 1961.

Cumings, J. N.: Abnormalities in lipid metabolism in two members of a family with Niemann-Pick disease. In: Cerebral Sphingolipidoses (Aronson, S. M., Volk, B. W., eds.), pp. 171—178. New York: Academic Press 1962.

Cutz, E., Lowden, J. A., Conen, P. E.: Ultrastructural demonstration of neuronal storage in fetal Tay-Sachs disease. J. Neurol. Sci. 21: 197—202, 1974.

Debré, R., Bertrand, I., Grumbach, R., Bargeton, E.: Maladie de Gaucher du nourrisson. Arch. franç. Pédiat. 8: 38—42, 1951.

De Marsh, Q. B., Kantz, J.: The submicroscopic morphology of Gaucher cells. Blood 12: 324—335, 1957.

Derry, D. M., Fawcell, J. S., Andermann, F., Wolfe, L. S.: Late infantile systemic lipidosis. Neurology (Minneap.) 18: 340—348, 1968.

Diezel, P. B.: Histochemische Untersuchungen an primären Lipoidosen: Amaurotische Idiotie, Gargoylismus, Niemann-Picksche Krankheit, Gauchersche Krankheit, mit besonderer Berücksichtigung des Zentralnervensystems. Virchows Arch. 326: 89—118, 1954.

Dolman, C. L., Chang, E., Duke, R. J.: Pathologic findings in Sandhoff disease. Arch. Path. 96: 272—275, 1973.

Donnelly, W. J. C., Sheahan, B. J., Rogers, T. A.: G_{M1}-gangliosidosis in Friesian calves. J. Path. 111: 173—180, 1973.

Eeg-Olofson, O., Kristensson, K., Sourander, P., Svennerholm, L.: Tay-Sachs disease; a generalized metabolic disorder. Acta pediat. scand. 55: 546—562, 1966.

Epstein, C. J., Brady, R. O., Schneider, E. L., *et al.*: In utero diagnosis of Niemann-Pick disease. Amer. J. hum. Genet. 23: 533—535, 1971.

Farrell, D. F., Baker, H. J., Herndon, R. M., Lindsey, J. R., McKhann, G. M.: Feline G_{M1}-gangliosidosis: Biochemical and ultrastructural comparisons with the disease in man. J. Neuropath. exp. Neurol. 32: 1—18, 1973.

Fredrickson, D. S., Sloan, H. R.: Sphingomyelin lipidoses: Niemann-Pick disease. In: The Metabolic Basis of Inherited Disease (Stanbury, J. B., Wyngarden, J. B., Fredricksen, D. S., eds.), Third Edition, Chapter 35. New York: McGraw-Hill 1972.

Friede, R. L., Allen, R. J.: Enzyme histochemical studies of Tay-Sachs disease. J. Neuropath. exp. Neurol. 23: 619—634, 1964.

Gonatas, N. K., Baird, H. W., Evangelista, I.: The fine structure of neocortical synapses in infantile amaurotic idiocy. J. Neuropath. exp. Neurol. 27: 39—49, 1968.

— Gonatas, J.: Ultrastructural and biochemical observations on a case of systemic late infantile lipidosis and its relationship to Tay-Sachs disease and gargoylism. J. Neuropath. exp. Neurol. 24: 318—340, 1965.

Gumbinas, M., Larsen, M., Mei Liu, H.: Peripheral neuropathy in classic Niemann-Pick disease. Neurol. 25: 107—113, 1975.

Haberland, C., Brunngraber, E. G.: Early infantile neurolipidosis with failure of myelination. A chemical and histopathological study. Arch. Neurol. (Chic.) 23: 481—488, 1970.

— Brunngraber, E., Witting, L., Brown, B.: The white matter in G_{M2}-gangliosidosis. A comparative histopathological and biochemical study. Acta neuropath. (Berl.) 24: 43—55, 1973.

Halliday, N., Deuel, H. J., Tragerman, L. J., Ward, W. E.: On the isolation of a glucose-containing cerebroside from spleen in a case of Gaucher's disease. J. Biol. Chem. 132: 171—180, 1940.

Hernandez, F., Bueno, M.: Infantile neurological Gaucher's disease in three siblings. An ultrastructural study. Virchows Arch. path. Anat. 360: 27—32, 1973.

Herrlin, K. M., Hillborg, P.: Neurologic signs in juvenile Gaucher's disease. Acta paediat. (Uppsala) 51: 137—154, 1962.

Heyne, K., von der Linde, J., Trubsbach, A.: Die Lungenerkrankung bei generalisierter G_{M1}-Gangliosidose. Helv. paediat. Acta 27: 591—600, 1972.

Hibbs, R. G., Ferrans, V. J., Cipriano, P. R., Tardiff, K. J.: A histochemical and electron microscopic study of Gaucher cells. Arch. Path. (Chic.) 89: 137—153, 1970.

Hillborg, P. O., Svennerholm, L.: Blood level of cerebrosides in Gaucher's disease. Acta paediat. (Uppsala) 49: 707—710, 1960.

Ho, M. W., Seck, J., Schmidt, D., *et al.*: Adult Gaucher's disease: Kindred studies and demonstration of a deficiency of acid β-glucosidase in cultured fibroblasts. Amer. J. hum. Genet. 24: 37—45, 1972.

Hsia, D. Y. Y., Naylor, J., Bigler, J. A.: The genetic mechanism of Gaucher's disease. In: Cerebral Sphingolipidoses (Aronson, S. M., Volk, B. W., eds.), pp. 327—342. New York: Academic Press 1962.

Jatzkewitz, H., Sandhoff, K.: On a biochemically special form of infantile amaurotic idiocy. Biochim. biophys. Acta 70: 354—356, 1963.

Jervis, G. A., Harris, R. G., Menkes, J. H.: Cerebral lipidosis of unclear nature. In: Cerebral sphingolipidoses (Aronson, S. M., Volk, B. W., eds.), pp. 101—123. New York: Academic Press 1962.

Jørgensen, L., Blackstad, T. W., Hallmark, W., Steen, J. A.: Niemann-Pick's disease. Report of a case with histochemical evidence of neuronal storage of acid glycolipids. Acta neuropath. (Berl.) 4: 90—106, 1964.

Juif, J.-G., Luckel, J.-C., Nußbaum, J.-L., *et al.*: La gangliosidose GM 2 avec déficit complet en β-N-acetyl-hexosaminidase ou maladie de Sandhoff. Arch. franç. Pédiat. 30: 29—43, 1973.

Kamoshita, S., Aron, A. M., Suzuki, K., Suzuki, K.: Infantile Niemann-Pick disease. Amer. J. Dis. Child. 117: 379—394, 1969.

Klenk, E.: Über die Natur der Phosphatide der Milz bei der Niemann-Pickschen Krankheit. Hoppe Seyler Z. Physiol. Chem. 229: 151—156, 1934.

— Über die Natur der Phosphatide und anderen Lipoide des Gehirns und der Leber bei der Niemann-Pickschen Krankheit. Hoppe Seyler Z. Physiol. Chem. 235: 24—36, 1935.

— Niemann-Picksche Krankheit und amaurotische Idiotie. Hoppe Seyler Z. Physiol. Chem. 262: 128—143, 1939.

— Über die Ganglioside des Gehirns bei der infantilen amaurotischen Idiotie vom Typ Tay-Sachs. Ber. dtsch. chem. Ges. 75: 1632—1636, 1942.

— Rennkamp, F.: Der Zucker im Cerebrosid der Milz bei der Gaucher-Krankheit. Z. physiol. Chem. 272: 272—280, 1942.

Klibansky, C., Saifer, A., Feldman, N. I., *et al.*: Cerebral lipids in a case of systemic G_{M2}-gangliosidosis of a late infantile type. J. Neurochem. 17: 339—346, 1970.

Landing, B. H., Silverman, F. N., Craig, J. M., *et al.*: Familial neurovisceral lipidosis. Amer. J. Dis. Child. 108: 503—522, 1964.

Lazarus, S. S., Vethamay, V. G., Schneck, L., Volk, B. W.: Fine structure and histochemistry of peripheral blood cells in Niemann-Pick disease. Lab. Invest. 17: 155—170, 1967.

— Wallace, B. J., Volk, B. W.: Neuronal enzyme alterations in Tay-Sachs disease. Amer. J. Path. 41: 579—591, 1962.

Ledeen, R., Salsman, K.: Structure of the Tay-Sachs' ganglioside. Biochemistry (Wash.) 4: 2225—2233, 1965.

— — Gonatas, J., Tachavy, A.: Structure comparison of the major monosialogangliosides from brains of normal human, gargoylism and late infantile systemic lipidosis. J. Neuropath. exp. Neurol. 24: 341—351, 1965.

Lee, R. E.: The fine structure of the cerebroside occurring in Gaucher's disease. Proc. nat. Acad. Sci. (U.S.A.) 61: 484—489, 1968.

— Balcerzak, S. P., Westerman, M. P.: Gaucher's disease. Amer. J. Med. 42: 891—898, 1967.

Levine, S., Hoenig, E. M.: Astrocytic gliosis of vascular adventitia in arachnoid membrane in infantile Gaucher's disease. J. Neuropath. exp. Neurol. 31: 147—156, 1972.

Lieb, H.: Cerebrosidspeicherung bei Splenomegalie, Typus Gaucher. Z. physiol. Chem. (Hoppe Seyler) 140: 305—313, 1924.

Lowden, J. A., Cutz, E., Conen, P. E., *et al.*: Prenatal diagnosis of G_{M1}-gangliosidosis. New Engl. J. Med. 288: 225—228, 1973.

— Callahan, J. W., Norman, M. G., *et al.*: Juvenile G_{M1}-gangliosidosis. Arch. Neurol. 31: 200—203, 1974.

Lynn, R., Terry, R. D.: Lipid histochemistry and electron microscopy in adult Niemann-Pick disease. Amer. J. Med. 37: 987—994, 1964.

MacBrinn, M. C., Okada, S., Ho, M. W., *et al.*: Generalized gangliosidosis: impaired cleavage of galactose from a mucopolysaccharide and a glycoprotein. Science 163: 946—947, 1969.

Maloney, A. F. J., Cumings, J. N.: A case of juvenile Gaucher's disease with intraneuronal lipid storage. J. Neurol. Neurosurg. Psychiat. 23: 207—213, 1960.

Martin, J.-J., Philippart, M., Van Hauwaert, J., *et al.*: Niemann-Pick disease (Crocker's group A). Late onset and pigmentary degeneration resembling Hallervorden-Spatz syndrome. Arch. Neurol. (Chic.) 27: 45—51, 1972.

Menkes, J. H., O'Brien, J. S., Okada, S., *et al.*: Juvenile G_{M2}-gangliosidosis. Arch. Neurol. (Chic.) 25: 14—22, 1971.

Mihatsch, M. J., Ohnacker, H., Riede, U. N., *et al.*: G_{M1}-gangliosidosis. Helv. paediat. Acta 28: 521—542, 1973.

Milunski, A., Littlefield, J. W., Kanfer, J. N., *et al.*: Prenatal genetic diagnosis. New Engl. J. Med. 283: 1370—1381; 1441—1447; 1498—1504, 1970.

Norman, R. M.: Niemann-Pick disease. In: Handbook of Clinical Neurology (Vinken, P. J., Bruyn, G. W., eds.), Vol. 10, pp. 484—508. Amsterdam: North Holland 1970.

— Gaucher's disease. In: Handbook of Clinical Neurology (Vinken, P. J., Bruyn, G. W., eds.), Vol. 10, pp. 509—531.

— Forrester, R. M., Tingey, A. H.: The juvenile form of Niemann-Pick disease. Arch. Dis. Child. 42: 91—96, 1967.

— Tingey, A. H., Newman, C. G. H., Ward, S.: Tay-Sachs disease with visceral involvement and its relation to gargoylism. Arch. Dis. Child. 39: 634—640, 1964.

— Urich, H., Lloyd, O. L.: The neuropathology of infantile Gaucher's disease. J. Path. Bact. 72: 121—131, 1956.

— — Tingey, H. H., Goodbody, R. A.: Tay-Sachs' disease with visceral involvement and its relationship to Niemann-Pick's disease. J. Path. Bact. 78: 409—421, 1959.

O'Brien, J.: Generalized gangliosidosis. J. Pediat. 75: 167—186, 1969.

O'Brien, J. S., Okada, S., Chen, A., Fillerup, D. L.: Tay-Sachs disease. Detection of heterozygotes by serum hexosaminidase assay. New Engl. J. Med. 283: 15—20, 1970.

— Stern, M. B., Landing, B. H., *et al.*: Generalized gangliosidosis. Amer. J. Dis. Child. 109: 338—346, 1965.

Okada, S., O'Brien, J. S.: Tay-Sachs disease: generalized absence of a Beta-D-N-acetylhexosaminidase component. Science 165: 698—700, 1969.

— McCrea, M., O'Brien, J. S.: Sandhoff's disease (G_{M2}-gangliosidosis type 2): Clinical, chemical, and enzyme studies in five patients. Pediat. Res. 6: 606—615, 1972.

— Veath, M. L., O'Brien, J. S.: Juvenile G_{M2}-gangliosidosis: partial deficiency of hexosaminidase A. J. Pediat. 77: 1063—1064, 1970.

Patton, V. M., Dekaban, S. S.: G_{M1}-gangliosidosis and juvenile cerebral lipidosis. Clinical, histochemical, and chemical study. Arch. Neurol. (Chic.) 24: 529—537, 1971.

Pilz, H., Jatzkewitz, H.: Dünnschichtchromatographische Bestimmungen von C_{18} und C_{24} Sphingomyelin in normalen und pathologischen Gehirnen einschließlich eines Falles von Niemann-Pickscher Erkrankung. J. Neurochem. 11: 603—611, 1964.

— Sandhoff, K., Jatzkewitz, H.: Eine Gangliosidstoffwechselstörung mit Anhäufung von Ceramid-lactosid, monosialo ceramid-lactosid und Tay-Sachs-gangliosid im Gehirn. J. Neurochem. 13: 1273—1282, 1966.

Roels, H., Quatacker, J., Kint, A., *et al.*: Generalized gangliosidosis—G_{M1} (Landing disease). II. Morphological study. Europ. Neurol. 3: 129—160, 1970.

Rosenberg, A.: The sphingolipids from the spleen of a case of lipidosis. In: Cerebral sphingolipidoses (Aronson, S. M., Volk, B. W., eds.), pp. 119—123. New York: Academic Press 1962.

Rouser, G., Feldman, G., Galli, C.: Fatty acid compositions of human brain lecithin and sphingomyelin in normal individuals, senile cerebral cortical atrophy, Alzheimer's disease, metachromatic leucodystrophy, Tay-Sachs and Niemann-Pick disease. J. Amer. Oil Chem. Soc. 42: 411—412, 1965.

Sachs, B.: A family form of idiocy, generally fatal, associated with early blindness (amaurotic family idiocy). J. nerv. ment. Dis. 23: 475—479, 1896.

Sacrez, R., Juif, J. G., Gigonnet, J. M., *et al.*: La maladie de Landing: ou idiotie amaurotique infantile précoce avec gangliosidose généralisée de type G_{M1}. Pediatrie 22: 143—162, 1967.

Samuels, S., Gonatas, N. K., Weiss, M.: Chemical and ultrastructural comparison of synthetic and pathologic membrane system. J. Cell Biol. 21: 148—152, 1964.

— Korey, S. R., Gonatas, J., *et al.*: Studies in Tay-Sachs disease. IV. Membranous cytoplasmic bodies. J. Neuropath. exp. Neurol. 22: 81—97, 1963.

Sandhoff, K., Andreae, U., Jatzkewitz, H.: Deficient hexosaminidase activity in an exceptional case of Tay-Sachs disease with additional storage of kidney globoside in visceral organs. Life Sci. 7: 283—288, 1968.

— Harzer, K., Wässle, W., Jatzkewitz, H.: Enzyme alterations and lipid storage in three variants of Tay-Sachs disease. J. Neurochem. 18: 2469—2489, 1971.

Schaffer, K.: Zur Pathogenese der Tay-Sachs'schen amaurotischen Idiotie. Neurol. Centralbl. 24: 386—392; 437—448, 1905.

Schairer, E.: Die Gehirnveränderungen beim Morbus Gaucher des Säuglings. Virchows Arch. path. Anat. 315: 395—406, 1948.

Scherer, H. J.: Die Ammonshornveränderungen bei der familiären amaurotischen Idiotie. Z. Neur. 138: 481—492, 1932.

Schneider, E. L., Ellis, W. G., Brady, R. O., *et al.*: Prenatal Niemann-Pick disease: Biochemical and histologic examination of a 19-gestational week fetus. Pediat. Res. 6: 720—729, 1972.

— — — Infantile (type II) Gaucher's disease: In utero diagnosis and fetal pathology. J. Pediat. 81: 1134—1139, 1972.

Schneider, P. B., Kennedy, E. P.: Sphingomyelinase in normal spleens and the spleens from subjects with Niemann-Pick disease. J. Lipid Res. 8: 202—209, 1967.

Seitelberger, F.: Über Gehirnbeteiligung bei der Gaucherschen Krankheit im Kindesalter. Arch. Psychiat. Nervenkr. 206: 419—440, 1964.

Severi, F., Magrini, U., Tettamanti, G., *et al.*: Infantile GM 1 gangliosidosis. Histochemical, ultrastructural and biochemical studies. Helv. paediat. Acta 26: 192—209, 1971.

Singer, H. S., Nankervis, G. A., Schafer, I. A.: Leukocyte beta-galactosidase activity in the diagnosis of generalized $G_{M\,1}$-gangliosidosis. Pediatrics 49: 352—361, 1972.

Sloan, H. R., Uhlendorf, B. W., Jacobsen, C. B., *et al.*: β-galactosidase in tissue culture derived from human skin and bone marrow: enzyme defect in $G_{M\,1}$-gangliosidosis. Pediat. Res. 3: 532—537, 1969.

Snyder, P. D., Jr., Krivit, W., Sweeley, C. C.: Generalized accumulation of neutral glycosphingolipids with G_{M2} ganglioside accumulation in the brain. J. Lipid Res. 13: 128—136, 1972.

Stern, J.: The induction of ganglioside storage in nervous system cultures. Lab. Invest. 26: 509—514, 1972.

Suzuki, K., Suzuki, K., Chen, G. C.: Morphological, histochemical and biochemical studies on a case of systemic late infantile lipidosis (generalized gangliosidosis). J. Neuropath. exp. Neurol. 27: 15—38, 1968.

— — Kamoshita, S.: Chemical pathology of G_{M1}-gangliosidosis. J. Neuropath. exp. Neurol. 28: 25—73, 1969.

— — Rapin, I., *et al.*: Juvenile G_{M2}-gangliosidosis: Clinical variant of Tay-Sachs disease or a new disease. Neurology (Minneap.) 20: 190—204, 1970.

Suzuki, Y., Crocker, A., Suzuki, K.: G_{M1}-gangliosidosis. Correlation of clinical and biochemical data. Arch. Neurol. (Chic.) 24: 58—64, 1971.

— Jacob, J. C., Suzuki, K., *et al.*: G_{M2}-gangliosidosis with total hexosaminidase deficiency. Neurology (Minneap.) 21: 313—328, 1971.

— Suzuki, K.: Partial deficiency of hexosaminidase component A in juvenile G_{M2}-gangliosidosis. Neurology (Minneap.) 20: 848—851, 1970.

Svennerholm, L.: The chemical structure of normal human brain and Tay-Sachs gangliosides. Biochem. biophys. Res. Commun. 5: 436—441, 1962.

— Sourander, P.: Investigations on brain autopsy material in lipidoses. Proc. 5th Int. Congr. Neuropath. Zürich. Excerpta Med. Foundation, Amsterdam 1966, pp. 342—349.

Tanaka, Y., Brecher, G., Fredrickson, D. S.: Cellules de la maladie de Niemann-Pick et de quelques autres lipoidoses. Nouv. Rev. franç. Hémat. 3: 5—16, 1963.

Tay, W.: Symmetrical changes in the region of the yellow spot in each eye of an infant. Trans. ophthal. Soc. U.K. 1: 55—57, 1881.

Terry, R. D., Korey, S. R.: Membranous cytoplasmic granules in infantile amaurotic idiocy. Nature 188: 1000—1002, 1960.

— Weiss, M.: Studies in Tay-Sachs disease. II. Ultrastructure of the cerebrum. J. Neuropath. exp. Neurol. 22: 18—55, 1963.

Themann, H., Diekmann, L., v. Bassewitz, D. B.: Die Feinstruktur der menschlichen Leber bei generalisierter Gangliosidose G_{M1}. Beitr. path. Anat. 140: 194—211, 1970.

Trams, E. G., Brady, R. O.: Cerebroside synthesis in Gaucher's disease. J. clin. Invest. 39: 1546—1550, 1960.

Uzman, L. L.: The lipoprotein of Gaucher's disease. Arch. Path. (Chic.) 51: 329—339, 1951.

Vidailhet, M., Neimann, N., Grigon, G., *et al.*: Maladie de Sandhoff (gangliosidose A GM 2, de type 2). Etude clinique, biochimique et anatomo-pathologique. Arch. franç. Pédiat. 30: 45—60, 1973.

Vogt, H.: Familiäre amaurotische Idiotie, histologische und histopathologische Studien. Arch. Kinderheilk. 51: 1—35, 1909.

Volk, B. W., Adachi, M., Schneck, L., *et al.*: G_5-ganglioside variant of systemic late infantile lipidosis. Arch. Path. (Chic.) 87: 393—403, 1969.

— Wallace, B. J.: The liver in lipidosis. Amer. J. Path. 49: 203—226, 1966.

Wallace, B. J., Schneck, L., Kaplan, H., Volk, B. W.: Fine structure of the cerebellum of children with lipidoses. Arch. Path. (Chic.) 80: 466—486, 1965.

— Volk, B. W., Lazarus, S. S.: Fine structural localization of acid phosphatase activity in neurons of Tay-Sachs disease. J. Neuropath. exp. Neurol. 23: 676—692, 1964.

— — Schneck, L., Kaplan, H.: Fine structural localization of two hydrolytic enzymes in the cerebellum of children with lipidoses. J. Neuropath. exp. Neurol. 25: 76—96, 1966.

Wolfe, L. S., Callahan, J., Fawcett, J. S., *et al.*: G_{M1}-gangliosidosis without chondrodystrophy or visceromegaly. B-galactosidase deficiency with gangliosidosis and the excessive excretion of a keratan sulfate. Neurology (Minneap.) 20: 23—44, 1970.

Wolman, M.: A histochemical study of various forms of cerebral lipidoses. J. clin. Path. 15: 324—327, 1962.

Zeman, W., Dyken, P.: Neuronal ceroid-lipofuscinosis (Batten's disease): Relationship to amaurotic family idiocy? Pediatrics 44: 570—583, 1969.

37. Ceroid Lipofuscinosis; Miscellaneous Lipidoses

Neuronal Ceroid Lipofuscinosis. This disease, like Tay-Sachs disease, was initially recognized by its fundoscopic manifestations (Batten, 1903). In the first report on its cerebral lesions Spielmeyer (1905) noticed the pigmentary nature of some of the material deposited in the neurons and thought that the disease differed from Tay-Sachs disease in its later onset and longer duration. Vogt (1909), on the other hand, was more impressed with the similarities in the symptomatology and in the neuronal changes of his cases with Tay-Sachs disease and thought that both were fundamentally similar. His interpretation was to prevail for half a century, and neuronal ceroid lipofuscinosis was classified as late infantile, juvenile or adult forms of amaurotic idiocy. The evolution of the unitary concept of amaurotic idiocies and their eventual separation into different disease entities are discussed in the first paragraphs of Chapter 36.

Batten (1914) on reporting additional cases summarized the clinicopathologic features of ceroid lipofuscinosis, which he called "juvenile progressive cerebral degeneration" to distinguish it from Tay-Sachs disease. His definition of the disease remains valid to this day; later additions pertain mainly to the characteristics of the material deposited in the neurons and to the widespread affectation of viscera. According to Batten the disease has its onset in late infancy or youth, and the length of its course varies greatly; there is no racial preference. Main manifestations are loss of intellectual capacities, of vision, and motor disturbances; the symptoms may develop concurrently or successively, and there may be considerable intervals between the appearance of one manifestation and the other. Convulsions are common. Retinal changes involve degeneration of the macula for some, retinitis pigmentosa for others, or there may be no retinal changes at all.

The differences between Batten disease and infantile amaurotic idiocy (Tay-Sachs disease) have been emphasized repeatedly over the years, but these observations did not prevail over the unitary concept that amaurotic idiocy is a single nosologic entity: Sjögren (1931) on reviewing 115 cases of juvenile amaurotic idiocy found not one for whom Tay-Sachs disease had occurred in the same family. Klenk (1939) observed no increase of the Tay-Sachs glycolipid, which he later identified with ganglioside, for juvenile cases of "amaurotic idiocy" although there was much increase in the infantile cases. Wyburn-Mason (1943) stressed the different fundoscopic manifestation which, along with the different age of onset and clinical course, suggested to him that Tay-Sachs and Batten diseases were two unrelated entities.

The recent reclassification of juvenile amaurotic idiocy as gangliosidosis and the concurrent elaboration of its enzymatic defects as well as its electron microscopic features greatly reinforced the concept that the so-called infantile amaurotic idiocy differs, in principle, from most of the so-called late infantile or juvenile amaurotic idiocies, and the unitary classification was no longer tenable. Zeman and Dyken (1969) introduced the name "neuronal ceroid lipofuscinosis", a modification of the term "diffuse lipofuscinosis of the nervous system" (Pallis *et al.*, 1967) to separate Batten disease from the gangliosidoses. The term is gaining general acceptance, and neuronal ceroid lipofuscinosis is now considered the most common one among the various diseases previously lumped under the designation "amaurotic idiocy" (Gordon *et al.*, 1972).

The chemical identification of neuronal ceroid lipofuscinosis is still in evolution. Klenk's (1939) original observation that neuronal ceroid lipofuscinosis differs from the gangliosidoses in the absence of a significant increase in cerebral gangliosides was reconfirmed in many studies (Duffy *et al.*, 1968; Zeman and Dyken, 1969; Herman *et al.*, 1971; Haberland *et al.*, 1972; and others); also, there is no hexosaminidase deficiency. A variety of other laboratory studies, reviewed by Ricoy-Campo and Bruens (1970), yielded no observations of specific diagnostic significance. Two fractions of different density, ceroid and lipofuscin, were obtained on isolation of the lipopigments from the brain tissue. Both were rich in metal ions, though differing in their relative concentration. The content of copper, calcium and iron was higher in ceroid than in lipofuscin; also, ceroid was unstable upon removal of the cations (Siakotos *et al.*, 1972). Research toward the understanding of the causes of ceroid-lipofuscin accumulation has been directed toward the metabolism of vitamin E because of the well known relationship between vitamin E deficiency and ceroid deposition. Recent data, however, implicate a peroxidase deficiency in granulocytes as a possible cause of pigment accumulation (Armstrong *et al.*, 1974). A deficiency of peroxidase was also found in English setters affected by ceroid lipofuscinosis, and the activity of this enzyme was reduced in the heterozygos carriers of this canine form of the disease (Patel *et al.*, 1974). A number of lysosomal hydrolases were found to be hyperactive (Nevalainen *et al.*, 1973), a feature common to many lysosomal diseases.

Examination of series of patients in terms of the enzyme defect can be expected to disclose, in the near future, whether neuronal ceroid lipofuscinosis is a single disease with various ages of onset, or a group of different conditions producing similar tissue changes. The former assumption is consistent with the observation that both the juvenile and the adult forms of the disease have been known to occur in the same family (Zeman and Hoffman, 1962). Furthermore, deficient leukocyte peroxydase has been found in a family with Kuf disease (Armstrong *et al.*, 1974). Within the frame of present knowledge, it appears that ceroid lipofuscinosis may manifest in several forms distinguished by their ages of onset, symptoms, or length of course; all forms have similar light microscopic neuronal changes. The subclassifications proposed by Zeman and Siakotos (1973) and Dekaban and Herman (1974) are basically alike except for the significance attributed to the fine structure of the neuronal deposits (Table 7).

Late infantile onset of neuronal ceroid lipofuscinosis, after the second year of life, is characterized by a rapidly progressive course involving convulsions, blindness and severe dementia; retinal changes vary. The age of onset, however, is only a relative criterion in distinguishing ceroid lipofuscinosis from G_{M2}-gangliosidosis: G_{M2}-gangliosidosis is mostly of infantile onset, but it also occurs in a juvenile form. Ceroid lipofuscinosis, on the other hand, is mostly late infantile or juvenile, but it may, on occasion, begin during the first year of life and take a particularly violent course (Haltia *et al.*, 1973). Onset of neuronal ceroid lipofuscinosis during the second half of the first decade—the juvenile form—usually presents with initial blindness accompanied by the fundoscopic changes of retinitis pigmentosa. There is a much slower progression of mental deterioration and a late development of dementia. The adult form may manifest with psychiatric symptoms or with neurologic disturbances which may include choreoathetosis and myoclonus. Mental deterioration is slight or absent, and there are no seizures or retinal changes. Neuronal ceroid lipofuscinosis is commonly transmitted in an autosomal recessive pattern without racial predilection. Boehme *et al.* (1971) described an exceptional family with autosomal dominant transmission.

In addition to the main subtypes of neuronal ceroid lipofuscinosis listed above, there have been attempts at defining other subentities in terms of symptomatology or of light or electron microscopic findings, but their differentiation from the forms described earlier remains a matter of conjecture. Seitelberger *et al.* (1966), elaborating on earlier observations, delinated a myoclonic variant of cerebral lipidosis characterized by myoclonus and unusually large, nodular deposits in the neurons of the basal ganglia. Elfenbein (1968) described a case characterized by extrapyramidal manifestations and exceptional variance in the electron microscopic features of the cytosomes, which he called "familiar dystonic lipidosis". A case of myoclonic variant was shown to have uniform accumulation of all four major gangliosides (Bartsch, 1970).

Corresponding to the variance in clinical courses, there is much variance in the gross appearance of the brain in neuronal ceroid lipofuscinosis. Atrophy may be minimal or absent, particularly for the adult cases having a short course. For others moderate to exceptionally severe atrophy may

Table 7. *Subclassification of Neuronal Ceroid Lipofuscinosis* (Childhood, Juvenile and Adult Lipidosis)

Type	Age of Onset; Course; Duration	Neurologic Signs	Ocular Changes	Cerebral Changes
		Classification of Zeman and Siakotos, 1973		
Jansky-Bielschowsky	2–4 years (as late as 20); rapidly progressive; from less than 1 to about 6 years	Onset with convulsions, consistently blindness and complete dementia	Optic atrophy, sometimes retinitis pigmentosa and macular degeneration	Severe brain atrophy
Spielmeyer-Sjøgren	4–8 years (as early as 1 year); slowly progressive; average duration 11 years	Onset with blindness; dementia late and moderately severe	Retinitis pigmentosa, macular degeneration	Commensurate with duration of illness
Kuf	After 20 years; slowly progressive; lasts from 5 to 30 years	Onset with mental changes, occasional convulsions; blindness absent; mental changes vary, often minimal	Usually absent	Moderate, depending on duration
		Classification of Dekaban and Herman, 1974		
1 A	2–6 years; rapid progression; lasts 3–6 years	Rapid mental and motor deterioration, spasticity, seizures, myoclonic jerks, protracted impairment of vision	Pigmentary degeneration and macula changes	Ubiquitous neuronal deposits. EM: Uniform inclusions containing convoluted paired membranes (multilamellar cytosomes)
1 B	Identical to 1 A except for electron microscopic data			EM; Pleomorphic bodies with stacked or concentric delicate membranes similar to those in gangliosidoses
2	7 to 10 years; slow progression; lasts 5–12 years	Rapid development of blindness, slow mental deterioration, infrequent seizures	Marked pigmentary degeneration of macula and peripheral retina	Laminar accentuation of neuronal deposits. EM: Cytosomes with focal densities, short linear segment "fingerprints"
3	Past 11 years	Myoclonus, choreoathetosis, moderate mental deterioration, no spasticity, mental disturbances mild	None	Deposits prevail in basal ganglia, cerebellum and brain stem. EM: Similar to lipofuscin

cause marked reduction in brain weight, ventricular distension, and shrinkage of the cerebral cortex which assumes a yellowish-brown color (Fig. 131). There is often an associated atrophy of the cerebellar hemispheres, but the cerebellum remains completely intact for other cases. The consistency of the tissue is increased throughout. The degree of atrophy is particularly severe

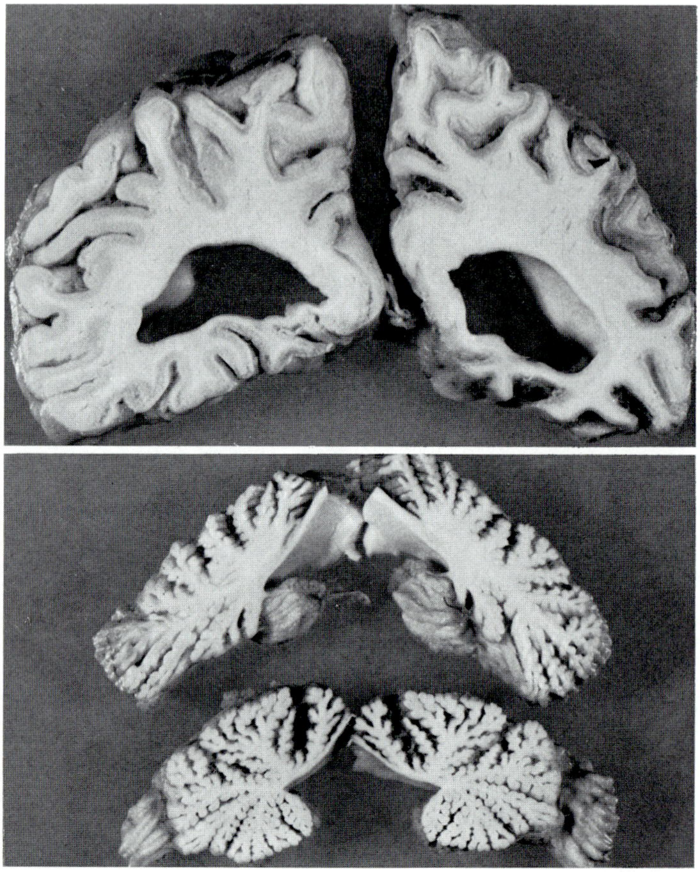

Fig. 131. Severe cerebral and cerebellar cortical atrophy in neuronal ceroid lipofuscinosis

in early infantile cases; the severity of neuronal devastation may well be augmented by the convulsions which commonly accompany this form of the disease. Neuronal ceroid lipofuscinosis differs from the gangliosidoses in that the brain is not enlarged, atrophy prevailing by far, and in the relative preservation of the white matter which does not show the leukodystrophic changes seen in the gangliosidoses.

Microscopic examination reveals widespread neuronal storage of an eosinophilic, slightly pigmented granular material which shows a strong yellow autofluorescence in ultra violet light, is strongly PAS positive, stains with Sudan dyes and many other stains characteristic of lipofuscin (Fig. 132). The material is insoluble in common lipid solvents and persists quantitatively in paraffin sections, contrary to the behavior of the material accumulating in neurons in the gangliosidoses. Gangliosides, also, are strongly acidic, staining metachromatic and having affinity for colloidal iron, features which are absent in ceroid lipofuscinosis (Wolman, 1962).

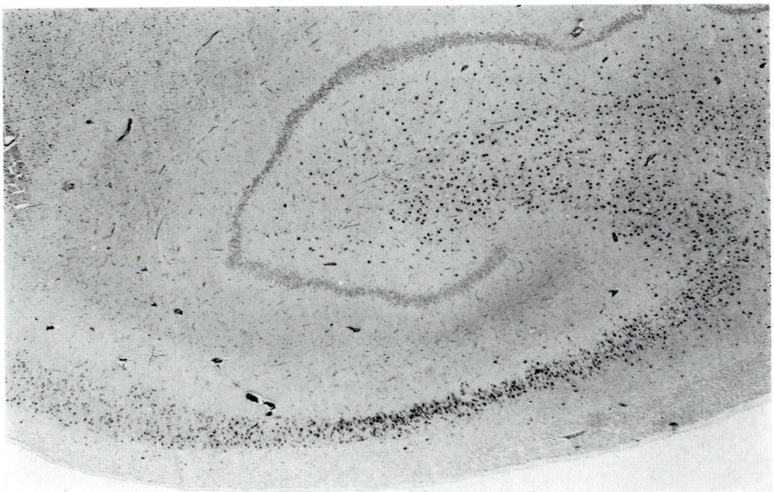

Fig. 132. Neuronal ceroid lipofuscinosis; preferential storage of PAS-positive material in the resistant sector and the endplate of the Ammon's horn, similar to the pattern in G_{M2}-gangliosidosis; PAS ×15

The deposition of ceroid lipofuscin in the late infantile form of the disease is virtually ubiquitous; more discrete patterns, such as a laminar preponderance of storage in the cerebral cortex or a predilection for basal ganglia, may be seen in the juvenile or the adult forms or in the myoclonic variant. There are also regional differences in the morphology of the neuronal deposits which are finely granular for many portions of gray matter but show a tendency to coalesce to larger globules or inclusion body-like masses in pallidum, subthalamic nucleus, substantia nigra, dentate nucleus and other brain stem nuclei. This feature has been emphasized in attempts to delineate a myoclonic variant of the disease (Seitelberger *et al.*, 1966; Ricoy Campo and Bruens, 1970).

The storage of abnormal material is associated with neuronal destruction and reactive gliosis. Pigment granules released from decayed neurons are incorporated by macrophages. Neuronal destruction, however, does not specifically relate to the extent of storage which rarely reaches the extent seen in gangliosidoses and other neurolipidoses, and does not cause extreme degrees of distension or ballooning of the cells (Fig. 133). Furthermore, certain types of neurons appear to be quite susceptible to damage in the absence of excessive storage, including particularly small granule cells like those in the olfactory bulb, the outer retinal layers, and the upper layers of the cerebral cortex. Metabolic dysfunction, therefore, appears to be more important than the mechanical damage induced by storage. The coexistence of progressive sclerosing cortical atrophy from repeated convulsions (Chapter 10) may further accentuate neuronal loss, and this factor may well explain the difference in the degree of atrophy between the late infantile and the adult cases. In extreme cases loss of cortical neurons may reach sufficient severity to induce status spongiosus of the tissue. The extent of neuron loss in the cerebellar cortex varies, or it may be absent altogether. Chemical and histochemi-

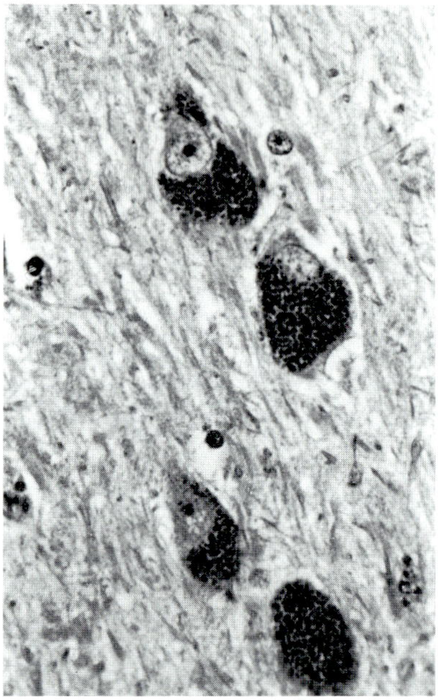

Fig. 133. Neuronal ceroid lipofuscinosis. Deposition of coarse granular PAS-positive material in neuronal perikarya; cell bodies are not—or only moderately—distended; PAS ×440

cal examination of the hemispheric white matter discloses deposition of triglycerides and cholesterol in macrophages, consistent with an active degeneration of fibers as well as the storage of lipofuscin-like material in glia cells (Edgar and van Bogaert, 1967). Retinal involvement in ceroid lipofuscinosis differs from that in the gangliosidoses in that there is a primary degeneration of the neuroepithelium, rather than one of the ganglion cell layer, as first emphasized by Stock (1908).

Neuronal ceroid lipofuscinosis involves widespread deposition of lipofuscin-like material in viscera including myocardium, liver, spleen, lymph nodes and renal collecting tubules, as well as many other tissues (Sjövall, 1934; Kristensson *et al.*, 1965; Kristensson and Sourander, 1966). Its occurrence in the thyroid gland was emphasized by Dayan and Trickey (1970); peripheral nerve lesions including segmental demyelination were described by Kristensson *et al.* (1967). The visceral material shows yellow autofluorescence in ultra violet light and stains positive with Sudan black and PAS. It may

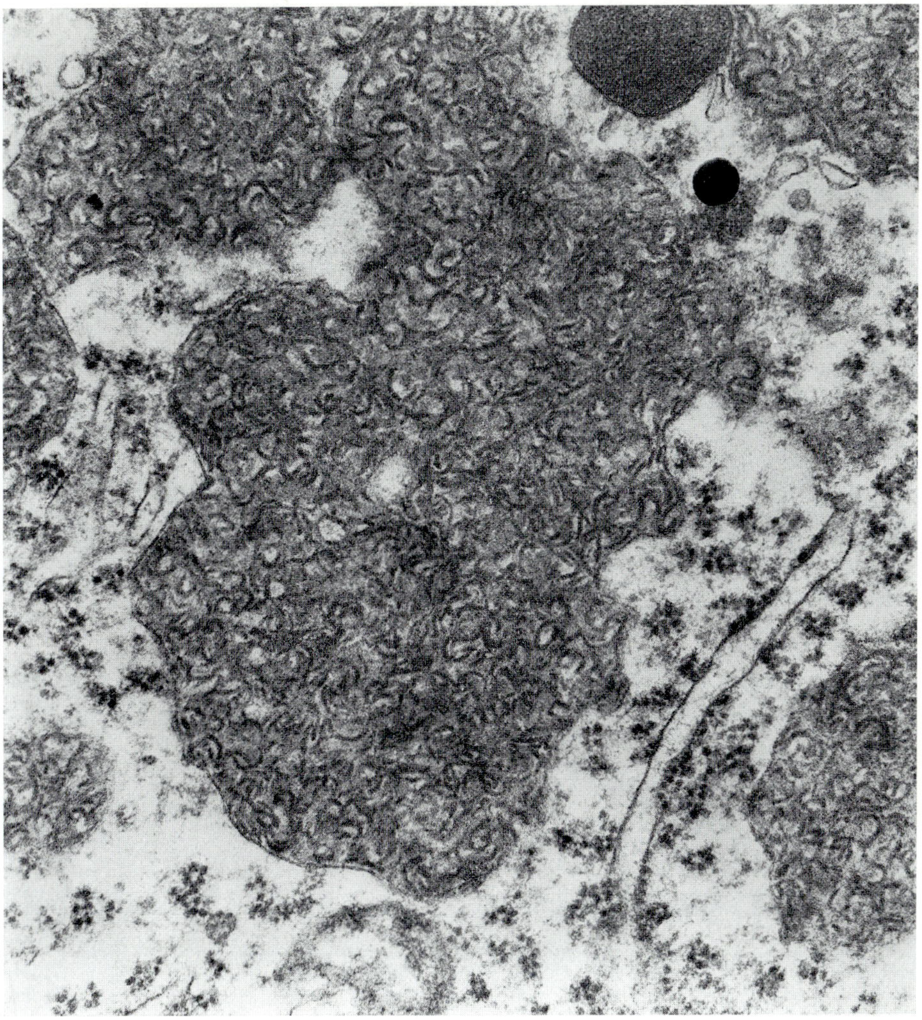

Fig. 134. Neuronal ceroid lipofuscinosis; curvilinear bodies (courtesy of Dr. Carpenter)

be overlooked because of its less severe accumulation than in neurons, never causing the affected cells to bulge; also, there is greater variation in staining properties than for neurons.

An extraordinary variety of cytosomes has been found in neurons and in viscera on electron microscopic examination. Several types have been identified and appear to be related to the age at which neuronal ceroid lipofuscinosis develops (Elfenbein and Cantor, 1969). Other investigators, however, have thought that the various forms of cytosomes are merely phases in their development, the endstage being particles resembling lipofuscin (Donahue *et al.*, 1966; Sluga and Majdezki, 1967; Zeman and Dyken, 1969). Dekaban and Herman (1974), who prefer the terms childhood, juvenile or

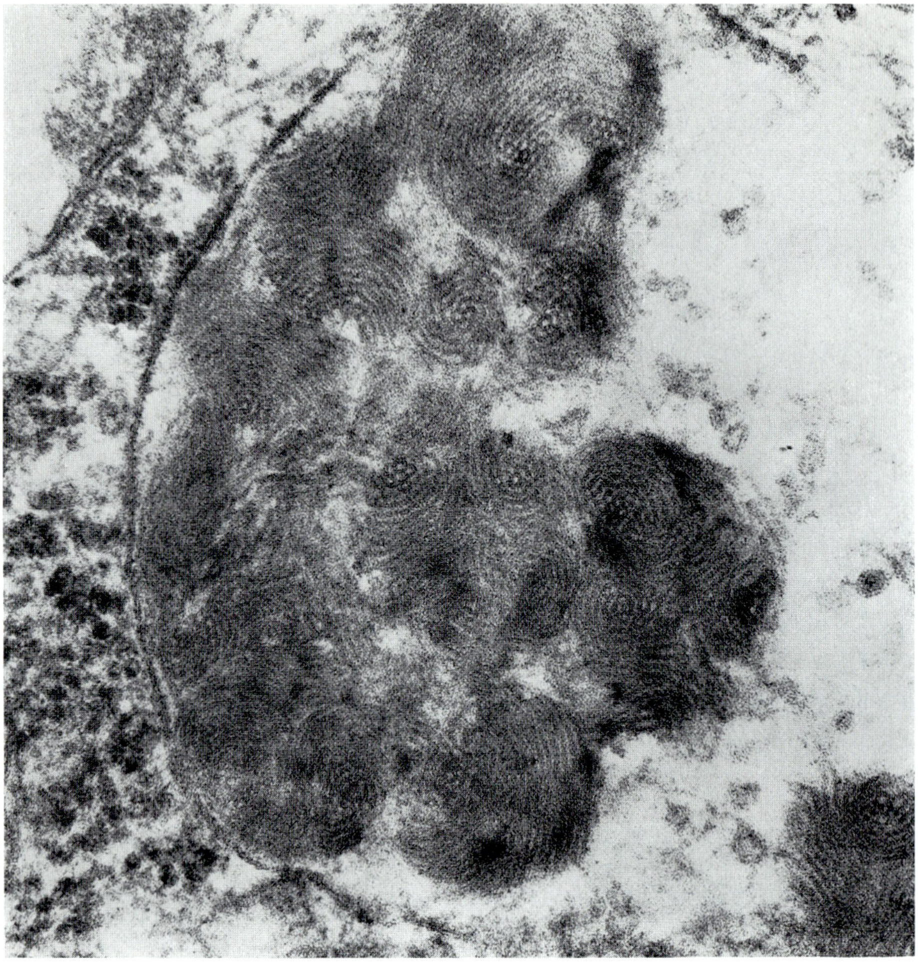

Fig. 135. Neuronal ceroid lipofuscinosis, 15½ years, onset age 6 years, fingerprint inclusions (courtesy Dr. Carpenter)

adult cerebral lipidosis, subclassify the disease according to the fine structure of cytosomes, and the following is a modified presentation of their scheme: 1. Uniform spherical globules and aggregates of globules bounded by a unit membrane and filled with a finely granular material are seen in the infantile form (Rapola and Haltia, 1973). 2. Some cytosomes consist of membrane-bounded dense bodies containing abundant short segments of round, oval or tubular profiles (Fig. 134), described as pleomorphic multilocular bodies (Zeman and Donahue, 1963), curvilinear bodies (Duffy, 1968), granular osmophilic deposits with membrane fragments (Sluga and Majdezki, 1967), or multilammellal cytosomes (Gonatas *et al.*, 1968). 3. In some cases of early onset a variety of pleomorphic bodies combining the feature of membranous cytoplasmic bodies, zebra bodies and irregular lamellal deposits were reported

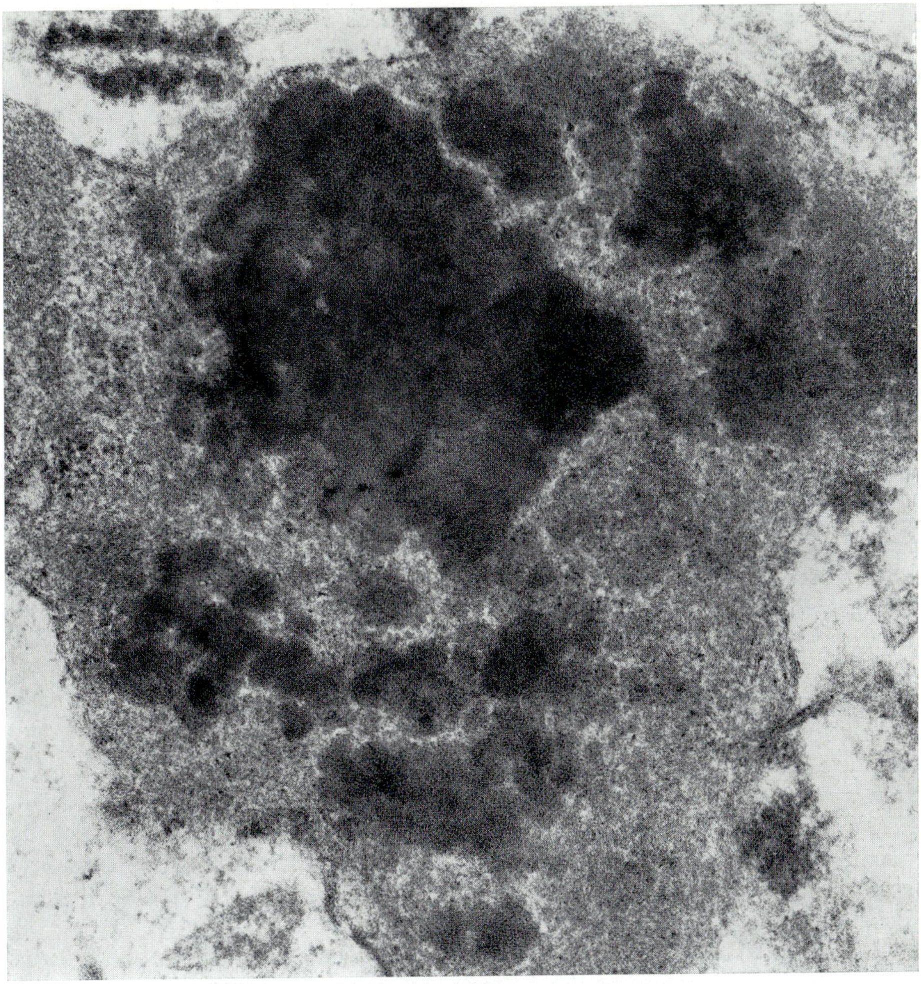

Fig. 136. Neuronal ceroid lipofuscinosis, 18 years, onset age 8 years, granular osmophilic deposits (courtesy Dr. Carpenter)

(Elfenbein, 1968; Dekaban and Herman, 1974). 4. Inclusions of greater electron density having a fingerprint-like internal structure (Fig. 135) were observed in cases of juvenile onset, in association with structures similar to curvilinear bodies or with particles having a structure like that of lipofuscin (Suzuki *et al.*, 1968; Gonatas *et al.*, 1969). 5. The inclusions observed in the adult form of neuronal ceroid lipofuscinosis show the greatest similarity to lipofuscin (Fig. 136). They consist of dense bodies of extremely variable shapes and have a dense, finely granular matrix; some vary from lipofuscin in having membranous or crystalloid internal structures; others show membranous inclusions reminiscent of various other types of cytosomes or miniature membranous cytoplasmic bodies (Chou and Thompson, 1970; Boehme *et al.*, 1971; Kornfeld, 1972). Inclusions of these types are seen not only in neurons, but in glia and endothelial cells as well (Richardson and Bornhofen, 1968; Gonatas *et al.*, 1968), and in the cells of the myenteric plexus (Elsner and Prensky, 1969).

In some cases all cytosomes were remarkably similar in structure, while others exhibited considerable pleomorphy, no two cytosomes being exactly alike (Elfenbein, 1968). Different types of cytosomes may coexist in the same cell, and even one given cytosome may be composed of components having different structure (Sluga and Majdezki, 1967; Herman *et al.*, 1971; Towfighi *et al.*, 1973). Such observations were interpreted as indicative of an evolution from one type of cytosome to another. However, in cases in whom the cytosomes were studied at various phases in the progression of the disease their structure remained unchanged over a period of 5 or 6 months (Duffy *et al.*, 1968; Herman *et al.*, 1971). Cytosomal structure, thus, has been thought to be representative of the age of the neurons at which the metabolic defect first becomes manifest, rather than as phases of an evolutionary process (Elfenbein and Cantor, 1969). The cytosomes were shown to contain variable acid phosphatase activity (Towfighi *et al.*, 1973); it decreased with increasing size of the cytosomes, which was interpreted as development of residual bodies from lysosomes that had exhausted their enzyme supply (Ishii and Gonatas, 1971).

Electron microscopic examination of viscera disclosed cytosomes of the same type as those found in neurons, such as in biopsies of peripheral nerves, skeletal muscle and skin (Carpenter *et al.*, 1972; Joosten *et al.*, 1973), as well as in circulating lymphocytes (Witzleben, 1972). In cases in which the fine structure of the cytosomes in nerve cells was compared with that in viscera, they were generally of similar type (Duffy *et al.*, 1968; Dolman and Chang, 1972). Furthermore, in the 8 cases of Carpenter *et al.* (1972) those of late infantile onset had curvilinear cytosomes in the viscera, those of juvenile onset, fingerprint cytosomes, which corresponds to the observations made in cerebral tissue.

Unclassified Processes Previously Considered Variants of Amaurotic Idiocy. The dismantling of the unitary concept of amaurotic idiocies has left no niche for certain rare conditions previously considered its variants, in particular the so-called congenital form and the pigment variant. No chemical data are presently available for the classification of these processes.

The so-called congenital form of amaurotic idiocy was observed in 3 girls among 9 siblings studied by Norman and Wood (1941) and by Brown *et al.* (1954). The afflicted infants were microcephalic and died from a progressive debilitating disease within 2 months after birth. The brains were small and firm, and microscopic examination disclosed neurons distended with lipid granules; needle-shaped crystals of cholesterol were found in the subcortical white matter, and there was also massive deposition of lipids in rounded cells, particularly in astrocytes. Severe atrophy was found in the cerebellar cortex. In the case reported by Brown *et al.* (1954) the cerebral cholesterol content was nearly four times normal. The case reported as congenital amaurotic idiocy by Hagberg *et al.* (1965) is of doubtful attribution; the brief gross description of the cerebral lesions strongly suggests hydranencephaly.

Another group of cases of uncertain classification (Jervis, 1952; Moschel, 1954; Zeman and Scarpelli, 1958) has been referred to as the "pigment variant of amaurotic idiocy" (Seitelberger, 1962). This group appears to run a protracted course, with death occurring at a juvenile or young adult age. The cerebral lesions combine the features of a lipidosis with abnormal pigmentation of the basal ganglia. The aspects of the lipidosis vary from case to case and were considered consistent with amaurotic idiocy (Jervis, 1952), or mucopolysaccharidosis (Zeman and Scarpelli, 1958), or the adult form of neuronal ceroid lipofuscinosis (Jakob and Kolkmann, 1973). Abnormal brownish pigmentation affects the basal ganglia, particularly the nucleus pallidus and the reticular part of the substantia nigra, in a pattern similar to that in Hallervorden-Spatz disease. Microscopically there is a granular pigment, which is nonlipidic and gives a strong reaction for iron, in the astrocytes and diffuse throughout the tissue; no dystrophic axons were described for these cases. In view of the differences among individual cases, particularly regarding the features of the lipidosis, there appears to be reasonable doubt as to the classification of this group as a nosologic entity.

Cephalin Lipidosis. Baar and Hickmans (1956) described a sibship of 7 members in whom 3 were affected by a slowly progressive mental deterioration starting at 1$^1/_2$ year of age. Autopsy findings in 2 sibs that had died at 5 and 4 years respectively showed widespread lipid storage in neurons, particularly in the cerebral cortex, and large numbers of foam cells arranged in nests in the spleen, liver and bone marrow, and, occasionally, in kidneys. Significant increases in cephalin, identified as inosamine phosphatide, were found in spleen, liver and brain.

Wolman Disease. The disease described as "generalized xanthomatosis" by Wolman (Abramov *et al.*, 1956) has so far been reported for 18 patients tabulated by Patrick and Lake (1973, review). The onset of symptoms usually occurs after several weeks of apparently normal postnatal development, beginning with vomiting, diarrhea and failure to gain weight. The abdomen becomes distented from hepatosplenomegaly and there is enlargement of lymph nodes. Lymphocytes, neutrophils and monocytes show a vacuolation of their cytoplasm from deposition of lipid droplets, but serum lipid levels are not elevated. Radiologic examination discloses adrenal enlargement with punctate mineralization, a feature which, in the context of the other symptoms, is pathognomonic of the disease. There are usually no signs of central nervous system involvement. The disease leads to death before the 6th month of age, but milder courses were also observed.

Chemical analyses of the viscera disclosed an excess of lipids, mostly triglycerides and free and esterified cholesterol (Crocker *et al.*, 1965; Konno *et al.*, 1966; Marshall *et al.*, 1969; Kyriakides *et al.*, 1970). The metabolic pathway common to the degradation of these compounds is the cleavage of their ester linkages, and a deficiency of acid esterase (lipase) has been demonstrated as the cause of the disease (Patrick and Lake, 1969; Lake and Patrick, 1970) and was confirmed by other investigators. Reduced acid esterase activity is found in the heterozygous carriers of the disease (Patrick and Lake, 1973).

General autopsy findings disclose widespread disposition of lipidladen histiocytes in liver, spleen, lymph nodes, bone marrow and lamina propria of the intestinal mucosa, being maximum in the duodenum (Abramov, 1956; Crocker *et al.*, 1965; Marshall *et al.*, 1969) as well as in many other tissues (Guazzi *et al.*, 1968). The cytoplasm of the histiocytes contains PAS negative, sudanophilic lipids, fatty acid crystals and cholesterol. Hepatic parenchymal cells are distended with foamy deposits; hepatic parenchymal necrosis with interstitial fibrosis and cirrhosis may ensue. Electron microscopic examination of hepatic cells discloses membrane-bounded vacuoles, the membrane having acid phosphatase activity, surrounding homogeneous lipid droplets (Lake and Patrick, 1970). Also, histochemical tests for E 600 resistant esterase were negative. The enlarged adrenal glands are of normal shape, firm and bright yellow. The superficial layers of the cortex show normal architecture, but the inner portion shows loss of cellular architecture with a haphazard disposition of foamy, lipid-laden cells, some of which are multinucleated. There is necrosis and disintegration of cells leading to focal mineralization. The adrenal medulla is spared.

Neuropathologic examination disclosed no evidence of neuronal lipid storage for most cases, although foamy histiocytes or lipid droplets were seen in the perivascular spaces and in leptomeninges (Crocker *et al.*, 1965; Marshall *et al.*, 1969). Lipid deposition is also seen in the stroma of the choroid plexus (Guazzi *et al.*, 1968). In the case reported by Kahana *et al.* (1968) moderate foamy cytoplasmic changes were seen in Purkinje cells and more severe alterations of the same type in the myenteric plexus and the sympathetic ganglia. Guazzi *et al.* (1968) report deposition of sudanophilic lipids, diffusely throughout the tissue as well as in perivascular crowding, and an associated diffuse gliosis in the cerebral hemispheric white matter, findings, however, which are difficult to interpret in a 4-month-old child (Chapter 1). Chemical determinations in brain tissue disclosed a mild accumulation of triglycerides and changes in fatty acid composition of lipids suggestive of a disturbance in myelination (Eto and Kitagawa, 1970).

References

Abramov, A., Schorr, S., Wolman, M.: Generalized xanthomatosis with calcified adrenals. Amer. J. Dis. Child. 91: 282—286, 1956.

Armstrong, D., Dimmitt, S., Van Wormer, D. E.: Studies in Batten disease. I. Peroxidase deficiency in granulocytes. Arch. Neurol. (Chic.) 30: 144—152, 1974.

— — Boehme, D. H., *et al.*: Leukocyte peroxidase deficiency in a family with Kuf's disease. Science 186: 155—156, 1974.

Baar, H. S., Hickmans, E. M.: Cephalin-lipidosis. A new disorder of lipid metabolism. Acta med. scand. 155: 49—64, 1956.

Bartsch, G. G.: Glycolipid abnormalities in a myoclonic variant of late infantile amaurotic idiocy. J. Lipid Res. 11: 241—247, 1970.

Batten, F. E.: Cerebral degeneration with symmetrical changes in the maculae in two members of a family. Trans. ophthal. Soc. U.K. 23: 386—390, 1903.

— Family cerebral degeneration with macular change (so-called juvenile form of family amaurotic idiocy). Quart. J. Med. 7: 444—454, 1914.

Boehme, D. H., Cottrell, J. C., Leonberg, S. C., Zeman, W.: A dominant form of neuronal ceroid-lipofuscinosis. Brain 94: 745—760, 1971.

Brown, N. J., Carver, B. D., Dodgson, M. C. H.: A second case in the family of congenital cerebral lipidosis resembling amaurotic idiocy. Arch. Dis. Child. 29: 48—54, 1954.

Carpenter, S., Karpati, G., Andermann, F.: Specific involvement of muscle, nerve, and skin in late infantile and juvenile amaurotic idiocy. Neurology (Minneap.) 22: 170—186, 1972.

Chou, S. M., Thompson, H. G.: Electron microscopy of storage cytosomes in Kuf's disease. Arch. Neurol. (Chic.) 23: 489—501, 1970.

Crocker, A. C., Vawter, G. F., Neuhauser, E. B. D., Rosowsky, A.: Wolman's disease: Three new patients with a recently described lipidosis. Pediatrics 35: 627—640, 1965.

Dayan, A. D., Trickey, R. J.: Thyroid involvement in juvenile amaurotic family idiocy (Batten's disease). Lancet 2: 296—297, 1970.

Dekaban, A. S., Herman, M. M.: Childhood, juvenile, and adult cerebral lipidoses. Are these different nosological entities? Arch. Path. (Chic.) 97: 65—73, 1974.

Dolman, C. L., Chang, E.: Visceral lesions in amaurotic familial idiocy with curvilinear bodies. Arch. Path. (Chic.) 94: 425—430, 1972.

Donahue, S., Zeman, W., Watanabe, I.: Electron microscopic observations in Batten's disease. In: Inborn Errors of Sphingolipid Metabolism (Aronson, S. M., Volk, B. M., eds.), pp. 3—22. Oxford: Pergamon 1966.

Duffy, P. E., Kornfeld, M., Suzuki, K.: Neurovisceral storage disease with curvilinear bodies. J. Neuropath. exp. Neurol. 27: 351—370, 1968.

Edgar, G. W. F., van Bogaert, L.: Anatomo-chemical study of the white matter in late infantile amaurotic idiocy. In: Inborn Disorders of Sphingolipid Metabolism (Aronson, S. M., Volk, B. W., eds.), pp. 75—91. Oxford: Pergamon 1967.

Elfenbein, I. B.: Dystonic juvenile idiocy without amaurosis. Johns Hopkins Med. J. 123: 205—221, 1968.

— Cantor, H. E.: Late infantile amaurotic idiocy with multilamellar cytosomes: An electron microscopic study. J. Pediat. 75: 253—264, 1969.

Elsner, B., Prensky, A. L.: Ultrastructure of rectal biopsies in juvenile amaurotic idiocy. Neurology (Minneap.) 19: 834—840, 1969.

Eto, Y., Kitagawa, T.: Wolman's disease with hypolipoproteinemia and acanthosis: Clinical and biochemical observations. J. Pediat. 77: 862—867, 1970.

Gonatas, N. K., Gambetti, P., Baird, H.: A second type of late infantile amaurotic idiocy with multilamellar cytosomes. J. Neuropath. exp. Neurol. 27: 371—389, 1968.

— — Tucker, S. H., *et al.*: Cytoplasmic inclusions in juvenile amaurotic idiocy. J. Pediat. 75: 796—805, 1969.

Gordon, N. S., Marsden, H. B., Noronha, M. J.: Neuronal ceroid lipofuscinosis (Batten's disease). Arch. Dis. Child. 47: 285—291, 1972.

Guazzi, G. C., Martin, J. J., Philippart, M., *et al.*: Wolman's disease. Europ. Neurol. 1: 334—362, 1968.

Haberland, C., Brunngraber, E. G., Witting, L. A., Hof, H.: Late infantile amaurotic idiocy (LIAI). Anatomochemical report of a case. Neurology (Minneap.) 22: 305—311, 1972.

Hagberg, B., Hultquist, G., Öhman, R., Svennerholm, L.: Congenital amaurotic idiocy. Acta paed. scand. 54: 116—131, 1965.

Haltia, M., Rapola, J., Santavuori, P.: Infantile type of so-called neuronal ceroid-lipofuscinosis. Histological and electron microscopic studies. Acta neuropath. (Berl.) 26: 157—170, 1973.

— — — Keränen, A.: Infantile type of so-called neuronal ceroid-lipofuscinosis, Part 2 (Morphological and biochemical studies). J. Neurol. Sci. 18: 269—285, 1973.

Herman, M. M., Rubinstein, L. J., McKhann, G. M.: Additional electron microscopic observations on two cases of Batten-Spielmeyer-Vogt disease (neuronal ceroid-lipofuscinosis). Acta neuropath. (Berl.) 17: 85—102, 1971.

Ishii, T., Gonatas, N. K.: The multilamellar cytosome in late infantile amaurotic idiocy. Acta neuropath. (Berl.) 19: 265—270, 1971.

Jakob, H., Kolkmann, F.-W.: Zur Pigmentvariante der adulten Form der amaurotischen Idiotie (Kufs). Acta neuropath. (Berl.) 26: 225—236, 1973.

Jervis, G. A.: Hallervorden-Spatz disease associated with atypical amaurotic idiocy. J. Neuropath. exp. Neurol. 11: 4—17, 1952.

Joosten, E., Gabreels, F., Stadhouders, A., *et al.*: Involvement of sural nerve in neuronal ceroid-lipofuscinoses. Neuropädiatrie 4: 98—110, 1973.

Kahana, D., Berant, M., Wolman, M.: Primary familial xanthomatosis with adrenal involvement (Wolman's disease). Pediatrics 42: 70—76, 1968.

Klenk, E.: Niemann-Picksche Krankheit und amaurotische Idiotie. Hoppe Seyler Z. physiol. Chem. 262: 128—143, 1939.

Konno, T., Fuijii, M., Watanuki, T., Koizumi, K.: Wolman's disease: The first case in Japan. Tohoku J. exp. Med. 90: 375—389, 1966.

Kornfeld, M.: Generalized lipofuscinosis (generalized Kufs' disease). J. Neuropath. exp. Neurol. 31: 668—682, 1972.

Kristensson, K., Olsson, Y., Sourander, P.: Peripheral nerve changes in Tay-Sachs and Batten-Spielmeyer-Vogt disease. A preliminary report. Acta path. microbiol. scand. 70: 630—632, 1967.

— Rayner, S., Sourander, P.: Visceral involvement in juvenile amaurotic idiocy. Acta neuropath. (Berl.) 4: 421—424, 1965.

— Sourander, P.: Occurrence of lipofuscin in inherited metabolic disorders affecting the nervous system. J. Neurol. Neurosurg. Psychiat. 29: 113—118, 1966.

Kyriakides, E. C., Filippone, N., Paul, B., *et al.*: Lipid studies in Wolman's disease. Pediatrics 46: 431—436, 1970.

Lake, B. D., Patrick, A. D.: Wolman's disease: Deficiency of E 600-resistant acid esterase activity with storage of lipids in lysosomes. J. Pediat. 76: 262—266, 1970.

Marshall, W. C., Ockenden, B. G., Fosbrooke, A. S., Cumings, J. N.: Wolman's disease. Arch. Dis. Child. 44: 331—341, 1969.

Moschel, R.: Amaurotische Idiotie mit einer besonderen Form von Pigmentablagerung. Dtsch. Z. Nervenheilk. 172: 102—110, 1954.

Nevalainen, T. J., Panelius, M., Riekkinen, P. J.: Neuronal ceroid-lipofuscinosis. Report of two cases with neurochemical and morphological observations. Europ. Neurol. 9: 298—314, 1973.

Norman, R. M., Wood, N.: A congenital form of amaurotic family idiocy. J. Neurol. Psychiat. (Chic.) 4: 175—190, 1941.

Pallis, C. A., Duckett, S., Pearse, A. G. E.: Diffuse lipofuscinosis of the central nervous system. Neurology (Minneap.) 17: 381—394, 1967.

Patel, V., Koppang, N., Patel, B., Zeman, W.: p-phenylnediamine-mediated peroxidase deficiency in English setters with neuronal ceroid-lipofuscinosis. Lab. Invest. 30: 366—368, 1974.

Patrick, A. D., Lake, B. D.: Deficiency of an acid lipase in Wolman's disease. Nature 222: 1067—1068, 1969.

— — Wolman's disease. In: Lysosomes and Storage Diseases (Hers, H. G., Van Hoof, F., eds.), pp. 453—473. New York: Academic Press 1973.

Rapola, J., Haltia, M.: Cytoplasmic inclusions in the vermiforme appendix and skeletal muscle in two types of so-called neuronal ceroid-lipofuscinosis. Brain 96: 833—840, 1973.

Richardson, M. E., Bornhofen, J. H.: Early childhood cerebral lipidosis with prominent myoclonus. Ultrastructural and histochemical studies of a cerebral biopsy. Arch Neurol. (Chic.) 18: 34—43, 1968.

Ricoy-Campo, J. R., Bruens, J. H.: Contribution critique à l'étude de la variante dite myoclonique des idioties amaurotiques familiales non gangliosidiques. J. Neurol. Sci. 10: 435—456, 1970.

Seitelberger, F., Jacob, H., Schnabel, R.: The myoclonic variant of cerebral lipidosis. In: Inborn Disorders of Sphingolipid Metabolism (Aronson, S. M., Volk, B. M., eds.), pp. 43—73. Oxford: Pergamon Press 1966.

— Simma, K.: Pigment variant of amaurotic idiocy. In: Cerebral Sphingolipidoses (Aronson, S. M., Volk, B. W., eds.), pp. 29—37. New York: Academic Press 1962.

Siakotos, A. N., Goebel, H. H., Patel, V., *et al.*: The morphogenesis and biochemical characteristics of ceroid isolated from cases of neuronal ceroid-lipofuscinosis. In: Sphingolipidoses (Volk, V. W., Aronson, S. M., eds.), pp. 53—61. New York: Plenum Press 1972.

Sjögren, T.: Die juvenile amaurotische Idiotie. Klinische und erblichkeitsmedizinische Untersuchungen. Hereditas 14: 197—426, 1931.

Sjövall, E.: Die Bedeutung der pathologisch-histologischen Veränderungen im Zentralnervensystem bei der juvenilen amaurotischen Idiotie. Verh. dtsch. Ges. Path. 27: 185—190, 1934.
Sluga, E., Majdezki, Th.: Zur Ultrastruktur des Speichermaterials von spätinfantiler amaurotischer Idiotie. Acta neuropath. (Berl.) 9: 254—272, 1967.
Spielmeyer, W.: Über familiäre amaurotische Idiotien. Neurol. Centralbl. 24: 620—621; 1131—1132, 1905.
Stock, W.: Über eine bis jetzt noch nicht beschriebene Form der familiär auftretenden Netzhaut-Degeneration bei gleichzeitiger Verblödung und über Pigment-Degeneration der Netzhaut. Klin. Mbl. Augenheilk. 5: 225—244, 1908.
Suzuki, J., Johnson, A. B., Marquet, E., Suzuki, K.: A case of juvenile lipidosis: Electron microscopic, histochemical and biochemical studies. Acta neuropath. (Berl.) 11: 122—139, 1968.
Towfighi, J., Baird, H. W., Gambetti, P., Gonatas, N. K.: The significance of cytoplasmic inclusions in late infantile and juvenile amaurotic idiocy. An ultrastructural study. Acta neuropath. (Berl.) 23: 32—42, 1973.
Vogt, H.: Familiäre amaurotische Idiotie, histologische und histopathologische Studien. Arch. Kinderheilk. 51: 1—35, 1909.
Witzleben, C. L.: Lymphocyte inclusions in late-onset amaurotic idiocy. Value as a diagnostic test and genetic marker. Neurology (Minneap.) 22: 1075—1078, 1972.
Wolman, M.: A histochemical study of various forms of cerebral lipidoses. J. clin. Path. 15: 324—327, 1962.
Wyburn-Mason, R.: On some anomalous forms of amaurotic idiocy and their bearing on the relationship of the various types. Brit. J. Ophthal. 27: 145—173, 193—206, 1943.
Zeman, W., Donahue, S.: Fine structure of the lipid bodies in juvenile amaurotic idiocy. Acta neuropath. (Berl.) 3: 144—149, 1963.
— Dyken, P.: Neuronal ceroid-lipofuscinosis (Batten's disease): Relationship to amaurotic family idiocy? Pediatrics 44: 570—583, 1969.
— Hoffman, J.: Juvenile and late forms of amaurotic idiocy in one family. J. Neurol. Neurosurg. Psychiat. 25: 352—362, 1962.
— Scarpelli, D. G.: The non-specific lesions of Hallervorden-Spatz disease. J. Neuropath. exp. Neurol. 17: 622—630, 1958.
— Siakotos, A. N.: The neuronal ceroid lipofuscinoses. In: Lysosomes and Storage Diseases (Hers, H. G., Van Hoof, F., eds.), Chapter 23, pp. 519—551. New York: Academic Press 1973.

38. Metachromatic Leukodystrophy (Sulfatase A Deficiency) and Multiple Sulfatase Deficiency

Metachromatic leukodystrophy was first described in adults. Alzheimer (1910) gave a brief abstract of a case which he characterized as a white matter disease with destruction of myelin and abundant, brightly metachromatic deposits in glia cells. Witte (1921) reported similar findings and recognized the accumulation of metachromatic granules in neuronal perikarya and in liver, kidney, gallbladder, anterior pituitary and testes; he suggested that *in vivo* diagnosis of the disease should be possible from metachromatic material excreted into the urine. Kaltenbach (1922) gave the first detailed description of the histopathology of the white matter lesions. These early descriptions of many of the essential microscopic features of metachromatic leukodystrophy had relatively little impact on its classification in subsequent reports, because the chemistry of metachromasia was not understood, and its significance for the classification of the disease was not realized. Hence, the first descriptions of metachromatic leukodystrophy in infants emphasized other, less specific, criteria such as its familial occurrence, the age of onset or rate of progression, the interpretation of the metachromatic deposits as "prelipoids", or a high degree of selectivity in the affectation of oligodendroglia. Brain and Greenfield (1950) defined the clinical features of the late infantile course of the disease and deserve the credit for identifying the metachromatic staining of the deposits as the key feature in classifying the disease. A tabulation of 68 case reports was published by Helmstaedt (1963).

Metachromasia in general refers to an altered staining of a tissue component, whereby the absorption spectrum of the dye-tissue complex differs from that of the original dye; thiazine dyes exhibit a characteristic change from blue to red. Lison (1935) attributed metachromasia to the binding of dye to strongly negatively charged acidic groups, especially sulphuric acid esters, and Michaelis and Granick (1945) suggested that the spectral change results from polymerization of the bound dye molecules. The significance of the metachromasia of the deposits found in metachromatic leukodystrophy was elucidated through the studies of Austin (1958, 1960), Jatzkewitz (1958) and Hagberg *et al.* (1960) showing abnormal accumulation of sulfatides in brain tissue as well as in other organs. It is now widely accepted that these sulfatides are responsible for the metachromatic staining. Metachromatic leukodystrophy, therefore, may be classified as a neurolipidosis—that is, an abnormal accumulation of lipids in the tissue (Austin, 1960), or as a leukodystrophy, in that the brunt of the damage is borne by the myelinated fibers in the white matter or by their sheath cells respectively.

The next breakthrough in the understanding of the disease was the discovery of the deficiency of a specific enzyme involved in sulphate hydrolysis. Indeed, metachromatic leukodystrophy was the first lipidosis, or leukodystrophy, for which a specific enzyme deficiency was identified. Patients suffering from metachromatic leukodystrophy have lower than normal or absent arylsulfatase A activity in the gray and white matter of the brain as well as in liver, kidney and body fluids (Austin *et al.*, 1963). Subnormal activity of arylsulfatase A is also found in the heterozygos carriers of the afflicted families (Bass *et al.*, 1970; Taniguchi and Nanba, 1970; Kaback and Howell, 1970). Sulfatases are hydrolytic enzymes splitting sulfate from sulfate linkages. Sulfatase A and B are lysosomal enzymes distinguishable electrophoretically and with selective inhibitors. The term arylsulfatase refers to the enzyme's activity toward a synthetic aromatic substrate, nitrocatechole sulfate. Mehl and Jatzkewitz (1968) demonstrated that the naturally occurring substrate of arylsulfatase A is cerebroside sulfate. The preponderance of available evidence indicates that excess sulfatides accumulate in metachromatic leukodystrophy because of the deficiency in cerebroside sulfatase, or arylsulfatase A, respectively.

Clinical Course. Metachromatic leukodystrophy is a genetically determined disease, being transmitted by an autosomal recessive gene; there is no evidence of racial or sex predilection. The disease may manifest at any age, from infancy to adult life, but the late infantile course accounts for approximately two-thirds of all cases (Holländer, 1964). It typically has its onset between 12 and 18 months, practically never before the 9th month, the preceding postnatal development being normal. The first manifestations may suggest a peripheral neuropathy, with clumsiness in walking, weakness, hypotonia and reduced or absent tendon reflexes. Neuropathic changes may be the only manifestations (de Silva and Pearce, 1973), but they are commonly superseded by signs of central nervous system involvement including upper motor neuron signs, nystagmus or cerebellar signs. Progression of the disease leads to dementia, tonic seizures, optic atrophy and quadruparesis (Hagberg *et al.*, 1960), death occurring within 6 years (Holländer, 1964).

The rare juvenile course has an onset between 3 and 10 years. If the onset is during the second decade, the course of the disease resembles that in the adult, characterized by psychiatric symptoms or dementia, dyskinesias, and speech disturbances. For the adults the average age at onset is 29 years and the average duration 14 years (Austin *et al.*, 1968).

Diagnostic measures include examination of the urine sediment for metachromatic granules as a preliminary, nonspecific screening procedure. Increased amounts of sulfatides and reduced or absent arylsulfatase A are found in the urine (Austin *et al.*, 1966); the enzyme deficiency may be demonstrated in peripheral leukocytes, cultured skin fibroblasts, amniotic fluid and serum (Thunold, 1972, references; Beratis *et al.*, 1973). Microscopic examination of biopsies of cerebral cortex, kidney, dental pulp or rectum demonstrates sulfatide deposits, but a biopsy of peripheral nerves is the most convenient diagnostic technique (Thieffry and Lyon, 1959; Hagberg *et al.*, 1962).

Morbid Anatomy. Gross inspection of the brain in late infantile metachromatic leukodystrophy reveals only minor changes, although the brain is usually quite firm and may be enlarged and heavier than normal; atrophy with reduced weight is also observed. The cut surface may not reveal any discoloration of the white matter; the cerebral ventricles are normal or slightly dilated. Microscopic examination discloses a diffuse leukodystrophy, with paucity or absence of myelinated fibers. Maximum changes are seen in the centrum semiovale of the cerebral hemispheres, but there is also demyelination in cerebellar white matter and in various tracts of brain stem and cord. As a rule, the leukodystrophic changes are most marked in those fiber systems that have not attained their full myelination at birth. There are diffuse gradients in the intensity of the leukodystrophic process in the centrum semiovale, and the transitions between demyelinated and apparently normal portions are gradual. The process is often most intense in the periventricular tissue, diminishing toward the surface and sparing the subcortical U-fibers, but the latter is by no means consistent. There is no tendency to cavitation; inflammatory changes are absent. Oligodendroglia nuclei are completely absent from the demyelinated regions; fewer than normal nuclei may be seen in adjacent, apparently well myelinated white matter (Greenfield, 1933). Regional studies of the white matter with microassays demonstrate accumulation of sulfatides and loss of myelin lipids in portions that have a normal myelin density with conventional histological methods (Jatzkewitz *et al.*, 1964). Axis cylinders are relatively spared, but their density is reduced in the severely affected areas. There is proliferation of astrocytes; little, if any, neutral fat is found in the tissue or in macrophages. Metachromatic deposits are scattered throughout the tissue or are localized in the processes of astrocytes or within macrophages which may crowd within the perivascular spaces (Fig. 137). The greatest density of metachromatic deposits is seen in regions with complete demyelination. The deposits consist of irregular granular masses, 15 to 20 μ in diameter, which exhibit a characteristic golden-brownish metachromasia when stained with acid cresyl violet. The use of frozen sections is imperative as metachromasia is diminished or abolished by lipid extraction and/or changes

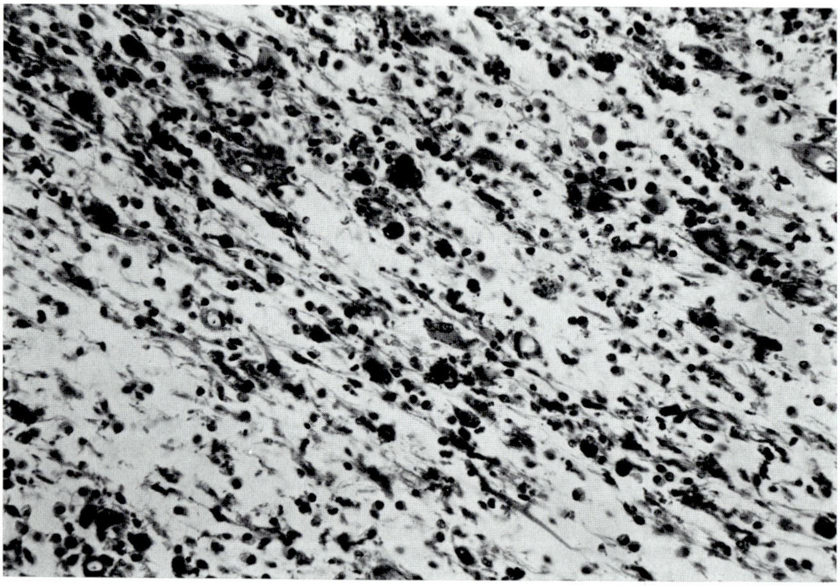

Fig. 137. Metachromatic leukodystrophy; granular metachromatic deposits in the demyelinated white matter; ×290

in the molecular structure of the deposits upon paraffin embedding. A mahagony-brown metachromasia is characteristic of the disease, to be distinguished from the nonspecific reddish metachromasia of myelin sheaths and other tissue structures (Hirsch and Peiffer, 1955). The tissue deposits and/or cerebroside sulfates also have an exceptionally strong affinity for acriflavin and acridine orange, emitting a golden-yellow fluorescence on microscopic examination in ultraviolet light (Holländer, 1963). The granules stain strongly with the periodic acid-Schiff reaction, which persists after treatment with lipid solvents (Norman *et al.*, 1960). Isolation of a highly purified fraction of metachromatic granules from brain tissue yielded equimolar amounts of cholesterol, galactolipids and phosphatides as well as relatively much chloroform-methanol insoluble residue; most of the galactolipids were sulfatides (Suzuki *et al.*, 1967).

The gray matter tends to be well preserved, and loss of neurons is generally slight or absent. The cerebellar cortex, however, may show a marked atrophy of the granular layer type (Chapter 31), with persistence of Purkinje cells, axonal torpedoes and dendrite swellings (Norman *et al.*, 1960). Metachromatic granular material is stored in neuronal perikarya, though rarely in sufficient amounts as to balloon the cell. Granules either occur diffusly throughout the cytoplasm or aggregated in one pole of the cell. There is a characteristic regional pattern in the affection of nuclear groups. Metachromatic deposits are found in the neurons of pallidum, thalamus, subthalamic nucleus, hypothalamus, lateral geniculate, amygdala, and dentate nucleus. The gray matter of the spinal cord and spinal ganglia are involved, and brain stem nuclei show a highly selective pattern of affection. The cerebral and cerebellar cortex, claustrum, putamen, caudate nucleus and certain brain stem nuclei tend to be spared (Abraham and Lampert, 1963). The regional selectivity of storage of metachromatic material in neurons distinguishes metachromatic leukodystrophy from many other lipidoses and carbohydrate storage diseases having a diffuse pattern of storage.

Deposition of metachromatic material in peripheral nerve is of particular significance for the clinical diagnosis of the disease. Metachromatic granules occur in the cytoplasm of Schwann cells as well as in macrophages, the latter being the more reliable diagnostic feature. Granules in Schwann cells accumulate preferentially in the paranuclear cytoplasm and at the nodes of Ranvier, as shown in teased fibers (Dayan, 1967) and with the electron microscope (Webster, 1962). Only a few fibers may be affected on light microscopic examination, but widespread affection of the Schwann cells of myelinated and nonmyelinated fibers is seen with the electron microscope. There is evidence of segmental demyelination and concurrent widespread remyelination.

Storage of metachromatic material outside the central nervous system involves liver, gallbladder, pancreatic islands, lymph nodes, kidney, adrenal glands and ovaries (Wolfe and Pietra, 1964). In the kidney the epithelia of convoluted tubules, the loops of Henle and the collecting tubules are involved and granular casts are seen in the tubular lumen. Deposition of metachromatic material in these organs is usually not associated with changes indicating cellular dysfunction, except for the gallbladder, which often has a thickened or fibrotic wall.

There are many reports on the fine structure of the metachromatic deposits (Aurebeck *et al.*, 1964; Toga *et al.*, 1972; Anzil *et al.*, 1973, references). The most highly organized type of inclusion is the prismatic (Fig. 138), consisting of piles of lipid leaflets stacked in columns or sheets separated by a matrix which probably contains mucopolysaccharides (Grégoire *et al.*, 1966; Résibois-Grégoire, 1967). Other inclusions consist of concentric layers of weakly osmophilic lamellar material. Both are found free in the cytoplasm. Still other inclusions of greater electron density consist of chaotic, densely osmophilic grains and particles and of variable amounts of randomly oriented aggregates of lamellar material. They are usually bound by a unit membrane, and their derivation from lysosomes is indicated by acid phosphatase activity (Grégoire *et al.*, 1966; Terry *et al.*, 1966). The latter is found particularly in the inclusion showing the least structural organization (Résibois, 1969).

Inclusions of various types occur not only in the central nervous tissue, where they involve oligodendroglia, astrocytes, macrophages and other elements, but also in peripheral nerves and kidneys, but the prismatic type is rare in the kidney. Concentric membranous inclusions are found in hepatic cells (Résibois, 1971). Intracerebral or epidural injection of sulfatides in rabbits induces cytosomes similar to those found in man (Anzil *et al.*, 1973).

Pathogenetic Considerations. The preponderance of evidence indicates that there is a direct causal relationship between the deficiency of arylsulfatase A, or cerebroside sulfatase activity, respectively, and the abnormal accumulation of cerebroside sulfates in metachromatic leukodystrophy. There is discussion, however, on the mode of induction of white matter lesions by the disease. Sulfatides are normal constituents of myelin sheaths; they are enriched in myelin fractions and increase in brain tissue concurrent with myelination. In rat brain sulfatase activity increases from birth to reach a maximum between 15 and 19 days, which corresponds to the period when incorporation of sulfate into sulfatides is at maximum (Austin *et al.*, 1968). Sulfatides, however, are not restricted to myelin; they are membrane lipids in general, including the membranes of cytoplasmic organelles. Thus, Malone and Conole (1969) demonstrated an increase in sulfatides in the plasma membranes of renal tubular cells in cases of metachromatic leukodystrophy.

The manifestation of a sulfatide lipidosis in terms of a leukodystrophy evidently is related to the high sulfatide content of myelin, and of plasma membranes in general, and to the derivation of the myelin lamellae from the plasma membranes of the sheath cells. Several specific pathogenetic mechanisms may be involved in the destruction of myelin: First, the abnormal lipid metabolism may cause the formation of a chemically abnormal myelin membrane which is more prone to disintegration than is normal myelin; secondly, the progressive accumulation of sulfatides in the sheath cells may interfere with their metabolism, causing the destruction of sheath cells or their inability to maintain the myelin sheaths. Evidence has been presented in favor of either hypothesis, but the latter one appears more likely. The formation of a chemically abnormal myelin was assumed by O'Brien (1964), based on an excess of cerebroside sulfate and a deficiency of cerebrosides in isolated myelin fractions. Electron microscopic observations on abnormalities in the structure of the myelin sheath, such as variation in the dense lines (Webster, 1962) or an abnormal looseness of myelin lamellae, appear to be consistent with O'Brien's concept; however, changes in the fine structure of sheaths were seen only on occasion; they were not observed by other investigators, and their interpretation was criticized (Terry *et al.*, 1966). The available electron microscopic data are more consistent with a structural normalcy of the myelin sheaths and a progressive impairment of sheath cell's metabolism by the intracellular accumulation of lipid material.

One may speculate that the deficiency of an enzyme involved in lipid degradation becomes more deleterious when myelination and the concurrent demand for myelin lipids subside. This assumption may explain the onset of symptoms at a time when many tracts are in advanced myelination, but there is as yet no satisfactory explanation for the great variance in the age

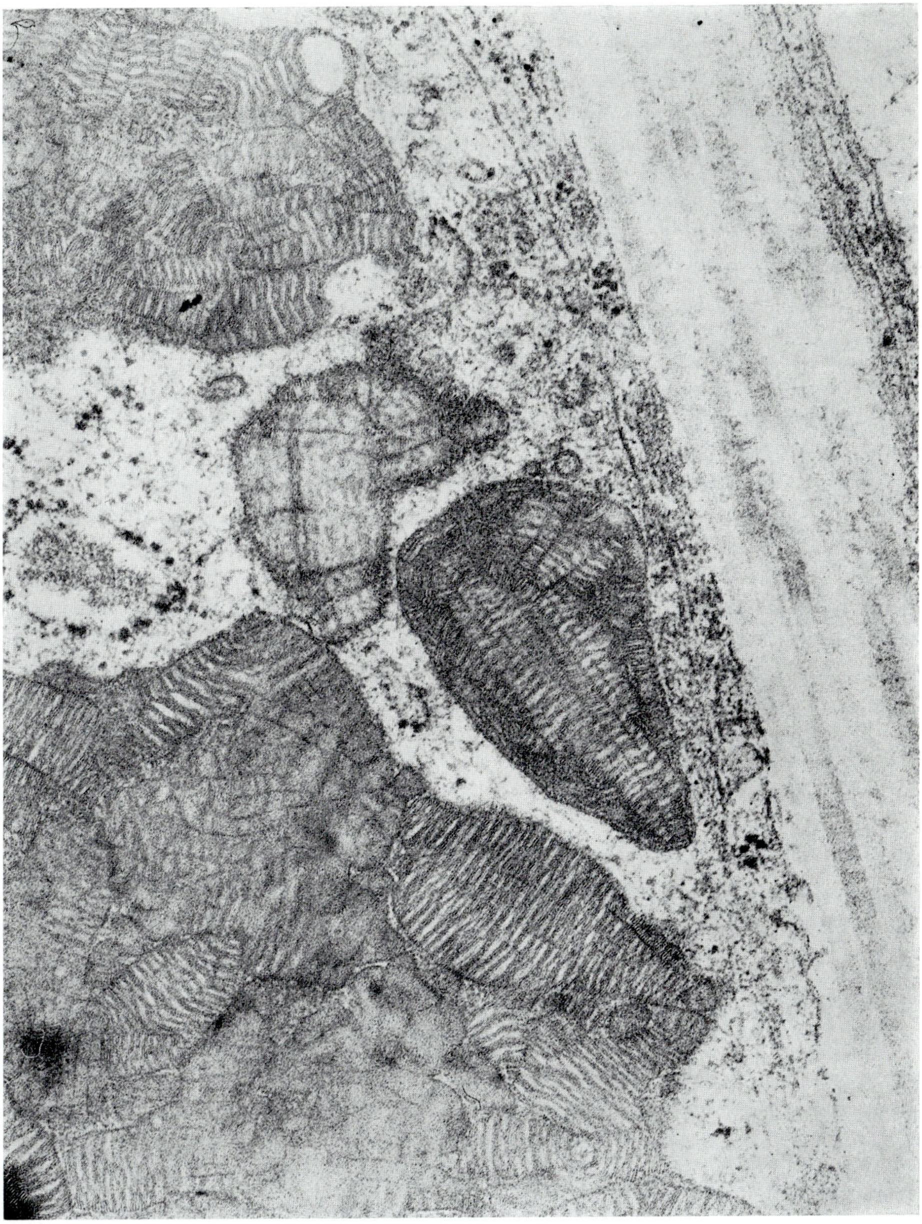

Fig. 138. Metachromatic leukodystrophy; prismatic cytoplasmic inclusions (courtesy of Drs. Anzil and Blinzinger)

of onset and the speed of progression of the disease. The deficiency of arylsulfatase A activity in urine was found to be less severe in the adult form (Stumpf and Austin, 1971), but determinations of sulfatase activity in organs (Mehl and Jatzkewitz, 1968) and leukocytes (Hirose and Bass, 1971) did not support the assumption that the adult course is simply a less severe degree of enzyme deficiency. Two components of arylsulfatase, A_1 and A_2, were shown by Suzuki and Mizuno (1974): both were deficient in the late infantile form of the disease, while only A_1 was missing in the juvenile form.

The deposition of sulfatides in various organs may be explained in terms of a spillover of the sulfatides released from the leukodystrophic brain tissue (Witte, 1921), or they may be manifestations of a general metabolic derangement. The renal deposition of sulfatides after cerebroside injection into normal rats observed by Hansson *et al.* (1967) is consistent with the first assumption; however, the renal deposits were few and inconsistent, and none were found by Austin (1963) upon subcutaneous injections of massive amounts of sulfatides. It is more likely that deposition of sulfatides in various organs is caused by the local sulfatase deficiency; it was shown that the sulfatides accumulating in peripheral nerves have a fatty acid composition similar to that of normal nerves but different from that of sulfatides in brain or kidney (Malone and Stoffyn, 1967).

Multiple Sulfatase Deficiency. Three sibs with a progressive neurologic disorder which combined elements of metachromatic leukodystrophy and of amaurotic idiocy were described by Mossakowski *et al.* (1961). The brains showed histologic features characteristic of metachromatic leukodystrophy as well as widespread neuronal storage of lipidic material, loss of neurons in cerebral and cerebellar cortex, and retinitis pigmentosa. The lipids accumulated in the neurons were considered gangliosides or a glycolipid intermediary between gangliosides and cerebrosides; those accumulated in the white matter, cerebrosides and cerebroside sulfuric esters. These cases and a similar one reported by Lüthy *et al.* (1966) and Bischoff and Ulrich (1967) defy definite classification in the absence of enzyme determinations, but they are rather similar to documented cases of multiple sulfatase deficiency.

The clinical manifestations of multiple sulfatase deficiency (Austin, 1973) are similar to those of late infantile metachromatic leukodystrophy, but there are, in addition, anomalies of bones such as depressed sternum and flaired ribs, broadened phalanges, and structural changes in vertebral bodies and metacarpals. Large basophilic to azurophilic granules are seen in lymphocytes. These are suggestive of multiple sulfatase deficiency when found in a patient having the clinical and laboratory findings of infantile metachromatic leukodystrophy.

Multiple sulfatase deficiency has been characterized biochemically by an absence of the lysosomal sulfatases A and B, and of at least one microsomal sulfatase, arylsulfatase C (Austin *et al.*, 1965; Harzer *et al.*, 1973). Hepatic β-galactosidase is also reduced to the same degree as in Hurler's syndrome. Chemical analysis of the brain (Bischel *et al.*, 1966) has shown an increase in sphingolipid sulfates (sulfatides), and cholesterol sulfate, and G_{M3}- and G_{M2}-gangliosides in the cerebral cortex, as well as an increase in sulfated acid polysaccharides (glucosaminoglycans). Pedigrees indicate an autosomal, recessive inheritance.

The morbid anatomy of the few documented cases shows atrophy of the cerebral and cerebellar cortices, with thickening and cloudiness of leptomeninges. There are changes in the white matter identical to those of metachromatic leukodystrophy. In addition, there is widespread neuronal storage of lipid material, particularly in the cerebral cortex. The neuronal material is finely granular, PAS positive and shows a slightly reddish-purple metachromasia.

References

Abraham, K., Lampert, P.: Intraneuronal lipid deposits in metachromatic leukodystrophy. Histochemical and topographic observations. Neurology (Minneap.) 13: 686—692, 1963.

Alzheimer, A.: Beiträge zur Kenntnis der pathologischen Neuroglia und ihrer Beziehungen zu den Abbauvorgängen im Nervensystem. Histol. Histopath. Arbt. Großhirnrinde (Nissl, Alzheimer) 3: 401—562, 1910.

Anzil, A. P., Blinzinger, K., Martinus, J.: Ultrastructure of the storage materials in metachromatic leucodystrophy peripheral neuropathy and in rabbit tissues after sulfatide application with special reference to pleated lamellar systems. J. Microscopie 18: 173—186, 1973.

Aurebeck, G., Osterberg, K., Blaw, M., *et al.*: Electron microscopic observations on metachromatic leucodystrophy. Arch. Neurol. (Chic.) 11: 273—288, 1964.

Austin, J. H.: Metachromatic form of diffuse cerebral sclerosis. II. Diagnosis during life by isolation of metachromatic lipids from urine. Neurology (Minneap.) 7: 716—723, 1957.

— Observations in metachromatic leucoencephalopathy. Trans. Amer. neurol. Ass. 83: 149—152, 1958.

— Metachromatic form of diffuse sclerosis. III. Significance of sulfatide and other lipid abnormalities in white matter and kidney. Neurology (Minneap.) 10: 470—483, 1960.

— Studies in metachromatic leukodystrophy. Arch. Neurol. (Chic.) 28: 258—264, 1973.

— Balasubramanian, A. S., Pattabiraman, T. N., *et al.*: A controlled study of enzymic activities in three human disorders of glycolipid metabolism. J. Neurochem. 10: 805—816, 1963.

— Armstrong, D., Fouch, S., *et al.*: Metachromatic leukodystrophy (MLD). VII. MLD in adults; diagnosis and pathogenesis. Arch. Neurol. 18: 225—240, 1968.

— — Shearer, L.: Metachromatic form of diffuse cerebral sclerosis. V. The nature and significance of low sulfatase activity: A controlled study of brain, liver and kidney in four patients with metachromatic leukodystrophy (MLD). Arch. Neurol. (Chic.) 13: 593—614, 1965.

— — — McAfee, D.: Metachromatic form of diffuse cerebral sclerosis. VI. A rapid test for the sulfatase A deficiency in metachromatic leukodystrophy (MLD) in urine. Arch. Neurol (Chic.) 14: 259—269, 1966.

Bass, N. H., Witmer, E. J., Dreifus, F. E.: A pedigree study of metachromatic leukodystrophy. Neurology (Minneap.) 20: 52—62, 1970.

Beratis, N. G., Aron, A. M., Hirschhorn, K.: Metachromatic leukodystrophy: Detection in serum. J. Pediat. 83: 824—826, 1973.

Bischel, M., Austin, J., Kemeny, M.: Metachromatic leukodystrophy (MLD). Arch. Neurol. (Chic.) 15: 13—28, 1966.

Bischoff, A., Ulrich, J.: Amaurotische Idiotie in Verbindung mit metachromatischer Leukodystrophie: Übergangsform oder Kombination? Acta neuropath. (Berl.) 8: 292—308, 1967.

Brain, W. R., Greenfield, J. G.: Late infantile metachromatic leucencephalopathy with primary degeneration of the interfascicular oligodendroglia. Brain 73: 291—317, 1950.

Dayan, A. D.: Peripheral neuropathy of metachromatic leucodystrophy: Observations on segmental demyelination and remyelination and the intracellular distribution of sulphatide. J. Neurol. Neurosurg. Psychiat. 30: 311—318, 1967.

de Silva, K. L., Pearce, J.: Neuropathy of metachromatic leucodystrophy. J. Neurol. Neurosurg. Psychiat. 36: 30—33, 1973.

Greenfield, J. G.: A form of progressive cerebral sclerosis in infants associated with primary degeneration of the interfascicular glia. J. Neurol. Psychopath. 13: 289—302, 1933.

Grégoire, A., Périer, O., Dustin, P.: Metachromatic leucodystrophy, an electron microscopic study. J. Neuropath. exp. Neurol. 25: 617—636, 1966.

Hagberg, B., Sourander, P., Svennerholm, L., Voss, H.: Late infantile metachromatic leucodystrophy of the genetic type. Acta Paediat. 49: 135—153, 1960.

— — Thorén, L.: Peripheral nerve changes in the diagnosis of metachromatic leucodystrophy. Acta Paediat., Suppl. 135: 63—71, 1962.

Hansson, H.-A., Olsson, Y., Sourander, P.: Experimental studies on the pathogenesis of leucodystrophies. III. Cellular accumulation of injected sulphatides in brain, peripheral nerve and kidney. Acta neuropath. (Berl.) 9: 134—140, 1967.

Harzer, K., Stinshoff, K., Mraz, W., Jatzkewitz, H.: The patterns of arylsulphatases A and B in human normal and metachromatic leucodystrophy tissues and their relationship to the cerebroside sulphatase activity. J. Neurochem. 20: 279—287, 1973.

Helmstaedt, E. R.: Über eine Beobachtung von metachromatischer Leukodystrophie. Dtsch. Z. Nervenkr. 184: 213—234, 1963.

Hirose, G., Bass, N. H.: Adult and late infantile metachromatic leucodystrophy: a comparative biochemical study. Neurology (Minneap.) 21: 443—443, 1971.

Hirsch, T. von, Peiffer, J.: Über histologische Methoden in der Differentialdiagnose von Leucodystrophien und Lipoidosen. Arch. Psychiat. (Berl.) 194: 88—104, 1955.

Holländer, H.: A staining method for cerebroside sulfuric esters in brain tissue. J. Histochem. Cytochem. 11: 118—119, 1963.

— Über metachromatische Leukodystrophie. II. Relation zwischen Erkrankungsalter und Verlaufsdauer. Arch. Psychiat. Nervenkr. 205: 300—305, 1964.

Jatzkewitz, H.: Zwei Typen von Cerebrosid-Schwefelsäureestern als sog. „Praelipoide" und Speichersubstanzen bei der Leukodystrophie Typ Scholz (metachromatische Form der Diffusen Sklerose). Hoppe Seyler Z. Physiol. Chem. 311: 279—282, 1958.

— Pilz, H., Holländer, H.: Biochemische und vergleichende histochemische Untersuchungen in umschriebenen Gebieten des Gehirns bei Fällen von adulter und infantiler metachromatischer Leukodystrophie. Acta neuropath. (Berl.) 4: 75—89, 1964.

Kaback, M. M., Howell, R. R.: Infantile metachromatic leukodystrophy. Heterozygote detection in skin fibroblasts and possible applications to intrauterine diagnosis. New Engl. J. Med. 282: 1336—1340, 1970.

Kaltenbach, H.: Über einen eigenartigen Markprozeß mit metachromatischen Abbauprodukten bei paralyseähnlichem Krankheitsbild. Z. Neurol. Psychiat. 75: 138—146, 1922.

Lison, L.: Etudes sur la métachromasie. Colorants metachromatiques et substances chromotropes. Arch. Biol. (Liege) 46: 599—668, 1935.

Lüthy, F., Ulrich, J., Regli, F., Isler, W.: Amaurotic idiocy with metachromatic change in the white matter? Proc. 5th Internat. Congr. Neuropath. 125—130, Excerpta Medica Foundation, Amsterdam 1966.

Malone, M. J., Conole, J.: Sulfatides and demyelination. Arch. Neurol. (Chic.) 21: 32—43, 1969.

— Stoffyn, P.: Peripheral nerve glycolipids in metachromatic leukodystrophy. Neurology (Minneap.) 17: 1033—1040, 1967.

— — Moser, H.: Structural studies on sulphatides in metachromatic leucodystrophy. J. Neurochem. 13: 1033—1036, 1966.

Mehl, E., Jatzkewitz, H.: Cerebroside 3-sulfate as a physiological substrate of arylsulfatase A. Biochim. biophys. Acta 151: 619—627, 1968.

Michaelis, L., Granick, S.: Metachromasy of basic dyestuffs. J. Amer. Chem. Soc. 67: 1212—1219, 1945.

Mossakowski, M., Mathieson, G., Cumings, J. N.: On the relationship of metachromatic leucodystrophy and amaurotic idiocy. Brain 84: 585—604, 1961.

Norman, R. M., Urich, H., Tingey, A. H.: Metachromatic leucencephalopathy: A form of lipidosis. Brain 83: 369—380, 1960.

O'Brien, J.: A molecular defect of myelination. Biochem. biophys. Res. Commun. 15: 484—490, 1964.

Pilz, H., Müller, D.: Studies on adult metachromatic leukodystrophy. Part 2. Biochemical aspects of adult cases of metachromatic leukodystrophy. J. Neurol. Sci. 9: 585—595, 1969.

Résibois, A.: Electron microscopic study of metachromatic leucodystrophy. III. Lysosomal nature of the inclusions. Acta neuropath. (Berl.) 13: 149—156, 1969.

— Electron microscopic studies of metachromatic leucodystrophy. IV. Liver and kidney alterations. Path. Europ. 6: 278—298, 1971.

Résibois-Grégoire, A.: Electron microscopic studies of metachromatic leucodystrophy. II. Compound nature of the inclusions. Acta neuropath. (Berl.) 9: 244—253, 1967.

Stumpf, D., Austin, J.: Metachromatic leucodystrophy. IX. Qualitative and quantitative differences in urinary arylsulfatase A in different forms of MLD. Arch. Neurol. (Chic.) 24: 117—124, 1971.

— Neuwelt, E., Austin, J., Kohler, P.: Metachromatic leukodystrophy (MLD). X. Immunological studies of the abnormal sulfatase A. Arch. Neurol. (Chic.) 25: 427—431, 1971.

Suzuki, K., Suzuki, K., Chen, G. C.: Isolation and chemical characterization of the metachromatic granules from a brain with metachromatic leukodystrophy. J. Neuropath. exp. Neurol. 26: 537—550, 1967.

— — Mizuno, Y.: Juvenile metachromatic leukodystrophy. Deficiency of an arylsulfatase A component. J. Pediat. 85: 823—824, 1974.

Taniguchi, N., Nanba, I.: Enzymatic abnormality of the carrier state in metachromatic leucodystrophy. Clin. chem. Acta 29: 375—379, 1970.

Terry, R. D., Suzuki, K., Weiss, M.: Biopsy study in 3 cases of metachromatic leucodystrophy. J. Neuropath. exp. Neurol. 25: 141—143, 1966.

Thieffry, S., Lyon, G.: Diagnostic d'un cas de leucodystrophic metachromique (type Scholz) par la biopsie d'un nerf périphérique. Rev. Neurol. (Paris) 100: 452—456, 1959.

Thunold, S.: Late infantile metachromatic leucodystrophy. Report of 2 cases and review of in vivo diagnostic tests. Beitr. path. Anat. 146: 322—331, 1972.

Toga, M., Bérard-Badier, M., Pinsard, N., Gambarelli, D., Hassoun, J., Tripier, M. F.: Etude clinique, histologique et ultrastructurale de quatre cas de leucodystrophie métachromatique infantile et juvénile. Acta neuropath. (Berl.) 21: 23—38, 1972.

Webster, H. de F.: Schwann cell alterations in metachromatic leukodystrophy: Preliminary phase and electron microscopic observations. J. Neuropath. exp. Neurol. 21: 534—554, 1962.

Witte, F.: Über pathologische Abbauvorgänge im Zentralnervensystem. Münch. med. Wschr. 68: 69—69, 1921.

Wolfe, H. J., Pietra, G. G.: The visceral lesions of metachromatic leukodystrophy. Amer. J. Path. 44: 921—930, 1964.

39. Globoid Cell Leukodystrophy

The credit for the recognition of globoid cell leukodystrophy is traditionally given to Krabbe (1916), who reported 2 sets of siblings and one sporadic case, 3 of the 5 with histologic data. Short descriptions of the cerebral lesions were published earlier by Bullard and Southard (1906) and by Beneke (1908). Krabbe considered his cases representative of a new form of diffuse sclerosis and cited Beneke's case as the only other similar observation. He emphasized that his cases differed from those described by Pelizaeus and Merzbacher by an early onset and relentless progress, from Tay-Sachs' disease by the absence of nerve cell changes, and from Schilder's encephalitis periaxialis diffusa by the early onset and familial occurrence. Krabbe described and illustrated the globoid cells and referred to them at one point as epithelial, but he did not emphasize them as a diagnostic feature. The pathognomonic significance of the globoid cells was recognized by Collier and Greenfield (1924) who stressed that the morphology of globoid cells and the absence of cytoplasmic osmophilia are quite unlike the features of the fatty macrophages of Wallerian degeneration; they introduced the term "globoid cell" which later became pathognomic and synonymous with Krabbe's disease.

The peculiar features of the globoid cells are suggestive of intracellular storage of a specific substance, which, on the basis of histochemical staining reactions was tentatively identified as cerebroside (Diezel, 1955). However, chemical analyses of brain tissue in several laboratories, reviewed by Austin (1963), showed in most instances a reduction rather than an increase in sphingolipids in the leukodystrophic white matter; globoid cell leukodystrophy, therefore, cannot be considered a cerebroside lipidosis in the gross, conventional sense. Several factors need to be considered in the interpretation of these chemical data. There is a severe depletion of myelin lipids high in cerebroside content; the phase reached in the progression of the disease differs among individual brains as well as among various portions of the white matter in a given brain; furthermore, the cell-bound sphingolipids seem to have altered solubility characteristics affecting their extractability from the tissue. In Austin's (1963 a) studies the most characteristic alteration in the lipid composition of the white matter consisted of an abnormally high ratio of cerebrosides to sulfatides. Fractionation of the tissue yielded 4 times as much cerebrosides as sphingomyelins in those fractions that had highest counts of globoid cells (Austin, 1963 b), corroborating the involvement of these cells in cerebroside storage.

The search for a specific enzymatic defect in globoid cell leukodystrophy initially focussed on cerebroside-sulphatide sulphotransferase, based on the increase in the cerebroside-sulphatide ratio. The activity of this enzyme was found to be reduced in the brain tissue, but this alteration cannot be considered a key feature of the disease as normal activity was found in kidneys. Suzuki and Suzuki (1970, 1971) demonstrated a profound deficiency of galactosecerebroside-β-galactosidase in brain, liver, spleen, serum, leukocytes and fibroblasts of patients with globoid cell leukodystrophy. Other lysosomal hydrolases splitting sphingolipids or other substrates are either slightly elevated or not decreased (Austin *et al.*, 1970). The deficiency of galactose-cerebroside-β-galactosidase is now considered the salient enzyme deficiency in globoid cell leukodystrophy. The disease is not restricted to man and was also reported for dogs (Frankhauser *et al.*, 1963; Fletcher *et al.*, 1966) and for cats (Johnson, 1970).

Clinical Course. Globoid cell leukodystrophy is an inherited disorder of autosomal recessive transmission. The most common course is early infantile, with onset of symptoms at 3 to 5 months, some of the infants being subnormal from birth. Stagnation in development induces hypersensitivity, irritability, frequent crying and stiffness of the limbs. The deterioration proceeds within several months to quadruparesis, opistotonus, extended and crossed legs, optic atrophy, and severe mental retardation. There may be episodes of unexplained high fever and tonic and clonic seizures. Death usually occurs within the first 2 years of life.

A delayed onset and protracted infantile course of the disease is less common. The existence of a juvenile form of globoid cell leukodystrophy having the onset of symptoms between 2 and 8 years was recently confirmed by the absence of galactocerebroside β-galactosidase (Hanefield *et al.*, 1973; Crome *et al.*, 1973); the first reported case (Bullard and Southard, 1906) and others tabulated by Crome *et al.* (1973) belong into this group. The occurrence of globoid cell leukodystrophy in adults has not been verified as yet;

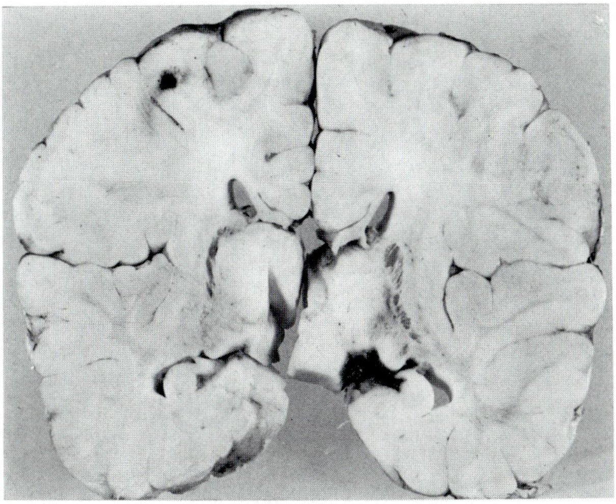

Fig. 139. Krabbe disease. The leukodystrophy has progressed to cavitation in the internal capsule; discoloration is evident throughout the rest of white matter

cases reported as such (Verhaart, 1931; Guillain *et al.*, 1941) are difficult to interpret.

Definite diagnosis of globoid cell leukodystrophy depends on demonstrating the absence of galactocerebroside galactosidase activity in the patients. Also, characteristic cellular inclusions may be shown in electron micrographs of peripheral nerve biopsies. Reduced enzyme activity is found in the heterozygous carriers of the disease (Suzuki and Suzuki, 1971). Globoid cell leukodystrophy may be diagnosed *in utero* from the deficient enzyme activity in cultured amniotic fluid cells obtained by amniocentesis (Suzuki *et al.*, 1971).

Morbid Anatomy. Gross inspection of the brain of patients with globoid cell leukodystrophy reveals a moderate to marked diffuse atrophy of cortical gyri and reduction in weight. All portions of the brain are unusually firm to the touch, as expressed in the old term "diffuse sclerosis". At the cut surface the white matter is discolored, grayish or pale-brownish, somewhat translucent and hardened; it may contain focal nests of opaque whitish tissue. A faint grayish discoloration is seen in less severely affected portions. The cerebral ventricles are enlarged, with firm walls. Discoloration is also evident in the cerebellar white matter. Hydrocephalic ventricular distension was described by Laxdal and Hallgrimsson (1974), but there were subependymal cavities suggestive of perinatal distress in this case.

On microscopic examination there is marked diminution or complete loss of myelin sheaths in the sclerotic white matter. The axis cylinders are destroyed although the loss of axons may be less severe or less widespread than the loss of myelin sheaths. All oligodendroglia cells have disappeared from the demyelinated tissue and are replaced by proliferated astrocytes at

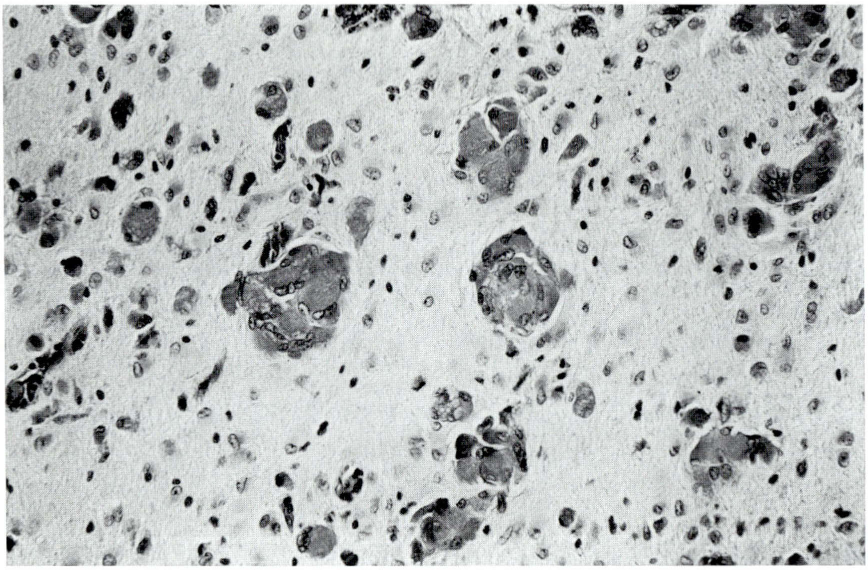

Fig. 140. Krabbe disease; nests of globoid cells in the demyelinated white matter; PAS ×200

times to an excessive degree. There is a corresponding diffuse fibrillary gliosis throughout the affected white matter which stains intensely in Holzer stains. There may be microcystic cavitation of the tissue in the most severely affected regions (Fig. 139).

The pathognomonic feature of the leukodystrophy consists of the accumulation of globoid cells (Fig. 140). These have rounded cytoplasmic bodies, 35 to 40 μ in diameter, and multiple peripherally situated nuclei which may be quite numerous being arranged in clusters or in rows along the cell surface. There are also smaller rounded cells with single nuclei. It has been suggested to distinguish the mononuclear "epitheloid" cells from the multinuclear "globoid" cells; another nomenclature calls the mononuclear types "globoid cells" and the multinuclear ones "globoid bodies". However, both types have identical fine structure (Suzuki and Grover, 1970) and are evidently closely related. Both types are called globoid cells in this text. The enlarged cytoplasmic bodies of the globoid cells have an almost clear or finely granular cytoplasm which is never foamy. Only a faint staining is obtained with sudan dyes or with osmication and there is no metachromasia. The cytoplasm stains diffusely with the periodic acid-Schiff reaction and the latter is quite resistant to common lipid solvents.

Globoid cells tend to aggregate in clusters or nests in the dystrophic white matter, sparing the gray matter. They are particularly abundant within perivascular spaces, encompassing the vessels with cuffs of tightly packed cells. The density of globoid cells is in a rough proportion to the intensity of active leukodystrophic changes, but the number of cells decreases in older lesions where the leukodystrophy has run its course.

The derivation of globoid cells has been the subject of much debate based on the interpretation of morphologic criteria discernible with the light microscope. Their derivation from mesodermal macrophages or from microglia is now widely accepted, based on the presence of high acid phosphatase activity, and on the absence of glial fibrils in electron micrographs (Nelson *et al.*, 1963). Their derivation from adventitial histiocytes and from splenic tissue was shown by experimental injection of cerebrosides (Austin, 1961; Austin and Lehfeldt, 1965). Cells resembling globoid cells are seen, occasionally, upon massive myelin destruction from various disease processes, presumably resulting from the ingestion of large amounts of cerebrosides from the disintegrating sheaths. In these instances, however, the cells concur with fat-laden macrophages and they usually do not progress beyond the mononuclear stage. Also, they do not mass to the extent seen in globoid cell leukodystrophy.

Globoid cell leukodystrophy may affect the entire cerebral white matter, though subject to regional differences in intensity. In the cerebral hemispheres the changes may diminish from the ventricles outwards and spare the subcortical fibers, or there may be gradients between cerebral lobes, *e.g.*, fronto-occipital. The optic tracts are commonly involved. The severity of affection of tracts in the brain stem and cord varies: The roots of cranial and spinal nerves are usually best preserved, while the long descending and ascending tracts, particularly the dorsal tracts and corticospinal tracts, are severely affected, at times to the extent of microcystic cavitation of the pyramids. Electron microscopic examination of the demyelinating fiber tracts reveals degenerative changes in axons, and collapse of myelin sheaths with abnormal pattern of lamination, degradation of myelin remnants in macrophages and astrocytic proliferation (Schochet *et al.*, 1969; Liu, 1970).

That the evolution of the white matter lesions commences *in utero* is evident from the presence of typical globoid cells with tubular inclusions in their cytoplasm in the spinal tracts of a fetus of 22 weeks gestation, when no comparable changes were present in the cerebral hemispheres (Ellis *et al.*, 1973). D'Agostino *et al.* (1963) suggested that globoid cells form from the ingestion of intra- and extracellular PAS positive material which may be seen in the absence of globoid cells in minimally affected tracts.

There is no evidence of lipid storage in neurons, and the gray matter is generally well preserved. In some instances there is loss of neurons in olives, pons, cerebellum and basal ganglia (D'Agostino *et al.*, 1963). These changes may be attributed to metabolic dysfunction, degeneration secondary to destruction of axons, or to convulsions that frequently accompany the disease.

The peripheral nerves were thought to be unaffected by globoid cell leukodystrophy prior to 1967. After the report of Sourander and Olsson (1967) a prolific number of publications attested to their common involvement, which was also found in dogs with globoid cell leukodystrophy (Kurtz and Fletcher,

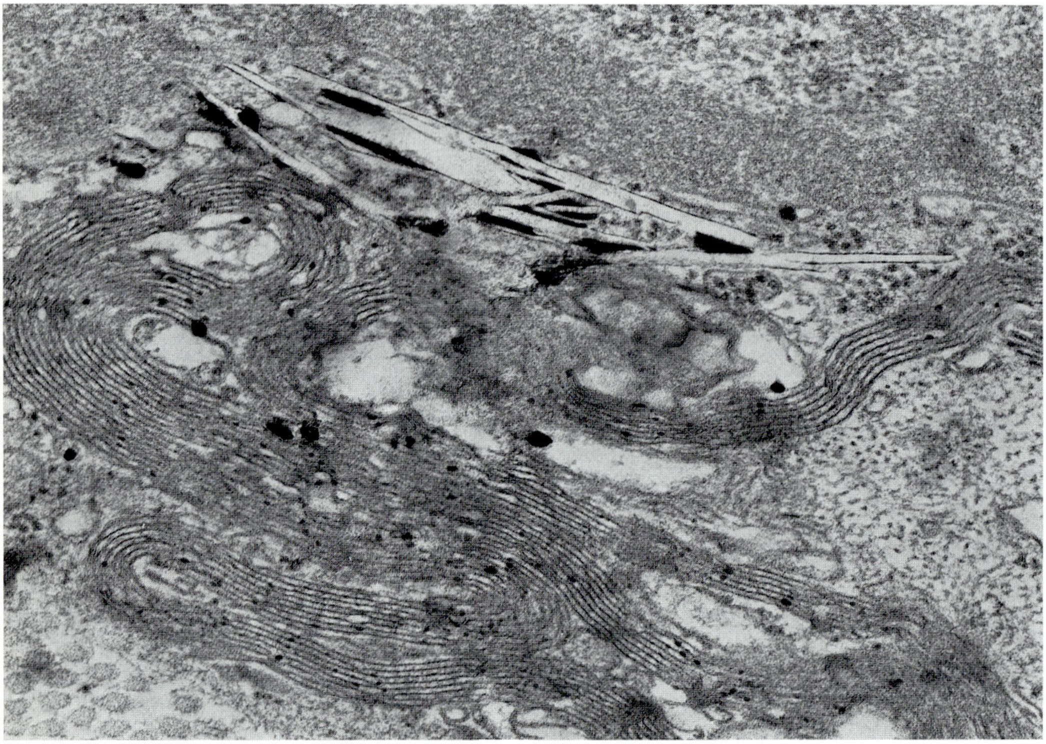

Fig. 141. Krabbe disease; cytoplasmic inclusions in Schwann cells in a peripheral nerve biopsy

1970). Light microscopic examination discloses degenerative changes in the axons and in myelin sheaths, with segmental demyelination in teased fiber preparations. There is endoneural fibrosis and perivascular accumulation of histiocytes, which, however, rarely progress to multinucleated forms. Ventral and dorsal roots are affected alike, and abnormal granular PAS positive lipid material is shown in Schwann cells and endoneural phagocytes (Lake, 1968; Sourander and Olsson, 1968; Dunn *et al.*, 1969). Tubular inclusions are seen with the electron microscope in Schwann cells and histiocytes (Bischoff and Ulrich, 1969). No evidence of peripheral nerve involvement was found for the juvenile form (Crome *et al.*, 1973).

The fine structure of abnormal deposits in central and peripheral nervous tissue is somewhat variable, generally consisting of gently curved, 250 to 500 Å wide tubular inclusions which may show 60 Å longitudinal striations

(Fig. 141). In cross sections they have a characteristic angular or crystalloid profile (Schochet *et al.*, 1969; Andrews and Cancilla, 1970; Suzuki and Grover, 1970; Liu, 1970; Shaw and Carlson, 1970). In addition there may be thinner, twisted tubules with a rectangular or oval profile similar to those found in Gaucher disease (Yunis and Lee, 1969). The tubular inclusions are most common within the globoid cells where most are freely dispersed throughout the cytoplasm, rarely membrane enclosed. They are less frequent in neuroglial elements of uncertain classification or in astrocytes (Yunis and Lee, 1969; Anzil *et al.*, 1972). In the peripheral nerves the inclusions are common in the cytoplasm of Schwann cells, and also in histiocytes.

Globoid cell leukodystrophy characteristically does not involve non-neural tissue. However, sparse, needle-like, tubular inclusions within lysosomes were seen in electron micrographs of bone marrow aspirates (Anzil *et al.*, 1972), and a finely granular material staining bluish-gray with toluene blue was noted in bulges of the cell membranes of epithelial cells in the urine sediment (Austin, 1962). Giant cells in lungs, spleen and lymph nodes were reported by Hager and Oehlert (1957), but there was coexistent chronic leptomeningitis, and the attribution of the granulomatous changes to the metabolic disorder is dubious. These negative observations, however, do not indicate that non-neural tissue lacks the potential for the formation of globoid cells, as the latter were produced by experimental injection of cerebrosides into the spleen (Austin and Lehfeldt, 1965).

Pathogenetic Considerations. Galactocerebroside β-galactosidase is a lysosomal enzyme (Bowen and Radin, 1968) hydrolyzing the galactose moyety from galactocerebrosides. Galactocerebrosides occur in selectively high concentration in myelin; they are practically nonexistent in brain before the onset of myelination and increase with its progress, with a corresponding rapid rise of cerebroside β-galactosidase activity (Bowen and Radin, 1969).

These data are consistent with the disturbances in myelin sheaths in galactosidase deficiency and with the restriction of the pathologic changes to nervous tissue. The details of the pathogenetic mechanism are still subject to study. There is evidence that a myelin of normal chemical composition is laid down initially by the sheath cells (Austin, 1963; Eto *et al.*, 1970). One may speculate that cerebrosides accumulate because of continued turnover of myelin lipids; accumulation may also be enhanced by a decreased demand for lipid upon advancing myelination as the most rapid incorporation of myelin lipids into the sheaths is known to occur during the initial phase of myelin formation. The accumulation of cerebrosides seems to interfere with the maintenance of the myelin sheaths, because of a progressive dysfunction of the sheath cells themselves or because of the globoid cells hindering the sheath cells (Eto *et al.*, 1970). The former explanation appears more likely: Fractionated tissue shows a lipid imbalance similar to that in the globoid cells in a fraction that contains 95 to 98 percent glia tissue (Austin, 1963 b). This is consistent with electron microscopic observations in peripheral nerves, where the abnormal inclusions are most common in the Schwann cells. If Wallerian degeneration is superimposed on leukodystrophy by experimental transection of nerves in leukodystrophic dogs, it can be shown that the proliferating Schwann cells contribute to the formation of globoid cells (Fletcher *et al.*, 1971). These data favor the concept that a cellular dysfunction is induced in the sheath cells by the accumulation of lipids in their cytoplasm, and that the destruction of myelin results from the dysfunction and destruction of the sheath cells. The oligodendroglia cells appear to be more sensitive to the disturbance than the Schwann cells.

The formation of the globoid cells is most probably induced by the release of large amounts of cerebrosides into the tissue and its uptake by histiocytes. Cells having all the features of globoid cells can be induced by injection of cerebrosides into the brain or spleen of experimental animals (Austin, 1963 a; Olsson *et al.*, 1966). Such cells show, on electron microscopic examination, tubular inclusions similar to those found in human globoid cell leukodystrophy (Suzuki, 1970). The response of histiocytes to cerebroside is lipid specific, as no comparable changes are induced by injection of sulfatides, a variety of other lipids, fatty acids, polysaccharides, or miscellaneous materials (Austin and Lehfeldt, 1965).

References

Andrews, J. M., Cancilla, P. A.: Cytoplasmic inclusions in human globoid cell leukodystrophy. Krabbe's disease. Arch. Path. (Chic.) 89: 53—55, 1970.

Anzil, A. P., Blinzinger, K., Mehraein, P., Dorn, G., Neuhauser, G.: Cytoplasmic inclusions in a child affected with Krabbe's disease (globoid leucodystrophy) and in the rabbit injected with galactocerebrosides. J. Neuropath. exp. Neurol. 31: 370—388, 1972.

Austin, J. H.: Recent studies in the metachromatic and globoid forms of diffuse sclerosis. Proc. Ass. Res. Nerv. Ment. Dis. 40: 189—219, 1962.

— Studies in globoid (Krabbe) leukodystrophy. I. The significance of lipid abnormalities in white matter in 8 globoid and 13 control patients. Arch. Neurol. (Chic.) 9: 207—231, 1963 a.

— Studies in globoid (Krabbe) leukodystrophy. II. Controlled thin-layer chromatographic studies of globoid body fractions in seven patients. J. Neurochem. 10: 921—930, 1963 b.

— Lehfeldt, D.: Studies in globoid (Krabbe) leukodystrophy. III. Significance of experimentally-produced globoid-like elements in rat white matter and spleen. J. Neuropath. exp. Neurol. 24: 265—289, 1965.

— Suzuki, K., Armstrong, D., Brady, R., Bachhawat, B. K., Schlenker, J., Stumpf, D.: Studies in globoid (Krabbe) leukodystrophy. V. Controlled enzymic studies in ten human cases. Arch. Neurol. (Chic.) 23: 502—512, 1970.

Beneke, R.: Ein Fall hochgradigster ausgedehnter Sklerose des Centralnervensystems. Arch. Kinderheilk. 47: 420—422, 1908.

Bischoff, A., Ulrich, J.: Peripheral neuropathy in globoid cell leukodystrophy (Krabbe's disease). Ultrastructural and histochemical findings. Brain 92: 861—870, 1969.

Bowen, D. M., Radin, N. S.: Properties of cerebroside galactosidase. Biochim. biophys. Acta 152: 599—610, 1968.

— — Cerebroside galactosidase: A method for determination and comparison with other lysosomal enzymes in developing brain. J. Neurochem. 16: 501—511, 1969.

Bullard, W. N., Southard, E. E.: Diffuse gliosis of the cerebral white matter in a child. J. nerv. ment. Dis. 33: 188—193, 1906.

Collier, J., Greenfield, J. G.: The encephalitis periaxialis of Schilder: Clinical and pathological study, with an account of two cases, one of which was diagnosed during life. Brain 47: 489—519, 1924.

Crome, L., Hanefeld, F., Patrick, D., Wilson, J.: Late onset globoid cell leucodystrophy. Brain 96: 841—848, 1973.

Cumings, J. N., Rozdilsky, J. N.: The cerebral lipid composition of the brain in six cases of Krabbe's disease. Neurology (Minneap.) 15: 177—183, 1965.

D'Agostino, A. N., Sayre, G. P., Hayles, A. B.: Krabbe's disease. Globoid cell type of leukodystrophy. Arch. Neurol. (Chic.) 8: 82—96, 1963.

Diezel, P. B.: Histochemische Untersuchungen an den Globoidzellen der familiären infantilen diffusen Sklerose vom Typus Krabbe. Virchows Arch. path. Anat. 327: 206—228, 1955.

Dunn, H. G., Lake, B. D., Dolman, C. L., Wilson, J.: The neuropathy of Krabbe's infantile cerebral sclerosis (globoid cell leucodystrophy). Brain 92: 329—344, 1969.

Ellis, W. G., Schneider, E. L., McCulloch, J. R., Suzuki, K., Epstein, C. J.: Fetal globoid cell leukodystrophy (Krabbe disease). Arch. Neurol. (Chic.) 29: 253—257, 1973.

Eto, Y., Suzuki, K., Suzuki, K.: Globoid cell leucodystrophy (Krabbe's disease) isolation of myelin with normal glycolipid composition. J. Lipid Res. 11: 473—479, 1970.

Fletcher, T. F., Kurtz, H. J., Low, D. G.: Globoid cell leukodystrophy (Krabbe type) in the dog. J. Amer. vet. med. Ass. 149: 165—172, 1966.

— — Stadlan, E. M.: Experimental Wallerian degeneration in peripheral nerves of dogs with globoid cell leukodystrophy. J. Neuropath. exp. Neurol. 30: 593—602, 1971.

Frankhauser, R., Luginbühl, H., Hartley, W. J.: Leucodystrophie vom Typus Krabbe beim Hund. Schweiz. Arch. Tierheilk. 105: 198—207, 1963.

Guillain, G., Bertrand, I., Gruner, J.: Sur un type anatomo-clinique spécial de leuko-encéphalite à nodule morulés gliogènes. Rev. Neurol. (Paris) 73: 401—414, 1941.

Hager, H., Oehlert, W.: Ist die diffuse Hirnsklerose des Typs Krabbe eine entzündliche Allgemeinerkrankung? Z. Kinderheilk. 80: 82—96, 1957.

Hanefield, F., Wilson, J., Crome, L.: Die juvenile Form der Globoidzelleukodystrophie. Mschr. Kinderheilk. 121: 293—293, 1973.

Johnson, K. H.: Globoid leucodystrophy in the cat. J. Amer. vet. med. Ass. 157: 2057—2064, 1970.

Krabbe, K.: A new familial infantile form of diffuse brain sclerosis. Brain 39: 74—114, 1916.

Kurtz, H. J., Fletcher, T. F.: The peripheral neuropathy of canine globoid-cell leukodystrophy (Krabbe-type). Acta neuropath. (Berl.) 16: 226—232, 1970.

Lake, B. D.: Segmental demyelination of peripheral nerves in Krabbe's disease. Nature 217: 171—172, 1968.

Laxdal, T., Hallgrimsson, J.: Krabbe's globoid cell leucodystrophy with hydrocephalus. Arch. Dis. Child. 49: 232—234, 1974.

Liu, H. M.: Ultrastructure of globoid leukodystrophy (Krabbe's disease) with reference to the origin of globoid cells. J. Neuropath. exp. Neurol. 29: 441—462, 1970.

Nelson, E., Aurebeck, G., Osterberg, K., Berry, J., Jabbour, J. T., Bornhofen, J.: Ultrastructural and chemical studies on Krabbe's disease. J. Neuropath. exp. Neurol. 22: 414—434, 1963.

Olsson, Y., Sourander, P., Svennerholm, L.: Experimental studies on the pathogenesis of leucodystrophies. I. The effect of intracerebrally injected sphingolipids in the rat's brain. Acta neuropath. (Berl.) 6: 153—163, 1966.

Schochet, S. S., Jr., Hardman, J. M., Lampert, P. W., Earle, K. M.: Krabbe's disease (globoid leukodystrophy). Arch. Path. (Chic.) 88: 305—313, 1969.

Shaw, C.-M., Carlson, C. B.: Crystalline structures in globoid-epithelioid cells: An electron microscopic study of globoid leukodystrophy (Krabbe's disease). J. Neuropath. exp. Neurol. 29: 306—319, 1970.

Sourander, P., Olsson, Y.: Morphological and lipid-histochemical studies on peripheral nerves in globoid cell leukodystrophy. Acta path. microbiol. scand. 70: 147—147, 1967.

— — Peripheral neuropathology in globoid cell leucodystrophy (Morbus Krabbe) 11: 69—81, 1968.

Suzuki, K.: Ultrastructural study of experimental globoid cells. Lab. Invest. 23: 612—619, 1970.

— Grover, W. D.: Krabbe's leukodystrophy (Globoid cell leukodystrophy). An ultrastructural study. Arch. Neurol. (Chic.) 22: 385—396, 1970.

— Schneider, E. L., Epstein, C. J.: In utero diagnosis of globoid cell leukodystrophy (Krabbe's disease). Biochem. biophys. Res. Commun. 45: 1363—1366, 1971.

— Suzuki, Y.: Globoid cell leucodystrophy (Krabbe's disease): Deficiency of galactose cerebroside β-galactosidase. Proc. nat. Acad. Sci. 66: 302—309, 1970.

Suzuki, Y., Suzuki, K.: Krabbe's globoid cell leukodystrophy: Deficiency of galactocerebrosidase in serum, leukocytes, and fibroblasts. Science 171: 73—75, 1971.
Verhaart, W. J. C.: A case of multiple sclerosis with an Indian in the Dutch Indies. Psychiatr. Bl. 35: 511—529, 1931.
Yunis, E. J., Lee, R. E.: The ultrastructure of globoid (Krabbe) leucodystrophy. Lab. Invest. 21: 415—419, 1969.

40. Adreno-Leukodystrophy and Its Relation to "Schilder Disease"

Clinicopathologic documentation of the concurrence of a sudanophilic leukodystrophy indistinguishable from "Schilder disease" with adrenal insufficiency was first reported by Siemerling and Creutzfeldt (1923). A review by Hoefnagel *et al.* (1962) found only 4 other cases, but the number increased rapidly in the subsequent literature (See *et al.*, 1971, references). The publication of a series of 9 cases by Powers and Schaumburg (1973) has focussed considerable interest on the disease, and it reopened the problem of its nosologic distinction from "Schilder disease", as discussed at the end of this chapter. A recent review of the literature (Powell *et al.*, 1975) accounts for about 50 cases.

A juvenile and an adult form of adrenoleukodystrophy may be distinguished. All of the recorded juvenile cases were male, half of them familial. Several pedigrees of afflicted families have been reported (Hoefnagel *et al.*, 1962; Strunk and Strunk, 1965; Schaumburg *et al.*, 1972), showing a sex-linked, recessive inheritance pattern. The clinical course is fairly uniform. Symptoms of adrenal insufficiency, such as bronzing of the skin, often precede the onset of neurologic disorder by several years; they are generally of slight degree. Most of the early descriptions are of this type. For others the onset of the neurologic disorder concurs with that of adrenal insufficiency, manifesting with gastrointestinal symptoms, weakness, lethargy or dehydration. Still other cases have no clinical symptoms of adrenal insufficiency. Six of the 9 cases with histologically documented adrenal changes of Powers and Schaumburg (1973) had no symptoms of adrenal insufficiency; in one adrenal insufficiency was evident from reduced levels of adrenal cortico-steroids only.

The onset of the neurologic disorder dates to after the 6th year of life, most commonly toward the end of the first decade. First signs often consist of a lack of progress in school, followed by the development of specific neurologic deficits, such as disturbances in vision, speech, various pareses which progress to increasing disability with spasticity, blindness, deafness, incontinence and, finally, to deep coma unless death intervenes earlier. Disturbances in affective behavior may develop during the progress of the disease; some patients have repeated, severe convulsions. The subacute, relentlessly progressive course lasts from 6 months to several years, on the average 21 months. The average age at death is 10 years (counting 32 cases with complete autopsy findings).

The adult course of the disease is less common, and few cases have been documented with autopsy findings (Powers *et al.*, 1974). The few known or presumed female cases were adults. For that described by Pilz (1973) the

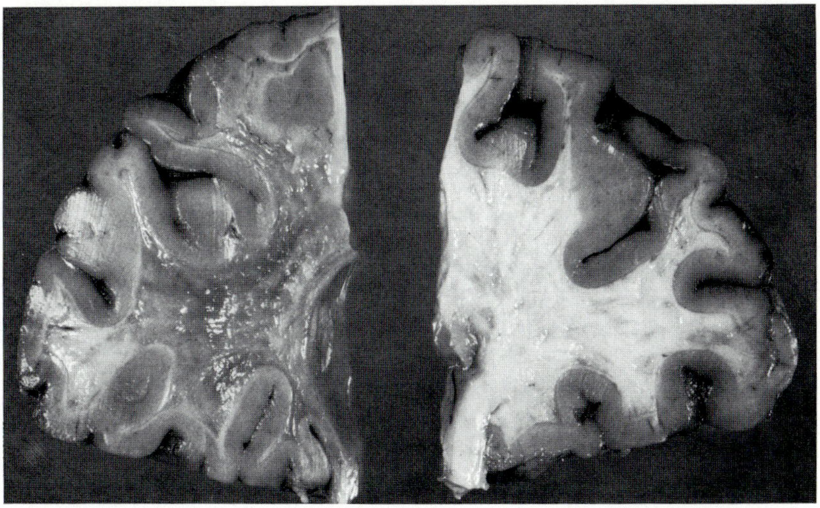

Fig. 142. White matter changes in adrenoleukodystrophy

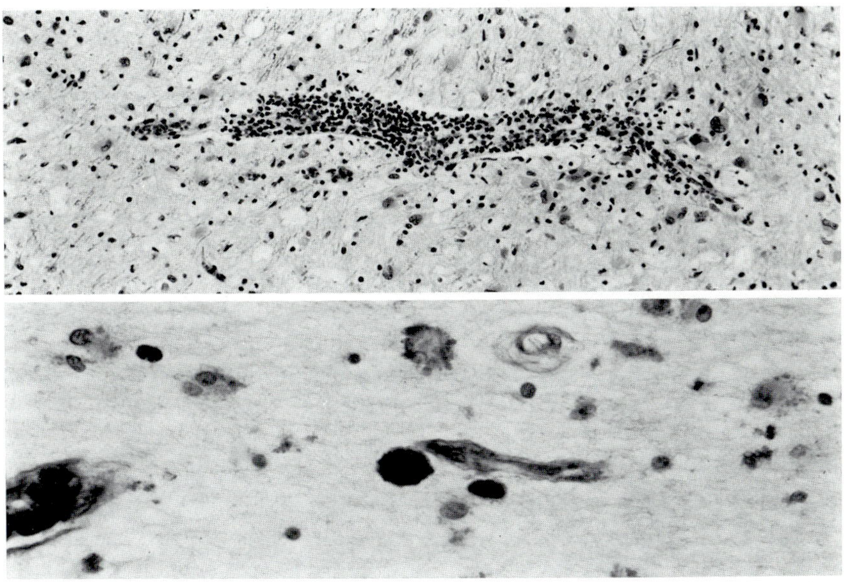

Fig. 143. Adrenoleukodystrophy. Lymphocytic cuffing in demyelinated white matter; ×110; strongly PAS-positive macrophages; ×300

adrenal insufficiency was diagnosed at the age of 36, and the neurologic disease started at 41 leading to death in 2 years.

Gross inspection of the brain in adreno-leukodystrophy discloses no change in hemispheric configuration. The cut surface shows large areas of demyelination in the hemispheric white matter; these are much softer than normal, brownish discolored, and often sunken below the cut surface (Fig. 142).

Extensive periventricular lesions cause dilation of the cerebral ventricles. The demyelination typically affects the centrum semiovale bilaterally, though without strict symmetry; it may begin in any of the cerebral lobes, most often parietal. Unilateral foci are uncommon, as the disease seems to extend rapidly across the midline, or else develops concurrently in symmetric foci. It eventually spreads throughout the entire centrum semiovale, sparing only the subcortical U fibers. There is no sharp boundary between the demyelinated portions and the adjacent white matter which may appear soft and discolored at some distance from the area of maximum demyelination.

Microscopic examination discloses a severe to complete loss of myelin in the affected areas. Relative sparing of the axis cylinders is seen in metallic impregnations, particularly at the progressing edges of the lesion, but axons are destroyed as well with increasing severity and/or duration of the disease process. The demyelinating tissue is filled with abundant macrophages, particularly near the edges of the lesions. Their foamy cytoplasm is filled with droplets of lipid material having histochemical staining reactions consistent with neutral fat and cholesterol esters. In addition, scattered strongly PAS-positive macrophages are found. Perivascular cuffing with lymphocytes is common (Fig. 143). Areas of demyelination may also extend into the brain stem, involving particularly the tegmentum of the pons. There is often complete secondary degeneration of the corticospinal tracts in the pyramids and in the spinal cord. Chemical analysis of the demyelinated white matter may reveal only slight alterations in lipid content (Aguilar *et al.*, 1967; Powell *et al.*, 1975) or a decrease in various lipids and an increase in cholesterol esters, consistent with a demyelinative process (See *et al.*, 1971); there is no evidence for an abnormal deposition of a specific type of lipid.

Atrophy of the adrenal glands is evident on gross inspection; it may be slight or the glands may be reduced to a fraction of a gram; in one case no glands could be found at all. Microscopic examination of glands with relatively slight changes shows disturbances in the architecture of the zona fasciculata and reticularis, the zona glomerulosa remaining intact. There are aggregates of ballooned cells (Fig. 144), some multinucleated, having a granular eosinophilic cytoplasm which may show a striated texture or microvacuolization (Powers and Schaumburg, 1973). More severe atrophy of the gland involves loss of the demarcation between the zona fasciculata and reticularis, or between all three zones, the cortex being reduced to a thin membrane a few cells thick. Nearly half of the cases have adenomatous nodular aggregates of swollen cortical cells, interpreted as signs of abortive regeneration (Farkas-Bargeton *et al.*, 1967). Lymphocytic infiltrates in the adrenal cortex are found in approximately one-fourth of cases. The adrenal medulla is not affected. There are no consistent changes in other endocrine organs, although a decrease in pituitary basophils and an interstitial cell tumor of the testes have been noted (Hoefnagel *et al.*, 1962; Aguilar *et al.*, 1967).

Electron microscopic examination of adrenals and Schwann cells (Powers and Schaumburg, 1974) and brain (Powell *et al.*, 1975) disclosed randomly oriented intracytoplasmic linear deposits or spicules consisting of two 25 Å wide electron dense lines separated by a clear space (Fig. 145), somewhat similar to the deposits in Krabbe disease.

The cause-effect relationship between adrenal changes and leukodystrophy is still obscure, as is the etiology of the disease. A defect in steroid metabolism is suggested by the data of Burton and Nadler (1974). It is unlikely that adrenal changes are secondary to the leukodystrophy as the symptoms of adrenal insufficiency often antedate those of the cerebral disorder by several years. Clinical data and the extent of cortical atrophy are also incon-

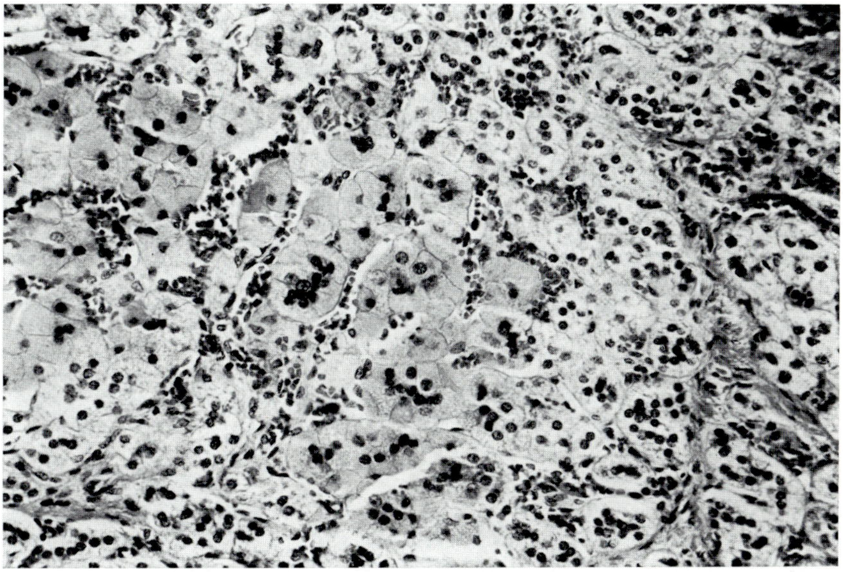

Fig. 144. Adrenoleukodystrophy; aggregates of distended cells, some multinucleated in the adrenal cortex; H & E $\times 200$

sistent with a secondary adrenal atrophy caused by steroid substitution therapy. It remains unclear whether the adrenal insufficiency predisposes to the development of a leukodystrophy, or whether adrenal insufficiency and leukodystrophy are concurrent but not necessarily interdependent manifestations of an unknown underlying metabolic or genetic disorder. The failure of arresting the leukodystrophy by adrenal substitution therapy would seem to favor the second interpretation.

Nosologic Considerations. The emergence of adreno-leukodystrophy as a well defined clinico-pathologic entity, and the realization that the symptoms of adrenal insufficiency are slight or even absent, reopens the cumbersome problem of the definition of "Schilder disease" and its distinction from other sudanophilic leukodystrophies. Many cases diagnosed as Schilder disease were probably adreno-leukodystrophy. Several of the reports on adreno-leukodystrophy cited above contain references to siblings that had been diagnosed earlier as diffuse sclerosis, Schilder disease, or a variant of Pelizaeus-Merzbacher disease. There are also pedigrees of familial, sex-linked sudanophilic leukodystrophies quite similar to those of adreno-leukodystrophy, but without reference to findings in the adrenals (Crome and Zapella, 1963; Schenk *et al.*, 1967). Hence, a brief reconsideration of the history and problems of defining Schilder disease is in order.

The first case reported by Schilder (1912) as "encephalitis periaxialis diffusa" does not fit the known features of adreno-leukodystrophy, in that the disease afflicted a 14-year-old girl. Future observations will have to document the exact type of relationship between affection of females and the course of adreno-leukodystrophy. None of the available pedigrees on adreno-leukodystrophy offer anatomically documented evidence of the type of involvement in female members of a given sibship. The second case reported by Schilder (1913) has been reinterpreted as an instance of metachromatic leukodystrophy, based on Schilder's comment on scattered, slightly metachromatic spherical deposits in the white matter adjacent to the zone of demyelination; however, his description is more suggestive of Buscaino bodies (Chapter 44) than of the deposits in metachromatic leukodystrophy. The earlier clinical and pathologic description of the same case by Haberfeld and Spieler (1910) makes reference to fairly dark pigmentation of the patient's skin and to the affectation of a sibling of undefined sex by a disease having a quite similar course. Considering, in addition, the age of onset and the duration of the disease, it seems likely that Schilder's second case was an instance of adreno-leukodystrophy. Marie and Foix (1914) later published a case of bilateral sclerosis of the occipital white matter in a girl who had come down with signs of diffuse sclerosis at age 18 but had recovered to survive for 10 years. The designation Schilder-Foix disease, therefore, was widely used in the French literature; but the case described by Marie and Foix is difficult to interpret, and its classification as a leukodystrophy or as a demyelinating disease has been challenged. The pertinent arguments and the historical development of the concept of Schilder disease in general were reviewed by Poser and van Bogaert (1956). The third case of "encephalitis periaxialis diffusa" was published by Schilder in 1924, after several similar cases had been reported by other authors. It pertains to a 37-year-old woman whose lesions may be identified retrospectively as a chronic encephalitis, possibly an instance of progressive sclerosing panencephalitis. It is evident, therefore, that the term "encephalitis periaxialis diffusa", or Schilder disease, had been applied to a heterogeneous group of diseases from the very start. It subsequently became synonymous with leukodystrophy, particularly in the Anglo-American literature; for example, Collier and Greenfield's (1924) classic description of globoid cell leukodystrophy is entitled "The Encephalitis Periaxialis Diffusa of Schilder", and the first description of spongy degeneration of the nervous system, likewise, referred to it as Schilder disease. There are also several instances for which sclerosing residual lesions of perinatal brain damage were erroneously reported as Schilder disease. With the recognition of metachromatic and globoid cell leukodystrophies, and of spongy degeneration, the name Schilder disease became redefined to apply to white matter diseases having sudanophilic breakdown products, but the subclassification of this group remains confusing and controversial. Many authors

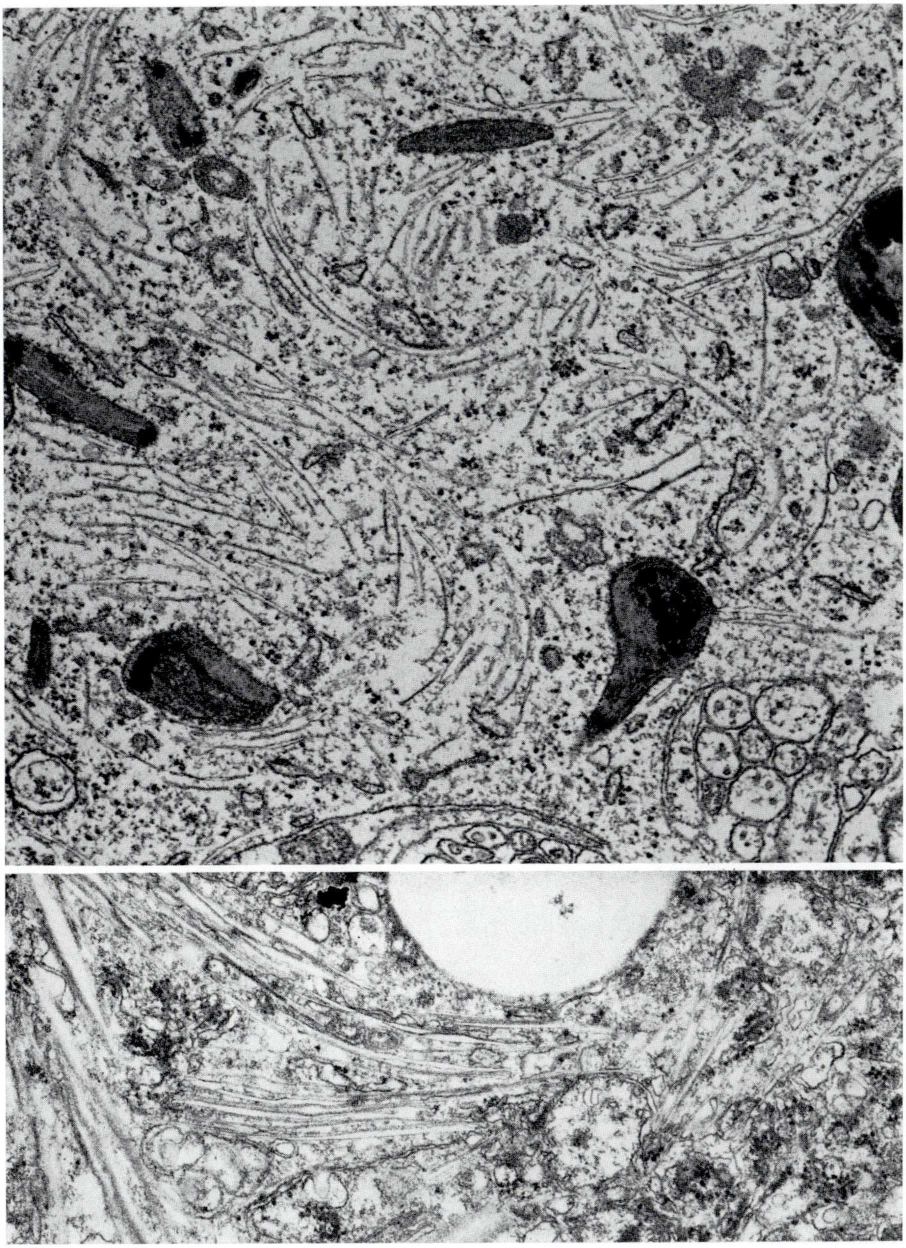

Fig. 145. Cytoplasmic inclusions in adrenoleukodystrophy. Top: white matter. Bottom: adrenal gland (courtesy Drs. Powell and Lampert)

consider Schilder disease a variant of multiple sclerosis, which tends to be more common in children (Poser and van Bogaert, 1956); Christensen *et al.* (1961), on the other hand, consider Schilder disease an exogenic sporadic type of demyelination found most often in adults. There is also a tendency to distinguish sporadic cases of "Schilder disease" from familial cases of "sudanophilic leukodystrophy", but all subclassifications remain arbitrary as there are no definite morphological criteria for the identification of subentities.

Since adreno-leukodystrophy was not widely recognized until recently, it is still difficult to assess its frequency and its relationship to what is generally called "Schilder disease". Adreno-leukodystrophy probably accounts for the substance of familial, sex-linked, sudanophilic leukodystrophies, as well as for some sporadic cases diagnosed as Schilder disease. Although the cerebral pathology of adreno-leukodystrophy is identical with Schilder disease, it seems best to reserve the latter term for sudanophilic demyelinating disease processes other than adreno-leukodystrophy. Continued attention to this group may eventually provide the criteria to show whether there are familial juvenile sudanophilic leukodystrophies other than adreno-leukodystrophy, or whether sporadic cases of massive sudanophilic demyelinating disease in children and young adults should be grouped as a variant of multiple sclerosis and other acquired demyelinating diseases of adulthood.

References

Aguilar, M. J., O'Brien, J. S., Taber, P.: The syndrome of familial leukodystrophy, adrenal insufficiency and cutaneous melanosis. In: Inborn Disorders of Sphingolipid Metabolism. Proc. 3rd Int. Symposium Sphingolipidoses (Aronson, S. M., Volk, B. W., eds.), pp. 149—166. London: Pergamon Press 1967.

Burton, B. K., Nadler, H. L.: Schilder's disease: Abnormal cholesterol retention and accumulation in cultivated fibroblasts. Pediat. Res. 8: 170—175, 1974.

Christensen, E., Melchior, J., Negri, S.: A comparative study of 16 cases of diffuse sclerosis with special reference to histopathological findings. Acta neurol. scand. 37: 163—208, 1961.

Collier, J., Greenfield, J. G.: The encephalitis periaxialis of Schilder: Clinical and pathological study, with an account of two cases, one of which was diagnosed during life. Brain 47: 489—519, 1924.

Crome, L., Zapella, M.: Schilder's disease (sudanophilic leucodystrophy) in five male members of one family. J. Neurol. Neurosurg. Psychiat. 26: 431—438, 1963.

Farkas-Bargeton, E., Sarrut, S., Philippart, M., Launay, C.: Démyélinisation du système nerveux central assocée à une atrophie cortico-surrénale. Rev. Neurol. (Paris) 117: 627—641, 1967.

Haberfeld, W., Spieler, F.: Zur diffusen Hirn-Rückenmarkssklerose im Kindesalter. Dtsch. Z. Nervenheilk. 40: 436—463, 1910.

Hoefnagel, D., Van den Noort, S., Ingbar, S. H.: Diffuse cerebral sclerosis with endocrine abnormalities in young males. Brain 85: 553—568, 1962.

Marie, P., Foix, C.: Sclérose intra-cérébrale centrolobaire et symétrique. Rev. Neurol. (Paris) 27: 1—16, 1914.

Pilz, P.: Kombination von Morbus Addison und Morbus Schilder bei einer 43jährigen Frau. Zbl. ges. Neurol. Psychiat. 208: 132—132, 1973.

Poser, C. M., van Bogaert, L.: Natural history and evolution of the concept of Schilder's diffuse sclerosis. Acta psychiat. neurol. scand. 31: 285—331, 1956.

Powell, H., Tindall, R., Schultz, P., *et al.*: Adrenoleukodystrophy: Electron microscopic findings. Arch. Neurol. 32: 250—260, 1915.

Powers, J. M., Schaumburg, H. H.: The adrenal cortex in adreno-leukodystrophy. Arch. Path. (Chic.) 96: 305—310, 1973.

— — Adrenoleukodystrophy: Similar ultrastructural changes in adrenal cortical and Schwann cells. Arch. Neurol. (Chic.) 30: 406—408, 1974.

Schaumburg, H. H., Richardson, E. P., Johnson, P. C., *et al.:* Schilder's disease. Sex-linked recessive transmission with specific adrenal changes. Arch. Neurol. (Chic.) 27: 457—460, 1972.

Schenk, V. W. D., Stam, F. C., Batenburg-Plenter, A. M.: A family with sudanophilic leucodystrophy. Acta neuropath. (Berl.) 9: 233—243, 1967.

Schilder, P.: Die Encephalitis periaxialis diffusa. Arch. Psychiat. 71: 327—356, 1924.

— Zur Frage der Encephalitis periaxialis diffusa (sogenannte diffuse Sklerose). Z. Neurol. Psychiat. 15: 359—376, 1913.

— Zur Kenntnis der sogenannten diffusen Sklerose (Über Encephalitis periaxialis diffusa). Z. Neurol. Psychiat. 10: 1—60, 1912.

See, G., Dayras, J.-Cl., Czernichow, P., Guesry, P.: Addison's disease and leukodystrophy. Clinical and anatomical study. Arch. franç. Pédiat. 28: 847—864, 1971.

Siemerling, E., Creutzfeldt, H. G.: Bronzekrankheit und sklerosierende Encephalomyelitis. Arch. Psychiat. 68: 217—244, 1923.

Strunk, P., Strunk, G.: Beitrag zur Klinik und Pathomorphologie orthochromatischer Leukodystrophien. Dtsch. Z. Nervenheilk. 186: 496—510, 1965.

van Bogaert, L., Edgar, G. H. F., Karcher, D.: Type orthochromatique (à substance soudanophile) diffus de la leucodystrophie familiale. Acta neuropath. (Berl.) 1: 289—307, 1961.

41. Pelizaeus-Merzbacher Disease, Cockayne Syndrome and Related Conditions

Pelizaeus (1885) reported a sibship afflicted with a chronic, debilitating neurologic disorder which had its onset in early infancy and took a protracted course to young or middle adult age. Fourteen members were eventually found to be afflicted in this sibship, and Merzbacher (1910) gave a detailed description of the neuropathologic findings in one. There was hypoplasia of the cerebral and cerebellar white matter with a patchy deficiency of myelin and interspaced sharply delineated islands of myelinated fibers. This pattern is traditionally described as "tigroid", although it is actually more similar to a leopard skin (Norman *et al.*, 1966). The disease afflicting the Pelizaeus sibship evidently represented a nosologic entity quite different from other known inherited neurologic conditions; yet, much difficulty was encountered later in defining what constitutes "Pelizaeus-Merzbacher disease". Its etiology and pathogenesis remain obscure, and there was so much variance in the course and morphologic findings for subsequent cases that their definition as an entity or as a loosely related group of diseases remains unclear. Consequently, the pertinent literature is highly controversial.

The "tigroid" pattern of myelin deficiency observed by Merzbacher has often been considered the morphologic hallmark of the disease, and the classification of the so-called adult cases of Pelizaeus-Merzbacher disease, in particular, rests entirely on this criterion. However, for the rapidly progressive connatal form described by Seitelberger (1954) there is a subtotal absence of myelin without the characteristic patchy pattern of persisting myelin islands. Other observations also deemphasize the pathognomonic significance of the "tigroid" pattern: Members of a given sibship may show it to different degrees; whereas, patchy deficiencies of myelin quite similar to those in Pelizaeus-Merzbacher disease have been found in dysmorphic syndromes, particularly in Cockayne syndrome, which evidently differ from Pelizaeus-Merzbacher disease. Diezel *et al.* (1965) tabulate two groups of lesions, based on the variance in myelin pattern: 1. Those with complete absence of myelin, as in the connatal type of Seitelberger and 2. those with irregular, patchy absence of myelin. They considered the sharply delineated perivascular islands of myelin described by Merzbacher characteristic of a given phase of the disease process rather than a constant, pathognomonic feature. Many authors classify Pelizaeus-Merzbacher disease among the sudanophilic leukodystrophies, but this classification is one of exclusion, eliminating all other types of leukodystrophies characterized by more specific tissue changes. The classification of Pelizaeus-Merzbacher disease as a sudanophilic leukodystrophy may also be criticized on the grounds that many cases show only minimal sudanophilic breakdown products. Zeman *et al.* (1964) proposed a rigid genetic definition of Pelizaeus-Merzbacher disease, accepting only those cases in whom a sex-linked transmission is associated with a characteristic clinical course; they deemphasized the significance of morphologic features in defining the disease. This approach singles out a homogenous nucleus of cases, but it leaves many others unclassified, including all sporadic cases. Moreover, the definition of the disease as a sex-linked disorder has to resort to auxiliary theories to explain the rare occurrences in whom female members of a sibship were afflicted. Jellinger and Seitelberger (1969), on the other hand, accept morphologic changes as the basis for classifying Pelizaeus-Merzbacher disease, of which they distinguish six forms: 1. The classical form described by Merzbacher, a sex-linked, recessive condition with infantile or late infantile onset and slow progression. 2. The connatal form, sex linked, recessive, with postnatal onset and rapid progression. 3. The adult form. 4. Cases transitional between groups 1 and 2, all of which are sporadic. 5. Variants transitional to sudanophilic leukodystrophies having more pronounced sudanophilic breakdown products. 6. Cockayne syndrome, representing a "symptomatic" form. Seitelberger (1970, review) provides a tabulation of pertinent case reports.

The present chapter is divided into two sections. The first one, on Pelizaeus-Merzbacher disease, includes inherited white matter diseases with a striking male predilection running an early infantile, fast course (connatal form) or a more protracted course (classical form). The second section refers to patchy demyelination of white matter associated with cerebral mineralization occurring as a component of several dysmorphic syndromes including Cockayne syndrome. Either of these two sections includes data on additional cases that do not fit the common mold and present with problems in classification. Not considered in this chapter is the so-called adult form of Pelizaeus-Merzbacher disease. The few pertinent observations (Löwenberg and Hill, 1933; Peiffer and Zerbin-Rüdin, 1963, case 1) pertain to patchy white matter lesions similar to those in the classical form, but of otherwise quite different features. The widely quoted dominant inheritance of the adult form rests on extremely rudimentary clinical data (Camp and Löwenberg, 1941).

Pelizaeus-Merzbacher Disease. The disorder manifests in early infancy with aimless, wandering eye movements and failure of the infant to develop normal head control, symptoms which are rather characteristic and were noted in many of the reported cases. They are followed by a lack of growth and development, the infants being underweight and microcephalic. Skeletal anomalies including osteoporosis and kyphoscoliosis develop later, either as a concurrent manifestation of the disease itself, or, more likely, as secondary effects of debilitation. In the connatal form, early infantile onset induces a relatively short course leading to death within a few years. The infants are terminally in a state of complete paresis, spasticity, incontinence and deep dementia. For the protracted or "classical" form an extremely drawn out course is characteristic and patients often live to adult life. The progression of the neurologic disabilities is more rapid during infancy and childhood and becomes arrested or very slow later on. Many of the cases of either group belong to identified sibships in whom a sex-linked transmission affects males. There appears to be no overlap or combination of the connatal and the protracted forms of the disease in a given sibship. There are also sporadic cases for whom similar clinical courses as well as cerebral lesions were found. Affliction of females is rare, but it has been observed in identified sibships as well as for sporadic cases.

Postmortem examination shows a brain smaller than normal, though without distinct cortical atrophy or sclerosis. At the cut surface the dusky, discolored white matter is poorly delineated from the gray matter. The volume of the white matter may be normal, particularly in the connatal form, but it is markedly reduced for the protracted form and there is atrophy of the corpus callosum and enlargement of the cerebral ventricles.

The connatal form was defined by Seitelberger (1954) who described its characteristic histopathologic features. The classification of a clinicopathologically similar case reported by Lüttge (1914) is doubtful as the author emphasizes a marked cytoplasmic disorganization of cortical neurons seen in silver impregnation, the significance of which is difficult to assess in retrospect. Myelin stains show a complete to subtotal absence of myelin sheaths in the white matter of the cerebral and cerebellar hemispheres, the brain stem and the spinal cord; only the roots of cranial and spinal nerves are myelinated. Irregularly disposed nests or small islands of myelinated fibers are found on scrutiny, but they are not a prevalent feature and vary in their extent from case to case.

In the protracted form there is a patchy absence of myelin mainly in the white matter of the centrum semiovale and the cerebellar hemispheres; islands of myelinated tissue persist, often in a perivascular arrangement, and may be sharply delineated or may blend gradually with the adjacent nonmyelinated white matter. There is no sparing of subcortical U fibers. The fiber tracts of basal ganglia, brain stem and cord may be completely preserved, or they may show a diffuse pallor, but they are usually devoid of patchy myelin defects. The intensity of the white matter changes varies over a wide range; the case 1 of Wicke (1938), for example, which belongs to an identified sibship with Pelizaeus-Merzbacher disease, had merely a diffuse pallor of the hemispheric white matter with occasional, small, more intensely staining islands of myelin. There are, on the other hand, cases which may be considered intermediary between the subtotal absence of myelin in the connatal form and the flaky pattern observed with the protracted course.

Contrary to other leukodystrophic processes, *e.g.*, adrenoleukodystrophy, there is generally good preservation of axis cylinders in metallic impregnation, a finding confirmed by the presence of tightly packed neurites in electron micrographs (Watanabe *et al.*, 1969). Indeed, the integrity of the axons appears to be a prerequisite for the occurrence of short segments of myelinated fibers in the white matter, as Merzbacher (1910) had postulated although he had succeeded only in staining the axons within the myelinated islands and not those in the adjacent, myelin-free tissue. Though axons survive in number, they are not entirely unaffected by the disease: axon counts in the pyramids indicated that fibers are either hypoplastic or less numerous than normal (Zeman *et al.*, 1964). Areas devoid of myelin show a marked reduction or total absence of oligodendroglia cells. There is a diffuse, moderate proliferation of astroglia, and the resultant increase in the density of glial fibers may cause, in the connatal form, a selective staining of the white matter in Holzer preparations.

Many cases, particularly those in the connatal group, show little or no evidence of active myelin breakdown, lipid-laden macrophages being sparse or absent. However, considerable variance in the intensity and distribution of sudanophilic products in the tissue has been recorded. There may be a dusting of astrocytes with fine lipid droplets, as well as lipid droplets in endothelial cells and macrophages (Bargeton-Farkas and Edgar, 1964). Due consideration has to be given, however, to the common occurrence of diffuse fatty deposits in the infantile white matter unrelated to cerebral disease (Chapter 5). Lipid-laden macrophages may be found scattered throughout the islands of persistent myelinated fibers, and histochemical examination of the lipids shows a prevalence of cholesterol and triglycerides (Diezel and Huth, 1963); such observations are consistent with an element of demyelination (Norman *et al.*, 1966).

The gray matter, particularly the cerebral cortex, is generally unaffected by the disease. In the cerebellum there may be focal or diffuse cortical atrophy; its type is not always well documented, and it was thought to be secondary to convulsions (Zeman *et al.*, 1964). However, diffuse atrophy of the granular layer type may occur, a type which has never been linked to convulsions or disturbances in oxygenation. The report of Thulin *et al.* (1968) documents an instance of granular cell ectopia and superficial fiber reorientation of the developmental type described in Chapter 31.

The coexistence of malformations with Pelizaeus-Merzbacher disease has been noticed in several instances, such as a small frontal area of abnormal cortical gyration in one of Seitelberger's (1964) cases or a typical polymicrogyria (Norman *et al.*, 1966). There are also several reports on leukodystrophic changes in severely malformed brains which defy classification. A sudanophilic leukodystrophy in a pachygyric brain (Norman *et al.*, 1962) is rather similar to a case reported as dysplastic gliosis (Kramer, 1956). A sister of the case of Norman *et al.* had, also, microcephaly, pachygyria and sudanophilic leukodystrophy, but there was, in addition, a peculiar flaky absence of myelin in the cerebral cortex and a granular layer atrophy of the cerebellum, reminiscent of the changes in Pelizaeus-Merzbacher disease (Norman *et al.*, 1967).

Cockayne Syndrome and Related Conditions. White matter changes similar to those in Pelizaeus-Merzbacher disease occur as a component of several dysmorphic syndromes, in particular that described by Cockayne (1936, 1946) for a brother and a sister afflicted with a syndrome of dwarfism, retinal atrophy and blindness. Cockayne syndrome is a familial disorder of sex-independent transmission consistent with an autosomal recessive inheritance (Macdonald *et al.*, 1960). The infants usually have a normal history of gestation and delivery, and the first signs of the disease manifests at about 6 months of age with a photo-sensitive dermatitis. Growth retardation, dwarfism and kyphosis develop by the 2nd year of life, and there is microcephaly, prognatism of the maxilla, mental retardation, retinitis pigmentosa, optic atrophy and slowly progressive signs of upper motor neuron disease and cerebellar dysfunction. Characteristic facial features include a pre-aged appearance, a beak-shaped nose, and a dermatitis in butterfly distribution over cheeks and nose. The disease progresses slowly and may extend over several decades with a terminal state of blindness, deafness and paralysis. Functional disturbances include abnormalities in renal function, in glucose metabolism, and hyperlipoproteinemia; no chromosomal abnormalities have been found.

Neuropathologic findings for a case of Cockayne syndrome were described by Moossy (1967) and compared with several earlier reports on similar neuropathologic findings. The brain was markedly micrencephalic (460 gm) with cortical atrophy, reduction in the volume of white matter and ventricular dilation. On microscopic examination there was a patchy, irregular deficiency of myelin interspaced with islands of preserved myelin, most marked in the hemispheric white matter and not sparing the subcortical U fibers. The second characteristic alteration consisted of granular mineralization of capillaries and pericapillary parenchyma in the cerebral cortex and the striatum. Mineralization of Purkinje dendrites may also occur (Rowlatt, 1969). There was an increase in lipofuscin in neuronal perikarya and a cerebellar cortical atrophy of the granular layer type. A peripheral neuropathy with loss of myelin and relative preservation of axis cylinders has been described recently for patients with Cockayne syndrome (Moosa and Dubowitz, 1970; Srivastava *et al.*, 1974). General autopsy findings (Rowlatt, 1969) included thickening of the basement membrane of glomeruli and Bowman's membrane, and tubular calcification, splenic fibrosis, and atrophy of ovaries and pituitary gland.

The brothers described as Pelizaeus-Merzbacher disease by Lüthy and Bischoff (1961) were probably Cockayne syndrome, as there was retinitis pigmentosa, dwarfism, testicular atrophy, mineralization in the basal ganglia, and atrophy of the cerebellar granular layer. Other cases now widely accepted as instances of Cockayne syndrome had been reported under the name "microcephaly with cerebral calcification" (Horanyi-Hechst and Meyer, 1939; Jervis, 1954; Norman and Tingey, 1966); the attribution of these cases to Cockayne syndrome is based on the white matter changes and the mineralization, although description of the rest of the dysmorphic syndrome is rudimentary. Cases 1 and 2 of Hallervorden (1950), reported as postmeningoencephalitic syndrome, also seem to represent instances of Cockayne syndrome. On the other hand, the combination of microcephaly with cerebral calcifications has also been described as the result of secondary scarred lesions, such as the presumably postencephalitic defects described by Dennis and Alvord (1961), or the postanoxic lesions described by Young and Courville (1961). Widespread, patchy mineralization in the 7-month-old infant described by D'hoore and Gullotta (1971) was associated with multiple cavities highly suggestive of periventricular infarcts (Chapter 4).

Neuropathologic changes in a syndrome similar to, but not identical with, Cockayne syndrome were reported by Martin *et al.* (1971) for brothers afflicted with noncongenital microcephaly, a peculiar facies with strikingly large ears, severe mental retardation, a progressive optic atrophy and spasticity with choreoathetoid movements. Retrognatism, lack of senile features and spindle shaped fingers were emphasized as differing from Cockayne syndrome. The micrencephalic brain showed patchy deficiency of myelin and severe granular layer atrophy of the cerebellum, but the abnormal mineralization seen in Cockayne syndrome was absent. Gamstorp (1972) discussed the possible relations of Cockayne syndrome to leprechaunism (Donohue syndrome)—stunted children with little subcutaneous adipose tissue, a hairy skin, widely set eyes and low set large ears. The neuropathology of leprechaunism is still undefined.

Melchior *et al.* (1960) report two families in whom members of either sex were affected by a progressive, deteriorating neurologic disease. The onset of symptoms dated to infancy or childhood, and the extremely protracted course led to death in adult life in a state of spasticity and contractures. Retinitis pigmentosa was described for members of the first family and microcephaly for members of the second. Neuropathologic data for one member of each family showed massive, confluent mineralization in the basal ganglia, particularly in the putamen, in the depth of sulci and the cerebral cortex, and in cerebellar cortex and white matter. No deficiency of myelin in the white matter is mentioned. These two families show certain resemblances to Cockayne syndrome, but they differ in many other aspects. The cerebral mineralization, in particular, was focally more intense and confluent, leading to tissue destruction, resembling the changes customarily described as "Fahr disease" in adults, rather than those in Cockayne syndrome. Cerebral changes similar to those described by Melchior *et al.* (1960) were found by the present author in a 2-year-old boy who died from lymphoblastic anemia. There had been no clinical evidence of neurological disease except for seizures and coma prior to death; there were 3 normal siblings and an inquiry disclosed no evidence of familial disease. Intense, granular perivascular and parenchymal mineralization was found in the putamina and in the depth of sulci of the frontal cortex as well as in subjacent white matter; in the latter there was also a diffuse pallor in myelin stains. Dentate nucleus and cerebellar cortex were normal. A unilateral sclerosis of the Ammon's horn with subtotal loss of cells in the fascia denta, Sommer's sector and the endplate was the only other change in this difficult to classify case.

Pathogenetic Considerations. The etiology, pathogenesis, and even the precise nosologic definition of the diseases described in the present chapter are obscure. Pelizaeus-Merzbacher disease has been thought to be a disturbance in glycerophosphatide metabolism (Seitelberger, 1957), but subsequent chemical studies revealed only changes consistent with a reduction in myelin. The interpretation of the white matter changes in Pelizaeus-Merzbacher disease hinges, to a considerable extent, on whether the deficiency of myelin results from a primary failure in myelin formation, as originally proposed by Merzbacher (1910), or from the destruction of myelin sheaths, as proposed by Spielmeyer (1923). Identification of this basic mechanism is also crucial for the classification of Pelizaeus-Merzbacher disease among sudanophilic, myelinoclastic leukodystrophies or as a category of its own. Poser (1961) attempted to distinguish all leukodystrophies from the demyelinating processes, postulating that leukodystrophies are the result of disturbed myelin formation, or "dysmyelination", in contrast to the myelinoclastic processes. However, the newer insights into the pathogenesis of metachromatic and of globoid cell leukodystrophy (Chapters 38, 39) are inconsistent with his concept. Evidence has been presented, on the other hand, that the lesions described in the present chapter, particularly those of Pelizaeus-Merzbacher disease, may indeed be dysmyelinative in nature. Electron microscopic examination of a frontal biopsy taken at the age of 6 months from a patient with a pedigree of Pelizaeus-Merzbacher disease showed complete absence of compact myelin sheaths in cortex and white matter (Watanabe *et al.*, 1969). A biopsy from a 14-week-old patient (Watanabe *et al.*, 1973) disclosed numerous redundant myelin sheaths presenting as "myelin balls" whose continuity with myelin sheath was uncertain. There were also cytoplasmic inclusions in oligodendroglia cells composed of lamellae encircling a central vacuole which contained floccules of ribosome-like material. Scattered macrophages were also observed. Schneck *et al.* (1971) found only occasional myelinated fibers in a biopsy of a 3½-year-old boy; membrane-bound, vacuolated lipid bodies were seen in the cytoplasm of oligodendroglia cells, but the latter lacked the concentric lamellae described by Watanabe *et al.* (1973). Density gradient centrifugation showed no measurable amounts of myelin in this brain; myelin lipids were markedly reduced and the proportions of lipid fractions were similar to those before the onset of myelin formation. The authors attribute the disease to a failure in myelin formation, perhaps from a failure in the proliferation of oligodendroglia cells.

Diseases consistent with "dysmyelination" were also observed in laboratory animals: The quaking mutant of mice, an autosomal recessive disorder, showed concentrations of cerebral sphingo- and phospholipids comparable to those found in controls at an early stage of myelination; at the age of 65 days cerebroside levels were only 10 percent of normal (Hogan and Joseph, 1970). The enzymatic capacity for cerebroside biosynthesis in the mutant is depressed up to 65 percent (Costantino-Ceccarini and Morell, 1971). These chemical deficiencies are consistent with electron microscopic data showing thin, hypoplastic myelin sheaths in which the number of myelin lamellae is approximately one-half that of normal axons of comparable size (Samorajski *et al.*, 1970). There are also anomalies in sheath structure such as distortions and disruptions of myelin sheaths, redundant sheaths as well as round or lamellar inclusions in oligodendroglia cytoplasm (Berger, 1971; Wisniewski and Morell, 1971). These morphologic and chemical features in quaking mice are in many regards similar to those in Pelizaeus-Merzbacher disease.

One may speculate, in conclusion, that the white matter lesions in the various human disease processes described in the present chapter are alike because they have similar pathogenetic mechanisms in common. The patchy myelin deficiency, or persistence of myelin islands, once thought diagnostic of Pelizaeus-Merzbacher disease may well be a phenotype of a lesion caused by a variety of etiologic agents. Perhaps an analogy may be drawn to the granular layer atrophy of the cerebellum, which is caused by a great variety of infectious, physical, toxic or metabolic agents which have in common that they are capable of interfering with cell proliferation in the fetal superficial granular layer of the cerebellar cortex. There is experimental evidence to show that myelination of a central tract may be interferred with if the proliferating oligodendroglia cells are destroyed by X-irradiation (Beal and Hall, 1974). Experiments of this type provide important leads for the understanding of dysmyelinative disease processes.

References

Bargeton-Farkas, E., Edgar, G. W. F.: Anatomo-chemical study on a case of congenital sudanophilic leucodystrophy. Acta neuropath. (Berl.) 3: 578—587, 1964.

Beal, J. A., Hall, J. L.: A light microscopic study of the effects of X-irradiation on the spinal cord of neonatal rats. J. Neuropath. exp. Neurol. 33: 128—143, 1974.

Berger, B.: Quelques aspects ultrastructuraux de la substance blanche chez la souris quaking. Brain Res. 25: 35—53, 1971.

Camp, D. D., Löwenberg, K.: An American familiy with Pelizaeus-Merzbacher disease. Arch. Neurol. Psychiat. (Chic.) 45: 261—264, 1941.

Cockayne, E. A.: Dwarfism with retinal atrophy and deafness. Arch. Dis. Child. 11: 1—8, 1936.

— Dwarfism with retinal atrophy and deafness. Arch. Dis. Child. 21: 52—54, 1946.

Costantino-Ceccarini, E., Morell, P.: Quaking mouse: *In vitro* studies of brain sphingolipid biosynthesis. Brain Res. 29: 75—84, 1971.

Dennis, J. P., Alvord, E. C.: Microcephaly with intracerebral calcification and subependymal ossification. J. Neuropath. exp. Neurol. 20: 412—426, 1961.

D'hoore, E., Gullotta, F.: Entmarkungsprozeß mit Hirnverkalkungen bei einem mikrocephalen Säugling. Cockayne-Syndrom? Acta neuropath. (Berl.) 18: 311—316, 1971.

Diezel, P. B., Fritsch, H., Jakob, H.: Leukodystrophie mit orthochromatischen Aufbaustoffen. Ein Beitrag zur Pelizaeus-Merzbacherschen Krankheit. Virchows Arch. path. Anat. 338: 371—394, 1965.

— Huth, K.: Pelizaeus-Merzbachersche Erkrankung mit familiären Befall. Dtsch. Z. Nervenheilk. 184: 264—287, 1963.

Gamstorp, I.: Donahue's syndrome—Leprechaunism—Cockayne's syndrome. A report of two patients and discussion of the relation between Donahue's syndrome and Cockayne's syndrome. Europ. Neurol. 7: 26—33, 1972.

Hallervorden, J.: Über diffuse symmetrische Kalkablagerungen bei einem Krankheitsbild mit Microcephalie und Meningoencephalitis. Arch. Psychiat. 184: 579—600, 1950.

Hogan, E. L., Joseph, K. C.: Composition of cerebral lipids in murine leucodystrophy: The quaking mutant. J. Neurochem. 17: 1209—1214, 1970.

Horanyi-Hechst, B., Meyer, A.: Diffuse sclerosis with preserved myelin islands. J. ment. Sci. 85: 22—28, 1939.

Jellinger, K., Seitelberger, F.: Pelizaeus-Merzbacher disease. Transitional form between classical and co-natal (Seitelberger) type. Acta neuropath. (Berl.) 14: 108—117, 1969.

Jervis, G. A.: Microcephaly with extensive calcium deposits and demyelination. J. Neuropath. exp. Neurol. 13: 318—329, 1954.

Kramer, W.: Dysgenetic gliosis of the brain. A case of macrogyria. J. Neuropath. exp. Neurol. 15: 471—484, 1956.

Löwenberg, K., Hill, T. S.: Diffuse sclerosis with preserved myelin islands. Arch. Neurol. Psychiat. (Chic.) 29: 1232—1245, 1933.

Lüthy, F., Bischoff, A.: Die Pelizaeus-Merzbacher-Krankheit. Acta neuropath. (Berl.) 1: 113—134, 1961.

Lüttge: Über einen besonderen histologischen Befund aus dem Gebiete der frühinfantilen familiären Erkrankungen des Nervensystems. Dtsch. Z. Nervenheilk. 50: 30—35, 1914.

Macdonald, W. B., Fitch, K. D., Lewis, I. C.: Cockayne's syndrome. A heredofamiliar disorder of growth and development. Pediatrics 25: 997—1007, 1960.

Martin, J. J., Deberdt, R., Philippart, M., Van Acker, K. J., Hooft, C.: Peculiar dysmorphic syndrome with orthochromatic leucodystrophy. Discussion of its relationship with Cockayne's syndrome and Pelizaeus-Merzbacher's disease. Acta neuropath. (Berl.) 18: 224—233, 1971.

Melchior, J. C., Benda, C. E., Yakovlev, P. I.: Familial idiopathic cerebral calcifications in childhood. J. Dis. Child. 99: 787—803, 1960.

Merzbacher, L.: Eine eigenartige familiär-hereditäre Erkrankungsform (Aplasia axialis extracorticalis congenita). Z. Neurol. Psychiat. 3: 1—38, 1910.

Moosa, A., Dubowitz, V.: Peripheral neuropathy in Cockayne's syndrome. Arch. Dis. Child. 45: 674—677, 1970.

Moossy, J.: The neuropathology of Cockayne's syndrome. J. Neuropath. exp. Neurol. 26: 654—660, 1967.

Norman, R. M., Tingey, A. H.: Syndrome of micrencephaly, strio-cerebellar calcifications, and leucodystrophy. J. Neurol. Neurosurg. Psychiat. 29: 157—163, 1966.

— — Harvey, P. W., Gregory, A. M.: Pelizaeus-Merzbacher disease: a form of sudanophil leucodystrophy. J. Neurol. Neurosurg. Psychiat. 29: 521—529, 1966.

— — Valentine, J. C., Danby, T. A.: Sudanophil leucodystrophy in a pachygyric brain. J. Neurol. Neurosurg. Psychiat. 25: 363—369, 1962.

— — — Hislop, H. J.: Sudanophil leucodystrophy: a study of intersib variation in the form taken by the demyelinating process. J. Neurol. Neurosurg. Psychiat. 30: 75—82, 1967.

Peiffer, J., Zerbin-Rüdin, E.: Zur Variationsbreite der Pelizaeus-Merzbacherschen Krankheit. Acta neuropath. (Berl.) 3: 87—107, 1963.

Pelizaeus, F.: Über eine eigentümliche Form spastischer Lähmung mit Cerebralerscheinungen auf hereditärer Grundlage (Multiple Sklerose). Arch. Psychiat. 16: 698—710, 1885.

Poser, C. M.: Leukodystrophy and the concept of dysmyelination. Arch. Neurol. (Chic.) 4: 323—332, 1961.

Rowlatt, V.: Cockayne's syndrome. Report of a case with necropsy findings. Acta Neuropath. 14: 52—61, 1969.

Samorajski, T., Friede, R. L., Reimer, P. R.: Hypomyelination in the quaking mouse. A model for the analysis of disturbed myelin formation. J. Neuropath. exp. Neurol. 24: 507—523, 1970.

Schneck, L., Adachi, M., Volk, B. W.: Congenital failure of myelinization: Pelizaeus-Merzbacher disease? Neurology (Minneap.) 21: 817—824, 1971.

Seitelberger, F.: Die Pelizaeus-Merzbachersche Krankheit. Wien. Z. Nervenheilk. 9: 228—289, 1954.

Seitelberger, F.: Histochemie und Klassifikation der Pelizaeus-Merzbacherschen Krankheit. Wien. Z. Nervenheilk. 14: 74—83, 1957.
— Pelizaeus-Merzbacher disease. In: Handbook of Clinical Neurology (Vinken, P. J., Bruyn, G. W., eds.), Vol. 10, Chapter 10, pp. 150—202. Amsterdam: North Holland Publ. Co. 1970.
Spielmeyer, W.: Der anatomische Befund bei einem zweiten Fall von Pelizaeus-Merzbacherscher Krankheit. Zbl. Neurol. Psychiat. 32: 202—203, 1923.
Srivastava, R. N., Gupta, P. C., Mayekar, G., Roy, S.: Cockayne's syndrome in two sisters. Acta paediat. scand. 63: 461—464, 1974.
Thulin, B., McTaggart, D., Neubuerger, K. T.: Demyelinating leukodystrophy with total cortical cerebellar atrophy. Arch. Neurol. (Chic.) 18: 113—122, 1968.
Watanabe, I., McCaman, R., Dyken, P., Zeman, W.: Absence of cerebral myelin sheaths in a case of presumed Pelizaeus-Merzbacher disease. Electron microscopic and biochemical studies. J. Neuropath. exp. Neurol. 28: 243—256, 1969.
— Patel, V., Goebel, H. H., *et al.*: Early lesions of Pelizaeus-Merzbacher disease: Electron microscopic and biochemical study. J. Neuropath. exp. Neurol. 32: 313—333, 1973.
Wicke, R.: Ein Beitrag zur Frage der familiären diffusen Sklerosen einschließlich der Pelizaeus-Merzbacherschen Krankheit und ihre Beziehungen zur amaurotischen Idiotie. Z. Neurol. 162: 741—766, 1938.
Wiśniewski, H., Morell, P.: Quaking mouse: Ultrastructural evidence for arrest of myelinogenesis. Brain Res. 29: 63—73, 1971.
Young, E. F., Courville, C. B.: "Familial" central cerebral calcification in infancy. Report of two cases in siblings. Bull. Los Angeles Neurol. Soc. 26: 198—208, 1961.
Zeman, W., Demyer, W., Falls, H. F.: Pelizaeus-Merzbacher disease. A study in nosology. J. Neuropath. exp. Neurol. 23: 334—354, 1964.

42. Alexander Disease and Related Conditions

Alexander (1949) described previously unrecorded morphologic changes in the brain of a 16-month-old boy who had suffered from progressive mental deterioration and enlargement of the head since the age of 7 months. Postmortem examination disclosed a leukodystrophy and an abundance of rod-shaped eosinophilic deposits which are now generally recognized as Rosenthal fibers. The deposits were found throughout the tissue, with particular predilection for the pial and vascular interfaces of the nervous parenchyma. Alexander considered the disease a "progressive fibrinoid degeneration of fibrillary astrocytes".

Alexander disease is uncommon, and only scattered observations have been reported. Herndon *et al.* (1970) quote 10 infantile cases with clinical and morphologic findings similar to those by Alexander. Several other reports suggest that the early infantile disease described by Alexander is merely one manifestation of a group, or spectrum, of disease processes having diffuse deposition of Rosenthal fibers as a common denominator. Hence, three types are distinguished in the present text: Cases of early infantile onset and rapid progression; those of delayed or juvenile onset and protracted course; and, thirdly, instances of widespread occurrence of Rosenthal fibers in the brains of adults, either as the sole pathologic finding or associated with other disease processes. All three groups have in common that Rosenthal fibers occur widespread throughout the CNS, in distinction from their focal occurrence in gliotic, scarred, or neoplastic lesions affecting the periventricular, subependymal tissue, as discussed later in this chapter.

Cases with Onset in Early Infancy. Alexander disease in early infancy manifests during the first months of life, or it may present from birth. The infants show mental and neurologic deterioration, often with spasticity, some having a history of repeated seizures. Enlargement of the head is common, leading to a clinical diagnosis of hydrocephalus. The course is progressive, and death often occurs before the second year, but it may be delayed for more than a decade. Ten of the 11 cases listed by Herndon *et al.* (1970) were male; no familial occurrences have been recorded as yet.

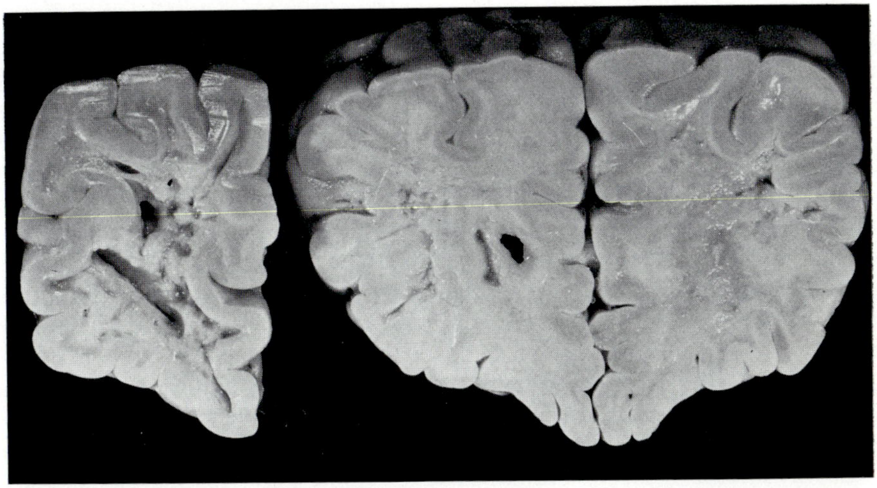

Fig. 146. Cavitation of frontal white matter in Alexander disease

Gross examination of the brain discloses increased size and a normal convolutional pattern. A diffuse discoloration of the hemispheric white matter is seen at the cut surface, and there may be softening of the tissue which may reach the degree of cavitation (Fig. 146), most often in the deep portions of the frontal lobes. The cerebral ventricles are not enlarged, the increase in brain weight being due to an increase in the tissue mass. Hydrocephalic distension of the ventricular system was noted in some instances and was attributed to coexistent obstruction of CSF flow at the foramina of Monro or at the aqueduct.

Microscopic features characteristic of the disease consist of widespread deposition of abnormal structures having the tinctorial, histochemical, and electron microscopic features of Rosenthal fibers and of a diffuse demyelination of white matter (Fig. 147). These two changes may coexist in the same portions of the brain, but their relationship is not consistent, neither in intensity nor in regional distribution. The disposition of Rosenthal fibers is generally more widespread than are the demyelinating changes in white matter. The latter are most pronounced in the centrum semiovale of the cerebral hemispheres, often at maximum intensity in the deep portions of the frontal lobes. Loss of myelin staining may extend up to the cortex, or it may diminish in intensity toward the cortex with variable sparing of U fibers. There is no sharp delineation of the affected zones and transitions to normal tissue are gradual. The less severely affected portions of white matter show typical demyelination of the persisting axons and sparsity of oligodendroglia. Rarefication of axons may occur, however, in severely affected portions of white matter, particularly near and within areas of cavitation. Reactive gliosis and signs of myelinoclastic activity are slight or absent; in particular, there is very little microglial activity and macrophages with deposits of neutral fat are sparse or absent. The case of Sherwin and Berthrong (1970) is exceptional in its sudanophilia as well as in the incorporation of eosinophilic deposits into the perikarya of swollen astrocytes. The demyelination is most marked in the cerebral hemispheres; involvement of other portions of cerebral white matter varies. There may be diffuse demyelination of cerebellar hemispheric white matter, and various fiber tracts of the brain stem may show diffuse pallor; affection is usually least pronounced in the long tracts of the spinal cord.

The diagnostic feature of the disease consists of the deposition of an abundance of homogeneous eosinophilic masses forming elongated tapered rods, up to 30 μ in length. These accumulate preferentially at all the interfaces between the neuroectodermal parenchyma and its mesodermal investments. They line all subpial surfaces of the central nervous system extending into the tissue cuffing the perivascular spaces. Most deposits are oriented in register approximately perpendicular to the interface, which results in palisading at the surface of brain or in a radial arrangement of the deposits around cross sections of blood vessels. The inner surface of the glia-Schwann cell border in the roots of cranial and spinal nerves is coated with a layer of deposits continous with the pial surface of the nerve roots. In addition to crowding at interfaces the deposits are also scattered throughout the tissue. They may be seen in the pineal gland but tend to be absent from the leptomeninges, the choroid plexus, and the adventitia or the walls of the blood vessels. The surface of the cerebellar molecular layer may be spared or affected less severely than other surfaces of brain tissue.

The staining and morphology of the eosinophilic deposits are the same as those of Rosenthal fibers in glial scars or in piloid astrocytomas, the only difference being their widespread occurrence off the ventricular surface and their crowding at interfaces. The deposits stain intensely with myelin stains or the Smith Dietrich reaction; they stain blue with Holzer stain, purple with PTAH, brownish to bright red with Masson trichrome. Staining with the periodic acid-Schiff reaction is usually slight but varies in intensity. The deposits do not stain for iron, calcium, mucin, DNA, or amyloid, but they are positive with various reactions for proteins (Wohlwill *et al.*, 1959; Friede, 1964). On light microscopic examination most deposits appear to be in interstitial tissue spaces, but some can be located in the processes of glial cells, particularly in Holzer stains or in silver impregnations for astroglia. Schlote (1966) showed that the fine structure of the deposits in Alexander disease is the same as that of Rosenthal fibers. This observation was confirmed repeatedly (Schochet *et al.*, 1968; Herndon *et al.*, 1970) and led to the wide acceptance of their identity with Rosenthal fibers. Electron micrographs show

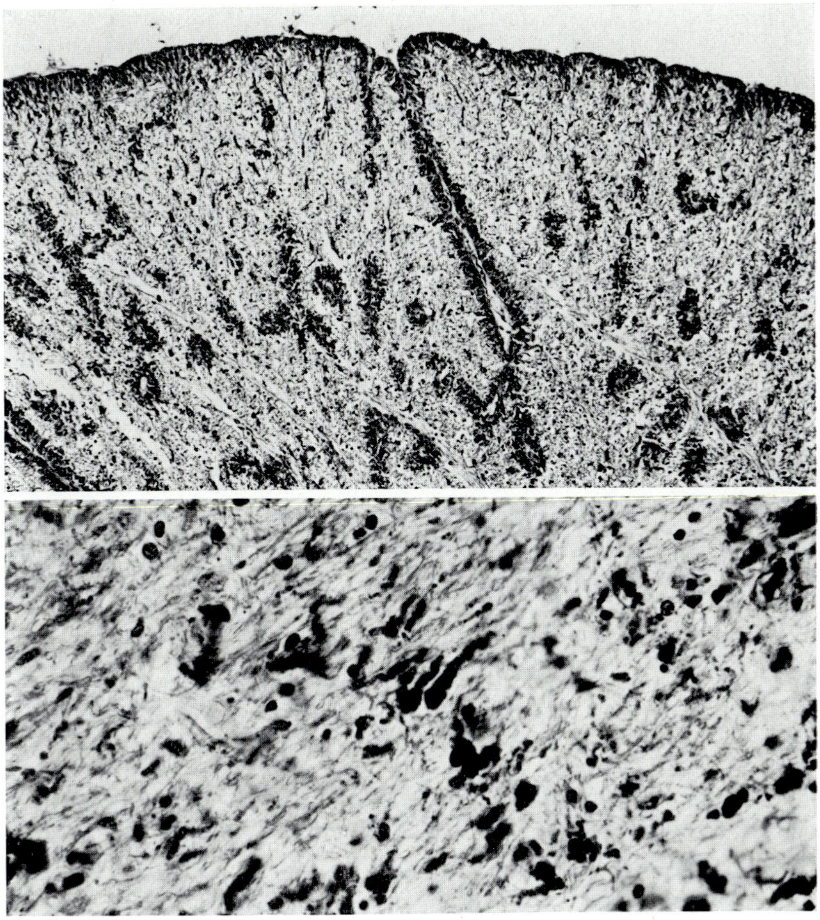

Fig. 147. Alexander disease. Top: characteristic subpial and perivascular accumulation of Rosenthal fibers Klüver-Barrera, ×100. Bottom: random disposition of Rosenthal fibers in white matter, Weigert's stain ×350

masses of granular dense osmophilic material surrounded by aggregates of tightly packed glial filaments displacing other cytoplasmic organelles (Fig. 148). The filaments project into the granular masses and may appear slightly thickned near the point of contact. Deposits of this type are found within the cytoplasm of glial cells variously identified as being astrocytes, abnormal astrocytes, or spongioblasts.

Cases of Late Onset and Protracted Course. Cases reported by Vogel and Hallervorden (1962) and Rewcastle (1966) showed progressive neurologic signs at 7 and 14 years respectively, the course of the disease extending over many years; enlargement of the head was absent. Brain weight was reduced in the case of Vogel and Hallervorden. Widespread deposition of Rosenthal fibers throughout the brain was associated with leukodystrophic changes which, generally, were less severe than in infantile cases. Because of the small number of available observations there is still insufficient delineation of the clinicopathologic features of this variant of the disease; the striking similarity of the morphologic changes to those observed in infants justifies classification as Alexander disease of late onset.

Diffuse Formation of Rosenthal Fibers in the Brains of Adults. Mastri and Sung (1973) reported 4 adults, 19 to 82 years old, in whom Rosenthal fibers were found widely distributed in brain stem, paraventricular tissue and spinal cord, with crowding along interfaces. Their density varied regionally, tending to be maximum in the brain stem. There were no demyelinating changes, and no clinical syndrome could be attributed to the presence of Rosenthal fibers. In other, similar cases widespread Rosenthal fibers coexisted in the brains of adults with other apparently unrelated lesions. The case reported by Seil *et al.* (1968) had a clinical course similar to multiple sclerosis, beginning at the age of 34 and progressing to death 13 years later. The brain showed widespread distribution of Rosenthal fibers associated with multiple cavitated lesions in cerebral and cerebellar white matter; Rosenthal fibers were inconsistent and variable at the edges of the cavitated lesions.

In other instances diffuse or focal depositions of Rosenthal fibers coexisted with typical plaques of multiple sclerosis (Herndon *et al.*, 1970). Ule (1972) reported a combination of neuraxonal dystrophy and widespread Rosenthal fibers in a 24-year-old man who suffered from slow, progressive neurogenic muscle atrophy from the age of 4 years.

Pathogenetic and Nosologic Considerations. The etiology of Alexander disease is unknown at present, and information on its nature is based mainly on conjecture. Alexander's attribution of the eosinophilic deposits to degenerative changes in astrocytes remained a matter of debate until electron microscopic studies identified the deposits with Rosenthal fibers. Rosenthal fibers are generally accepted to be the product of retrogressive changes in glia cells, particularly in astrocytes, and the basic defect in Alexander disease appears to be a widespread affliction of astrocytic glia cells.

Focal formation of Rosenthal fibers is a well known feature of gliotic, scarred lesions of subependymal tissue including chronic ependymitis or syringomyelia; it also commonly occurs in the juvenile piloid astrocytomas arising near the midline, or in focal paraneoplastic gliosis. The disposition to formation of Rosenthal fibers appears to be present, to some extent, in normal subependymal glia; its more widespread occurrence with greater intensity may cause Alexander disease.

Some authors considered Alexander disease a primary leukodystrophy inducing secondarily abnormal eosinophilic deposits in the tissue (Wohlwill *et al.*, 1959). This interpretation is not likely as the deposition of Rosenthal fibers is more widespread than the demyelinating changes, and as it may occur in the absence of the latter. There is still uncertainty, however, as to the precise nature of the relation between Rosenthal fiber formation and demyelination, especially since the astroglial cells afflicted by the disease are not directly involved in the formation of myelin sheaths.

At the present state of knowledge it appears to be most advantageous to reserve the eponym Alexander disease to the early infantile and juvenile

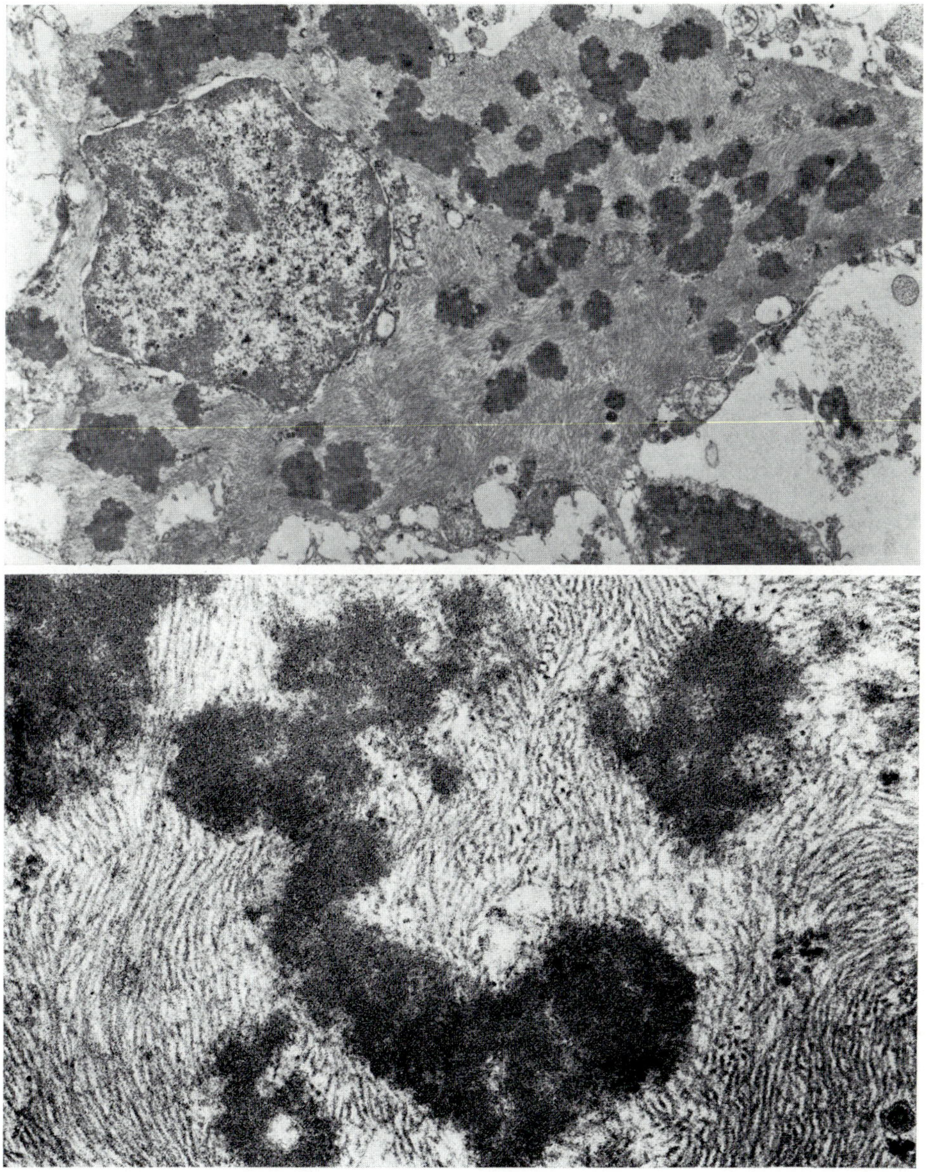

Fig. 148. Alexander disease. Fine structure of Rosenthal fibers in astrocytes (courtesy Dr. Schochet).

cases in whom widespread formation of Rosenthal fibers is associated with demyelination of white matter and a progressive neurologic disorder. It has been suggested that widespread deposition of Rosenthal fibers in the brains of adults without corresponding clinical manifestations and in the absence of other tissue changes may represent a *forme fruste* of Alexander disease, but classification remains tentative, pending identification of specific cellular or biochemical defects.

References

Alexander, W. S.: Progressive fibronoid degeneration of fibrillary astrocytes associated with mental retardation in a hydrocephalic infant. Brain 72: 373—381, 1949.

Friede, R. L.: Alexander's disease. Arch. Neurol. (Chic.) 11: 414—422, 1964.

Herndon, R. M., Rubinstein, L. J., Freeman, J. M., Mathieson, G.: Light and electron microscopic observations on Rosenthal fibers in Alexander's disease and in multiple sclerosis. J. Neuropath. exp. Neurol. 29: 524—551, 1970.

Mastri, A. R., Sung, J. H.: Diffuse Rosenthal fiber formation in the adult: A report of four cases. J. Neuropath. exp. Neurol. 32: 424—436, 1973.

Rewcastle, B.: Presentation to the Canadian Association of Neuropathologists, 1966. Cited in Herndon *et al.*, 1970.

Schlote, W.: Rosenthalsche „Fasern" und Spongioblasten im Zentralnervensystem. II. Elektronenmikroskopische Untersuchungen. Beitr. path. Anat. 133: 461—480, 1966.

Schochet, S. S., Jr., Lampert, P. W., Earle, K. M.: Alexander's disease. A case report with electron microscopic observations. Neurology (Minneap.) 18: 543—549, 1968.

Seil, J. J., Schochet, S. S., Jr., Earle, K. M.: Alexander's disease in an adult. Arch. Neurol. (Chic.) 19: 494—502, 1968.

Sherwin, R. M., Berthrong, M.: Alexander's disease with sudanophilic leukodystrophy. Arch. Path. (Chic.) 89: 321—328, 1970.

Ule, G.: Progressive neurogene Muskelatrophie bei neuroaxonaler Dystrophie mit Rosenthalschen Fasern. Acta neuropath. (Berl.) 21: 332—339, 1972.

Vogel, F. S., Hallervorden, J.: Leukodystrophy with diffuse Rosenthal fiber formation. Acta neuropath. (Berl.) 2: 126—143, 1962.

Wohlwill, F. J., Bernstein, J., Yakovlev, P.: Dysmyelinogenic leukodystrophy. Report of a case of a new, presumably familial type of leukodystrophy with megalobarencephaly. J. Neuropath. exp. Neurol. 18: 359—383, 1959.

43. Axon Dystrophies

One may assume that infantile neuraxonal dystrophy (Seitelberger disease)—once its chemical background becomes better understood—will be classified among the inherited metabolic defects. There are, however, other forms of axon dystrophy which clearly do not qualify as inherited metabolic diseases, like those associated with normal or premature aging or with toxic or nutritional derangements. Furthermore, a nonspecific swelling of axons upon local injury is a very common tissue response seen with a great variety of lesions. All these types of swollen axons are morphologically similar, particularly on light microscopic examination. It was considered advantageous, therefore, to review neuraxonal dystrophy within a general frame of classification of axon swellings.

Two basic types of axon swellings may be distinguished: Reactive and dystrophic. Not considered in this context are the distensions of the tips of growing or regenerating fibers which are considered normal aspects of growth rather than pathologic disturbances. Reactive axon swellings are defined as those developing in response to local injury to normal nerve fibers. They usually present as drop- or club-shaped distensions of the stumps of disrupted fibers, and it is common to see them at the edges of focal lesions, particularly if fibers of large caliber are severed. Reactive axon swellings also occur in the form of spindle shaped, varicose, or irregular local distensions of axons in the absence of loss of continuity, either at some distance from a main lesion, or in lesions that are not of sufficient severity to cause tissue disintegration. Dystrophic axon swellings are thought to be the product of a metabolic or degenerative process that afflicts the axon itself. They may occur in the absence of any other tissue change or in altered tissue, but in the latter case it is unlikely that the tissue changes are the causes of the axon swellings. Dystrophic axons tend to occur in a widespread distribution, or in a systemic pattern, or they may afflict certain fiber systems selectively. Also, they show a preference for involving the most distal segments of the fibers.

It may be seen from these definitions that the classification of axon swellings rests more on the circumstances of their occurrence and the assessment of their tissue environment than on the morphology exhibited by the swellings themselves. Indeed, reactive and dystrophic axon swellings are rather similar under the light microscope, save for a greater variance in the texture and stainability of the axoplasm of the latter. The differences are somewhat more pronounced under the electron microscope: In reactive axon swellings there is an abnormal crowding of axoplasmic organelles including mitochondria, membranous dense bodies, endoplasmic reticulum and vesicles. The same organelles may be seen in dystrophic axon swellings, but there is, in addition, a considerable variety of other abnormal structures such as patches of electron dense material derived from degenerating mitochondria, multigranular bodies from glycogen deposition in mitochondria, large vacuoles, aggregates of tubular rings and layered loops of membranes (Lampert, 1967). Lampert also distinguishes two additional types of axon swellings, the degenerative, which may be considered forms of disintegration of reactive swellings, and the regenerative swellings, which are identical with the end clubs of sprouting nerve fibers.

Reactive Axon Swellings. The experimental induction, the histochemistry and the fine structure of reactive axon swellings have been studied extensively, particularly in peripheral nerves. Swelling of the stumps of experimentally transected nerve fibers commences upon injury and progresses to a maximum within approximately 3 to 8 days. Both the proximal and the distal stumps swell, but the swelling is more extensive and more lasting in the proximal stump. The myelin sheaths of the swollen fibers first become distended and attenuated then disintegrate. The swollen axis cylinder disintegrates into droplets of axoplasm which eventually disappear; concurrently, regenerative fibers sprout into the defect from the proximal stump. Reactive axon swellings develop independently of fiber caliber in nonmyelinated as well as in myelinated fibers, but they are usually more conspicuous and more lasting for thick fibers.

Although these experimental observations are pertinent to human tissue as well, one needs to be cautious in extrapolating from experimental observations to human autopsy material. The presence of reactive axon swellings in the latter is often considered *prima facie* evidence of an *in vivo* lesion. Lindenberg and Freytag (1970), however, found swollen and vacuolated axons near tears of the pyramids at the pontomedullary junction and near tears of cranial nerve roots produced by fatal traumatic hyperextension of the head. Their findings suggest that axon swellings may develop supravitally, at least under certain favorable conditions, an observation which is confirmed by the well established fact that axon swellings develop in the stumps of fibers in excised nerve segments during incubation *in vitro*. While the pathologist needs to be aware of the possibility of supravital redistribution of axoplasm in autopsy or biopsy material, resultant changes are generally slight and are evident only on scrutiny. An abundance of greatly distended axons certainly indicates their *in vivo* development, mostly in lesions a few days to one week old; swollen axons may also be seen near lesions which must be considered much older, and they may even be mineralized, such as near the periventricular infarcts in newborns.

Purkinje cells show peculiar types of swellings of their dendrites or axons. The dendritic swellings in the molecular layer are commonly referred to as asteroid bodies, the swollen axons in the granular layer as torpedoes (Chapter 31). The classification of torpedoes as either reactive or dystrophic swellings is uncertain. Their reactive nature is suggested by their nonspecific occurrence with a variety of acquired cerebellar cortical lesions. However, torpedoes occur in the cerebellar atrophy that accompanies neuraxonal dystrophy, and they have been considered dystrophic in this context.

Axon Dystrophies — Subclassification. Dystrophic axon swellings occur in man under a variety of clinico-pathologic conditions which may be subclassified as follows: 1. Age-dependent axon dystrophy; 2. precocious age-dependent axon dystrophy; 3. neuraxonal dystrophy; 4. Hallervorden-Spatz disease. These four categories overlap to some degree, but most observations are easily assigned to one or the other. Their indiscriminate pooling tends to confuse clinico-pathologic disease concepts and is to be discouraged.

Age-dependent axon dystrophy consists of the accumulation of swollen axons in certain fiber tracts of normal subjects as a result of aging. In precocious age-dependent axon dystrophy the same changes develop at an earlier age or with exceptional intensity in patients suffering from certain chronic diseases. Both lesions are clinically asymptomatic; they are classified in this text as "axonal" rather than "neuraxonal" dystrophy, because neither shows evidence of abnormalities in the neuronal perikarya. The term "neuraxonal" dystrophy is reserved for the progressive neurologic disorders characterized pathologically by widespread occurrence of dystrophic axon swellings in association with neuronal lesions. The distinction between infantile neuraxonal dystrophy and infantile occurrence of Hallervorden-Spatz disease is based mainly on the topographic distribution of the swollen axons, as discussed in greater detail below.

The classification of axonal dystrophies given above limits the term to diseases for which dystrophic axons are the dominant or sole feature of the pathologic process. It excludes the occasional scattering of swollen axons seen in a variety of degenerative white matter diseases, particularly in those involving a progressive degeneration of tracts. Certain experimental intoxications also induce dystrophic axon swellings, though of a different type than those found in human diseases. Iminodiproprionitrile intoxication, for example, results in distension of the proximal segments of axons (Slagel and Hartmann, 1965).

Age-Dependent Axon Dystrophy. Age-dependent axon dystrophy consists of the progressive accumulation of dystrophic axon swellings in the terminal portion of the tractus gracilis and in the nucleus gracilis of normal subjects. Several other fiber systems may be affected, though always less severely than nucleus and tractus gracilis. Age-dependent axon dystrophy was described first by Newberne *et al.* (1960) who observed it in 40 percent of dogs older than 4 years, but rarely in dogs less than 1 year old. It was observed later in most of the common laboratory animals. Axon dystrophy in the tractus and nucleus gracilis is a normal feature of aging in man. Sung (1964), Fujisawa (1967), and Jellinger and Jirásek (1971) obtained somewhat different frequencies for age groups, but their data concur in showing the near constant presence of dystrophic axons beyond the age of 70, their absence before the age of 10, or sparsity during the first two decades of life. Swollen axons also scatter through the tractus and nucleus cuneatus, or into other nuclei in the caudal medulla oblongata (Fig. 149). They are also found in the substantia nigra, though not nearly as often as in the nucleus gracilis; most subjects in the 50-year age group had swellings in the nucleus gracilis, but only 40 percent had swellings in the substantia nigra (Jellinger and Jirásek, 1971). Still fewer swellings are seen in the pallidum; their occurrence has been emphasized to support the concept of premature aging in Hallervorden-Spatz disease.

Dystrophic axon swellings in the nucleus gracilis present as sharply delineated masses of proteinaceous material; their shape varies with the plane of cutting, circular in cross section, varicose or fusiform in longitudinal sections. The swellings are commonly eosinophilic, but tinctorial features vary and some are basophilic. The axoplasm is usually homogenous or slightly granular; it may be vacuolated or show a central condensation or a concentric structure. Disintegration of the swellings is indicated by the presence of vacuolar spaces in the tissue, some of which contain shrunken cytoplasmic remnants. There is little or no loss of neurons in the adjacent tissue, and glial changes are minimal or absent.

Electron microscopic studies reveal that the swellings often involve the terminal presynaptic portions of the fibers. The distended axis cylinder is crowded with axoplasmic organelles, as described above. The crowding of organelles commences proximal to the fiber ending and increases gradually along the distal portion of the tractus gracilis, as shown by a gradual increase in the axoplasmic density of mitochondrial enzymes (Friede and Knoller, 1964).

Precocious Age-Dependent Axon Dystrophy. Abnormal intensification of

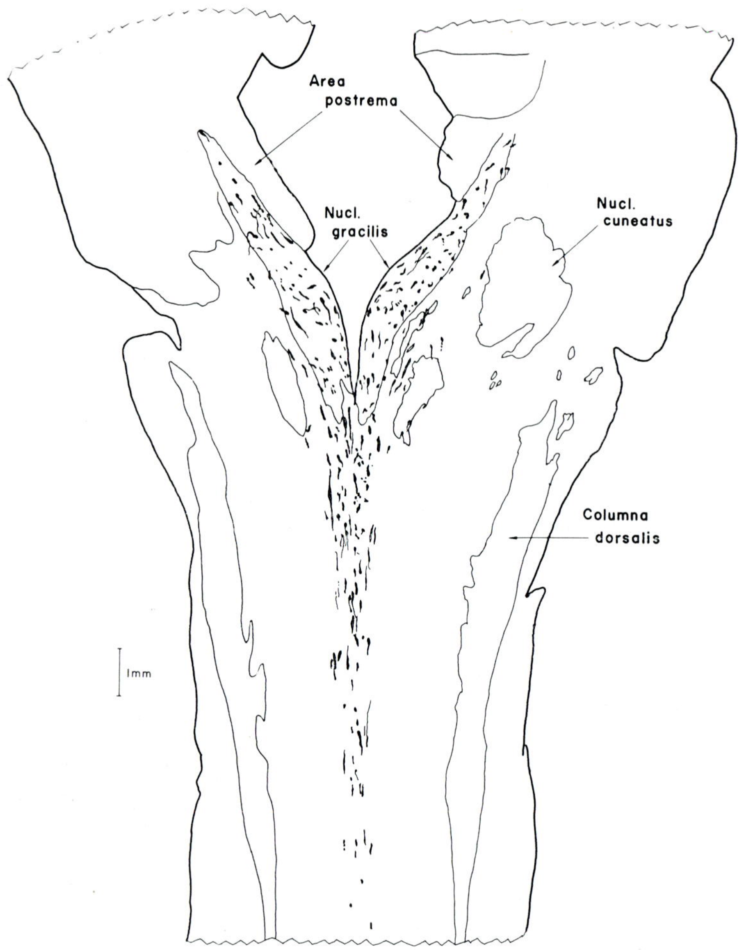

Fig. 149. Camera lucida drawing of longitudinal section through the cervicomedullary junction of a dog, cut in a bitemporal plane. The distribution of all discernible axon swellings is shown, demonstrating their predominance in the terminal portion of the tractus gracilis and within the nucleus gracilis (Friede and Knoller, 1964)

age-dependent axon dystrophy was observed by Sung (1964) in children and young adults suffering from mucoviscidosis, age 6 to 22 years. The same changes were observed in infants with biliary atresia, age 6 to 28 months (Sung and Stadlan, 1966). Precocious axon dystrophy affects mainly the nucleus gracilis (Fig. 150), but it is also seen less intensely in the nucleus cuneatus and the descending trigeminal root, rarely in other nuclear groups. Its microscopic features are the same as described for age-dependent axon dystrophy. Whether other general disease processes are capable of enhancing the development of age-dependent axon dystrophy is debatable. Excessive numbers of axon swellings may be found in alcoholics or in patients with nonalcoholic hepatic disease. However, a statistically significant excess was found for the 20 to 50 years age group only, and none existed at higher ages (Jellinger and Jirásek, 1971).

The experimental induction of axon dystrophy by vitamin E deficiency in rats figured prominently in the interpretation of precocious axon dystrophy. In the studies of Pentschew and Schwarz (1962) swollen axons were found in the nucleus gracilis of vitamin E deficient rats, as well as in the fasciculus cuneatus, the sensory fifth nerve nucleus, Lissauer's zone and the tractus solitarius; there were no significant changes in the respective neuronal

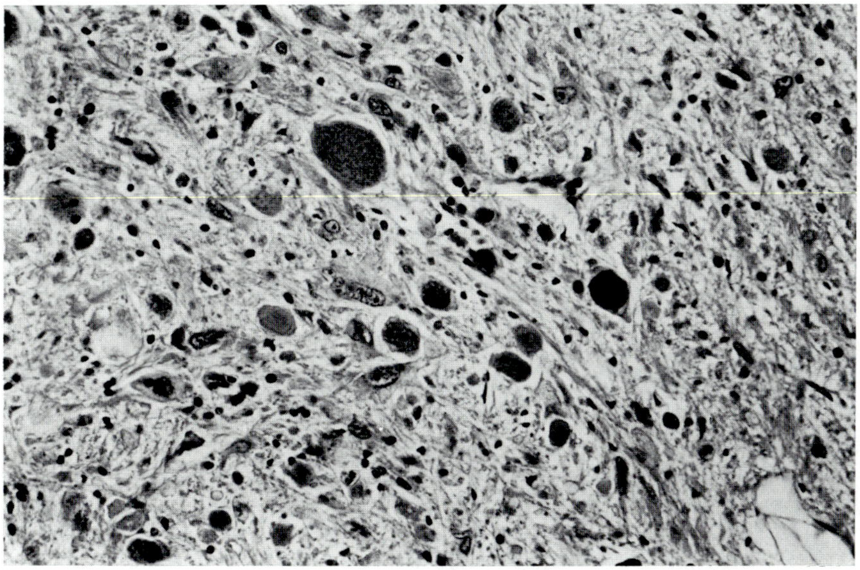

Fig. 150. Precocious axon dystrophy in the nucleus gracilis of a child with biliary atresia; H & E ×225

perikarya. Similar, though less abundant, swollen axons were also seen in the nucleus gracilis of control rats. The fine structure of these axons corresponds to those of dystrophic axons in general (Lampert *et al.*, 1964). The axon dystrophy in vitamin E deficient rats is more similar to precocious age-dependent axon dystrophy than to neuraxonal dystrophy even though vitamin E deficiency induces, in rats, a neurologic syndrome of ataxia, hyperalgesia and hypoestesia. Blakemore and Cavanagh (1969) also suggest that precocious axon dystrophy may be precipitated in rats by the "dying back" neuropathy induced by p-bromophenylacetylurea.

Infantile Neuraxonal Dystrophy (Seitelberger Disease). Seitelberger's (1952) initial impression of this disease process was that of a storage disease, but its pathognomonic relationship to swollen axons was soon recognized in subsequent studies. The now widely accepted term "infantile neuraxonal dystrophy" was introduced by Cowen and Olmstead (1963) and is a modification of Seitelberger's term "proteid neuraxonal dystrophy".

The disease begins most often by the end of the first year, usually between the 6th month and the 2nd year following a normal postnatal development; in some infants there are symptoms from birth on. An arrest of normal development and lack of spontaneous movements are followed by a slowly progressing deterioration with nondevelopment or loss of speech, abnormalities of walk and posture, nystagmus, strabism, and diminished visual acuity or blindness with optic atrophy. Flaccid or spastic paresis develop, with deterioration to complete motor disability and deep dementia. Involuntary movements are an uncommon feature of the disease process, in contrast to their frequency in infantile Hallervorden-Spatz disease. Some of the infants have repeated convulsions. Death occurs between 1 and 10 years for many. Familial occurrence appears to be associated with a more severe course of the disease, approximately half of the reported rapidly progressing cases being familial. Sex preference varies depending on the type of subclassification; there is a slight female preference for all reported cases of neuraxonal dystrophy; the familial cases show a female preponderance of 2 to 1.

A more protracted course of neuraxonal dystrophy leads to death during the second decade; it is sometimes, though variably, associated with onset of symptoms after the 2nd year of life. This milder form of the disease is mostly sporadic, familial occurrence being uncommon. The first description of a respective case is that of Rabinowicz and Wildi (1957), and a tabulation of later reports is given by Gilman and Barrett (1973). The morbid anatomy of these cases often features abnormal pigmentation of the basal ganglia, which is absent for most, but not all, of the rapidly progressive cases. Abnormal pigmentation, however, is not strictly correlated with the time of onset or with the course of the disease: The case described by Thilbault (1972) had symptoms from the age of 12 years on, and death occurred at the age of 38 years. The brain showed neuraxonal dystrophy with widespread spheroids and cerebellar atrophy, but there was no abnormal pigmentation in the basal ganglia.

Gross inspection of the brain in infantile neuraxonal dystrophy is usually nonconclusive, except for the frequent presence of cerebellar atrophy. The most characteristic microscopic features of the disease are: widespread occurrence of spheroids, cerebellar atrophy, and deposition of lipids and/or pigment in the basal ganglia in association with abnormal myelin patterns.

The term spheroids is widely used for the axon swellings of neuraxonal dystrophy to avoid the implication that axons are the only type of cell process involved in the production of swellings. The spheroids consist of accumulations of proteinaceous material, spherical or elongate, sharply delineated, and varying in size, many 20 to 60 μ in diameter, though others are much smaller and the largest ones may be more than twice that size. There is variance in tinctorial features and in texture, presumably as an indication of the progression of degenerative changes. Many spheroids contain slightly eosinophilic, finely granular material, and occasionally stain paler at their periphery. Others are coarsely granular or contain clefts, coarse vacuoles, or a concentric or radial internal structure; the latter type has been referred to as "spike ball" bodies. Variance in texture is accompanied with variance in staining ranging from eosinophilic to amphophilic or basophilic. Empty microcystic spaces and spaces containing shrunken residua of spheroids suggest that progressive degeneration of spheroids leads to their eventual disintegration. An abundance of empty spaces makes the neuropil of the affected nuclei appear spongy. The development and degeneration of spheroids elicit little astrocytic glial response; a rare microglial nodule may form about a spheroid.

Spheroids are argyrophilic, but the argyrophilia is often less pronounced in the center than at the periphery. The main advantage of silver impregnations is the demonstration of continuity of spheroids with axons or other cell processes in sections cut parallel to their axes. The histochemical reactions of spheroids have been studied extensively in hopes of identifying storage of a specific chemical compound. No characteristic histochemical feature has emerged, however, the reactions indicating a proteinaceous material containing complex lipids and carbohydrates (Cowen and Olmstead, 1963; and many others), as well as increased activities of several oxydative enzymes (Huttenlocher and Gilles, 1967). These histochemical features evidently are representative of the accumulation within the spheroids of axoplasm containing variable proportions of normal or abnormal axoplasmic organelles. Electron micrographs disclose distended cell processes, some enveloped by stretched, thinned, distended myelin sheaths. They are crowded with mitochondria and endoplasmic reticulum, as well as with focal aggregates of tubular filamentous material, densely packed fibrils, cyrstalloid formations, osmophilic bodies, multivesicular bodies and abnormal membranous aggregates (Kamoshita *et al.*, 1968; Hedley-Whyte *et al.*, 1968; Toga *et al.*, 1970; and others).

Preponderance of evidence indicates that most spheroids develop from axons, particularly from their terminal presynaptic portions as shown repeatedly in cortical biopsies. Swellings also develop more proximal, including the course of fibers through the white matter. There are also light microscopic observations on spheroid formation from swollen dendrites, such as from the dendrites of large spinal motor neurons or of Purkinje cells in the atrophic cerebellum. Some investigators emphasize a preponderance, generally, of spheroid formation from the proximal segments of axons, but this appears to be more characteristic of Purkinje cells than of neurons in general.

The regional distribution of spheroids in the brain is characterized by their preponderance in gray matter. Any portion of the nervous system may be involved, but changes tend to be most severe in various nuclear groups of the tegmentum of the brain stem and in the dorsal half of the cervical spinal cord. Fewer spheroids are found in the cerebellar nuclei and cerebellar cortex, and they are scattered in the basal ganglia without specific topographic preference. Spheroids tend to be inconspicuous in the cerebral cortex. There are, instead, numerous, small, pale eosinophilic bodies, 10 to 15 μ in size and often of angular shape, in the neuropil or attached to neuronal surfaces. In electron micrographs they correspond to altered presynaptic endings and were thought to be a type of degeneration characteristic of certain types of synapses (Hedley-Whyte *et al.*, 1968). Altered synaptic endings may be found in abundance in electron micrographs even if no changes were discernible with the light microscope (Herman *et al.*, 1969; Sandbank *et al.*, 1970). Neuraxonal dystrophy also involves the peripheral nervous system, and swollen axons with crowded organelles are seen in the myenteric plexus (Kamoshita *et al.*, 1968; Haberland *et al.*, 1972) and in the terminal branches of motor fibers in the skeletal muscle. Electron microscopic examination of muscle biopsies has been suggested for the clinical diagnosis of the disease (Berard-Badier *et al.*, 1971; Sengel and Stoebner, 1972).

The atrophy of the cerebellum may involve either the entire cortex or portions thereof. It is usually seen in its endstages with loss of Purkinje cells and the granular layer, shrinkage of the molecular layer, and persistence of Bergmann-glia cells which undergo reactive proliferation. There is pallor of the white matter in myelin stains, most marked in the folia and diminishing toward the deeper portions of white matter. Dendritic swellings (asteroid bodies) in the molecular layer and axon swellings (torpedoes) in the granular layer may be seen in persisting Purkinje cells. The changes are like those seen in the cerebellar atrophy caused by other metabolic disease (Chapter 31). Jellinger and Seitelberger (1968) suggested that the cerebellar changes develop during the initial phase of the disease, based on their findings in a 6-month-old boy in whom the cerebellar changes dominated the lesions. Absence of Purkinje cells associated with widespread spheroid formation was also seen in a girl stillborn at term, in whom neuraxonal dystrophy coexisted with osteoporosis (Fitch *et al.*, 1973). The cerebellar atrophy in human neuraxonal dystrophy is similar to the cerebellar atrophy associated with widespread axon dystrophy in the inherited boggler syndrome in the deer mouse (Vandermeer and Barto, 1969).

The basal ganglia show deposition of fine lipid droplets throughout the tissue or contained within macrophages. This change tends to be maximum in striatum and pallidum which may appear tightly crammed with lipid droplets in frozen sections and spongy after the extraction of the lipids during tissue processing. Histochemical methods suggest that the lipids are mostly neutral fat and cholesterol esters (Cowen and Olmstead, 1963). There is a light brown, finely granular PAS positive pigment consistent with lipofuscin. Neuronal density in the thalamus and basal ganglia is reduced, and the small cells of the striatum may be affected more than the large cells. There is also a reduced density of myelinated fibers in the lenticular nucleus, particularly in the pallidum, in a pattern reminiscent of "status dysmyelinisatus" (Chapter 8). Neither lipid deposition nor abnormal myelin patterns correspond in intensity to the local extent of spheroid formation. Abnormal pigmentation of the basal ganglia may occur, on occasion, in rapidly progressing courses but is seen more often in cases with protracted courses. In these the nucleus pallidus and the red zone (pars reticularis) of the substantia nigra may show a grossly visible yellowish discoloration. Microscopically, there are finely granular or larger mulberry shape concretions of an iron-containing pigment having a brownish to greenish color in hematoxylin eosin stains. There is also a diffuse iron staining throughout the tissue, and fine grains of pigment are scattered throughout the neuropil or are concentrated in glia cells, outlining their processes.

In addition to the changes described above, there may be diffuse pallor or degeneration of various fiber systems, most strikingly of the corticospinal tracts, the dorsal spinal tracts, spino-cerebellar tracts and the optic system. Loss of myelinated fibers corresponds to a decrease in cerebrosides in biochemical studies, but there is no evidence for the accumulation of an abnormal lipid or carbohydrate (Haberland *et al.*, 1972). A variety of other lesions were reported for infants suffering from neuraxonal dystrophy, such as status marmoratus of the basal ganglia, micronodular mineralization (Chapter 1), or diffuse fatty change of white matter (Chapter 5); these are to be considered coincidental rather than related to neuraxonal dystrophy. The general autopsy discloses, in some cases, clusters of histiocyte-like cells with large eosinophilic cytoplasmic bodies in the spleen, lymph nodes, thyroid and other organs. They have been interpreted as a neurovisceral form of neuraxonal dystrophy, but this concept is not supported by biochemical data.

Hallervorden-Spatz Disease of Infantile Onset. The classification of infantile neuraxonal dystrophy as a nosologic entity or as a juvenile form of Hallervorden-Spatz disease has been a matter of debate. Both disease processes have the occurrence of dystrophic axons in common, and there is overlap of other features as well, particularly in terms of abnormal pigmentation of the basal ganglia. Hence, most authors consider neuraxonal dystrophy and Hallervorden-Spatz disease related conditions, or even opposite ends of a spectrum in the manifestations of one and the same disorder. The final test of these interpretations will come with the discovery of the basic nature of the disease process; any subclassification short of this knowledge remains tentative, and a given case may fall into different subtypes depending on the criterion used for subclassification. Gilman and Barrett (1973) distinguished three groups according to the distribution of axon swellings and the presence of pigmentation: 1. Widespread spheroids without abnormal pigmentation, 2. widespread spheroids with abnormal pigmentation of basal ganglia, 3. spheroids and abnormal pigmentation confined to the basal ganglia. Their paper and that of Richter (1972) should be consulted for a listing of case reports beyond those quoted in this text. The first two types of Gilman and Barrett's classification are considered here under Neuraxonal Dystrophy, the third under Hallervorden-Spatz Disease.

The morbid anatomy of Hallervorden-Spatz disease in adults, with a list of autopsy cases, was reviewed by Dooling *et al.* (1974). Its occasional onset in infancy (Eicke, 1940; Bischoff and Regli, 1963; Indravasu and Dexter, 1968) is of interest in the present text in regard to the overlap between these cases and infantile neuraxonal dystrophy. Reported instances of infantile Hallervorden-Spatz disease had neurologic disturbances dating to early infancy, occasionally to birth, with a protracted course, death occurring later than the 10th year of life or in early adulthood. The clinical course was often associated with severe dystonic phenomena, induced by slowness of development and a progressive neurologic disorder involving disturbances of gait and speech, tremor, leading to spasticity and, finally, opistotonus.

The morbid anatomy is similar to that of Hallervorden-Spatz disease in adults showing excessive pigmentation of the red zone of the substantia nigra which appears larger than normal to the naked eye as well as in sections stained with myelin stains. A similar discoloration is seen in the pallidum. Microscopic changes are most pronounced in the pallidum and in the red zone of the substantia nigra where there is loss of neurons and gliosis associated with great numbers of spheroids. The electron microscopic features of the spheroids are indistinguishable from those in infantile neuraxonal dystrophy (Defendini *et al.*, 1973), adding evidence to the intrinsic similarity between the two disease manifestations. Contrary to neuraxonal dystrophy, the tissue changes are restricted to or prevail in the basal ganglia, and cell loss outside of the latter is slight. However, spheroids may be found beyond the affected nuclei and the cerebellum may show variation in Purkinje cell density or cortical atrophy. Only minimal alterations are present in the cerebral cortex. It seems appropriate, on the grounds of the available evidence, to consider Hallervorden-Spatz disease a localized form of neuraxonal dystrophy.

References

Bischoff, A., Regli, F.: Die Hallervorden-Spatzsche Krankheit. Arch. Psychiat. Nervenkr. 204: 589—602, 1963.

Berard-Badier, M., Gamberelli, D., Pinsard, N., *et al.:* Infantile neuroaxonal dystrophy or Seitelberger's disease. II. Peripheral nerve involvement: Electron microscopic study in one case. Acta neuropath. (Berl.) Suppl. V: 30—39, 1971.

Blakemore, W. F., Cavanagh, J. B.: "Neuroaxonal dystrophy" occurring in an experimental "dying back" process in the rat. Brain 92: 789—804, 1969.

Cordy, D. R., Richards, W. P., Bradford, G. E.: Systemic neuraxonal dystrophy in Suffolk sheep. Acta neuropath. (Berl.) 8: 113—140, 1967.

Cowen, D., Olmstead, E. V.: Infantile neuroaxonal dystrophy. J. Neuropath. exp. Neurol. 22: 175—236, 1963.

Defendini, R., Markesbery, W. R., Mastri, A. R., Duffy, P. E.: Hallervorden-Spatz disease and infantile neuroaxonal dystrophy. Ultrastructural observations, anatomical pathology and nosology. J. Neurol. Sci. 20: 7—23, 1973.

Dooling, E. C., Schoene, W. C., Richardson, E. P.: Hallervorden-Spatz syndrome. Arch. Neurol. (Chic.) 30: 70—83, 1974.

Eicke, W. J.: Neue Beobachtungen über die Hallervorden-Spatzsche Krankheit. Arch. Psychiat. Nervenkr. 11: 514—546, 1940.

Fitch, N., Carpenter, S., Lahance, R. C.: Prenatal axonal dystrophy and osteoporosis. Arch. Path. (Chic.) 95: 297—301, 1973.

Friede, R. L., Knoller, M.: Proximo-diatal increase in enzymic activity in the dorsal spinal tracts. J. Neurochem. 11: 679—686, 1964.

Fujisawa, K.: A unique type of axon alteration, so-called axonal dystrophy as seen in Goll's nucleus of 277 cases of controls. Acta neuropath. (Berl.) 8: 255—275, 1967.

Gilman, S., Barrett, R. E.: Hallervorden-Spatz disease and infantile neuroaxonal dystrophy. Clinical characteristics and nosological considerations. J. Neurol. Sci. 19: 189—205, 1973.

Haberland, C., Brunngraber, E. G., Witting, L. A.: Infantile neuroaxonal dystrophy. Neuropathological and biochemical study of a case. Arch. Neurol. (Chic.) 26: 391—402, 1972.

Hedley-Whyte, E. T., Gilles, F. H., Uzman, B. G.: Infantile neuroaxonal dystrophy. A disease characterized by altered terminal axons and synaptic endings. Neurol. (Minneap.) 18: 892—906, 1968.

Herman, M. M., Huttenlocher, P. R., Bensch, K. G.: Electron microscopic observations in infantile neuroaxonal dystrophy. Report of a cortical biopsy and review of the recent literature. Arch. Neurol. (Chic.) 20: 19—34, 1969.

Huttenlocher, P. R., Gilles, F. H.: Infantile neuroaxonal dystrophy: Clinical, pathologic and histochemical findings in a family with 3 affected siblings. Neurology (Minneap.) 17: 1174—1184, 1967.

Indravasu, S., Dexter, R. A.: Infantile neuroaxonal dystrophy and its relationship to Hallervorden-Spatz disease. Neurology (Minneap.) 18: 693—699, 1968.

Jellinger, K., Jirásek, A.: Neuroaxonal dystrophy in man: Character and natural history. Acta neuropath. (Berl.) Suppl. V: 3—16, 1971.

— Seitelberger, F.: Infantile neuroaxonale Dystrophie. Frühform mit bevorzugtem Kleinhirnbefall. Acta neuropath. (Berl.) 10: 123—131, 1968.

Kamoshita, S., Neustein, H. B., Landing, B. H.: Infantile neuroaxonal dystrophy with neonatal onset. Neuropathologic and electron microscopic observations. J. Neuropath. exp. Neurol. 27: 300—323, 1968.

Lampert, P., Blumberg, J. M., Pentschew, A.: An electron microscopic study of dystrophic axons in the gracile and cuneate nuclei of vitamin E-deficient rats. J. Neuropath. exp. Neurol. 28: 60—77, 1964.

Lampert, P. W.: A comparative electron microscopic study of reactive, degenerating, regenerating, and dystrophic axons. J. Neuropath. exp. Neurol. 26: 345—368, 1967.

Lindenberg, R., Freytag, E.: Brainstem lesions characteristic of traumatic hyperextension of the head. Arch. Path. (Chic.) 90: 509—515, 1970.

Newberne, J. W., Robinson, V. B., Estill, L., Brinkman, D. C.: Granular structures in brains of apparently normal digs. Amer. J. vet. Res. 21: 782—786, 1960.

Pentschew, A., Schwarz, K.: Systemic axonal dystrophy in vitamin E deficient adult rats. With implication in human neuropathology. Acta neuropath. (Berl.) 1: 313—334, 1962.

Rabinowicz, T., Wildi, E.: Spastic amaurotic axonal idiocy. A familial juvenile form of a lipo-glyco-protidic thesaurismosis including a pallidal siderosis. In: Cerebral Lipoidoses (Cumings, J. N., ed.), pp. 34—47. Springfield, Ill.: Thomas 1957.

Richter, E.: Ein Beitrag zur infantilen neuro-axonalen Dystrophie. Vergleich der histopathologischen Befunde und des klinischen Bildes mit der Hallervorden-Spatzschen Krankheit. Z. Neurol. 201: 160—195, 1972.

Sandbank, U., Lerman, P., Geifman, M.: Infantile neuroaxonal dystrophy: Cortical anoxic and presynaptic changes. Acta neuropath. (Berl.) 16: 342—352, 1970.

Seitelberger, F.: Eine unbekannte Form von infantiler lipoidspeichernder Krankheit des Gehirns. Proc. First Int. Congr. Neuropath., Rome 3: 323—333, 1952, Rosenberg and Sellier, Torino.

Sengel, A., Stoebner, P.: Intérêt de la biopsie neuro-musculaire dans le diagnostic de la dystrophie neuro-axonale infantile. Etude ultrastructurale de 3 cas dont 2 familiaux. Acta neuropath. (Berl.) 21: 109—216, 1972.

Slagel, D. E., Hartmann, H. A.: The distribution of neuroaxonal lesions in mice injected with iminodipropionitrile with special reference to the vestibular system. J. Neuropath. exp. Neurol. 24: 599—620, 1965.

Sung, J. H.: Neuroaxonal dystrophy in mucoviscidosis. J. Neuropath. exp. Neurol. 23: 567—583, 1964.

— Stadlan, E. M.: Neuraxonal dystrophy in congenital biliary atresia. J. Neuropath. exp. Neurol. 25: 118—120, 1966.

Thilbault, J.: Neuroaxonal dystrophy. A case of nonpigmented type and protracted course. Acta neuropath. (Berl.) 21: 232—238, 1972.

Toga, M., Berard-Badier, M., Bambarelli-Dubois, D.: La dystrophie neuroaxonale infantile ou maladie de Seitelberger. Etude clinique, histologique et ultrastructurale de deux observations. Acta neuropath. (Berl.) 15: 327—350, 1970.

Vandermeer, J., Barto, E.: Axonal dystrophy in a deer mouse (peromyscus maniculatus) with an inherited ataxia and tremor. J. Neuropath. exp. Neurol. 28: 257—266, 1969.

Woodward, J. C., Collins, G. H., Hessler, J. R.: Feline hereditary neuraxonal dystrophy. Amer. J. Path. 74: 551—566, 1974.

44. Spongy Degeneration of the Central Nervous System and Other Forms of Spongy Myelinopathy

The hereditary infantile disease known as spongy degeneration of the central nervous system of the van Bogaert-Bertrand type belongs to a group of conditions characterized by a microvacuolar, spongy state affecting predominantly, but not exclusively, the white matter. Sponginess of the tissue, or status spongiosus, as revealed by the light microscope, is not a specific type of tissue alteration. Taken on its own merit, it is an arbitrary criterion for the classification of disease entities. However, the status spongiosus of spongy degeneration of the van Bogaert-Bertrand type was shown on electron microscopic examination to be the result of a specific alteration in the fine structure of myelin, consisting of accumulation of large pockets of fluid between the lamellae of the sheaths. This change needs to be distinguished from the splitting of lamellae without outpouching of the sheaths as a preparative artefact or with retrogressive changes in the sheaths. Intramyelinic fluid accumulation, or spongy myelinopathy, is shared by the otherwise heterogeneous diseases described in the present chapter.

There is presently no clear-cut etiologic distinction between the diseases described in this chapter and those in the next (Chapter 45) on disturbances of intermediary metabolism. The etiology of spongy degeneration of the van Bogaert-Bertrand type is unknown, and future studies may well realize its derivation from a disturbance of the intermediary metabolism. There are, on the other hand, several known disturbances of intermediary metabolism, such as maple syrup urine disease, glycinosis and others (Chapter 45) which produce light microscopic changes in the brain that are quite similar to those in familial spongy degeneration. Indeed, some case reports on spongy degeneration may well have been unrecognized disturbances of amino acid metabolism. The fine structure of the status spongiosus in disturbances of amino acid metabolism has not been studied with the electron microscope as yet; if such data become available, they may well disclose a spongy myelinopathy, in which case these disturbances of amino acid metabolism would have to be considered along with the conditions described in the present chapter.

In spite of these uncertainties, spongy myelinopathy was considered the most reliable feature for classifying the diseases described in this chapter. Spongy myelinopathy is clearly different from the lesions produced by other leukodystrophic processes. The fact that it can be produced by more than one disease implies a similarity in pathogenesis, the same mechanism apparently being triggered by different agents. To set a frame of reference, the chapter is prefaced with a brief review of the fine structure of status spongiosus in general, including pertinent tissue artefacts.

Fine Structure and Classification of Status Spongiosus. The term "status spongiosus" in neuropathology designates a rarefied, loose, microvacuolar appearance of the tissue regardless of its causes. By convention, the term "spongy degeneration" became applied to status spongiosus of the white matter, while the term "spongiform encephalopathy" usually denotes a disease process causing status spongiosus in the gray matter; both terms are, strictly speaking, synonymous. Jellinger and Seitelberger (1970) make a distinction between a "spongy state" from loss of tissue and "spongy alteration" from the swelling and vacuolization of cells; however, their classification is difficult to apply at the light microscopic level. The review of the fine structure of status spongiosus by Adornato and Lampert (1971) shows that a spongy, microvacuolar texture of the tissue seen in light microscopic examination may result from the accumulation of fluids in entirely different tissue compartments—that is intracellular, extracellular or intramyelinic. Vacuolization of white matter may also result from autolysis or from supravital or preparatory tissue artefacts.

Intracellular fluid accumulation occurs most commonly in astrocytes, affecting their perikaryon and processes as well as their perivascular footplates. Distension of the latter produces the perivascular loosening of tissue structure often seen in routine preparations of edematous or normal brains. Swelling of astrocytes develops very rapidly postmortem, faster than in any other cell type, and it is responsible for the "watery" appearance of the cytoplasm on electron microscopic examination. Swelling of astrocytes is also a characteristic feature of brain edema. Oligodendroglia cells are less prone to swelling when examined with the electron microscope, although they commonly show an "empty" perinuclear halo in light microscopic preparations, resulting from supravital or postmortem changes. Swelling of oligodendroglia usually does not cause status spongiosus, except in certain experimental intoxications such as 6-amino-nicotinamide poisoning. Status spongiosus of the gray matter may be caused by swelling of neuronal elements, in the form of focal clearings of neuronal cytoplasm, of membrane-bounded vacuoles within the perikarya, or in the vacuolization of pre- or postsynaptic neuronal processes. Neuronal swelling appears to be the cause of the sponginess of the gray matter in the "spongy encephalopathies" caused by slow virus infection, including Creutzfeldt-Jakob disease, kuru, scrapie and mink encephalopathy. Neuronal changes may also produce status spongiosus of the white matter, such as in the form of focal axonal swellings of optic fibers in acute glaucoma. Extracellular accumulation of fluid causes status spongiosus in edematous white matter, such as in the vasogenic type of brain edema from altered vascular permeability in experimental cold injury, intracranial neoplasms, lead poisoning and inflammations, or from the seepage of CSF into the periventricular white matter in chronic hydrocephalus. Status spongiosus from intramyelinic accumulation of fluids is common to the diseases described in the present chapter.

These *in vivo* alterations of the fine structure of tissue need to be distinguished from the loosening of tissue texture from postmortem autolysis in poorly preserved specimens, and, also, from the more characteristic vacuolar artefacts of white matter of normal or diseased brains, commonly referred to as Buscaino (1929) bodies. Buscaino bodies need to be recognized as nonspecific, non-diagnostic artefacts, even though their derivation from premortem anoxia, agonal changes, postmortem autolysis, or techniques of fixation and tissue storage are not entirely clear. They present as oval or grape-shaped vacuoles which may be filled with basophilic, moderately metachromatic material. The latter is often dissolved upon tissue processing, leaving only an empty, smooth-walled cavity approximating 50 to 60 μ in diameter. Electron microscopic examination shows the Buscaino bodies filled with a debris of jumbled lamellar fragments derived from disintegrated myelin sheaths. Autolysis or Buscaino bodies cause tissue changes that may interfere with the assessment of spongy degeneration, particularly in poorly preserved brains.

Spongy Degeneration of the Central Nervous System (van Bogaert-Bertrand Type). Spongy degeneration of the central nervous system was established as a clinical and pathologic entity by van Bogaert and Bertrand (1949) in a report of a family of Polish jews in whom 3 infants were afflicted by a progressive, fatal neurologic disease. The pedigree of this family was later supplemented by van Bogaert (1963). The earlier report of Globus and Strauss (1928) may have been of the same condition, and certainly that of Canavan (1931) after whom the disease is sometimes named. Her case was reexamined and included in the series of 7 cases by Banker *et al.* (1964); these authors researched its family and found that two other infants had been afflicted by a similar disease. Reviews of the literature include the monographs of van Bogaert and Bertrand (1967) and Jellinger and Seitelberger (1970). The quotations in the following text are based on the recent review by Adachi *et al.* (1973), listing 94 reported cases, 72 histologically verified.

Spongy degeneration of the central nervous system typically manifests in early infancy, although a small number of connatal and juvenile cases have been reported. In the prevalent infantile form of the disease normal birth and early postnatal development is followed, after a few months of life, by an arrest in development, with sluggishness, hypotonia and inability to control the head. Concurrently, a progressive enlargement of the head sets in, being a rather characteristic feature of the disease. The generalized hypotonia subsequently gives way to attacks of hyperextension resembling decerebrate and decorticate posturing and, finally, persistent hypertonia and spasticity. Choreoathetoid movements and myoclonic episodes are common. There is failure to respond to visual stimuli, and the eyes show episodic saccadic movements. Fundoscopy shows pale discs. There is a progressive deterioration extending over several years, death usually occurring near the age of 4.

The disease runs in families, affecting both sexes with equal frequency; genetic studies indicate an autosomal recessive inheritance pattern. Most of the early reports concern families of jewish extraction, many of whom can be traced to the Vilna-Kovno region of Lithuania and Poland and the Wolhynia region of the Western Ukraine. However, non-jewish families of a variety of ethnic backgrounds were described with increasing frequency in later reports and comprise approximately one-fourth of the known cases.

The clinical course tends to be rather stereotype, but certain variances have been observed. In the protracted course the infants may survive beyond the 5th year of life with corresponding modifications in their cerebral lesions (Adachi and Volk, 1968). A connatal form of spongy degeneration has also been described, with hypotonia and lethargy from birth on or developing shortly after birth, inducing a rapid deterioration leading to death within a few weeks (Sacks *et al.*, 1965). The classification of the connatal form remains problematic as no amino acid studies had been done, and as the clinical and pathologic findings are very similar to those observed in disturbances in amino acid metabolism (Chapter 45).

A juvenile course of spongy degeneration was observed in only a few instances, all of whom were sporadic and of non-jewish extraction. The onset of the neurologic disorder occurred after age 5, and survival was to late adolescence. There was a progressive cerebellar syndrome, with tremor and ataxia, mental deterioration, loss of vision, deafness and general spasticity. Fundoscopy showed optic atrophy and retinitis pigmentosa; no enlargement of the head occurs with this form of the disease (Jellinger and Seitelberger, 1969, 1970).

The cerebral lesions of spongy degeneration vary somewhat with the course of the disease. In the infantile form there is an initial enlargement of the brain without anomalies of its outer surface markings. Brain weight is increased by a factor of 1.55 during the first 20 months of life, with little or no enlargement of the cerebral ventricles. Upon longer survival the increase in cerebral volume is less marked, as atrophy of the white matter develops with ensuing ventricular enlargement; the brain weight returns to approximately normal values by the 30th month. The brain may be atrophic and lighter than normal in the protracted course of the disease or in its juvenile form. The cut surface of the cerebral hemispheres shows a poor delineation of gray and white matter; the latter is soft, edematous, gelatinous or translucent, particularly in the subcortical portions which may be deeply sunken below the cut surface. There is no tendency to cavitation. Atrophy of optic nerves may be evident. The white matter of the cerebellar hemispheres is similarly affected and there may be slight atrophy of the cerebellar cortex. Brain stem and spinal cord appear pale, but otherwise without distinct alterations. The rest of the autopsy is noncontributory.

The most obvious light microscopic feature consists of an abundant vacuolization of the tissue having a predilection for certain portions of white matter and the cerebellar cortex (Fig. 151). The vacuoles are tightly crowded, rounded or oval, 5 to 100 μ in diameter; they are optically empty, and no abnormal contents are demonstrable with histochemical reactions in frozen or in paraffin-embedded sections. There is no consistent topographic relation between vacuoles and other tissue elements; glial or neuronal perikarya may occasionally border their edges, and nerve fibers may curve around their periphery. The long axes of the vacuoles tend to be oriented parallel to the prevailing course of fibers in the white matter.

The vacuolization of the tissue in the cerebral hemispheres is maximum at the junction of cortex and subcortical white matter. It involves the deeper cortical layers, diminishing toward the surface. Sponginess also diminishes toward the depth of white matter with least affection of the periventricular tissue. The subcortical tissue is devoid of myelin sheaths. Oligodendroglia nuclei may be present in normal numbers in the initial phase of the disease, but their number diminishes with its progression. Axons, likewise, are initially spared, being demonstrable near the vacuoles with silver impregnation. Scattered axonal swellings may be seen on scrutiny (Kamoshita *et al.*, 1967), evidently indicating a secondary axonal destruction rather than a concurrent primary axon dystrophy (Chapter 43). There is little or no evidence of myelin breakdown in the form of neutral fat or lipid-laden macrophages. Proliferation of astroglia with reactive hypertrophy is seen in the affected tissue; fibrillary gliosis in Holzer stains tends to be slight or absent initially, but it may become intense upon complete loss of myelin. Vacuolization of the tissue also involves the internal capsule, the fornix and the corpus callosum, although these fiber systems are generally less severely affected than the subcortical white matter and show no absence of myelin sheaths. Sponginess may also involve the optic nerve, and certain nuclear groups rich in myelinated fibers, such as pallidum, thalamus, or dentate nuclei.

The cerebellar white matter exhibits changes similar to those described above; there is also involvement of the cerebellar cortex by excessive vacuolization at the boundary of the molecular and granular layers, that is at the same level where postmortem autolytic changes are common in poorly preserved brains. Excessive sponginess at this interface may cleave the molecular layer from the granular layer, the intervening space being bridged by thin strands of tissue [1]. Cleavage occurs below the perikarya of the Purkinje cells which remain attached to the inner surface of the molecular layer along with many of the Bergmann-glia nuclei. The displacement of the Purkinje cells away from the granular layer is often erroneously described as displacement into the molecular layer, a change characteristic of granular layer aplasia (Chapter 31) which does not occur in spongy degeneration. No changes are evident in the perikarya of the Purkinje cells. The intensity of vacuolization diminishes in the cerebellar granular layer; the molecular layer is usually spared.

Involvement of the various fiber tracts of brain stem and spinal cord varies but, generally, tends to be less severe than that of cerebellar and cerebral hemispheric white matter. There may be a diffuse pallor in myelin stains, particularly in cases of protracted course. Marked vacuolization of fiber tracts in brain stem and cord has been described for cases that were considered the connatal form of the disease. No sponginess is evident in peripheral nerves. Vacuolated histiocytes in the perineural tissue and segmental axonal swellings reported by Suzuki (1968) were not seen by others (Adornato *et al.*, 1972).

The neuronal population of gray matter remains unaffected in the infantile course of the disease, but a marked proliferation of astroglia is seen, particularly in the cerebral cortex and the basal ganglia. These cells resemble Alzheimer type II glia cells (Chapter 45) in their nuclear features and in the absence of cytoplasm, as observed with the light microscope. Their nuclei are abnormally large, variably shaped, having sparsely distributed nuclear chromatin and a well defined nuclear membrane, but no intranuclear deposits

[1] Many authors describe this zone of cleavage as "lamina dissecans", but this term is better reserved for the type of lamination characteristic of fetal cerebellar cortex (Chapter 1).

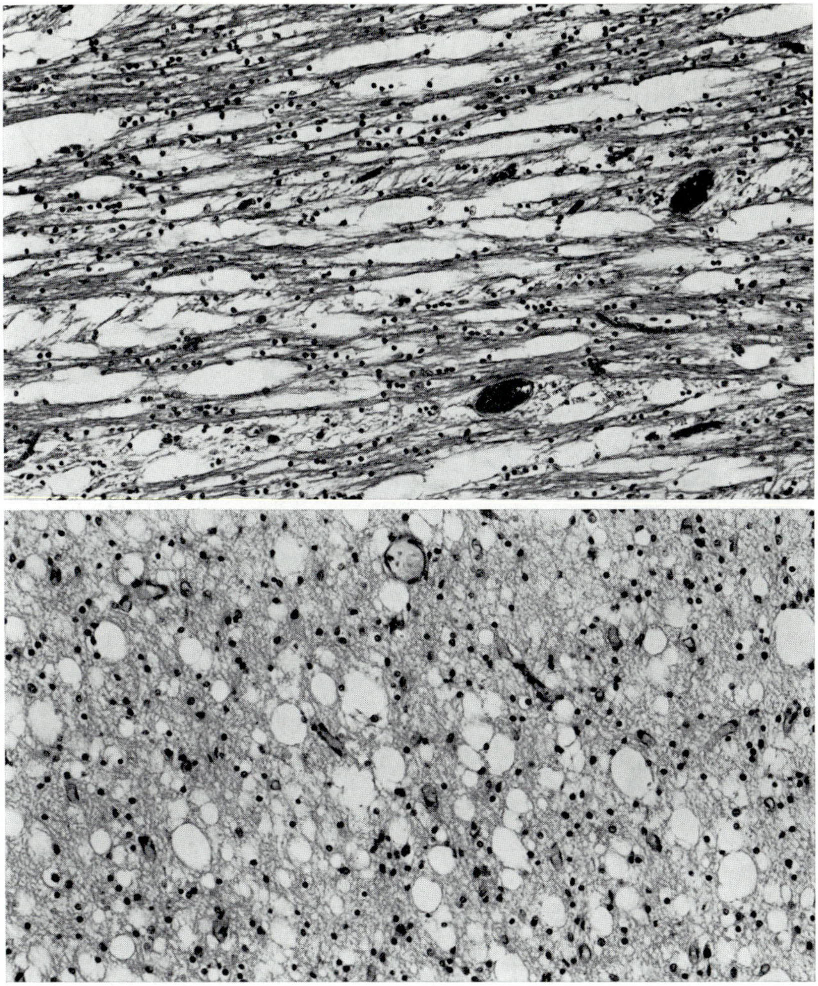

Fig. 151. Spongy degeneration—van Bogaert-Bertrand type. Top: Vacuoles in the white matter have their axes parallel to the course of fibers. Bottom: Spongy state of the subcortical white matter; PAS $\times 225$

of glycogen. These cells are most conspicuous in the cerebral cortex, and their nuclei may form pairs or clusters if proliferation is marked. They are also seen in the subcortical white matter and in the basal ganglia, while they are generally absent from the nuclear groups of brain stem and cord. They are not prevalent in the spongy portions of white matter, where nonspecific reactive astrocytes are more common.

The protracted course of the disease is associated with more widespread, extensive vacuolization which extends throughout the cerebral cortex and is accompanied with loss of neurons. Adachi and Volk (1968) also describe, in addition to Alzheimer type II glia, occasional abnormally large, bizarre, pleomorphic glial nuclei, 45 to 75 μ in diameter, having a finely dispersed nuclear chromatin and no visible cytoplasm. Except for being somewhat smaller, they resemble Alzheimer type I glia. Their derivation from Alzheimer type II glia is a matter of conjecture. The cerebral changes in the juvenile form of the disease are similar to those in the protracted course, showing widespread demyelination of the centrum semiovale and of the corpus callosum and extreme sponginess and atrophy of the tissue (Jellinger

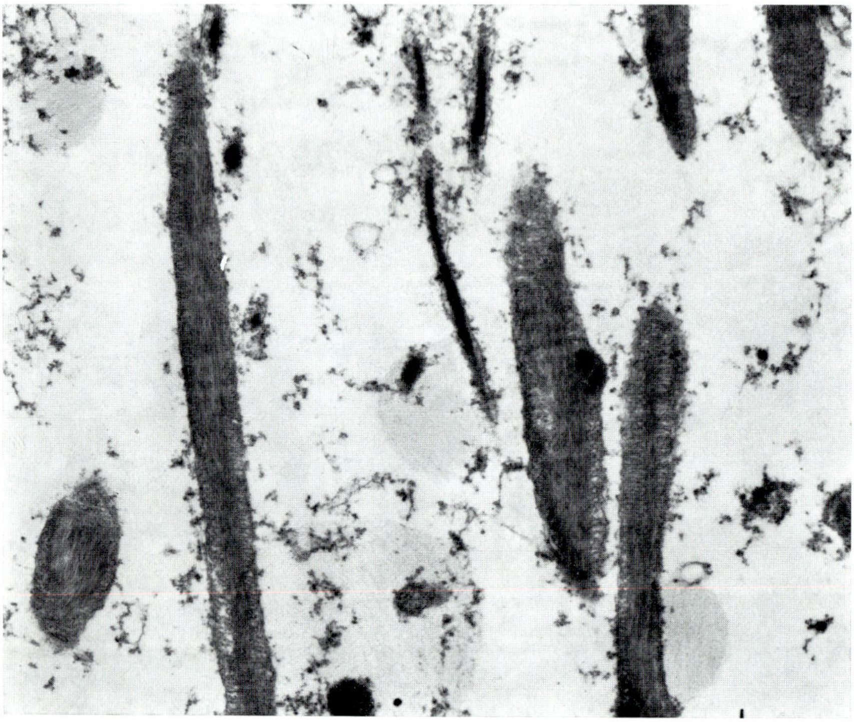

Fig. 152. Spongy degeneration; mitochondrial changes (courtesy of Dr. Lampert)

and Seitelberger, 1969). In addition, axonal dystrophy may be found in the striato-nigral system, presumably representing a precocious, age-dependent axon dystrophy (Chapter 43).

Electron microscopic examination reveals that two types of alterations in fine structure cause the sponginess of the tissue, that is, intramyelinic accumulation of fluid and excessive swelling of astrocytes (Adachi *et al.*, 1966; Adornato *et al.*, 1972; and others). The fine structural changes observed in the protracted course of the disease (Gambetti *et al.*, 1969) are essentially the same as those in the infantile course.

The swollen astrocytes have enlarged nuclei with sparse chromatin granules and prominent nucleoli. Their "watery" cytoplasm contains enormously elongated abnormal mitochondria, which may reach 15 μ in length (Fig. 152). No mitochondrial changes are seen in cells other than astrocytes. The mitochondria contain a central core of a striated or filamentous matrix composed of fine granules arranged in chains. The mitochondrial cristae are formed by abnormal infoldings of the inner mitochondrial membrane, presenting in profiles resembling buds, bridges or contorted segments.

The intramyelinic accumulation of fluid forms huge cystic spaces that do not contain electron dense material and are lined with layers of myelin leaflets which are continuous with the sheaths of adjacent nerve fibers (Fig. 153).

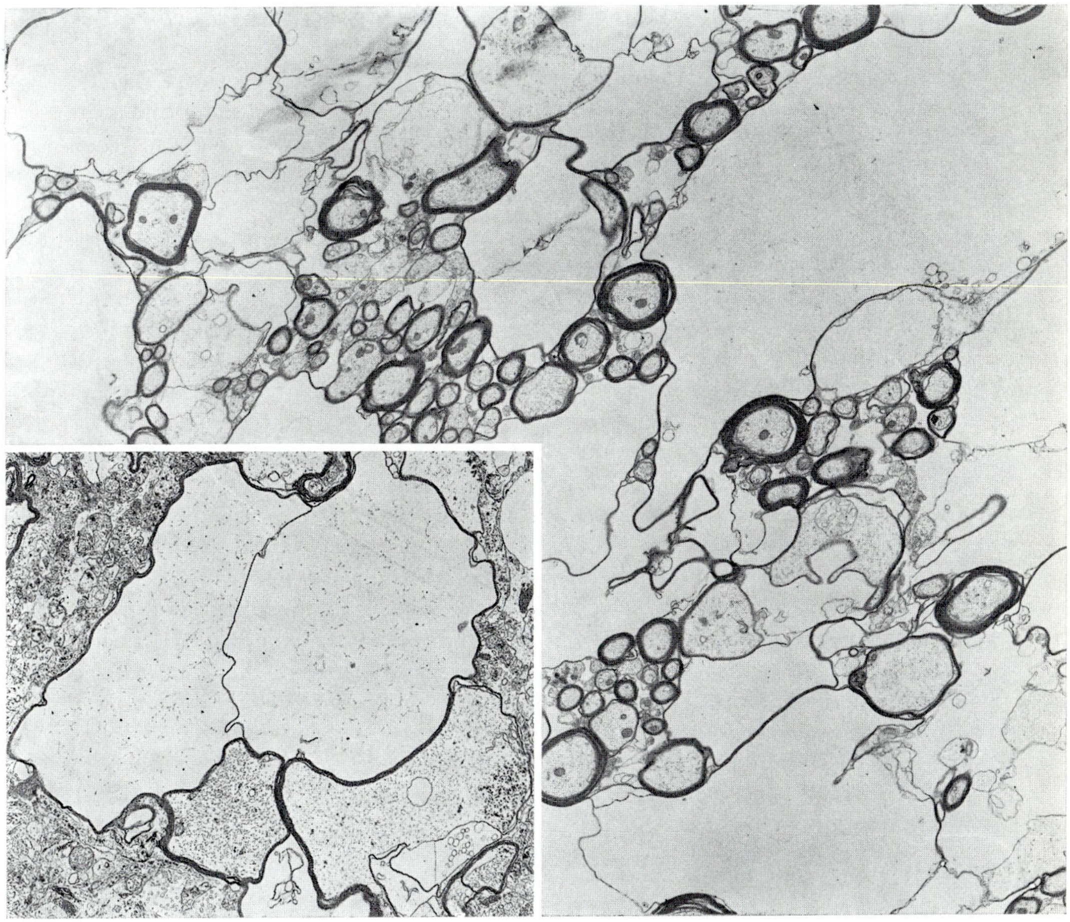

Fig. 153. Spongy myelinopathy; large vacuoles form from splitting of myelin sheaths and intramyelinic fluid accumulation. From an infant with hexachlorophene encephalopathy. Inset: Experimental hexachlorophene encephalopathy in the rat (courtesy of Dr. Lampert)

The vacuoles form from the splitting of the sheaths between two major dense lines at the level of the intermediary dense line. There may be multiple vacuoles within a given sheath. Secondary rupture of the myelin leaflets results in communication between the vacuoles and the extracellular space.

Pathogenetic Considerations. Although electron microscopic data contributed greatly to the understanding of spongy changes in the tissue, there is still incomplete understanding of the mutual interrelations between the various tissue alterations. The increase in the volume and in the weight of the brain during the early phase of the disease corresponds to an increase in water content (Blackwood and Cumings, 1954; Lees and Folch-Pi, 1961; Zu Rhein *et al.*, 1960; Kamoshita *et al.*, 1968). The increased water content had been attributed to chronic edema with secondary demyelination; it had also been postulated that a deficiency in myelination results from a primary failure in myelin formation (Blackwood and Cumings, 1954), or else, from a demyelinative process with accumulation of abnormal products of small molecular weight (Wolman, 1958). The electron microscopic demonstration of a specific type of intramyelinic edema, or spongy myelinopathy, suggests that this alteration is intimately related to the deficiency in myelin. Chemical analysis of isolated myelin (Kamoshita *et al.*, 1968) showed changes in composition thought to be characteristic of myelin in the process of undergoing destruction due to external nonspecific causes. These data, and the obvious destruction of myelin subsequent to its formation in the juvenile form of the disease, suggest strongly that spongy myelinopathy causes the destruction of myelin sheaths. It cannot be ruled out, on the other hand, that myelin formation may be hindered or abrogated if spongy myelinopathy develops while myelin formation is still in progress.

The fact that spongy myelinopathy is also induced by various neurotoxic agents suggests that all these processes have a common pathogenetic mechanism, apparently in the form of a loosening of the adhesion of myelin leaflets at the level of the intermediate dense line. The latter is continuous with the extracellular fluid compartment and provides a path for the diffusion of electron dense markers from the fluid encompassing the nerve fiber (Revel and Hamilton, 1969; Hall and Williams, 1971). Further, studies of the mechanism of the expansion of myelin sheaths in swollen fibers strongly suggest that the myelin leaflets may move over each other at the level of the intermediate dense line (Friede and Martinez, 1970; Friede and Miyagishi, 1972). These observations are consistent with a preferential splitting of sheats at the level of the intermediate dense line; however, the causes of this splitting as well as those responsible for the normal adhesion of myelin leaflets are still unknown.

The relations between the abnormalities in astrocytes and the spongy myelinopathy are likewise unknown. The abnormalities in astrocytic mitochondria and the similarity of the proliferating astrocytes to the Alzheimer type II glia cells of hepatic encephalopathy are suggestive of a metabolic derangement; moreover, there is a striking similarity between spongy degeneration and the cerebral lesions in disturbances of amino acid metabolism. However, no specific metabolic defect has been identified for spongy degeneration. An impairment in mitochondrial ATPase activity, suggested on the basis of histochemical stains (Adachi *et al.*, 1966), was not confirmed by enzyme assays (Adornato *et al.*, 1972). Increased calcium content of the tissue (Sacks *et al.*, 1965) has been attributed to a preparative artefact (Kamoshita *et al.*, 1968). The significance of abnormal elevation in urinary copper and zinc reported by Zu Rhein *et al.* (1960) is unclear.

Hexachlorophene Myelinopathy. Hexachlorophene myelinopathy was described by Powell *et al.* (1973) as a lesion caused in premature infants by repeated cutaneous application of hexachlorophene, which had been widely used as a germicidal agent in neonatal care. Hexachlorophene myelinopathy is of particular interest in that its lesions are readily reproducible in newborn rats, as well as in tadpoles (Webster *et al.*, 1974).

Premature infants appear to be more sensitive to hexachlorophene toxicity than infants of more than 32 weeks gestation, and repeated exposure appears to be necessary for inducing the cerebral changes; no specific clinical symptomatology has been described. Microscopic changes consist of vacuolization of myelinated tracts, most marked in the brain stem and including the medial longitudinal fascicle, medial lemniscus and superior cerebellar peduncle. There is no characteristic glial response in the affected tracts. Intralamellar cystic spaces within the myelin sheaths, similar to those in spongy degeneration, were found on electron microscopic examination (Powell *et al.*, 1973). Older infants are not entirely immune to hexachlorophene myelinopathy, as shown for a 2-year-old boy wo died following ingestion of large amounts of hexachlorophene (Martinez *et al.*, 1974).

Experimental hexachlorophene encephalopathy develops in rats after 2 weeks dietary exposure to the agent. The brain is grossly edematous, but there is no evidence of abnormal vascular permeability on injection of methylene blue. Microscopic examination discloses a marked status spongiosus of the white matter; intramyelinic fluid accumulation is seen with the electron microscope (Lampert *et al.*, 1973).

Neurotoxic Spongy Degeneration. Vacuolar degeneration of the white matter due to intramyelinic accumulation of fluid is caused by several neurotoxic agents other than hexachlorophene. These experimental intoxications may serve as a model for the understanding of at least certain aspects of spongy degeneration in man.

Intoxication of rats with triethyl tin induces a reversible neurologic syndrome of progressive weakness. Cerebral changes consist of an edema of the white matter of brain and spinal cord in the absence of neuronal changes in gray matter (Magee *et al.*, 1957). Electron microscopic examination of the white matter reveals intramyelinic accumulation of fluid, with splitting of the myelin sheaths at the level of the intermediate dense line, absence of affection of oligodendroglia cells, and a mild swelling of the astrocytes; no evidence of increased permeability of the blood brain barrier was found upon injection of methylene blue into the blood stream (Aleu *et al.*, 1963). Experimental triethyl tin intoxication, indeed, represents a milestone in the understanding of spongy myelinopathy, in that the intramyelinic type of fluid accumulation was first observed in this model.

Feeding of isonicotinic acid hydracide ("isoniazid", used in the treatment of tuberculosis) to immature pekin ducks induces a neurologic syndrome of tremors and trunk ataxia; isoniazid also has similar toxicity in dogs or in chickens (Carlton, 1967). Pathologic changes consist of a spongy change and demyelination, affecting preferentially the cerebellar white matter, as well as proliferation of astroglia resembling Alzheimer type II glia cells. Axonal changes are not a predominant feature, but beaded axis cylinders are seen in the affected tissue and torpedoes in the axons of Purkinje cells (Carlton and Kreutzberg, 1966; Carlton, 1967). The spongy change of the white matter was initially interpreted as resulting from liquefaction of astrocytes (Kreutzberg and Carlton, 1967), but electron microscopic examination disclosed a typical spongy myelinopathy with intramyelinic fluid accumulation (Lampert and Schochet, 1968; Rein *et al.*, 1968; Wegener *et al.*, 1968).

Spongy degeneration of cerebellum and brain stem and fine structural changes of spongy myelinopathy are also produced by feeding cuprizone to mice. This intoxication also produces giant mitochondria and proliferation of smooth endoplasmic reticulum in hepatocytes (Suzuki and Kikkawa, 1969).

References

Adachi, M., Schneck, L., Cara, J., Volk, B. W.: Spongy degeneration of the central nervous system (van Bogaert and Bertrand type; Canavan's disease). A review. Human Path. 4: 331—347, 1973.

— Volk, B. W.: Protracted form of spongy degeneration of the central nervous system (van Bogaert and Bertrand type). Neurology (Minneap.) 18: 1084—1092, 1968.

— Wallace, B. J., Schneck, L., Volk, B. W.: Fine structure of spongy degeneration of the central nervous system (van Bogaert and Bertrand type). J. Neuropath. exp. Neurol. 25: 598—616, 1966.

Adornato, B., Lampert, P.: Status spongiosus of nervous tissue. Electron microscopic studies. Acta neuropath. (Berl.) 19: 271—289, 1971.

Adornato, B. T., O'Brien, J. S., Lampert, P. W., Roe, T. F., Neustein, H. B.: Cerebral spongy degeneration of infancy. A biochemical and ultrastructural study of affected twins. Neurology (Minneap.) 22: 202—210, 1972.

Aleu, F. P., Katzman, R., Terry, R. D.: Fine structure and electrolyte analyses of cerebral edema induced by alkyl tin intoxication. J. Neuropath. exp. Neurol. 22: 403—413, 1963.

Banker, B. Q., Robertson, J. T., Victor, M.: Spongy degeneration of the central nervous system in infancy. Neurology (Minneap.) 14: 981—1001, 1964.

Blackwood, W., Cumings, J. N.: A histological and chemical study of three cases of diffuse cerebral sclerosis. Neurol. Neurosurg. Psychiat. 17: 33—49, 1954.

Buscaino, V. M.: La zolle distegratione a grappolo nell encephalo di conigli. Riv. Path. nerv. ment. 34: 382—409, 1929.

Canavan, M. M.: Schilder's encephalitis periaxialis diffusa. Report of a case in a child aged sixteen and one-half month. Arch. Neurol. Psychiat. (Chic.) 25: 299—308, 1931.

Carlton, W. W.: Neural toxicity of isonicotinic acid hydrazide (isoniazid) for chickens. Avian Dis. 11: 241—254, 1967.

— Iproniazid-induced encephalopathy in ducklings and chicks. Exp. Molec. Path. 7: 133—144, 1967.

— Kreutzberg, G.: Isonicotinic acid hydrazide-induced spongy degeneration of the white matter in the brains of pekin ducks. Amer. J. Path. 48: 91—105, 1966.

Friede, R. L., Martinez, A. J.: Analysis of axon-sheath relations during early Wallerian degeneration. Brain Res. 19: 199—212, 1970.

— Miyagishi, T.: Adjustment of the myelin sheath to changes in axon caliber. Anat. Rec. 172: 1—14, 1972.

Gambetti, P., Mellman, W. J., Gonatas, N. K.: Familial spongy degeneration of the central nervous system (van Bogaert-Bertrand disease). An ultrastructural study. Acta neuropath. (Berl.) 12: 103—115, 1969.

Globus, J. H., Strauss, I.: Progressive degenerative subcortical encephalopathy. Arch. Neurol. Psychiat. (Chic.) 20: 1190—1228, 1928.

Hall, S. M., Williams, P. L.: The distribution of electron-dense tracers in peripheral nerve fibres. J. Cell Sci. 8: 541—555, 1971.

Jellinger, K., Seitelberger, F.: Juvenile form of spongy degeneration of the CNS. Acta neuropath. (Berl.) 13: 276—281, 1969.

— Seitelberger, F.: Spongy degeneration of the nervous system in infancy. Current Topics Path. 53: 90—160, 1970.

Kamoshita, S., Rapin, I., Suzuki, K., Suzuki, K.: Spongy degeneration of the brain. A chemical study of two cases including isolation and characterization of myelin. Neurology (Minneap.) 18: 975—985, 1968.

— Reed, G. B., Aguilar, M. J.: Axonal dystrophy in a case of Canavan's spongy degeneration. Neurology (Minneap.) 17: 895—898, 1967.

Kreutzberg, G. W., Carlton, W. W.: Pathogenetic mechanism of experimentally-induced spongy degeneration. Acta neuropath. (Berl.) 9: 175—184, 1967.

Lampert, P., O'Brien, J., Garrett, R.: Hexachlorophene encephalopathy. Acta neuropath. (Berl.) 23: 326—333, 1973.

Lampert, P. W., Schochet, S. S.: Electron microscopic observations on experimental spongy degeneration of the cerebellar white matter. J. Neuropath. exp. Neurol. 27: 210—220, 1968.

Lees, M. B., Folch-Pi, J.: A study of some human brains with pathological changes. In: Chemical Pathology of the Nervous System, pp. 75—82. New York: Pergamon Press 1961.

Magee, P. N., Stoner, H. B., Barnes, J. M.: The experimental production of oedema in the central nervous system of the rat by triethyl tin compounds. J. Path. Bact. 73: 107—124, 1957.

Martinez, A. J., Boehm, R., Hadfield, M. G.: Acute hexachlorophene encephalopathy: Clinico-neuropathological correlation. Acta Neuropath. 28: 93—104, 1974.

Powell, H., Swarner, O., Gluck, L., Lampert, P.: Hexachlorophene myelinopathy in premature infants. J. Pediat. 82: 976—981, 1973.

Rein, H., Kolkmann, F.-W., Sil, R., Ule, G.: Zur Feinstruktur der INH-encephalopathie der Ente. Klin. Wschr. 46: 1060—1061, 1968.

Revel, J.-P., Hamilton, D. W.: The double nature of the intermediate dense line in peripheral nerve myelin. Anat. Rec. 163: 7—16, 1969.

Sacks, O., Brown, W. J., Aguilar, M. J.: Spongy degeneration of white matter. Canavan's sclerosis. Neurology (Minneap.) 15: 165-171, 1965.

Suzuki, K.: Peripheral nerve lesion in spongy degeneration of the central nervous system. Acta neuropath. (Berl.) 10: 95—98, 1968.

— Kikkawa, Y.: Status spongiosus of CNS and hepatic changes induced by cuprizone hexanone oxalydihydrazone. Amer. J. Path. 54: 307—325, 1969.

van Bogaert, L.: Familial spongy degeneration of the brain (Complementary study of the family R). Acta psychiat. scand. 39: 107—113, 1963.

— Bertrand, I.: Sur une idiotie familiale avec dégénérescence spongieuse du névraxe. Acta Neurol. Psychiat. 8: 572—587, 1949.

— — Spongy Degeneration of the Brain in Infancy. Amsterdam: North Holland Publishing Company 1967.

Webster, H., de F., Ulsamer, A. G., O'Connell, M. F.: Hexachlorophene induced myelin lesions in the developing nervous system of Xenopus tadpoles: Morphological and biochemical observations. J. Neuropath. exp. Neurol. 33: 144—163, 1974.

Wegener, K., Kolkmann, F.-W., Rein, H.: Autohistoradiographische Untersuchungen zur Frage der Bluthirnschrankenfunktion bei experimentell ausgelösten spongiösen Encephalopathien. Virchows Arch. path. Anat. 345: 352—364, 1968.

Wolman, M.: The spongy type of diffuse sclerosis. Brain 81: 243—247, 1958.

Zu Rhein, G. M., Eichman, P. L., Puletti, F.: Familial idiocy with spongy degeneration of the central nervous system of van Bogaert-Bertrand type. Neurology (Minneap.) 10: 998—1006, 1960.

45. Diseases of Intermediary Metabolism

Metabolic Astrocytosis. Several metabolic diseases of adulthood, particularly hepatic coma, hepatolenticular degeneration and uremia, produce a peculiar type of glial proliferation known as "metabolic astrocytosis", or glia cells of Alzheimer type II. Metabolic astrocytosis as a consequence of acquired hepatic diseases has been defined mostly through the studies of Adams and Foley (1953) and Victor *et al.* (1965). It consists of an increase in the number and size of astrocytic nuclei which may appear in pairs or in clusters if proliferation is intense. The nuclei enlarge significantly and may reach nearly twice their normal size; they are distinctly vesicular with a

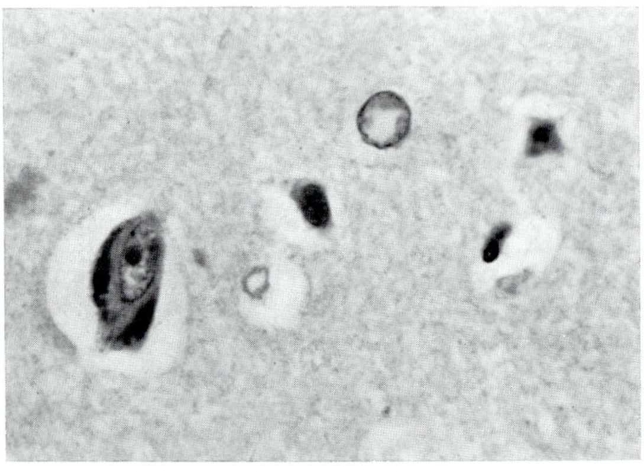

Fig. 154. Vesicular enlargement of astrocyte nucleus in metabolic astrocytosis; H & E ×600

prominent nuclear membrane encompassing a watery, empty-appearing nucleoplasm which may contain sparse chromatin particles resembling nucleoli (Fig. 154). Staining reactions for glycogen show usually single intranuclear inclusions in many of the nuclei, varying in size from small grains to larger than a nucleolus. The cytoplasmic bodies of the astrocytes are not discernible on light microscopic examination except for an occasional tuft of lightly stained cytoplasm; hence, the term "naked glial nuclei". No fibrillary gliosis is seen in Holzer stains.

Metabolic astrocytosis affects the gray matter, preferentially the basal ganglia and the cerebral cortex; it is less marked in other regions, *e.g.*, the cerebellar nuclei, Bergmann-glia or the pons, and is usually not discernible in the white matter. There are no characteristic changes of the neuronal population, although metabolic astrocytosis may coexist with parenchymal lesions attributable to hepatic encephalopathy, or to disturbances of oxygen or glucose supply, respectively.

The development of metabolic astrocytosis in the course of postnecrotic hepatic cirrhosis usually requires hepatic coma or precoma lasting for several days; it does not develop upon a precipitous onset of hepatic failure. The metabolite causing metabolic astrocytosis has not been identified with certainty, but current thinking centers on ammonia being at least a main factor;

support for this concept comes from the recent data of Cavanagh and Kyu (1971).

Metabolic astrocytosis having the same features as in adult brains is readily identified in children or infants older than 1 to 2 years. Little attention has been paid to the difficulties in assessing metabolic astrocytosis at an earlier age, although the problem is of some importance in the interpretation of the cerebral changes induced by congenital disturbances of amino acid metabolism. In the present author's experience metabolic astrocytosis is either absent or difficult to identify in infants dying at an age of less than 6 months from acquired destructive hepatic disease. At this age it apparently does not manifest with the same intensity as in older infants; also, several aspects of normal glial development resemble metabolic astrocytosis: Relatively large, vesicular glial nuclei without discernible cytoplasm can be seen in the white matter encompassing the periventricular matrix tissue, in the myelinating white matter, and in the cerebral cortex and basal ganglia where they occur in the absence of hepatic disease or of evident metabolic derangement. These developing glial nuclei are characterized by a sparse, though uniformly distributed chromatin, and they do not attain the excessive enlargement and the "empty" vesicular appearance characteristic of Alzheimer type II glia cells.

Metabolic astrocytosis can be identified in babies approximately 6 months old, but there may be only a few enlarged nuclei of Alzheimer type II among many others for which no changes are evident. Glycogen stains are of limited help, as nuclear glycogen inclusions, if present at all, are much less common and much smaller than in adults. These observations suggest that the newborn brain does not have the same potential for developing metabolic astrocytosis, as it has for developing nonspecific reactive astrocytic proliferation near destructive lesions, a tissue response which is well developed at the time of birth (Chapter 11). Certain inconsistencies in the literature regarding the presence of metabolic astrocytosis in connatal metabolic diseases, especially in hyperammonemia, are probably explained on this basis.

Disturbances of Amino Acid Metabolism, General Comments. Urinary excretion of amino acids is physiologic in premature infants and during the neonatal period. Pathologic aminoacidurias may be divided into two general classes: In the first, the so-called "spillover", or "overflow", aminoacidurias, there is an abnormal discharge of amino acids into the blood stream. Serum concentrations of amino acids may be elevated, and the latter are excreted into the urine on exceeding the renal threshold. Nonthreshold aminoacidurias pertain to amino acids normally occurring in intracellular intermediary metabolism for which there is no renal threshold; these are excreted in the urine in the absence of significant elevations of plasma levels. "Overflow" aminoacidurias are either acquired, such as from severe hepatic injury or from the infusion of large amounts of protein hydrolysates, or result from inborn errors of amino acid metabolism. The second class of aminoacidurias results from renal lesions which may be nonspecific, or may involve specific defects in the reabsorption of one or of a given group of amino acids; serum levels of amino acids are not increased.

Only the inborn errors of amino acid metabolism are reviewed here as they nearly always cause severe cerebral dysfunction and demonstrable lesions in the brain. Many are rare and of relatively recent discovery, and their neuropathology has not been studied extensively. However, several pathologic features are common to diseases in this general class, such as sponginess of the white matter, a deficiency in myelin, and a diffuse or "metabolic" gliosis. These changes tend to be most pronounced in the disturbances of aliphatic amino acids, less intense in disturbances of aromatic amino acids, and have not been reported for hyperammonemia from deficiencies of the initial steps of the urea cycle.

The status spongiosus of the white matter in disturbances of amino acid metabolism is quite similar to that in spongy degeneration of the van Bogaert-Bertrand type (Chapter 44). Indeed, several investigators reporting on the cerebral lesions of disturbances of amino acid metabolism emphasize that some of the cases may have been diagnosed erroneously as "spongy degeneration". Martin and Schlote (1972) mention that the lesions which they observed in arginosuccinic aciduria were quite similar to those in the congenital form of spongy degeneration described earlier by one of them without amino acid determinations.

Sponginess, delayed myelination and gliosis are difficult to assess in young infants, and features normal for age or nonspecific alterations commonly seen in the brains of young infants were often reported as lesions. These aspects are briefly reviewed to draw attention to the pitfalls in the assessment of the neuropathology of disturbances of amino acid metabolism. The often claimed delay of myelination is frequently not substantiated with description of the specific fiber systems affected, or with data on the gestational as well as the postnatal age of the infant. Many disturbances of amino acid metabolism lead to death in early infancy, when the cerebral hemispheric white matter is unmyelinated or incompletely myelinated. The difficulties in identifying a delay in myelination are therefore much greater than for spongy degeneration of the van Bogaert-Bertrand type which has a later onset and a longer course. Lipid chemical analysis may be of value in substantiating disturbances in myelin formation. The fine structural correlate of the status spongiosus in disturbances of amino acid metabolism has not yet been determined with the aid of the electron microscope. Application of this technique can be expected to disclose whether the sponginess is due to a spongy myelinopathy (Chapter 44) or to other causes. The degree of tissue preservation is also an important factor in assessing changes in the newborn. The extreme softness of many newborn brains and their tendency to "flow apart" with consequent loosening of the tissue structure are often thought to be normal features caused by the high water content of immature nerve tissue. However, newborn brains removed and fixed within approximately 2 hours after death are quite firm and slice easily, which attests to much greater rapidity of autolytic softening than for adult brains.

A sudanophilic myelinoclastic process has been described for some disturbances of amino acid metabolism without reference to the diffuse fatty change which is a common feature of the white matter of young infants (Chapter 5). The intensity of diffuse change is known to vary considerably from case to case, which renders it very difficult to assess sudanophilic myelin breakdown at this age, particularly if there are neither macrophages nor well defined lesions. Micronodular mineralization of the basal ganglia (Chapter 1) is another nonspecific alteration that has been described for disturbances of amino acid metabolism. Maldevelopment of neurons or of gray matter is also often cited, but the reports include reference to features normal for age, such as a persistent superficial granular layer in the cerebellum or an immature cerebral cortical architecture. Scattering of neuronal perikarya in the subcortical white matter is a developmental trait (Chapter 29) that is often reported as evidence of maldevelopment for brains having questionable, marginal, or ill defined lesions. Most descriptions of microgyria, polymicrogyria or pachygyria in disturbances of amino acid metabolism refer to subjective interpretations of gyral surface pattern without microscopic documentation of abnormal cortical architecture. Verified cortical malformations are sufficiently rare to consider them coincidental.

The arrangement of the following text is based on the molecular structure of the affected amino acids: The disturbances of aromatic amino acids, described first, include phenylketonuria, hyperprolinemia and tyrosinemia; they are followed by disturbances of aliphatic amino acids including, among others, maple syrup urine disease and sulfated amino acids; disturbances of the urea cycle are described last.

Phenylketonuria (Phenylpyruvic Oligophrenia). Fölling (1934) discovered the urinary excretion of large amounts of phenylpyruvic acid in 9 imbecile patients, 6 of whom were pairs of siblings. His report was a milestone in being the first on a specific metabolic defect as the cause of mental retardation, and it stimulated extensive research in this field.

Phenylketonuria is asymptomatic in the immediate postnatal period because of the protection of the fetus by the maternal liver. Vomiting during the first weeks of life is a frequent early manifestation. If the disease goes untreated, retarded mental development becomes apparent after the first half year and is often severe to the degree of idiocy (Jervis, 1937). Approximately one-third of the patients develop seizures before the 10th year of life; electroencephalographic anomalies are recorded for a majority even when there are no seizures. Patients characteristically show a fair complexion, blue eyes, pale skin and blond hair. There is a tendency to develop excema. Growth is stunted with a stooped posture and rigidity. Microcephaly was marked in 54 percent and mild in 21 percent of Paine's (1957) series. Life expectancy is reduced by intercurrent diseases. Some patients show marginal or normal intellectual development in spite of the presence of the metabolic defect.

The frequency of the disease in the general North American population has been estimated at 4 per 100,000 (Jervis, 1937), and similar frequencies were found for other populations of European origin; the disease is less common or absent in populations of jewish, negro or indian extraction. It is inherited in an autosomal recessive pattern; no mental deficit or urinary excretion of phenylalanine compounds are found in the heterozygous sibs. A moderate prevalence of females has been recorded in many small series, but it was not substantiated in larger materials. It is of interest, nonetheless, that there is a sex-dependent difference in the response to phenylalanine load (Blau *et al.*, 1973).

A new manifestation of phenylketonuria has been brought about by the improvement of life expectancy upon dietary treatment. Infants born to phenylpyruvic mothers are small for gestation and microcephalic with retarded psychomotor development; other congenital malformations have been observed as well (Stevenson and Huntley, 1967). No neuropathologic data have been reported as yet for these second generation patients.

Phenylpyruvic oligophrenia is due to a deficiency in phenylalanine hydroxylase, the enzyme necessary for the conversion of phenylalanine to tyrosine (Jervis, 1953; Udenfriend and Bessman, 1953); the enzyme occurs only in hepatic tissue. Tyrosine is the precursor for the formation of catecholamines, thyroxine, and melanin. The capacity for phenylalanine hydroxylation is absent or less than 10 percent of normal in phenylpyruvic patients; serum phenylalanine increases from normal values below 2 mg% to 20 to 60 mg%, and a similar increase occurs in the CSF. Phenylalanine tolerance tests in the asymptomatic heterozygous carriers of the disease reveal an abnormally high and persistent blood level of the amino acid (Hsia *et al.*, 1956; Berry *et al.*, 1957) and an increased urinary excretion of aromatic acids derived from phenylalanine (Blau *et al.*, 1973).

Phenylpyruvic patients excrete phenylalanine and various degradation products in the form of phenylpyruvic acid, phenyl lactic acid and phenyl acidic acid, as well as indole compounds and other metabolites. An olive green color is obtained upon adding iron chloride to the urine; the specific Guthrie test is based on the inhibition of the growth of the bacillus subtilis by phenylalanine. Early recognition of the disease is mandatory for preventing cerebral dysfunction by a dietary regime of low phenylalanine. Reviews of the biochemistry of the disease were given by, among others, Crome and Pare (1960) and Knox (1972).

The most consistent neuropathologic feature of phenylketonuria is micrencephaly; the brain is reduced in size and weight without specific anomalies in cortical development or cortical atrophy. The volume of the white matter appears to be reduced more than that of gray matter and the ventricles may be moderately dilated. There are no characteristic microscopic lesions in the gray matter, except for glial scars and defects attributable to postconvulsive necrosis. Microscopic changes of the white matter are absent for a majority of patients, *e.g.*, 10 of the 17 cases reviewed by Crome and Pare (1960). White matter changes observed first by Alvord *et al.* (1950) include sponginess of the centrum semiovale, the optic tracts, and certain tracts of the brain stem associated with irregular, indistinct areas of poor myelinization which the authors attributed to insufficient myelin formation. Malamud (1966), on reviewing a series of 8 cases, proposed an age-dependent variation in the manifestations of the disease; young patients tend to show focal status spongiosus of the white matter with little or no evidence of myelin breakdown. Adults may show, in addition, demyelinative lesions having more intense gliosis and large amounts of neutral fat: There are irregular, shadowy patches of pallor with indistinct boundaries, the myelin defect ranging from mild to complete.

There is no selective sparing of the subcortical U fibers. While there is very little neutral fat in regions showing spongy state only, there may be numerous macrophages and marked gliosis in the myelin defects. Cases were also reported having myelinoclastic lesions resembling those of Schilder disease with large areas of complete destruction of myelin, relative sparing of axons and sudanophilic breakdown products. Hypopigmentation of the substantia nigra and nucleus coerulus described by Fellman (1958) was not observed by others. Martin and Schlote (1972) tabulated the available autopsy observations.

Lipid chemical analysis of phyenylketonuric brains shows increase in water content and decrease in cerebrosides and cholesterol, consistent with a defect in myelin. Absence of esterified cholesterol in most cases indicates absence of active myelin destruction (Crome *et al.*, 1962; Prensky *et al.*, 1968). Changes in the fatty acid composition of the white matter lipids were considered suggestive of a disturbance in the synthesis of long chain fatty acids (Gerstl *et al.*, 1967; Cumings *et al.*, 1968). Studies of purified myelin gave below normal yields but without evidence of an abnormal composition of the myelin lipids (Shah *et al.*, 1972).

The white matter changes of phenylketonuric brains have been interpreted as either insufficient production of myelin or as its secondary destruction during adult life. Neither of these interpretations can be eliminated on the basis of the available chemical data, nor are they mutually exclusive. Phenylalanine and its primary degradation products are relatively nontoxic to myelinating nerve fibers in cultures of cerebellar tissue, but the indole compounds have considerable toxicity (Silberberg, 1967). There is general agreement that the white matter changes are an unlikely substrate of the mental retardation. Metabolic effects impeding nervous function include a competitive inhibition of the transport of other essential amino acids into cells by high tissue levels of phenylalanine, or the inhibitory effects of phenylalanine metabolites on various enzymes. Phenylalanine or its degradation products are known to inhibit 5-hydroxytryptophan-decarboxylase and glutamic acid decarboxylase as well as tyrosinase, thus causing hypopigmentation and reducing the concentrations of the neural transmitter substances serotonin and γ-amino-butyric acid. The relative significance of these various effects in producing mental retardation is still not clearly understood.

Hyperprolinemia. Hyperprolinemia is a rare hereditary disease of infancy or childhood characterized by elevated plasma concentrations of proline and by excretion of proline, as well as of hydroxyproline and glycine in the urine. Two types of hyperprolinemia are distinguished on the basis of different defects in the pathway of proline degradation; Type I is due to a deficiency of proline oxidase, type II of Δ-pyrroline-5-carboxylate dehydrogenase. Mental retardation may occur with either type, and type II has been found associated with convulsions. Type I may be associated with renal disease, but the association appears to be fortuitous, the renal disease being inherited independently of the hyperprolinemia (Scriver and Efron, 1972).

Neuropathologic observations are scanty. Efron (1966) reports absence of the ventral portion of the inferior olivary nucleus and diffuse neuronal loss in the cortex for one case. Sponginess of the cerebral and cerebellar white matter and perivascular accumulation of granules of unspecified nature was described for another (Woody *et al.*, 1969).

Tyrosinemia. Elevated blood tyrosine levels and urinary excretion of large amounts of tyrosine and tyrosyl compounds occur as part of a syndrome of hepatosplenomegaly, nodular hepatic cirrhosis, and vitamin D resistant rickets (La Du and Gjessing, 1972, review). The disease leads to death in early infancy or childhood, although survival to young adult age has been observed. Neuropathologic observations refer to metabolic astrocytosis (Perry *et al.*, 1965). Martin and Schlote (1972) found no Alzheimer type II glia but observed status spongiosus at the cortex-white matter border with a slight delay in myelination.

Hyperpipecolactemia. Gatfield *et al.* (1968) reported an infant with a progressive neurologic disease, hepatomegaly and hepatic fibrosis, in whom there was an accumulation of pipecolic acid, a cyclic amino acid derived from lysine. The brain showed multiple foci of demyelination affecting particularly cerebellar white matter and brain stem; cristalline intracellular accumulations of abnormal lipidic material were observed in the lesions.

Maple Syrup Urine Disease (Branch Chain Ketonuria). Maple syrup urine disease (Menkes *et al.*, 1954) derives its name from the characteristic maple syrup or caramel-like odor of the urine. The disease characteristically manifests by about the 4th day of life with vomiting, lethargy, muscular hypertonicity and convulsions. Rapid deterioration may lead to death during the first week of life, or during infancy; mental retardation becomes manifest upon longer survival. The disease is inherited in a pattern suggestive of autosomal recessive transmission.

Maple syrup urine disease is caused by a deficiency in the oxydative decarboxylation of the branch chain amino acids leucine, isoleucine and valine, and their respective keto acids; their breakdown normally proceedes through a series of four enzymatic reactions to yield isovaleric, alpha-methyl-butyric, and isobutyric acid. The metabolic block in oxidative decarboxylation causes the accumulation of the branch chain amino acids, their keto acids as well as alloisoleucine in body fluids.

The brain of young infants with maple syrup urine disease is enlarged, edematous, and may be quite heavy for age (Menkes *et al.*, 1965). Microscopic examination discloses a generalized status spongiosus of the white matter of brain and spinal cord; however, there is sparing of those portions of the hemispheric white matter in which myelination has not yet started. Sponginess may also affect basal nuclei, particularly the pallidum, because of its concentration of myelinated fibers (Fig. 155). The amount of myelin in the affected fiber systems appears to be reduced, but no sudanophilic breakdown products are seen. Marked astrocytic gliosis has been found in the spongy white matter, and overgrowth of "naked" glia nuclei was observed in the cerebral cortex (Crome *et al.*, 1961; Menkes *et al.*, 1965). Diezel and Martin (1964) described proteinaceous crystals in frozen sections of unfixed or alcohol-fixed tissue, but Martin and Schlote (1972) consider these common tissue artefacts. Silberman *et al.* (1961) described a severe deficiency of myelin, with sponginess of cerebral and cerebellar hemispheres, reactive astrocytosis and reduced numbers of oligodendroglia, in two infants that had lived to 9 months and less severe deficiencies in infants 13 and 20 months old; they thought that the difference in the intensity of the lesions implied a delay in myelination rather than a variation in the severity of the disease. Lipid chemical examinations of frontal white matter confirmed the reduction in myelin content in terms of an increased water content and a reduction in

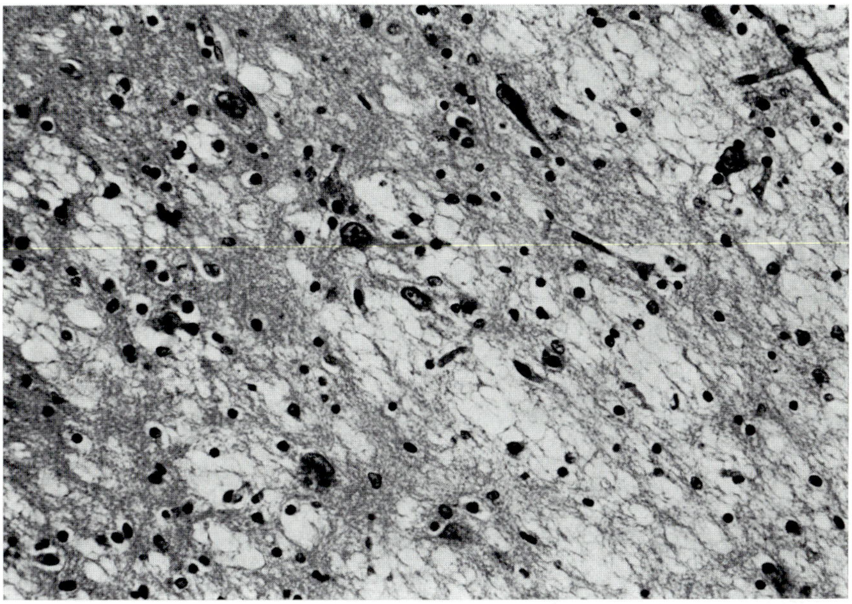

Fig. 155. Status spongiosus affecting mainly the bundles of myelinated fibers in the pallidum in a case of maple syrup urine disease; H & E ×225

cerebrosides and proteolipid proteins, changes that were interpreted as diminished myelin synthesis (Prensky *et al.*, 1968). Patients that had undergone dietary treatment showed no deficiency in myelin and a minimal sponginess of the white matter (Menkes and Solcher, 1967).

Oast House Disease. The urinary excretion of α-hydroxy-butyric acid in a phenylketonuric baby who lived to the age of 10 months was described by Smith and Strang (1958). The urine had a characteristic "oast house" (a kiln used to dry hops, malt or tobacco) or burned sugar odor. A brief reference to a widespread defect in myelination is given in the pathologic description.

Hyperglycinemia. Urinary excretion of glycine occurs in the absence of elevated serum levels of glycine in several syndromes including selective defects in renal tubular reabsorption of glycine, or as a secondary feature associated with other disturbances of amino acid metabolism such as hyperprolinemia, or in mercury intoxication. These conditions are of no concern to infantile neuropathology. Hyperglycinuria with hyperglycinemia (Childs *et al.,* 1961) is a disturbance of amino acid metabolism presenting as a severe neonatal disease with vomiting, acidosis and ketonuria. Other symptoms include periodic thrombocytopenia, neutropenia, agammaglobulinemia, numerous infections, developmental failure and osteoporosis. The disease is probably genetically determined, but its inheritance pattern is not established; it commonly leads to death in early infancy.

Neuropathologic reports on four cases by Rushton (1968) and on one each by Diezel and Martin (1966) and Anderson (1969) agree in showing marked status spongiosus of the white matter affecting only its myelinated portions without predilection for the immediate subcortical zone. The extent of myelination was thought to be reduced; however, lipid analysis of white matter in two cases gave equivocal data (Prensky *et al.,* 1968). Lipid-filled glia cells of the type seen in diffuse fatty change of the white matter (Chapter 5) have been reported and were thought to be characteristic of the disease. There are no comments on abnormal astroglial proliferation in these reports.

Homocystinuria. Homocystinuria is a rare inborn error in the metabolism of sulfated amino acids (Gerritsen *et al.,* 1962; Carson and Neill, 1962). The biochemical error consists of an inability to metabolize homocysteine, an intermediary of methionin metabolism, with excessive urinary excretion of homocystine. There is no renal threshold for this amino acid. The disease is caused by deficient activity of cystathionine synthethase (Mudd *et al.,* 1964). Approximately 20 cases have been described until 1965; the disease is probably inherited in autosomal recessive pattern (White *et al.,* 1965).

Clinical manifestations vary from severe to mild and the disease is compatible with survival to adulthood. Mental retardation, convulsions, ectopia lentis, and sparse hair are common features, resembling Marfan syndrome.

Neuropathologic manifestations of homocystinuria fall into two categories, vascular and parenchymal. The vascular and thromboembolic cerebral lesions are described in Chapter 12. The parenchymal lesions in the brain of a 1-year-old boy consisted of status spongiosus of the white matter including that of the spinal cord and proliferation of large astrocytic nuclei with little cytoplasm in the cerebral cortex (Chou and Waisman, 1965); the authors also report "polymicrogyria" but there were no histologic anomalies in the cortex.

Sulfite Oxidase Deficiency. This disease was described by Irreverre *et al.* (1967) for an infant who developed within 9 months extreme mental and physical retardation and opistotonus. There were dislocated ocular lenses and the urine contained large amounts of S-sulfo-L-cysteine, sulfite and thiosulfate. A deficiency of sulfite oxidase was found in liver, kidney and brain. This enzyme is responsible for the oxydation of sulfite to inorganic sulfate, being the terminal link in the degradation of sulfur-containing amino acids.

Neuropathologic examination of the brain of this infant (Rosenblum, 1968) disclosed loss of myelin, axonal depletion and gliosis of the white matter with multiple cystic lesions in the deep white matter, basal ganglia and cerebellum. The relation of the lesions, which resemble perinatal multilocular cystic encephalopathy (Chapter 11), to the metabolic disorder was not clear.

Diseases of the Urea (Krebs Henseleit) Cycle. Ammonia, the end product of intermediary nitrogen metabolism is excreted in the mammalian organism in the form of urea. Urea is synthesized through five major sequential steps known as the urea cycle. The enzymes involved in the urea cycle are found in many tissues, except for arginase which is found in liver only. The rate-limiting steps in the urea cycle are the first, third and fourth; whereas, ornithine transcarbamylase and arginase have higher activities.

Hereditary disorders of the urea cycle occur in the form of deficiencies of a given enzyme and may be associated with reduced activities of others. Assays of all five enzymes in liver biopsy are used for diagnosis. The metabolic blocks result in accumulation of the corresponding intermediary metabolites: hyperammonemia is produced by deficiencies of the first two steps of the urea cycle, carbamylphosphate synthethase (1), or ornithine transcarbamylase (2); citrullinemia results from deficiency in arginosuccinate synthetase (3); arginosuccinic acid accumulates from argino succinase (4) deficiency; the two latter deficiencies may also induce hyperammonemia. No arginase (5) deficiency has been identified so far. None of these enzyme deficiencies abolish the formation of urea, either because of partial enzyme defects or because of the availability of alternate pathways.

Hyperammonemia manifests in early infancy with symptoms attributable mainly to ammonia intoxication, that is vomiting, alkalosis, a semicomatous state and protein intolerance. The disease may result in death in early infancy or may produce mental retardation. Hyperammonemia from carbamylphosphate synthethase deficiency was reported to be associated with spongy degeneration of brain stem nuclei and basal ganglia (Hommes *et al.*, 1969). The neuropathologic changes of this patient, who had died at $7^1/_2$ months, and of two sibs who had died at 4 weeks were reported in detail by Ebels (1972). Severe loss of neurons was found in the cerebral cortex, and there was cavitation affecting particularly the subcortical white matter in a pattern interpreted as ulegyria. A deficiency of myelin and gliosis were found throughout the hemispheric white matter. Thalamus and portions of the putamen were affected, but the pallidum, subthalamic nucleus and Ammon's horn were spared. The pons showed a deficiency of myelin in a poorly delineated region in its central portion. Sponginess was observed in the inferior colliculus and the superior olivary nucleus. There was no metabolic astrocytosis.

Hyperammonemia from ornithine transcarbamylase deficiency appears to be associated with quite variable degrees of destruction of cerebral tissue. A cerebral cortical biopsy taken at 8 months showed disorganization, astrocytic gliosis and lipophages (Levin *et al.*, 1969). Hopkins *et al.* (1969) describe a mild enlargement of astrocytic nuclei and chromatolytic changes in neurons in an 18-month-old infant. Bruton *et al.* (1970) report two cases who had died before they reached the age of 8 years. No destructive lesions were found in one; the other had severe atrophy of the entire hemispheric walls, loss of cortical architecture and gliosis, and neuronal loss in the basal ganglia. Metabolic astrocytosis was present in both. In three cases of hyperammonemia studied by the present author, neither parenchymal lesions nor metabolic astrocytosis was present. All had died during the first month of life. The limited number of observations on hyperammonemia suggests great variance in the extent of damage which seems to afflict the neurons more than the white matter.

Citrullinemia had been observed in mentally retarded children, but no neuropathologic reports are available.

Arginosuccinic aciduria (Allan *et al.*, 1958) may manifest in early infancy or in childhood with mental retardation, epilepsy, ataxia, friable hair or liver disease. There is much variance in symptomatology and in the severity of the disease. Baumgartner *et al.* (1968) report rather equivocal cerebral changes for an infant that had died on the 9th day. Solitare *et al.* (1969) described an 8-month-old girl in whom they found poor myelination in the deep cerebellar and cerebral white matter, the pyramidal tract, internal capsule and anterior commissure. Metabolic astrocytosis was found in the gray matter.

Subacute Necrotizing Encephalomyelopathy (Leigh Disease). Subacute necrotizing encephalomyelopathy was described under this name by Leigh (1951). The cerebral changes of "breast milk intoxication" described by Tanaka (1934) may presumably represent the same disease, but they could also refer to infantile beriberi. Verhaart's (1938) cases are also often quoted in historical reviews although the lesions described are more similar to infantile bilateral striatal necrosis (Chapter 9). Subacute necrotizing encephalomyelopathy was originally considered rare; however, 65 cases verified at autopsy have been reported in the 20 years since Leigh's report. The review of Montpetit *et al.* (1971) tabulates 53 of these. Jellinger and Seitelberger (1970) give a detailed account of the disease.

The disease begins after a normal postnatal development during the first 2 years of life and takes a rapidly progressive course which lasts between one half and less than 4 years for most cases. The onset of the disease rarely dates to the immediate postnatal period. For other cases there is a protracted course lasting from 5 to 15 years; these are thought to represent a juvenile form by some authors, but neither symptomatology nor lesions afford a clear-cut distinction from the infantile cases. An adult form of Leigh disease has been described repeatedly, and Sipe (1973) tabulated 6 cases; there is still too much variance in clinical and pathologic features among these to permit a clear definition of the characteristics of the adult course.

Leigh disease is frequently familial, particularly for the cases with onset in early infancy; 55 afflicted families are known at present. Both sexes are affected by the disease, with a 3 : 2 male preference. The symptomatology varies. Initial problems may present with poor feeding and vomiting, and respiratory difficulties are common. There are signs of retardation, arrest and regression of psychomotor development. Neurologic symptoms point toward the brain stem, including nystagmus, strabism, bizarre eye movements, pupillary changes or paresis of various eye muscles. Optic atrophy is less common. Disturbances of gait and dystonic phenomena lead to paresis, hypotonus and mental retardation, often accompanied with seizures.

The morbid anatomy of Leigh disease resembles that of Wernicke polioencephalopathy, particularly in the histologic features of the lesions, but there are striking differences in their regional distributions. The most consistent localization of the lesions is in the brain stem, where they are visible with the naked eye as grayish, softened and slightly sunken zones in the tissue, occurring bilaterally although not with absolute symmetry. There is some preference for gray matter, but the lesions are not confined to it, and their borders meander across gray and white matter without respecting territories. They are generally sharply delineated from the adjacent tissue. Microscopic examination discloses marked sponginess of the tissue with a preferential rarefication of the neuropil (Fig. 156). Although neurons are destroyed even-

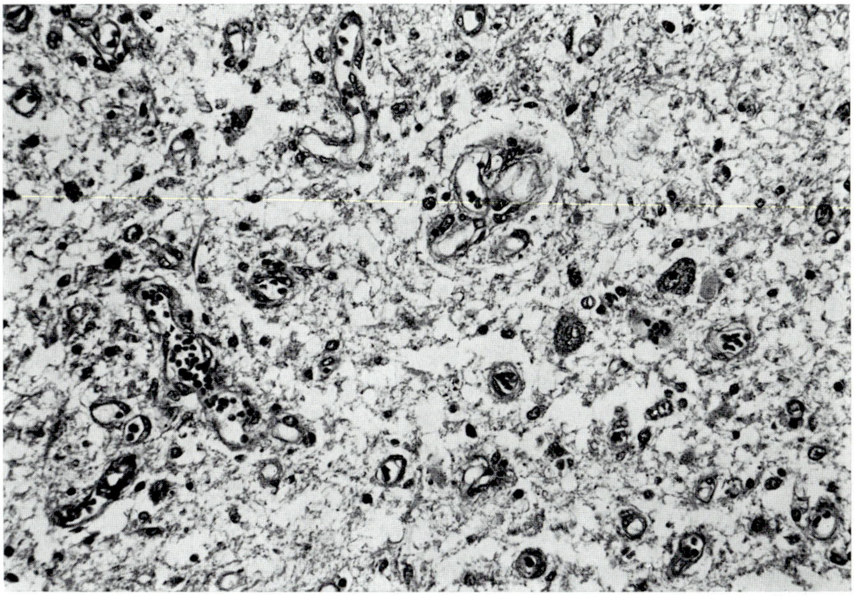

Fig. 156. Leigh disease. Sponginess of the tissue, vascular proliferation and persistent neurons in a tegmental lesion; H & E ×250

tually, they appear to be more resistant to the disease, as evident from scattered neuronal perikarya in the rarefied spongy tissue. Involvement of the white matter causes loss of myelin; degenerative changes of sheaths, such as irregularities or ballooning, are seen where the lesions are still in progress. Axons eventually become destroyed as well. An abundance of lipid-laden macrophages is seen in the active lesions, becoming more sparse later on. Although extravasations of polymorphonuclear leukocytes or lymphocytic cuffing have been described, they are not a characteristic feature of the lesions. The changes in the blood vessels, which show endothelial swelling or marked endothelial proliferation, are one of the most characteristic features of the disease. The cellular, dilated, tortuous vessels are quite prominent throughout the lesions; there may be an actual increase in vascular density. The hemorrhagic manifestations usually seen in Wernicke encephalopathy are absent.

Lesions of this type affect particularly midbrain and pons, most frequently in the tegmentum, periaqueductal gray matter and the posterior colliculi.

The basis pontis is often spared, but involvement of the substantia nigra is quite common, contrary to its sparing in Wernicke disease. Lesions in the medulla oblongata show a predilection for the floor of the fourth ventricle and the inferior olivary nuclei. In the cerebellum there is common involvement of the dentate nucleus and the white matter, less commonly of the cortex or the cerebellar peduncles. Involvement of the basal ganglia most frequently affects the putamen, with symmetrical necrosis reminiscent of that seen in infantile bilateral striatal necrosis (Chapter 9); lesions are also found in pallidum and caudate nucleus and may involve the centrum semiovale and optic nerve. Thalamic involvement is uncommon and sparing of the mammillary bodies is typical, although the latter were affected in rare instances (Kamoshita *et al.*, 1968). Lesions in the spinal cord present as Wallerian degeneration of descending tracts as well as independent lesions of gray and white matter; the dorsal tracts are commonly affected in the form of oval midline lesions or of larger lesions spreading in butterfly fashion. Involvement of peripheral nerves is an inconsistent feature; demyelination and axonal fragmentation was observed by Reye (1960), Namiki (1965) and others but was not found by several authors who had searched for it.

Of particular interest are the rare cases of exceptionally early onset and rapid course, such as that of Lewis (1965), who had symptoms from birth and died at 9$^{1}/_{2}$ weeks, and that of Tom and Rewcastle (1962), who had died at 14 weeks without clear data on the clinical course. Both infants showed prominent vascular endothelial proliferation and sponginess of brain stem and cord, but the lesions were less well defined than in older infants; lipid-laden macrophages were sparse and neuronal involvement varied; foamy cytoplasmic changes were described by Lewis. Gliosis was mild. No involvement of basal ganglia was observed in these infants.

Most pathogenetic assumptions on Leigh disease have clustered around some type of disturbance of thiamine metabolism, as proposed by Feigin and Wolf (1954). These assumptions are based on the similarity of the lesions to those of Wernicke encephalopathy, as well as on laboratory data showing elevated concentrations of lactate, pyruvate, or alanine, consistent with a block in pyruvic acid metabolism.

Available evidence does not favor the assumption of a dietary thiamine deficiency. There is no evidence of malnutrition, and medication of thiamine is without any or without lasting beneficiary effect; normal blood levels of thiamine have also been observed. The neuropathology of dietary thiamine deficiency in infancy is too little known to permit comparison of the pattern of lesions. The case of infantile beriberi described by Davis and Wolf (1958) had fatty degeneration of heart, liver and kidney and cerebral lesions similar to those of Wernicke encephalopathy involving the walls of the third ventricle, the mammillary bodies and several brain stem nuclei. Documentation of the regional pattern of lesions is incomplete in the case described by Cochrane *et al.* (1961).

A malfunction of thiamine-dependent enzymes pyruvate dehydrogenase, α-ketoglutarate dehydrogenase and transketolase may result in the accumulation of the metabolites proximal to those reactions. Although elevated levels of lactate, pyruvate and α-ketoglutarate have been observed, they are not consistent, and various mechanisms may enter in their interpretation. No conclusive evidence for a deficiency of thiamine-dependent enzymes has been accumulated (Greenhouse and Schneck, 1968).

A deficiency in pyruvate carboxylase was observed by Hommes *et al.* (1968) and Grover *et al.* (1972). Pincus *et al.* (1969) reported an absence of thiamine triphosphate in brain tissue and found a factor, probably a glycoprotein, in the blood and serum which inhibits the synthesis of thiamine triphosphate by the thiamine pyrophosphate adenosine triphosphate phosphotransferase (Cooper *et al.*, 1969).

Chronic Lactic Acidosis. Lactic acidosis may develop as a metabolic manifestation of a variety of functional and pathologic disorders. Apart from these, a condition characterized by recurrent bouts of severe lactic acidosis was described by Hartmann *et al.* (1962), but the metabolic background of this disturbance is still not understood. Neuropathologic lesions in a sibship with congenital lactic acidosis were reported by Farkas-Bargeton *et al.* (1971). A diffuse reduction of myelination was found in cerebral and cerebellar hemispheric white matter, and there were also subependymal cysts, but the latter were rather similar to those developing subsequent to subependymal hemorrhages (Chapter 2).

References

Adams, R. D., Foley, J. M.: Neurological complications of liver disease. Ass. Res. nerv. Dis. Proc. 32: 198—237, 1953.

Allan, J. D., Cusworth, D. C., Dent, C. E., Wilson, V. K.: A disease probably hereditary, characterized by severe mental deficiency and a constant gross abnormality of amino acid metabolism. Lancet 1: 182—187, 1958.

Alvord, E. C., Stevenson, L. D., Vogel, F. S., Engle, R. L.: Neuropathologic findings in phenyl-pyruvic oligophrenia (phenyl-ketonuria). J. Neuropath. exp. Neurol. 9: 298—310, 1950.

Anderson, J. M.: Spongy degeneration in the white matter of the central nervous system in the newborn: pathological findings in three infants, one with hyperglycinaemia. J. Neurol. Neurosurg. Psychiat. 32: 328—337, 1969.

Baumgartner, R., Scheidegger, S., Stadler, G., Hottinger, A.: Argininbernsteinsäure-Krankheit des Neugeborenen mit letalem Verlauf. Helv. paediat. Acta 23: 77—106, 1968.

Berry, H., Sutherland, B., Guest, G. M.: Phenylalanine tolerance test on relatives of phenylketonuric children. Amer. J. hum. Genet. 9: 310—316, 1957.

Blau, K., Summer, G. K., Newsome, H. C., Edwards, C. H., Mamer, O. A.: Phenylalanine loading and aromatic acid excretion in normal subjects and heterozygotes for phenylketonuria. Clin. chim. Acta 45: 197—205, 1973.

Bruton, C. J., Corsellis, J. A. N., Russell, A.: Hereditary hyper-ammonaemia. Brain 93: 423—434, 1970.

Carson, N. A., Neill, D. W.: Metabolic abnormalities detected in survey of mentally backward individuals in Northern Ireland. Arch. Dis. Child. 37: 505—513, 1962.

Cavanagh, J. B., Kyu, M. H.: Type II Alzheimer change experimentally produced in astrocytes in the rat. J. Neurol. Sci. 12: 63—75, 1971.

Childs, B., Nyham, W. L., Borden, M., Bard, L., Cooke, R. E.: Idiopathic hyperglycinemia and hyperglycinuria: a new disorder of amino acid metabolism. Pediatrics 27: 522—538, 1961.

Chou, S.-M., Waisman, H. A.: Spongy degeneration of the central nervous system. Case of homocystinuria. Arch. Path. (Chic.) 79: 357—363, 1965.

Cochrane, W. A., Collins-Williams, C., Donohue, W. L.: Superior hemorrhagic polioencephalitis (Wernicke's disease) occurring in an infant. Pediatrics 28: 771—777, 1961.

Cooper, J. R., Itokawa, Y., Pincus, J. H.: Thiamine triphosphate deficiency in necrotizing encephalomyelopathy. Science 164: 72—73, 1969.

Crome, L.: The association of phenylketonuria with leucodystrophy. J. Neurol. Neurosurg. Psychiat. 25: 149—153, 1962.

— Dutton, G., Ross, C. F.: Maple syrup urine disease. J. Path. Bact. 81: 379—384, 1961.

— Pare, C. M. B.: Phenylketonuria. J. ment. Sci. 106: 862—883, 1960.

— Tymms, V., Woolf, L. I.: A chemical investigation of the defects of myelination in phenylketonuria. J. Neurol. Neurosurg. Psychiat. 25: 143—148, 1962.

Cumings, J. N., Grundt, I. K., Yanagihara, T.: Lipid changes in the brain in phenylketonuria. J. Neurol. Neurosurg. Psychiat. 31: 334—337, 1968.

Davis, R. A., Wolf, A.: Infantile beriberi associated with Wernicke's encephalopathy. Pediatrics 21: 409—420, 1958.

Diezel, P. B., Martin, K.: Die Ahornsirupkrankheit mit familiärem Befall. Virchows Arch. path. Anat. 337: 425—445, 1964.

— — Hyperglycinämie (Glycinose) mit familiärer idiopathischer Hyperglycinurie. Dtsch. med. Wschr. 91: 2249—2254, 1966.

Ebels, E. J.: Neuropathological observations in a patient with carbamylphosphatesynthetase deficiency and in two sibs. Arch. Dis. Child. 47: 47—51, 1972.

Efron, M. L.: Disorders of proline and hydroxyproline metabolism. In: The Metabolic Base of Inherited Disease (Stanbury, J. B., Wyngaarden, J. B., Fredrickson, D. S., eds.), Chapter 18. New York: McGraw-Hill 1966.

Farkas-Bargeton, E., Goutières, F., Richardet, J. M., Thieffry, S., Brissaud, H. E.: Leucoencéphalopathie familiale associée à une acidose lactique congénitale. Acta neuropath. (Berl.) 17: 156—168, 1971.

Feigin, I., Wolf, A.: A disease in infants resembling chronic Wernicke's encephalopathy. J. Pediat. 45: 243—263, 1954.

Fellman, J. H.: Epinephrine metabolites and pigmentation in the central nervous system in a case of phenylpyruvic oligophrenia. J. Neurol. Neurosurg. Psychiat. 21: 58—62, 1958.

Fölling, A.: Über Ausscheidung von Phenylbrenztraubensäure in den Harn als Stoffwechselanomalie in Verbindung mit Imbezillität. Hoppe Seyler Z. Physiol. Chem. 227: 169—176, 1934.

Gatfield, P. D., Taller, E., Hinton, G. G., Wallace, A. C., Abdelnour, G. M., Haust, M. D.: Hyperpipecolactemia: A new metabolic disorder associated with neuropathy and hepatomegaly. Canad. Med. Ass. J. 99: 1215—1233, 1968.

Gerritsen, T., Vaughn, J. G., Waisman, H. A.: Identification of homocystine in urine. Biochem. biophys. Res. Commun. 9: 493—496, 1962.

Gerstl, B., Malamud, N., Eng, L. F., Hayman, B. S.: Lipid alterations in human brains in phenylketonuria. Neurology (Minneap.) 17: 51—57, 1967.

Greenhouse, A. H., Schneck, S. A.: Subacute necrotizing encephalomyelopathy. A reappraisal of the thiamine deficiency hypothesis. Neurology (Minneap.) 18: 1—9, 1968.

Grover, W. D., Auerbach, V. H., Patel, M. S.: Biochemical studies and therapy in subacute necrotizing encephalomyelopathy (Leigh's syndrome). J. Pediat. 81: 39—44, 1972.

Hartmann, A. F., Wohltman, H. J., Pukerson, M. L., Wesley, M. E.: Lactate metabolism: Studies of a child with a serious congenital deviation. J. Pediat. 61: 165—180, 1962.

Hommes, F. A., de Groot, C. J., Wilmink, C. W., Jonxis, J. H. P.: Carbamylphosphate synthetase deficiency in an infant with severe cerebral damage. Arch. Dis. Child. 44: 688—693, 1969.

— Polman, H. A., Reerink, J. D.: Leigh's encephalomyelopathy: an inborn error of gluconeogenesis. Arch. Dis. Child. 43: 423—426, 1968.

Hopkins, I. J., Connelly, J. F., Dawson, A. G., Hird, F. J. R., Maddison, T. G.: Hyperammonemia due to ornithine transcarbamylase deficiency. Arch. Dis. Child. 44: 143—148, 1969.

Hsia, D. Y., Driscoll, K. W., Troll, W., Knox, W. E.: Detection by phenylalanine tolerance tests of heterozygous carriers of phenyl ketonuria. Nature 178: 1239—1240, 1956.

Irreverre, F., Mudd, S. H., Heizer, W. D., Laster, L.: Sulfite oxidase deficiency: Studies of a patient with mental retardation, dislocated ocular lenses, and abnormal urinary excretion of S-sulfa-L-cysteine, sulfite and thiosulfate. Biochem. Med. 1: 187—217, 1967.

Jellinger, K., Seitelberger, F.: Subacute necrotizing encephalomyelopathy (Leigh). Erg. inn, Med. Kinderhkd. 29: 155—219, 1970.

Jervis, G. A.: Phenylpyruvic oligophrenia. Arch. Neurol. Psychiat. (Chic.) 38: 944—963, 1937.

— Phenylpyruvic oligophrenia: deficiency of phenylalanine oxydising system. Proc. Soc. exp. Biol. Med. 82: 514—515, 1953.

Kamoshita, S., Aguilar, M. J., Landing, B. H.: Infantile subacute necrotizing encephalomyelopathy. Amer. J. Dis. Child. 116: 120—129, 1968.

Knox, W. E.: Phenylketonuria. In: The Metabolic Basis of Inherited Disease (Stanbury, J. B., Wyngaarden, J. B., Fredrickson, D. S., eds.), pp. 266—295, Chapter 11. New York: Blackiston, McGraw-Hill 1972.

La Du, B. N., Gjessing, L. R.: Tyrosinosis and tyrosinemia. In: The Metabolic Base of Inherited Disease (Stanbury, J. B., Wyngaarden, J. B., Fredrickson, D. S., eds.), Chapter 12, pp. 296—307. New York: McGraw-Hill 1966.

Leigh, D.: Subacute necrotizing encephalomyelopathy in an infant. J. Neurol. Neurosurg. Psychiat. 14: 216—221, 1951.

Levin, B., Abraham, J. M., Oberholzer, V. G., Burges, E. A.: Hyperammonaemia: a deficiency of liver ornithine transcarbamylase. Arch. Dis. Child. 44: 152—161, 1969.

Lewis, A. J.: Infantile subacute necrotizing encephalopathy. Canad. med. Ass. J. 93: 878—881, 1965.

Lewis, P. D., Miller, A. L.: Arginosuccinic aciduria. Brain 93: 413—422, 1970.

Malmud, N.: Neuropathology of phenylketonuria. J. Neuropath. exp. Neurol. 25: 254—268, 1966.

Martin, J.-J., Schlote, W.: Central nervous system lesions in disorders of amino-acid metabolism. A neuropathological study. J. Neurol. Sci. 15: 49—76, 1972.

Menkes, J. H., Hurst, P. L., Craig, J. M.: New syndrome: Progressive familial infantile cerebral dysfunction associated with an unusual urinary substance. Pediatrics 14: 462—467, 1954.

— Philippart, M., Fiol, R. E.: Cerebral lipids in maple syrup disease. J. Pediat. 66: 584—594, 1965.

— Solcher, H.: Maple syrup disease. Effects of dietary therapy on cerebral lipids. Arch. Neurol. (Chic.) 16: 486—491, 1967.

Montpetit, V. J. A., Andermann, F., Carpenter, S., *et al.:* Subacute necrotizing encephalomyelopathy. A review and study of two families. Brain 94: 1—30, 1971.

Mudd, S. H., Finkelstein, J. D., Irreverre, F., Laster, L.: Homocystinuria: an enzymatic defect. Science 143: 1443—1445, 1964.

Namiki, H.: Subacute necrotizing encephalomyelopathy. Case report with special emphasis on associated pathology of peripheral nervous system. Arch. Neurol. (Chic.) 12: 98—107, 1965.

Paine, R. S.: The variability in manifestations of untreated patients with phenylketonuria. Pediatrics 20: 290—302, 1957.

Perry, T. L., Hardwick, D. F., Dixon, G. H., Dolman, C. L., Hansen, S.: Hypermethionemia: a metabolic disorder associated with cirrhosis, islet cell hyperplasia, and renal tubular degeneration. Pediatrics 36: 236—250, 1965.

Pincus, J. H., Itokawa, Y., Cooper, J. R.: Enzyme-inhibiting factor in subacute necrotizing encephalopathy. Neurology (Minneap.) 19: 841—845, 1969.

Prensky, A. L., Carr, S., Moser, H. W.: Development of myelin in inherited disorders of amino acid metabolism. Arch. Neurol. (Chic.) 19: 552—558, 1968.

Reye, R. D. K.: Subacute necrotizing encephalomyelopathy. J. Path. Bact. 79: 165—173, 1960.

Rosenblum, W. I.: Neuropathologic changes in a case of sulfite oxidase deficiency. Neurology (Minneap.) 18: 1187—1196, 1968.

Rushton, D. I.: Spongy degeneration of the white matter of the central nervous system associated with hyperglycinuria. J. clin. Path. 21: 456—462, 1968.

Scriver, C. R., Efron, M. L.: Disorders of proline and hydroxyproline metabolism. In: The Metabolic Basis of Inherited Disease (Stanbury, J. B., Wyngaarden, J. B., Fredrickson, D. S., eds.), Chapter 16, pp. 351—369. New York: McGraw-Hill 1972.

Shah, S. N., Peterson, N. A., McKean, C. M.: Lipid composition of human cerebral white matter and myelin in phenylketonuria. J. Neurochem. 19: 2369—2376, 1972.

Silberberg, D. H.: Phenylketonuria metabolites in cerebellum culture morphology. Arch. Neurol. (Chic.) 17: 524—529, 1967.

Silberman, J., Dancis, J., Feigin, I.: Neuropathological observations in maple syrup urine disease. Arch. Neurol. (Chic.) 5: 351—363, 1961.

Sipe, J. C.: Leigh's syndrome: The adult form of subacute necrotizing encephalomyelopathy with predilection for the brainstem. Neurology (Minneap.) 23: 1030—1038, 1973.

Smith, A. J., Strang, L. B.: An inborn error of metabolism with the urinary excretion of α-hydroxy-butyric acid and phenylpyruvic acid. Arch. Dis. Child. 33: 109—113, 1958.

Solitare, G. B., Shih, V. E., Nelligan, D. J., Dolan, T. F., Jr.: Arginosuccinic aciduria: clinical, biochemical, anatomical, and neuropathological observations. J. ment. Defic. Res. 13: 153—170, 1969.

Stevenson, R. E., Huntley, C. C.: Congenital malformations in offspring of phenylketonuric mothers. Pediatrics 40: 33—45, 1967.

Tanaka, T.: So-called breast milk intoxication. Amer. J. Dis. Child. 47: 1286—1298, 1934.

Tom, M. I., Rewcastle, N. B.: Infantile subacute necrotizing encephalopathy. Neurology (Minneap.) 12: 624—628, 1962.

Udenfriend, S., Bessman, S. P.: The hydroxylation of phenylalanine and antipyrine in phenylpyruvic oligophrenia. J. Biol. Chem. 203: 961—966, 1953.

Verhaart, W. J. C.: Symmetrical degeneration of neostriatum in Chinese infants. Arch. Dis. Child. 13: 225—234, 1938.

Victor, M., Adams, R. D., Cole, M.: The acquired (non-Wilsonian) type of chronic hepatocerebral degeneration. Medicine 44: 345—396, 1965.

White, H. H., Rowland, L. P., Araki, S., Thompson, H. L., Cowen, D.: Homocystinuria. Arch. Neurol. (Chic.) 13: 455—470, 1965.

Woody, N. C., Snyder, C., Harris, J. A.: Hyperprolinemia: Clinical and biochemical family study. Pediatrics 44: 554—563, 1969.

Appendix

46. Involvement of the CNS in Certain Hematologic Diseases of Infancy and Childhood

Hemorrhagic Disease of the Newborn. A bleeding disposition in the newborn infant may result from: 1. thrombocytopenia, 2. vitamin K deficiency, 3. a temporary insufficiency in hepatic synthesis of coagulation factors because of immaturity or due to hepatic damage by anoxia or infectious diseases, and 4. inherited anomalies of the coagulation mechanism. Intracranial or cerebral hemorrhages may be caused by any of these disease processes. Their neuropathologic documentation for infants is scanty, but the available observations suggest that the type of bleeding does not vary significantly with the various etiologies. The most common form of intracranial bleeding in hemorrhagic diseases of the newborn appears to be subarachnoid hemorrhage, and the subsequent development of obstructive hydrocephalus has been described in several reports.

Pearson *et al.* (1964) reviewed 55 cases of neonatal thrombocytopenic purpura of the isoimmune type; intracranial hemorrhages were documented for 8, suspected for 4. They report two cases of their own, one of whom had subarachnoid hemorrhage, the other had developed hydrocephalus subsequent to hemorrhage. Willi (1951) mentions petechial hemorrhages in the brain, but there is no further documentation. Such petechiae are found in a random distribution throughout the cerebral tissue (Fig. 157), which is a point of distinction with the types of hemorrhages accompanying asphyctic distress in the premature (Chapter 2). A syndrome of congenital hypoplastic thrombocytopenia associated with microcephaly and cerebellar atrophy of the granular layer type (Chapter 31) was described for two brothers by Hoyerall *et al.* (1970).

Intracranial hemorrhage has been observed in infants following anticoagulation therapy of the mother during pregnancy. Gordon and Dean (1955) described twins; one was stillborn with a subarachnoid hemorrhage, the other had developed hydrocephalus and succumbed at the age of 35 days with an organizing blood clot at the base of the brain. A similar case, also developing hydrocephalus, was reported by von Sydow (1947).

Classic hemophilia rarely manifests with severe bleeding during the immediate perinatal period. Hartman and Diamond (1957) reviewed 94 pediatric patients with hemophilia and related hemophilic disorders; 7 percent had intracranial bleeding, two of them fatal. This incidence is similar to that in adulthood (Silverstein, 1960). The development of hydrocephalus subsequent to massive intracranial hemorrhage was observed in an infant with classic hemophilia (McCarthy and Coble, 1973) and for Willebrand's disease (Cooper *et al.*, 1971). The majority of hemorrhages are subdural or subarachnoid, but organized intracerebral hematomas may be found within the brain substance of hemophilic children. Hemorrhages in the spine are rare (Keely *et al.*, 1972); hematomyelia in a young adult was described by Schenk (1963).

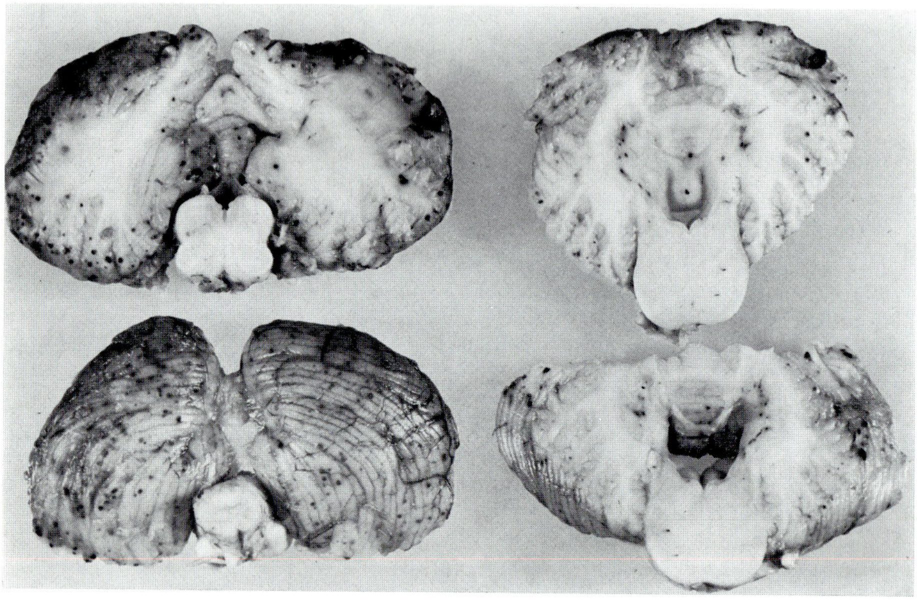

Fig. 157. Cerebellar petechiae in an infant with congenital thrombocytopenia

Hepatic immaturity or vitamin K deficiency have been implicated as etiologic factors in the common intraventricular and subarachnoid hemorrhages of asphyctic prematures (Chapter 2). This concept was supported by Willi (1951) and by Haupt (1965), who speculated that cerebral damage may cause disturbances in the coagulation mechanism which, in turn, may result in cerebral hemorrhages. These assumptions are difficult to reconcile with the pathologic manifestations of these hemorrhages; for example, with their rather stereotype origin from the stem or the main tributaries of the terminal vein, which implicates local pathogenetic factors rather than a diffuse bleeding tendency. Further, there is a consistent clinicopathologic correlation between these cerebral hemorrhages and asphyctic distress, indicating that disturbances of blood coagulation represent no more than a contributory pathogenetic factor of secondary importance (Chapter 2).

Erythrocyte Disorders. The most important contribution of various types of erythrocyte disorders to neonatal neuropathology is in terms of their causing hemolysis which may result in kernicterus if developing in the early postnatal period (Chapter 8).

Sickle cell disease is not a significant factor in neonatal neuropathology as the disease rarely manifests during the immediate postnatal period. In sickle cell disease the sixth amino acid of the beta peptide chain, glutamic acid, is replaced by either valine (HbS) or by lysine (HbC). Sickling of red blood cells under low oxygen conditions is attributed to the abnormal three-dimensional structure and relative insolubility of the abnormal hemoglobin molecule, impairing the ability of the red blood cells to mold their way through capillaries. Porter and Thurman (1963) reviewed 64 cases of sickle cell disease diagnosed during the first year of life; for none of them was death caused by cerebral lesions. Only 9 had manifested during the first 3 months and one of them had evidence of cerebral lesions. A most unusual complication of sickle cell disease was described by Veiga and Vaithianathan (1963): A white icteric premature infant had received an exchange transfusion from a donor with sickle trait and died with general intravascular sickling and focal infarcts in the brain.

Familial Lymphohistiocytosis (Erythrophagocytic or Hemophagocytic Lymphohistiocytosis or Reticulosis). Familial lymphohistiocytosis was described by Reese and Levy (1951) for 2 infant sisters suffering from a systemic illness which they considered Letterer-Siwe disease. Farquhar and Claireaux (1952) in their report on 2 siblings recognized the disease as a nosologic entity and called it familiar hemophagocytic reticulosis. Several similar names have been proposed in subsequent case reports, including "familiar erythrophagocytic lymphohistiocytosis" (MacMahon *et al.*, 1963) or familiar lymphohistiocytosis. Bell *et al.* (1968) reviewed 15 published cases and added 2 of their own. Several additional case reports have appeared since then, and their number can be expected to increase rapidly with wider recognition of the disease.

Familial lymphohistiocytosis manifests in early infancy, often presenting within the first 4 months of life, or in childhood. A progressive general disease with remittant temperatures and hepatosplenomegaly leads to rapid deterioration and death within weeks or months. Hematologic anomalies include a pancytopenia with typical mononuclear cells. Manifestations of CNS affection are common, particularly in the form of a lymphocytic meningitis, or in terms of specific neurologic deficits or seizures. CNS involvement was exclusive in the 4 sibs reported by Price *et al.* (1971), and they considered this sufficient basis for a separate classification of the cases although the histopathology otherwise was identical to generalized lymphohistiocytosis.

Gross inspection of the brain may not disclose any significant alterations, or there may be meningeal opacity from infiltrates. Necrotizing lesions of random disposition are seen at the cut surface, with a preference for the white matter. On microscopic examination there is an abundance of focal infiltrates in the leptomeninges and in the perivascular spaces of brain tissue and spinal cord (Fig. 158). The infiltrates also invade the brain parenchyma, causing necrotizing, destructive lesions. Lymphocytes and macrophages are the two main components of the infiltrates and either may prevail; it has been suggested that lymphocytes prevail initially, macrophages during the later phases. The cells are well differentiated and mitotic figures are uncommon. The most

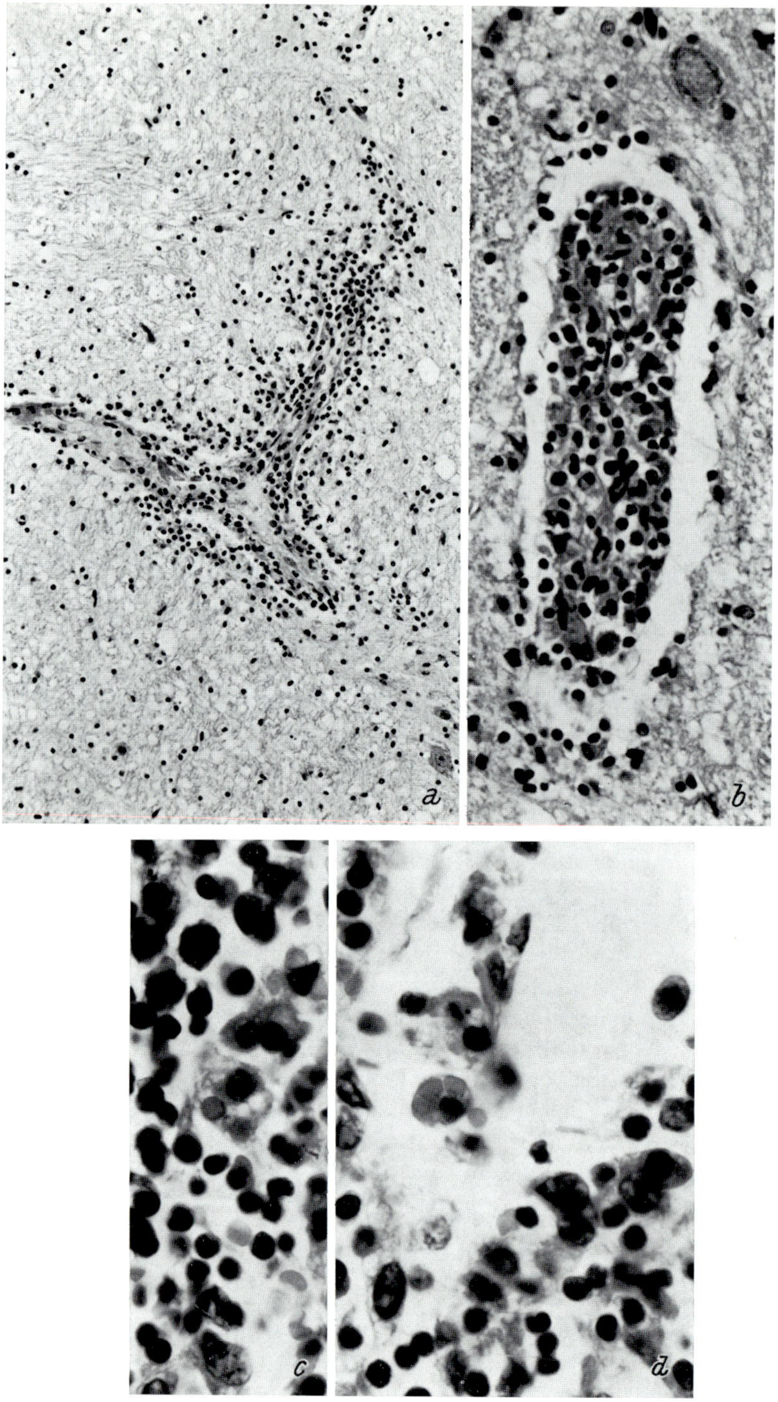

Fig. 158. Lymphohistiocytosis. A and B: Perivascular cerebral infiltrates; H & E ×115, ×320. C and D: Erythrophagocytosis in splenic macrophages; H & E ×600

characteristic feature of the disease is the inclusion into the macrophages of red blood cells (erythrophagocytosis) or lymphocytes (lymphophagocytosis). A given macrophage may contain a considerable number of either or both of these cells, which may be in excess of ten. The cytoplasm of the macrophages may be weakly positive with fat stains or with the PAS reaction. In addition to the macrophages exhibiting cytophagocytosis, there are also typical lipid-laden phagocytes, particularly within and at the edges of necrotizing lesions. Infiltrates of similar composition are found throughout the

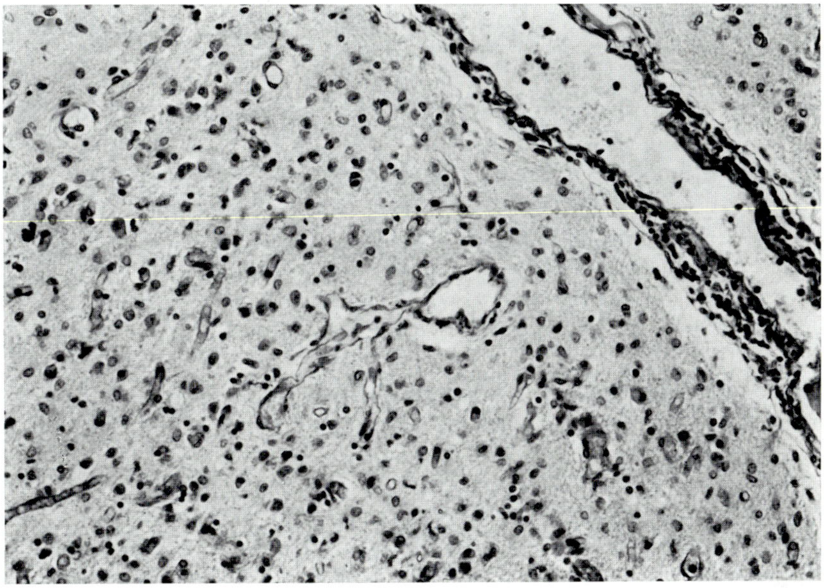

Fig. 159. Agammaglobulinemia: Loss of neurons, marked gliosis and sparse perivascular lymphocytic infiltrates in the tectum; ×180

rest of the body, particularly in parenchymal organs, bone marrow and lymph nodes.

The etiology of lymphohistiocytosis is unclear. The presence of well differentiated mature cell forms in the exudate and the scarcity of mitotic figures have been thought to indicate that the lesion is not basically neoplastic.

Hypo- and Agammaglobulinemia. Verhaart (1961) reported cerebral lesions in one of two brothers with hypogammaglobulinemia and lymphocytopenia. Both had developed a progressive neurologic syndrome and died before the age of 3 years. Widespread neuronal loss with reactive gliosis affected the nuclei of the brain stem, especially the substantia nigra and inferior olives. Similar cases have been reported subsequently. Dayan (1971) described 24 children with thymic alymphoplasia and humoral and cellular immune deficiencies. Extensive gliosis of the brain stem was found in 11, and a subacute polioencephalitis restricted to that region in 5. Most consistently affected were the quadrigeminal plate, basis pontis, tegmentum of the brain stem and the inferior olives. Only slight cerebellar involvement was noted, and no changes were seen in the cerebral cortex and basal ganglia. Microscopically there was a loss of neurons with marked reactive astroglial proliferation (Fig. 159) and patchy demyelination of the white matter. The cases having encephalitic changes showed nodular microglial proliferation. A more general dissemination of pathologic changes was reported by White *et al.* (1972); they describe a subacute nodular panencephalitis and lymphocytic infiltrates in the meninges compatible with a virus-induced encephalitis. Hanissian *et al.* (1972) reported a case in whom measles antigen was found in the brain tissue. The cerebral changes in hypo- and agammaglobulinemia are generally interpreted as being caused by a slow viral infection; attempts to support this interpretation with electron microscopic studies have demonstrated intranuclear particles considered consistent with viral origin.

Leukemia. A brief review of findings is included here even though the subject of neoplasia is beyond the scope of this text. Historical and clinical aspects of childhood leukemia were reviewed by Iversen (1966). Clinical manifestations of CNS involvement in order of decreasing frequency are: Blurring or loss of consciousness, cranial nerve involvement, paralysis of limbs, convulsions, headache, vomiting, nuchal rigidity and papilledema.

Moore *et al.* (1960) on reviewing the pathology of CNS leukemia in 117 cases, 54 of them children noted infiltrates in the dura mater in approximately two-thirds. This high frequency of dural involvement is consistent with the experience of the present author: some degree of dural infiltration is the most common feature of leukemia. Infiltrates are seen most often in the proximity of the superior sagittal sinus. Most of them are microscopic, but they may reach, on occasion, the extent of grossly visible masses of leukemic cells encompassing the sinus (Fig. 160); however, they have never been seen to obstruct the arachnoid granulations. The presence of leukemic infiltrates in the parietal dura is often heralded by thin, dull, barely vascularized neomembranes (Chapter 19). Microscopically the neomembranes may cover dura containing sparse infiltrates, or the neomembranes themselves may be infiltrated with leukemic cells. There may be concurrent recent hemorrhage into the neomembrane or into the subdural space.

Leptomeningeal infiltrates are much less common than dural infiltrates and were found in approximately one-third of the cases of Moore *et al.* (1960). The presence of leukemic leptomeningeal infiltrates is notoriously difficult to assess on gross inspection of the brain; they may be indiscernible to the naked eye, or arachnoid fibrosis may give the false impression of infiltrates. Thick infiltrates present as milky, opaque patches in the leptomeninges and may contain petechial hemorrhages. In extreme cases subarachnoid spaces and ventricles are completely filled up with leukemic cells (Fig. 161). The accumulation of leukemic cells in the subarachnoid spaces and, perhaps, reactive fibrosis, may impair the circulation of CSF, causing obstructive hydrocephalus with marked dilation of the cerebral ventricles.

Microscopic examination of minor meningeal infiltrates shows a haphazard focal scattering of leukemic cells in cranial and spinal arachnoid, often with a perivenous accentuation. Infiltrates may extend along the perivascular spaces deep into the brain tissue, forming perivascular cuffs without direct involvement of the nervous parenchyma. There may also be involvement of other structures bordering the CSF spaces such as the stroma of the choroid plexus, the nerve roots and their sleeves, the spinal ganglia, and the pituitary gland.

Leukemic infiltrates of the brain parenchyma are least common, occurring in less than 5 percent of cases. They are typically perivascular, usually with

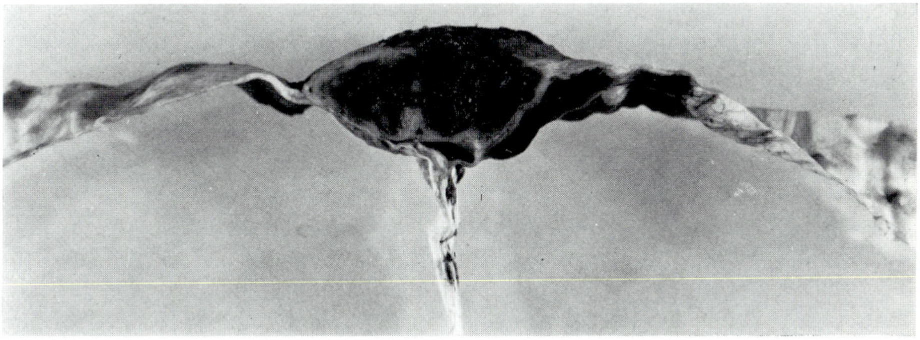

Fig. 160. Lymphoblastic leukemia, massive infiltrates of dura, occluding superior sagittal sinus

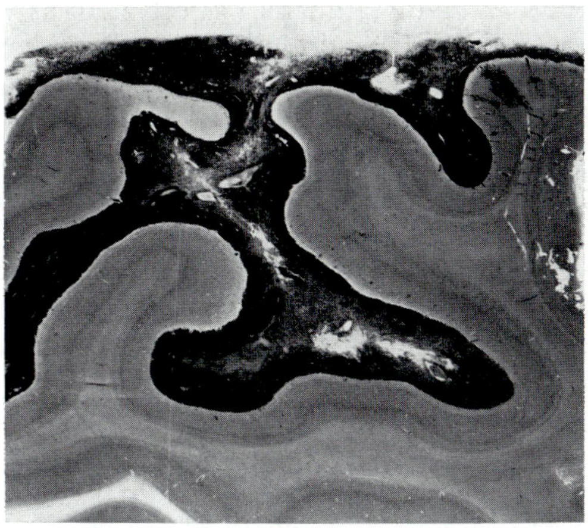

Fig. 161. Acute lymphoblastic leukemia; subtotal obliteration of subarachnoid spaces by dense blastic infiltrates; cresyl violet ×7

a characteristic gradient in the scattering of leukemic cells into the adjacent brain tissue; most do not present in the form of space occupying nodular lesions.

Aside from leukemic infiltrates, there are the lesions of complicating infectious diseases as well as leukemic hemorrhages. Intracranial hemorrhages complicating leukemia may present as intracerebral, subarachnoid and subdural hemorrhages, afflicting approximately one-fifth of the patients. Intracerebral hemorrhages are typically multiple with a preference for white matter; they may rupture into the inner or the outer CSF spaces. Freireich *et al.* (1960) reported the occurrence of these hemorrhages in direct proportion to the white cell count, but this relationship was recently challenged by Price and Johnson (1973). Microscopic examination of leukemic intracerebral hemorrhages shows leukocytes forming irregular or rounded masses among the erythrocytes. This feature has been interpreted as nodular proliferation of cells subsequent to leukostasis in blood vessels, and to intravascular proliferation and destruction of the vessels (Moore *et al.*, 1960). However, the separation of red and white cells is seen commonly in hematomas of nonleukemic patients, and the aggregates of leukemic cells may be a phenomenon of clot formation rather than true nodular proliferation. The above authors considered the subarachnoid hemorrhages of leukemic patients as being basically different from the intracerebral hemorrhages, the latter relating to thrombocytopenia rather than to high leukocyte counts.

Chediak-Higashi Disease. Chediak-Higashi disease was described in a number of independent original reports, the first of Beguez-Cesar (1943) of Cuba and of Steinbrinck (1948) of Breslau, Germany. The disease is now named after Chediak (1952) who described its clinical features as well as the abnormal granulations of the leukocytes and after Higashi (1954) who emphasized the appearance of the granules in peroxydase stains in his report on one of three afflicted siblings. Chediak-Higashi disease is now recognized as a rare autosomal recessive disease which affects man as well as the Aleutian mink (Leader *et al.*, 1963), the partial albino Hereford cattle (Padgett *et al.*, 1964) and the beige mouse (Lutzner *et al.*, 1967).

Manifestations of Chediak-Higashi disease include disturbances of pigmentation, with steel gray or light brown hair, photophobia, horizontal nystagmus, and pale ocular fundi (retinal albinism); there is a disposition to recurrent infections and fevers of occult origin. Anemia, leukopenia, thrombocytopenia as well as hepatosplenomegaly and lymphadenopathy are present, and jaundice or neurologic defects may develop during the course of the disease. Nearly all the circulating neutrophils contain multiple, large granules, up to 4 μ in diameter, which are peroxydase positive, stain greenish with the Romanowski stain, positive with sudan black and negative with PAS. The granules of eosinophils and basophils are abnormally large but have normal tinctorial features. Lymphocytes contain sparse azurophil granules which are positive for PAS and negative for sudan black and peroxydase. Consanguinity of parents was found for nearly half of the cases, and affection of siblings of either sex is common. The disease may take a rapidly progressive course from birth, or it may be quiescent at first having an accelerated terminal course. Death frequently intervenes before the 10th year of life.

The first account of neuropathologic changes in Chediak-Higashi disease by Donohue and Bain (1957) relates the presence of widespread encephalitic changes with focal or diffuse lymphocytic and histiocytic infiltrates, nodular microglial proliferation and various degrees of destructive lesions of white or gray matter. A chronic meningitis may be present. Lympho- and histiocytic infiltrates are seen in many organs throughout the body, and some authors have interpreted the former as lymphomas. The peripheral nerves may be involved with edema and focal swellings.

Sung *et al.* (1969) reported more specific neuropathologic alterations and reviewed the literature. They described multiple cytoplasmic inclusions having staining characteristics of lipofuscin granules, but larger, and having a tendency to clump to form compact masses; several types of inclusions may

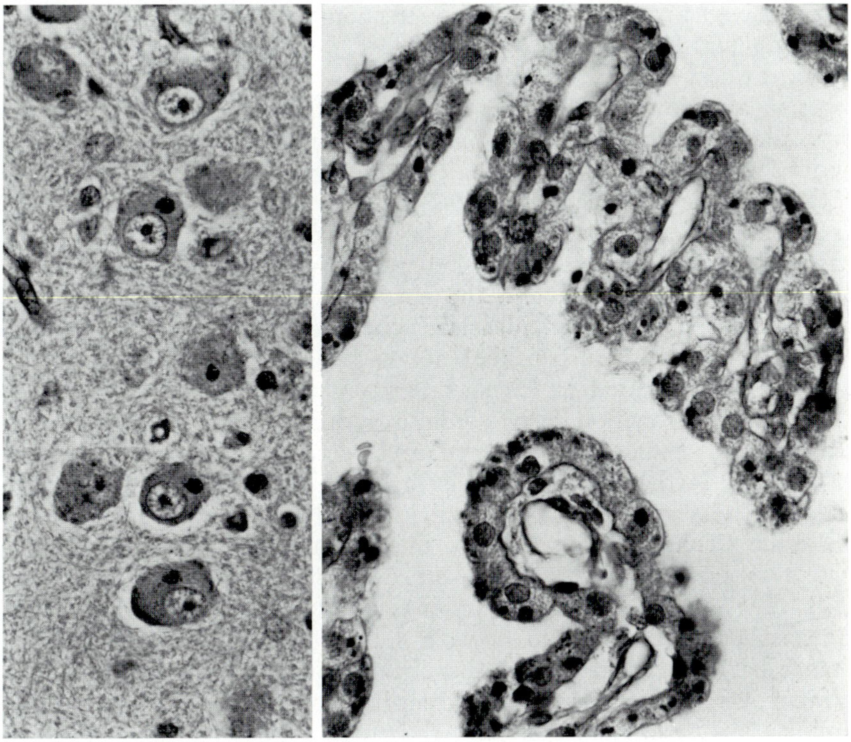

Fig. 162. Chediak-Higashi disease. Coarse PAS-positive inclusions in the neurons of the inferior olivary nucleus and in the choroid plexus epithelia; PAS ×440

be distinguished according to their size and configuration: Spherical inclusions may exceed the size of a nucleolus and even reach that of a nucleus. Glomerular inclusions have rather irregular size and shape. Small granular inclusions are like lipofuscin granules except for being coarser. The larger inclusions are strongly PAS positive, nonmetachromatic, and weakly positive with Ziehl-Neelsen and sudan dyes; they exhibit a strong autofluorescence in UV light.

Inclusions (Fig. 162) of these types occur in the neurons of the central and autonomic nervous system. Their similarity with lipofuscin granules is further accentuated by their tendency to increase with the patient's age and by their regional predilection for those nuclear groups that normally have a greater affinity for accumulating lipofuscin, *e.g.*, the inferior olivary nucleus. Large inclusions are also seen in the epithelia of the choroid plexus; much smaller inclusions occur in glial cells, satellite cells, endothelia or histiocytes. Pigmented nuclei, including the substantia nigra, show unusually large melanin granules which have a tendency to clump or form abnormally large aggregates.

Electron microscopic examination shows the inclusions to be formed by abnormally large, rounded or lobulated masses of finely granular material bounded by a single membrane; they may include lipid droplets or membranous fragments. The fine structure of these masses resembles lysosomes, and it is thought that they form from the confluence of abnormal lysosomes.

A peripheral neuropathy is often present in Chediak-Higashi disease, with lymphocytic and histiocytic infiltrates and focal demyelination. Chromatolytic changes in anterior horn motor neurons are likely secondary to the neuropathy. Electron microscopic examination reveals large homogenous granular inclusions consistent with abnormally large lysosomes in the cytoplasm of the Schwann cells (Lockman *et al.*, 1967).

No specific biochemical defect has been demonstrated for Chediak-Higashi disease. The light and electron microscopic changes are consistent with an anomaly of the lysosomes, and the abnormal granules seen with the light microscope were considered identical with giant lysosomes (White, 1966). Defective chemotaxis, bactericidial action and degranulation of leukocytes have been demonstrated in Chediak-Higashi disease. More direct evidence for lysosomal dysfunction derives from experiments demonstrating a retarded degradation of horseradish peroxydase by renal lysosomes (Prieur *et al.*, 1972), adding further evidence to the concept of an impairment in lysosomal digestive activity as the cause of Chediak-Higashi disease.

Chronic Granulomatous Disease of Childhood. Chronic granulomatous disease was described by Berendes *et al.* (1957) and Landing and Shirkey (1957). The disease is familiar and has marked male predilection without being absolutely restricted to boys; a sex-modified autosomal recessive inheritance has been suggested. A disposition for infections becomes manifest in infancy, with lymphadenitis, recurrent hepatosplenomegaly, skin infections, granulomatous or absceding lesions, recurrent pulmonary infiltrates, as well as with many other manifestations of chronic infection. Hypergammaglobulinemia, leukocytosis and elevated erythrocyte sedimentation rate are found in the blood. The disease takes a chronic progressive course leading to death in infancy or childhood for most cases. According to Holmes *et al.* (1966) the leukocytes are capable of phagocytosis of bacteria but they seem unable to kill and digest them. A wide variety of bacterial or fungal organisms have been isolated from the lesions, fungi becoming more common in the older children.

Autopsy discloses granulomatous lesions throughout parenchymal organs; these may be caseating, with numerous lymphocytes and plasma cells, or

---

Fig. 163. Chronic granulomatous disease of infancy. A: Multiple disseminated granulomatous lesions. B: Granuloma with numerous multinucleated giant cells encompassed by a dense fibrous capsule. The necrotic center contains numerous fungal hyphae; H & E ×45. C: Splenic tissue contains brownish pigmented macrophages; H & E ×375

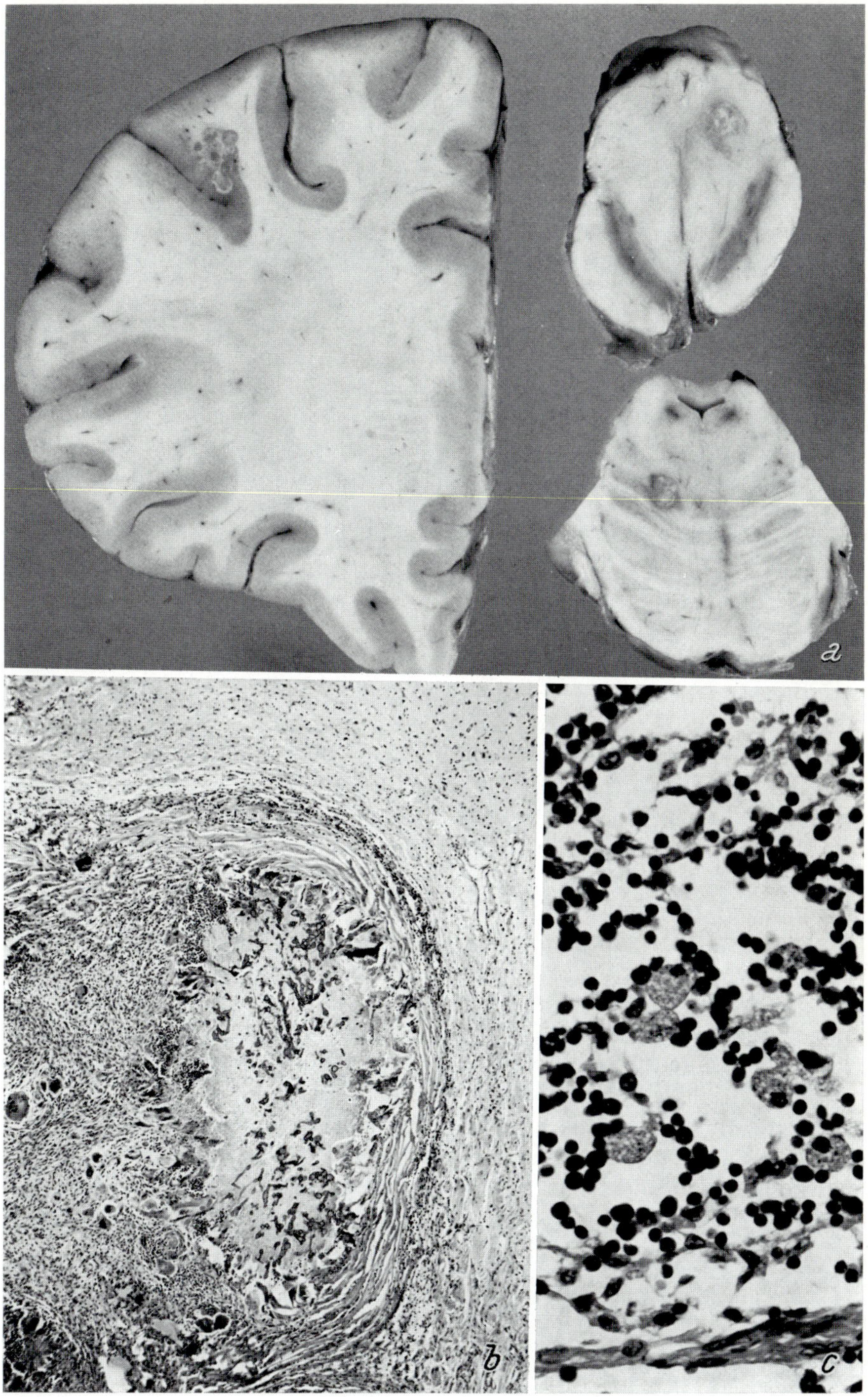

Fig. 163

epitheloid with leukocytes and multinucleated giant cells; fungi may be seen in the latter. An unusual feature are pigmented, lipid-laden histiocytes, which occur without strict correlation to the granulomatous lesions. Their examination with the electron microscope shows droplets of lipidic material in the cytoplasm (Bartman *et al.*, 1967).

Carson *et al.* (1965), in a series of 13 boys affected by the disease, found evidence of meningitis for 3; meningoencephalitis was present for one of 8 boys with autopsy records. There are, however, no specific descriptions of neuropathologic lesions in the literature. Thus, the following observation from the present author's material may be of interest; the case was remarkable for his survival to the age of 19 years.

The disease began at the age of 6 months with an abscess in the groin; the patient then had numerous hospital admissions because of various chronic granulomatous inflammations of skin and lungs from which various fungal and bacterial organisms including balstomyces, Hafnia, Aerobacter and Klebsiella were isolated. At the age of 18 he developed osteomyelitis of the calvaria, and pleocytosis, elevated protein and low glucose of the CSF. The ventricles were dilated and a ventriculostomy was placed. The final phase of the disease began 2 months prior to death with disturbances of consciousness, upward gaze and paresis of the right arm.

Neuropathologic examination disclosed a large epidural granuloma in the right parietal region, compressing the underlying hemisphere with severe hippocampal and cerebellar tonsillar herniations. The cerebral ventricles contained sparse purulent exudate and were relatively small, particularly the fourth, evidently because of chronic shunting. The foramina of Monroe were obstructed by irregular scar tissue. The cut surface of cerebral and cerebellar hemispheres showed numerous, firm, yellowish nodules, from less than 2 to about 10 mm in diameter (Fig. 163). On microscopic examination there were single or clustered miliary granulomata of fairly uniform structure. Each granuloma was encompassed by a dense connective tissue capsule with sparse chronic inflammatory infiltrates and reactive gliosis at its periphery. The inner surface of the capsule was lined with a monolayer of multinucleated giant cells which, in turn, encompassed the necrotic center, often containing masses of fungal hyphae. Some of the granulomas showed central infiltrates of polymorphonuclear leukocytes. Granulomas of this type were scattered throughout the cerebral and cerebellar hemispheres and the brain stem; in the midbrain a cluster of granulomas compressed the aqueduct. There was a relatively mild chronic ventriculitis, with gliosis, focal cuffing and subependymal nests of multinucleated giant cells. The epidural infiltrates, which had eroded and destroyed large portions of the calvaria, consisted of dense connective tissue with an abundance of necrotizing granulomata with multinucleated giant cells, epitheloid cells, and acute and chronic inflammatory infiltrates.

References

Bartman, J., Van de Velde, R. L., Friedmann, F.: Pigmented lipid histiocytes and susceptibility to infection: ultrastructure of splenic histiocytes. Pediatrics 40: 1000—1002, 1967.

Beguez-Cesar, A.: Neutropenia cronica maligna familiar con granulaciones atipicas de los leucocitos. Bol. Soc. Cub. Pediat. 15: 900—922, 1943.

Bell, R. J. M., Bradfield, A. J. E., Barnes, N. D., France, N. E.: Familial haemophagocytic reticulosis. Arch. Dis. Child. 43: 601—606, 1968.

Berendes, H., Bridges, R. A., Good, R. A.: A fatal granulomatosis of childhood. Minn. Med. 40: 309—312, 1957.

Carson, M. J., Chadwick, D. L., Brubaker, C. A., Cleland, R. S., Landing, B. H.: Thirteen boys with progressive septic granulomas. Pediatrics 35: 405—412, 1965.

Chediak, M.: Nouvelle anomalie leucocytaire de charactère constitutionel et familial. Nouv. Rev. franc. Hémat. 7: 362—367, 1952.

Cooper, H. A., Bowie, E. J. W., Bugert, E. O., Jr., Mellinger, J. F.: Hydrocephalus in child with von Willebrand's disease. Amer. J. Dis. Child. 121: 340—343, 1971.

Dayan, A. D.: Chronic encephalitis in children with severe immuno-deficiency. Acta neuropath. (Berl.) 19: 234—241, 1971.

Donohue, W. L., Bain, H. W.: Chediak-Higashi syndrome. Pediatrics 20: 416—430, 1957.

Farquhar, J. W., Claireaux, A. E.: Familial haemophagocytic reticulosis. Arch. Dis. Child. 27: 519—525, 1952.

Freireich, E. J., Thomas, L. B., Frei, E., Fritz, R. D., Forkner, C. E.: A distinctive type of intracerebral hemorrhages associated with "blastic crisis" in patients with leukemia. Cancer 13: 146—154, 1960.

Gordon, R. R., Dean, T.: Foetal deaths from antenatal anticoagulant therapy. Brit. med. J. 2: 719—721, 1955.

Hanissian, A. S., Jabbour, J. T., De Lamerens, S., Garcia, J. H., Horta-Barbosa, L.: Subacute encephalitis and hypogammaglobulinemia. Amer. J. Dis. Child. 123: 151—155, 1972.

Hartmann, J. R., Diamond, L. K.: Haemophilia and related haemorrhagic disorders. Practitioner 178: 179—190, 1957.

Haupt, H.: Störungen der Blutgerinnung infolge perinataler Hirnschädigung. Dtsch. med. Wschr. 90: 1473—1477, 1965.

Higashi, O.: Congenital gigantism of proxidase granules. Tohoku J. exp. Med. 59: 315—332, 1954.

Holmes, B., Quie, P. G., Windhorst, D. B., Good, R. A.: Fatal granulomatous disease of childhood. Lancet 1: 1225—1228, 1966.

Høyerall, H. M., Lamvik, J., Moe, P. J.: Congenital hypoplastic thrombocytopenia and cerebral malformations in two brothers. Acta paed. scand. 59: 185—191, 1970.

Iversen, T.: Leukaemia in infancy and childhood. Acta paediat. scand. Suppl. 106: 1—219, 1966.

Keely, M. L., Taylor, N., Chard, R. L., Fr.: Spinal cord compression as a complication of haemophilia. Arch. Dis. Child. 47: 826—827, 1972.

Landing, B. H., Shirkey, H. S.: A syndrome of recurrent infection and infiltration of viscera by pigmented lipid histiocytes. Pediatrics 20: 431—438, 1957.

Leader, R. W., Padgett, G. A., Gorham, J. R.: Studies of abnormal leukocyte bodies in the mink. Blood 22: 477—484, 1963.

Lockman, L. A., Kennedy, W. R., White, J. G.: The Chediak-Higashi syndrome: Electrophysiologic and electron microscopic observations on the peripheral neuropathy. J. Pediat. 70: 942—951, 1967.

Lutzner, M. A., Lowrie, C. T., Jordan, H. W.: Giant granules in leukocytes of the beige mouse. J. Hered. 58: 299—300, 1967.

MacMahon, H. E., Bedizel, M., Ellis, C. A.: Familial erythrophagocytic lymphohistiocytosis. Pediatrics 32: 868—879, 1963.

McCarthy, J. W., Coble, L. L.: Intracranial hemorrhage and subsequent communicating hydrocephalus in a neonate with classical hemophilia. Pediatrics 51: 123—124, 1973.

Moore, E. W., Thomas, L. B., Shaw, R. K., Freireich, E. J.: The central nervous system in acute leucemia. Arch. intern. Med. 105: 451—468, 1960.

Padgett, G. A., Leader, R. W., Gorham, J. R., O'Mary, C. C.: The familial occurrence of the Chediak-Higashi syndrome in mink and cattle. Genetics 49: 505—512, 1964.

Pearson, H. A., Shulman, N. R., Marder, V. J., Cone, T. E.: Isoimmune neonatal thrombocytopenic purpura. Blood 23: 154—177, 1964.

Porter, F., Thurman, W. G.: Studies of sickle cell disease. Amer. J. Dis. Child. 106: 35—42, 1963.

Price, D. L., Woolsey, J. E., Rosman, N. P., Richardson, E. P.: Familial lymphohistiocytosis of the nervous system. Arch. Neurol. (Chic.) 24: 270—283, 1971.

Price, R. A., Johnson, W. W.: The central nervous system in childhood leukemia. I. The arachnoid. Cancer 31: 520—533, 1973.

Prieur, D. J., Davis, W. C., Padgett, G. A.: Defective function of renal lysosomes in mice with Chediak-Higashi syndrome. Amer. J. Path. 67: 227—240, 1972.

Reese, A. J. M., Levy, E.: Familial incidence of non-lipoid reticulo-endotheliosis (Letterer-Siwe disease). Arch. Dis. Child. 26: 578—581, 1951.

Schenk, W. D.: Hemorrhage in spinal cord with syringomyelia in a patient with hemophilia. Acta neuropath. (Berl.) 2: 306—308, 1963.

Silverstein, A.: Intracranial bleeding in hemophilia. Arch. Neurol. 3: 141—157, 1960.

Steinbrinck, W.: Über eine neue Granulationsanomalie der Leukozyten. Dtsch. Arch. klin. Med. 193: 577—581, 1948.

Sung, J. H., Meyers, J. P., Stadlan, E. M., Cowen, D., Wolf, A.: Neuropathological changes in Chediak-Higashi disease. J. Neuropath. exp. Neurol. 28: 86—118, 1969.

Veiga, S., Vaithianathan, T.: Massive intravascular sickling after exchange transfusion with sickle cell trait blood. Transfusion 3: 387—391, 1963.

Verhaart, W. J. C.: Polio-encephalopathy or masked encephalitis in familial hypogammaglobulinemia. J. Neuropath. exp. Neurol. 20: 380—385, 1961.

Von Sydow, G.: Hypopotrombinemi och hjarnskada hos barn till dikumarinbehandlad moder. Nordisk. Medicin 34: 1171—1172, 1947.

White, H. H., Kepes, J. H., Kirkpatrick, C. H., Schimke, R. N.: Subacute encephalitis and congenital hypogammaglobulinemia. Arch. Neurol. (Chic.) 26: 359—365, 1972.

White, J. G.: The Chediak-Higashi syndrome: a possible lysosomal disease. Blood 28: 143—156, 1966.

Willi, H.: Die Blutungskrankheiten des Neugeborenen. Erg. inn. Med. Kinderheilk. 2: 467—543, 1951.

Subject Index